T0302089

RECOMBINANT ANTIBODIES FOR IMMUNOTHERAPY

Recombinant Antibodies for Immunotherapy provides a comprehensive overview of the field of monoclonal antibodies (mAbs), a market that has grown tremendously in recent years. Twenty-four chapters by experienced and innovative authors cover the isolation of specific human mAbs, humanization, immunogenicity, technologies for improving efficacy, "arming" mAbs, novel alternative Ab constructs, increasing half-lives, alternative concepts employing non-immuno-globulin scaffolds, novel therapeutic approaches, a market analysis of therapeutic mAbs, and future developments in the field.

The concepts and technologies are illustrated by examples of recombinant antibodies being used in the clinic or in development. This book will appeal to both newcomers and experienced scientists in the field, biology and biotechnology students, research and development departments in the pharmaceutical industry, medical researchers, clinicians, and biotechnology investors.

Melvyn Little's research group at the German Cancer Research Center (DKFZ) in Heidelberg was one of the first to develop methods for making and screening antibody libraries. After co-founding Affitech (Oslo, Norway) in 1997, he left the DKFZ in 2000 to found Affimed Therapeutics, a biotechnology company in Heidelberg specializing in the isolation and engineering of human antibodies to treat various diseases, especially cancer. He has been an extracurricular professor of biochemistry at the University of Heidelberg since 1986.

RECOMBINANT ANTIBODIES FOR IMMUNOTHERAPY

Edited by

Melvyn Little

Affimed Therapeutics

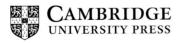

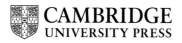

Shaftesbury Road, Cambridge CB2 8EA, United Kingdom

One Liberty Plaza, 20th Floor, New York, NY 10006, USA

477 Williamstown Road, Port Melbourne, VIC 3207, Australia

314–321, 3rd Floor, Plot 3, Splendor Forum, Jasola District Centre, New Delhi – 110025, India

103 Penang Road, #05–06/07, Visioncrest Commercial, Singapore 238467

Cambridge University Press is part of Cambridge University Press & Assessment, a department of the University of Cambridge.

We share the University's mission to contribute to society through the pursuit of education, learning and research at the highest international levels of excellence.

www.cambridge.org
Information on this title: www.cambridge.org/9780521887328

© Cambridge University Press & Assessment 2009

This publication is in copyright. Subject to statutory exception and to the provisions of relevant collective licensing agreements, no reproduction of any part may take place without the written permission of Cambridge University Press & Assessment.

First published 2009

A catalogue record for this publication is available from the British Library

Library of Congress Cataloging-in-Publication data
Recombinant antibodies for immunotherapy / edited by Melvyn Little.
     p. ; cm.
Includes bibliographical references and index.
ISBN 978-0-521-88732-8 (hardback)
1. Monoclonal antibodies – Therapeutic use. I. Little, Melvyn, 1945– II. Title.
[DNLM: 1. Immunotherapy – methods. 2. Antibodies, Monoclonal – therapeutic use.
3. Recombinant Proteins – therapeutic use. QW 940 R311 2009]

RM282.M65R43 2009
615´.37 – dc22   2008044201

ISBN   978-0-521-88732-8   Hardback

Cambridge University Press & Assessment has no responsibility for the persistence or accuracy of URLs for external or third-party internet websites referred to in this publication, and does not guarantee that any content on such websites is, or will remain, accurate or appropriate. Information regarding prices, travel timetables, and other factual information given in this work is correct at the time of first printing but Cambridge University Press & Assessment does not guarantee the accuracy of such information thereafter.

....

Every effort has been made in preparing this book to provide accurate and up-to-date information which is in accord with accepted standards and practice at the time of publication. Although case histories are drawn from actual cases, every effort has been made to disguise the identities of the individuals involved. Nevertheless, the authors, editors and publishers can make no warranties that the information contained herein is totally free from error, not least because clinical standards are constantly changing through research and regulation. The authors, editors and publishers therefore disclaim all liability for direct or consequential damages resulting from the use of material contained in this book. Readers are strongly advised to pay careful attention to information provided by the manufacturer of any drugs or equipment that they plan to use.

Contents

Color plates follow page xvi.

Contributors

Jan Terje Andersen
Department of Molecular Biosciences and
Centre for Immune Regulation
University of Oslo
Oslo, Norway

Kenneth D. Bagshawe
Department of Oncology
Imperial College London
London, U.K.

Matthew P. Baker
Antitope Ltd.
Babraham, Cambridge, U.K.

Claude Beltejar
Raven Biotechnologies
San Francisco, California, U.S.

Gerald Beste
formerly MedImmune Ltd.
Cambridge, U.K.
now Ablynx NV
Ghent, Belgium

Christophe Bourrilly
ABN AMRO Corporate Finance Ltd.
London, U.K.

Peter Brünker
Glycart Biotechnology (Roche Group)
Schlieren, Switzerland

Frank J. Carr
Antitope Ltd.
Babraham, Cambridge, U.K.

Aaron K. Chamberlain
Xencor
Monrovia, California, U.S.

Kerry A. Chester
CR UK Targeting & Imaging Group
Department of Oncology
UCL Cancer Institute
University College London
London, U.K.

Nigel S. Courtenay-Luck
Antisoma Research Ltd.
London, U.K.

Agamemnon A. Epenetos
Trojantec Ltd.
Nicosia, Cyprus

Claudia Fieger
Raven Biotechnologies
San Francisco, California, U.S.

Daron Forman
Tolerx
Cambridge, Massachusetts, U.S.

Yannick Gansemans
Algonomics NV
Gent-Zwijnaarde, Belgium

Gholamreza Hassanzadeh Ghassabeh
Laboratory of Cellular and Molecular
Immunology
Vrije Universiteit
and Department of Molecular and Cellular
Interaction
VIB
Brussels, Belgium

Sam P. Heywood
Antibody Research
UCB-Celltech
Slough, U.K.

David P. Humphreys
Antibody Research
UCB-Celltech
Slough, U.K.

Aya Jakobovits
Agensys, Inc.
Santa Monica, California, U.S.

David Jones
Antisoma Research Ltd.
London, U.K.

David J. King
formerly Medarex
Sunnyvale, California, U.S.
now AnaptysBio Inc.
San Diego, California, U.S.

Kathleen L. King
Raven Biotechnologies
San Francisco, California, U.S.

Ingo M. Klagge
MorphoSys AG
Martinsried/Planegg, Germany

Stefan Knackmuss
Affimed Therapeutics AG
Heidelberg, Germany

Christina A. Kousparou
Trojantec Ltd.
Nicosia, Cyprus

Ignace Lasters
Algonomics NV
Gent-Zwijnaarde, Belgium

Greg A. Lazar
Xencor
Monrovia, California, U.S.

Fabrice Le Gall
Affimed Therapeutics AG
Heidelberg, Germany

Jonathan Li
Raven Biotechnologies
San Francisco, California, U.S.

Tony W. Liang
Raven Biotechnologies
San Francisco, California, U.S.

Monica Licea
Raven Biotechnologies
San Francisco, California, U.S.

Melvyn Little
Affimed Therapeutics AG
Heidelberg, Germany

Deryk Loo
Raven Biotechnologies
San Francisco, California, U.S.

David Lowe
MedImmune Ltd.
Cambridge, U.K.

Helen L. Lowe
CR UK Targeting & Imaging Group
Department of Oncology
UCL Cancer Institute
University College London
London, U.K.

Jennie P. Mather
Raven Biotechnologies
San Francisco, California, U.S.

Devangi Mehta
Tolerx
Cambridge, Massachusetts, U.S.

Vera Molkenthin
Affimed Therapeutics AG
Heidelberg, Germany

Andrew Murphy
Regeneron
Tarrytown, New York, U.S.

Serge Muyldermans
Laboratory of Cellular and Molecular Immunology
Vrije Universiteit
and Department of Molecular and Cellular Interaction
VIB
Brussels, Belgium

Jurgen Pletinckx
Algonomics NV
Gent-Zwijnaarde, Belgium

Andreas Plückthun
Department of Biochemistry
University of Zürich
Zurich, Switzerland

Paul Ponath
Tolerx
Cambridge, Massachusetts, U.S.

Joe Ponte
Tolerx
Cambridge, Massachusetts, U.S.

Beverly Potts
Raven Biotechnologies
San Francisco, California, U.S.

Patricia Rao
formerly Tolerx
Cambridge, Massachusetts, U.S.
now Synta Pharmaceutical Corp.
Lexington, Massachusetts, U.S.

Michael Rosenzweig
Tolerx
Cambridge, Massachusetts, U.S.

Florian Rüker
Department of Biotechnology
University of Natural Resources
and Applied Life Sciences
Vienna, Austria

Dirk Saerens
Laboratory of Cellular and Molecular
Immunology
Vrije Universiteit
and Department of Molecular and Cellular
Interaction
VIB
Brussels, Belgium

José W. Saldanha
Division of Mathematical Biology
National Institute for Medical Research
Mill Hill, London, U.K.

Inger Sandlie
Department of Molecular
Biosciences and Centre for Immune Regulation
University of Oslo
Oslo, Norway

Surinder K. Sharma
CR UK Targeting & Imaging Group
Department of Oncology
UCL Cancer Institute
University College London
London, U.K.

Jessica Snyder
Tolerx
Cambridge, Massachusetts, U.S.

Peter Sondermann
Glycart Biotechnology (Roche Group)
Schlieren, Switzerland

Philippe Stas
Algonomics NV
Gent-Zwijnaarde, Belgium

Ross Stewart
MedImmune Ltd.
Cambridge, U.K.

Pablo Umaña
Glycart Biotechnology (Roche Group)
Schlieren, Switzerland

Herman Waldmann
formerly Tolerx
Cambridge, Massachusetts, U.S.
now Sir William Dunn School of Pathology
Oxford, U.K.

Carl Webster
MedImmune Ltd.
Cambridge, U.K.

Gordana Wozniak-Knopp
Department of Biotechnology
University of Natural Resources
and Applied Life Sciences
Vienna, Austria

Peter Young
Raven Biotechnologies
San Francisco, California, U.S.

Foreword

Antibodies were discovered in 1890 but remained on the periphery of the pharmaceutical industry for more than 100 years. Yet within the last 15 years, a succession of antibodies has been approved for therapy by the United States Food and Drug Administration (FDA). Unlike natural antibodies which are polyclonal and directed against infectious disease, almost all those approved by the FDA are monoclonal antibodies directed against human self-antigens and used for treatment of cancer and diseases of the immune system.

Two major breakthroughs proved necessary to launch this antibody revolution. The first breakthrough was rodent hybridoma technology in the 1970s. Antibodies could now be made against single antigens in complex mixtures and used to identify the molecular targets of disease. In some cases this allowed disease intervention by blocking the antigen or by killing a class of cells (such as cancer cells) bearing the antigen. However, hybridoma technology provided only part of the solution; the rodent antibodies proved immunogenic and often did not trigger human effector functions efficiently. The second breakthrough, in the 1990s, was protein engineering; its application allowed the creation of chimeric and humanized antibodies from rodent monoclonal antibodies; not only were these less immunogenic than rodent antibodies, but they more efficiently triggered human effector functions. These chimeric and humanized antibodies now account for the majority of the currently approved therapeutic antibodies.

Nevertheless the field continued to embrace new technologies and to spawn new approaches, most notably the development of genuine human antibodies in the 1990s. Human therapeutic antibodies were made by selection from highly diverse antibody repertoires displayed on filamentous phage, and then from mice transgenic with human antibody genes. The pace of innovation continued in the new millennium; antibodies were built from single domains, endowed with enhanced effector functions or prolonged serum half-life, and even tailored to bind antigen via engineered constant domains. Earlier approaches, for example those based on cytotoxic drugs or radio-immune conjugates, were also re-evaluated. In a field with few clinically validated targets and a thicket of intellectual property, technological innovation has offered freedom for new biotechnology companies to develop therapeutics based on antibodies or antibody mimics.

Recombinant Antibodies for Immunotherapy, edited by Professor Melvyn Little, covers both the fundamentals of the technology and the current state of its development and concludes with a section on novel therapeutic approaches and an overview of the market that has driven, and continues to drive, the field. The book promises to be an essential and most convenient guide to the field.

Sir Gregory Winter FRS
Deputy Director
Laboratory of Molecular Biology and MRC Centre for Protein Engineering
Cambridge, UK

Preface

The potential of antibodies as magic bullets for curing disease has excited the imagination of medical researchers ever since this phrase was first coined by Paul Ehrlich about a century ago. Seventy-five years after the publication of Ehrlich's side-chain theory to explain antibody-antigen reactions in 1900, Georges Köhler and César Milstein invented a means of cloning antibodies with defined specificity that paved the way for major advances in cell biological and clinical research. They were awarded the Nobel Prize in Medicine in 1984 for this ground-breaking research. In 1986, the first monoclonal antibody, the murine mAb OKT3 for preventing transplant rejection, was approved for clinical use, and although many other murine mAbs were subsequently investigated as therapeutic agents, most of them had a disappointing clinical profile largely due to their immunogenicity. This situation improved dramatically with the advent of techniques to humanize existing mAbs, followed by technologies that sought to imitate the generation of specific antibodies by the immune system *in vitro*. For example, the expression of antibody fragments in *E. coli* using bacterial leader sequences and the use of phage display and later ribosome display facilitated the selection of specific human antibodies from extremely large libraries. The process of somatic hypermutation to increase antibody affinity was mimicked by introducing random mutations. Another major advance for obtaining human antibodies was the creation of transgenic mice carrying a large part of the human antibody gene repertoire, which could be used to produce human antibodies by standard hybridoma technology. The success of these novel technologies resulted in a first generation of recombinant antibodies that now account for a large proportion of the market for biopharmaceuticals, with annual growth rates of almost 40%.

Therapeutic antibodies for cancer rely to a large extent on the recruitment of other elements in the immune system for their effect; very few of them function as magic bullets in the sense of "target and destroy." For example, although antibody binding to a specific epitope of a cell surface receptor can directly induce strong apoptotic signals, the effect is usually amplified by cross-linking of the antibody Fc domains through binding to Fc receptors on immune effector cells such as macrophages and natural killer cells. Concomitantly, the immune effector cells are activated by the engagement of the Fc receptors, resulting in an attack on the cells to which they are bound, a process known as antibody-dependent cell cytolysis (ADCC). The Fc domains can also activate the complement system, causing complement-dependent cytolysis (CDC). To what extent cell lysis is caused by direct binding and how much is due to the recruitment of immune effector cells and complement is difficult to quantify, especially in an *in vivo* system, and in many cases the mechanism of action of antitumor antibodies remains ill defined. For the action of most cytolytic antibodies, all three mechanisms are probably involved to a lesser or greater extent. Furthermore, recent findings suggest that ADCC also contributes to the efficacy of those antibodies that were previously thought to cause tumor regression solely by blocking the ligand-binding site of growth hormone receptors.

In the second generation of therapeutic recombinant antibodies now in various stages of development, novel techniques and creative antibody engineering have evolved to optimize pharmokinetic and pharmodynamic properties. For example, the affinity of antibody Fc domains for their receptors on immune effector cells or to complement has been improved by both random and targeted mutagenesis. Cell lines have also been generated for altering the glycosyl side chains on the Fc domains for better Fc-receptor binding. Algorithms and *in vitro* techniques have been devised for predicting immunogenicity and selecting the best variants. In addition, the cyto-toxic potential of antibodies and antibody fragments has been increased by arming them with toxins, radionuclides, or immune effector molecules such as cytokines. A large number of novel antibody formats ranging from single variable domains of approximately 13kDa to full-length antibodies with multiple variable domains of approximately 200kDa have been constructed to enable a variety of different func-tions. For example, bispecific antibodies for recruiting T cells to lyse tumor cells have been engineered without constant domains, thus reducing the risk of cytokine storms due to extensive cross-linking with Fc receptors. Finally, a variety of novel protein scaffolds are being investigated as alternatives to immunoglobulin fragments for the generation of libraries of highly diverse binding molecules that could result in novel therapeutic drugs. However, as nearly all of the alternative binding molecules are the same size as or even smaller than single immunoglobulin domain antibodies, their serum half-lives will probably have to be significantly extended using techniques such as pegylation or fusion to serum proteins such as albumin.

All of the recombinant antibody technologies just described are covered by the 24 articles in this book, written by recognized experts in their field, many of whom have pioneered important new techniques. Starting with a description of the technologies used to generate recombinant antibodies, the following chapters provide a fairly comprehensive overview, with examples and background information, on how anti-body efficacy is being improved by decreasing immunogenicity, increasing effector function through increased Fc-receptor binding, conjugating with cytolytic agents, using novel formats and scaffolds with multiple valencies and specificities, and increasing serum half-life. Several promising therapeutic approaches have been included, such as a novel method for selecting antibodies that specifically lyse tumor cells, the development of a recombinant antibody prodrug, and the use of novel recombinant antibodies that target T cells for the treatment of autoimmune disease. Last but not least, an attempt to forecast future developments in the field of ther-apeutic recombinant antibodies has been made on the basis of an excellent market analysis of this rapidly growing field.

M.L.

RECOMBINANT ANTIBODIES FOR IMMUNOTHERAPY

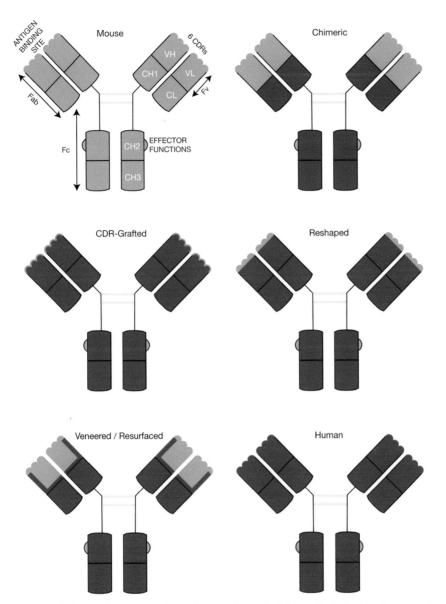

Figure 1.1. Schematic representations of mouse, humanized (chimeric, CDR-Grafted, reshaped, veneered/resurfaced) and human antibodies. Blue, mouse content; red, human content; yellow, disulphide bridges; green, carbohydrate moieties. VH, variable heavy domain; VL, variable light domain; CH1 to 3, constant heavy domains 1 to 3; CL, constant light domain; Fab, fragment antigen binding; Fc, fragment of crystallization; Fv, fragment variable.

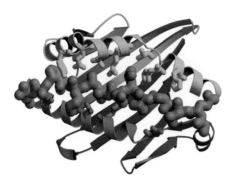

Figure 2.2. Top view of the HLA Class II DRB1*0101 binding groove, with α and β chains in blue and green, respectively, and the bound peptide in orange (PDB-code 1KLU).

(a) Asn-162

FcγRIII

Fucose

Fc

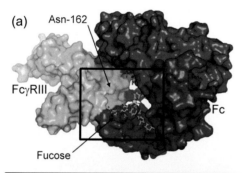

(b)

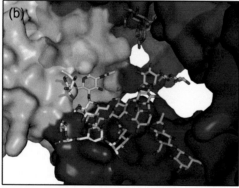

Figure 11.5. Model of the interaction of glycosylated FcγRIII with the Fc-fragment of IgG. **Top:** Clipping of the crystal structure of non-glycosylated FcγRIII expressed in *E. coli* (green) in complex with the Fc-fragment of native (fucosylated) IgG (PDB code 1e4k, red and blue) as indicated in the inset. The glycans attached to the Fc are shown as ball and sticks and colored accordingly. The fucose linked to the carbohydrate of the blue Fc-fragment chain is highlighted in red. **Bottom:** Model of the interaction between a glycosylated FcγRIII and the (non-fucosylated) Fc-fragment of IgG. In this model, the carbohydrates attached at Asn-162 of FcγRIII can thoroughly interact with the non-fucosylated IgG. The figure was created using the program PYMOL (www .delanoscientific.com).

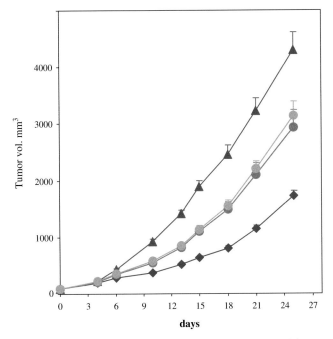

Figure 14.1. Efficacy of AS1409 in a PC3mm2 subcutaneous model.
▲ Phosphate-buffered saline
◆ huBC1-muIL-12 20μg × 7 daily doses
● huBC1 10μg & muIL-12 1.5μg × 7 daily doses
● muIL-12 1.5μg × 7 daily doses

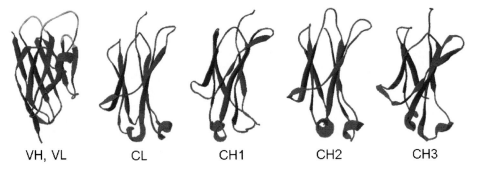

Figure 17.1. Ribbon presentation of the domains of an IgG1. Non-CDR loops are indicated in red, CDR loops in green, and the beta sandwich core in blue. The structures are aligned such that the N-terminal ends are on the top and the C-terminal ends are on the bottom.

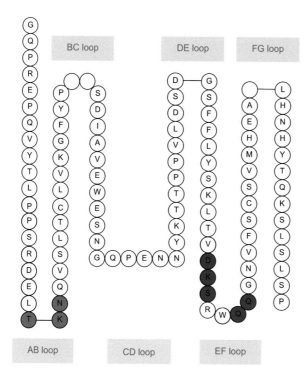

Figure 17.2. The fold of the CH3 domain of human IgG1 presented in perlchain form (Ruiz and Lefranc, 2002). Residues that were randomized in the CH3 libraries are indicated in blue and red, respectively.

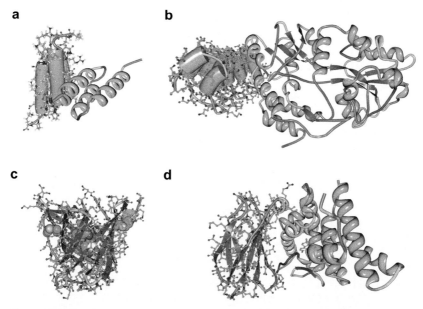

Figure 18.1. Representative structures of non-antibody binders in complex with their target. The figure attempts to emphasize the different secondary structures of the different scaffolds. Structures were obtained from the PDB. The selected binder is shown with its side chains, and helices as cylinders, the target without side chains and helices as ribbons. (a) Affibody in complex with its target, here another affibody (PDB ID 2B87), (b) DARPin in complex with Maltose Binding Protein (PDB ID 1SVX), (c) Anticalin in complex with fluorescein (shown as space filling model in the center); the two disulfide bonds of the libpocalin are also shown in space filling representation on the top left and top right (PDB ID 1N0S), (d) Monobody in complex with the human estrogen receptor alpha ligand-binding domain (PDB ID 2OCF).

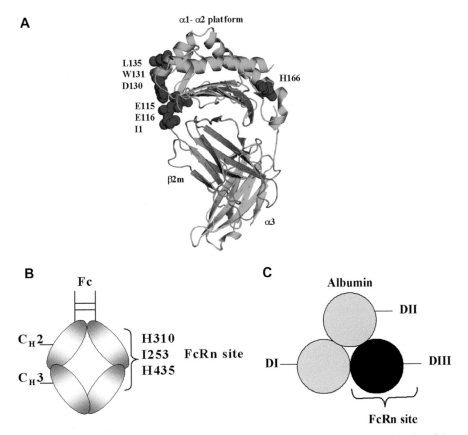

Figure 20.2. FcRn, IgG Fc, and albumin. (A) The crystal structure of shFcRn with the localization of the amino acids essential for IgG (E115, E116, D130, W131, and L135) and albumin (H166) binding highlighted. The heavy chain is shown in green and the β2m in orange. (B) IgG Fc. Amino acids (H310, H435 and I253) at the Fc elbow region involved in binding to FcRn are highlighted. (C) Albumin consists of three domains denoted DI, DII, and DIII. The putative FcRn binding site on DIII is in black. The figure in (A) was designed using pyMOL with the crystallographic data of the shFcRn crystal[12].

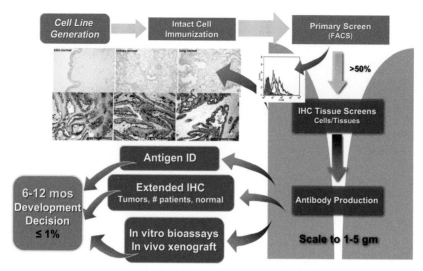

Figure 21.1. Raven antibody discovery platform. Raven-derived human tissue progenitor cell lines and cancer stem cell lines are used as input into the platform. Following immunization and hybridoma generation, the hybridoma supernatants are screened by flow cytometry – greater than 50% of hybridomas typically bind to the cell surface of the immunizing cell line and pass to the immunohistochemical tissue screens on a subset of human normal and tumor tissue samples. Hybridomas that pass this screen for differential expression on tumor tissues are scaled up to generate purified antibody for retesting and expanded immunohistochemistry, as well as antigen identification and bioactivity assays. This process filters out greater than 99% of the antibodies and yields a data package within 6 to 12 months to guide developmental decisions.

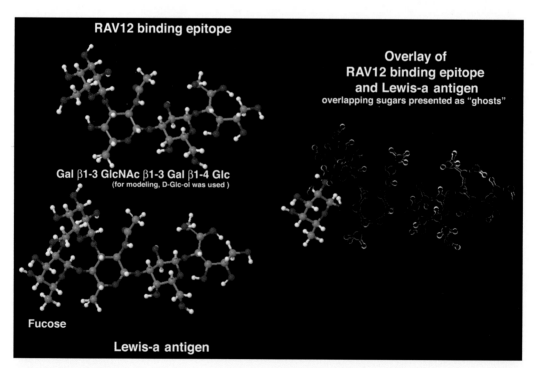

Figure 21.4. The RAAG12 glycotope, the target for the RAV12 antibody, is an N-linked carbohydrate distinct from known cancer glycotopes. The minimal RAV12 binding region encompasses Galβ1 – 3GlcNAcβ1 – 3Gal as determined using synthetic carbohydrate analogs. This epitope is similar to Lewis-a antigen, a member of the Lewis blood group antigens. As can be seen, the two structures are very similar (modeled Galβ1 – 3GlcNAcβ1 – 3Gal on top, as labeled, and modeled Lewis-a antigen on bottom, as labeled). The difference resides in the terminal α1–4 linked fucose found on the Lewis-a antigen. This is accentuated in the overlaid model shown on the right. The overlapping carbohydrate structures are "ghosted" out, highlighting the fucose, the difference between the two structures, and the structure that determines RAV12 specificity.

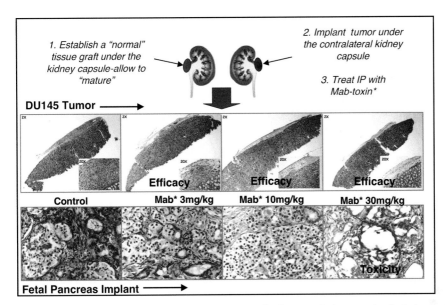

Figue 21.8. *In vivo* human tissue toxicology model. Human fetal pancreatic tissue was implanted under the renal capsule of athymic mice and allowed to mature for 5.5 months until it resembled that of the adult pancreas. 5 x 10^5 DU145 prostate tumor cells, which express the antigen of interest, were subsequently implanted under the contralateral renal capsule and allowed to establish for 2 days. The animals were then treated with a toxin-conjugated antibody twice weekly for 2 weeks, and the xenografts were analyzed histologically on day 16. Toxicity of the matured pancreatic tissue implant was observed at 30 mg/kg/dose, whereas antitumor efficacy was observed with doses as low as 3 mg/kg.

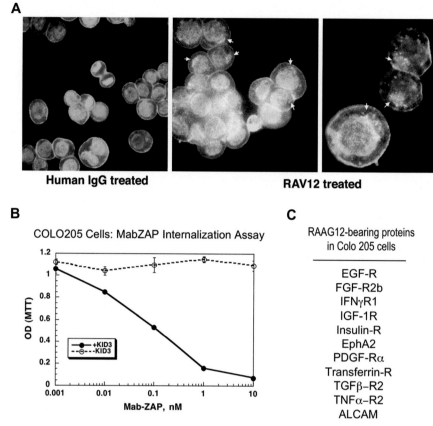

Figure 21.10. KID3 binds to RAAG12-bearing cell surface proteins and is rapidly internalized. **A:** COLO 205 tumor cells were treated with RAV12 antibody or human IgG for 48 hours (see figure label) then applied human IgG Fc was visualized by fluorescent microscopy. The treatment with RAV12, which binds strongly to the cell surface, results in capping and internalization of the RAV12 antibody (red, Cy3-conjugated antihuman IgG Fc – see arrows). Capping and internalization of RAV12 could be observed within 1 hour of antibody treatment. Capping and internalization was not observed in conditions where cells were treated with control human IgG. Unbound RAAG12 was stained using fresh KID3 antibody (green, FITC-conjugated anti-mouse IgG Fc) and is membrane specific on both RAV12 treated and untreated cells. **B:** *In vitro* internalization of KID3 antibody by COLO 205 tumor cells measured by internalization of a toxin-conjugated anti-mouse secondary antibody (mAb-ZAP). A differential decrease in cell viability in the KID3 condition relative to the control condition (no KID3 present), as measured by MTT, indicates antibody internalization. **C:** A partial list of cell surface proteins that are decorated with RAAG12 in COLO 205 cells.

PART I

HUMANIZED ANTIBODIES

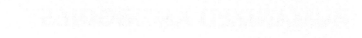

CHAPTER ONE

Humanization of Recombinant Antibodies

José W. Saldanha

Since 1890, when von Behring and Kitasato reported that animal antitoxin serum could protect against lethal doses of toxins in humans, antisera have been used to neutralize pathogens in acute disease as well as in prophylaxis. Antisera are also used *in vitro* as diagnostic tools to establish and monitor disease. However, antisera invariably induce an immune response resulting in joint pains, fevers, and sometimes life-threatening anaphylactic shock. Various proteins contribute to the immunogenicity, as the serum is a crude extract containing not only the antibodies against the disease-causing antigen (often at low concentration), but also other antibodies and proteins.

FULLY MOUSE TO FULLY HUMAN

In 1975, Köhler and Milstein (1975) at the Medical Research Council's (MRC) Laboratory of Molecular Biology in Cambridge (UK) reported their discovery of a way to produce custom-built antibodies *in vitro* with relative ease. They fused rodent antibody-producing cells with immortal tumor cells (myelomas) from the bone marrow of mice to produce hybridomas. A hybridoma combines the cancer cell's ability to reproduce almost indefinitely with the immune cell's ability to produce antibodies. Once screened to isolate the hybridomas yielding antibodies of the required antigen specificity and affinity – and given the right nutrients – a hybridoma will grow and divide, mass-producing antibodies of a single type (monoclonals). Nearly a century before, the German scientist Paul Ehrlich envisaged that such entities could be used as magic bullets to target and destroy human diseases, and hybridomas seemed like a production line of batch consistency for these magic bullets.

Although monoclonal antibodies (mAbs) from hybridoma technology have proved to be immensely useful scientific research and diagnostic tools, they have not completely fulfilled the possibilities inherent in Ehrlich's vision. The problems include identifying better antigenic targets of therapeutic value with which to raise mAbs; making useful fragments of mAbs that can be produced using microbial expression systems and are better, for instance, at penetrating solid cancerous tumors; and attaching toxic payloads, such as radioisotopes or immunotoxins, to the mAbs since animal antibodies are not as effective as human in recruiting the other cells of the immune system to complete their therapeutic function. The major hurdle has proven to be similar to that of antisera therapy – namely, that when animal mAbs are administered in multiple doses, the patient almost invariably raises an immune response to the mAbs causing attenuation of their biological activity and clinical symptoms similar to serum sickness and sometimes serious enough to endanger life. This anti-antibody response (AAR), also known as the human anti-mouse antibody response (HAMA) (Schroff et al., 1985) (since rodents are the most common source of animal mAbs), can develop shortly after initiation of treatment and precludes long-term therapy. The HAMA response can be of two types: anti-isotypic and anti-idiotypic. In actual fact, when the murine antibody OKT3 was administered to human patients, much of the resulting antibody response was directed to the variable domains, making it anti-idiotypic (Jaffers et al., 1986). Despite this difficulty, several murine antibodies or their Fab fragments have been approved for diagnostic and therapeutic use by the Food and Drug Administration (FDA) of the United States (Table 1.1A).

The obvious solution to overcome this hurdle would be to raise human mAbs to the therapeutic targets, but this has been difficult both practically and ethically using the route of immortalization of human antibody-producing cells. Human hybridomas, besides being difficult to prepare, are unstable and secrete low levels of mAbs of the IgM class with low affinity although *ex vivo* immunization and immortalization of human B cells is becoming possible (Li et al., 2006). Two other approaches to producing fully human mAbs from phage libraries (McCafferty et al., 1990) (see section titled "Phage Libraries" later in this chapter) or transgenic animals (Brüggemann et al., 1991) have been possible since the early 1990s, and a couple of these have been approved by the FDA (Table 1E): Humira (adalimumab) developed from a phage library for the treatment of rheumatoid arthritis, Crohn's disease, and plaque psoriasis; and Vectibix (panitumumab) obtained from a transgenic mouse and used in the treatment of colorectal cancer.

HUMANIZED ANTIBODIES

Chimeric Antibodies

In an effort to realize Ehrlich's dream of a magic bullet with high binding affinity, reduced immunogenicity (reduced AAR), increased half-life in the human body, and adequate recruitment of human effector functions, scientists have used techniques to design, engineer, and express mAbs from hybridoma technology to produce humanized antibodies. These approaches are possible because of the segmented structure of the antibody molecule, which allows functional domains carrying antigen-binding or effector functions to be exchanged (Figure 1.1: Mouse). One interpolative step between fully mouse and fully human antibodies is to construct a chimeric antibody by coupling the animal antigen-binding variable domains to human constant domains (Figure 1.1: Chimeric) (Boulianne et al., 1984; Morrison et al., 1984; Neuberger et al., 1985) and expressing the engineered, recombinant antibodies in myeloma cells. Transgenic animals have also been bred whose

TABLE 1.1. Antibody drugs approved by the Food and Drug Administration (FDA)

rINN[a]	Trade name	Antigen[b]	Therapeutic area[c]	Approval date (U.S.)	Isotype subtype[d]
A. MURINE					
Muromonab-CD3	Orthoclone OKT3	CD3	AIID	1986	mIgG2a
Tositumomab	Bexxar	CD20 radiolabel I-131	Onco	2003	mIgG2a
Arcitumomab	CEA-Scan	CEA radiolabel Tc-99m	Onco (D)	1996	mIgG1 (Fab)
Imciromab Pentetate	Myoscint	cardiac myosin radiolabel In-111	Card (D)	1996	mIgG2a (Fab)
Capromab Pendetide	Prostascint	PSMA radiolabel In-111	Onco (D)	1996	mIgG1
Technetium nofetumomab merpentan	Verluma	NR-LU-10 (40kd gp) radiolabel Tc-99m	Onco (D)	1996	mIgG2b (Fab)
Ibritumomab Tiuxetan	Zevalin	CD20 radiolabel Y-90/In-111	Onco	2002	mIgG1
B. CHIMERIC					
Cetuximab	Erbitux	EGFR	Onco	2004	hIgG1
Infliximab	Remicade	TNFα	AIID	1998	hIgG1
Abciximab	ReoPro	gpIIb/IIIa Receptor	Card	1994	hIgG1 (Fab)
Rituximab	Rituxan/MabThera	CD20	Onco	1997	hIgG1
Basiliximab	Simulect	CD25	AIID	1998	hIgG1
C. CDR-GRAFTED					
Eculizumab[e]	Soliris	Complement C5	PNH	2007	hIgG2/4
D. RESHAPED					
Bevacizumab	Avastin	VEGF	Onco	2004	hIgG1
Alemtuzumab	Campath	CD52	Onco	2001	hIgG1
Trastuzumab	Herceptin	HER2	Onco	1998	hIgG1
Ranibizumab	Lucentis	VEGF	Ophth	2006	hIgG1 (Fab)
Gemtuzumab Ozogamicin	Mylotarg	CD33 cytotoxic calicheamicin	Onco	2000	hIgG4
Efalizumab	Raptiva	CD11a	AIID	2003	hIgG1
Palivizumab	Synagis	RSV F	Infec	1998	hIgG1
Natalizumab[f]	Tysabri	integrin-α4	AIID	2004	hIgG4
Omalizumab	Xolair	IgE	Resp	2003	hIgG1
Daclizumab	Zenapax	CD25	AIID	1997	hIgG1
Tocilizumab	Actemra	IL-6R	CD	2005 (Japan)	hIgG1
E. HUMAN					
Adalimumab	Humira	TNFα	AIID	2002	hIgG1
Panitumumab	Vectibix	EGFR	Onco	2006	hIgG2

Note: Not all the murine antibodies are commercially available.

[a] rINN, recommended International Nonproprietary Name.

[b] CD, cluster of differentiation; CEA, carcinoembryonic antigen; PSMA, prostate specific membrane antigen; kd, kilodalton; gp, glycoprotein; EGFR, epidermal growth factor receptor; TNFα, tumor necrosis factor alpha; VEGF, vascular endothelial growth factor receptor; HER2, human epidermal growth factor receptor 2; RSV F, respiratory syncytial virus F protein; IgE, immunoglobulin E; IL-6R, interleukin 6 receptor.

[c] (D), diagnostic; AIID, arthritis, inflammation, immune disease; Onco, oncological disease; Card, cardiovascular disease; Ophth, ophthalmic disease; PNH, paroxysmal nocturnal hemoglobinuria; Infec, infectious disease; Resp, respiratory disease; CD, Castleman's disease.

[d] m, mouse; h, human; Fab, fragment antigen binding.

[e] Since Eculizumab (Soliris) used the structural (Chothia) loops for CDR-H1, it arguably contains backmutations and therefore is not strictly a pure CDR graft.

[f] Voluntary suspension in 2005; granted restricted approval 2006.

immune systems produce such chimeric antibodies (Jensen et al., 2007). Variations on this theme have also been attempted, for instance Lv et al. (2007) have recently attached a mouse single chain Fv (scFv) to the CH3 domain of human IgG1 using a redesigned human IgG1 hinge region resulting in what they call a bivalent "partial chimeric" antibody.

The main decision in producing a chimeric antibody is the choice of human constant regions (Figure 1.1: Mouse) that provide an isotype relevant to the desired biological function; IgG1 and IgG3 subtypes are most effective for complement and cell-mediated lysis-triggering effector cascades whereas IgG2 and IgG4 are preferred for target neutralization. In fact, most of the humanized antibodies on the market are of the IgG1 subtype (Table 1.1). In some cases, the effector functions of the constant regions are removed by modifying the Fc so that it does not bind its receptor, thereby minimizing T cell activation and cytokine release, and other modifications could also lead to IgG subtypes with better biological properties. Chimeric antibodies with the same antigen-binding domains fused to different subtypes of constant regions can show different binding affinities (Morelock et al., 1994) and also immunogenicity on repeated administration – the so-called human antichimeric antibody (HACA) response (Brüggemann et al., 1989). This HACA response varies depending on the chimeric antibody and therefore some have still been approved by the FDA (Table 1.1B).

CDR-Grafted Antibodies

Going one step further on the path between fully mouse and fully human antibodies, Greg Winter (Jones et al., 1986), also at the MRC's Cambridge Laboratory of Molecular Biology, realized that only the antigen-binding site from the human antibody (the tip of the variable domains) needed to be replaced by the antigen-binding site from the rodent antibody using genetic engineering techniques. Since the antigen-binding site consists mainly of the six complementarity determining region (CDR) peptide loops, only these were grafted into the human variable (V) regions (Figure 1.1: CDR-grafted). Antibodies generated this way are called CDR-grafted, and in some cases pure CDR-grafting can produce a humanized antibody with roughly the same antigen specificity and affinity as the original animal (usually mouse) antibody. The only choices required are which human V regions to graft the CDRs into and the isotype required to provide the desired biological function. The isotype choice is governed as for chimeric antibodies (see above), but the choice of human V regions is more demanding.

Choice of Human Variable Regions

The early literature on humanization showed a preference for the same human V regions, known as the "fixed frameworks" approach. Usually REI for the variable light (VL) and NEW or KOL for the variable heavy (VH) were chosen since their three-dimensional structures had been solved. This was the case for the

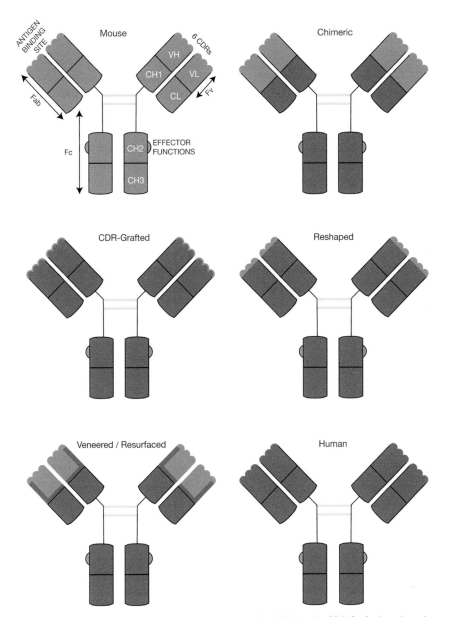

Figure 1.1. Schematic representations of mouse, humanized (chimeric, CDR-Grafted, reshaped, veneered/resurfaced) and human antibodies. Blue, mouse content; red, human content; yellow, disulphide bridges; green, carbohydrate moieties. VH, variable heavy domain; VL, variable light domain; CH1 to 3, constant heavy domains 1 to 3; CL, constant light domain; Fab, fragment antigen binding; Fc, fragment of crystallization; Fv, fragment variable. [See color plate.]

humanized antibody, Campath (Alemtuzumab) (Riechmann et al., 1988) for the treatment of B cell chronic lymphocytic leukemia and later for Actemra (Tocilizumab) (Sato et al., 1993), which is licensed in Japan for the treatment of Castleman's disease and rheumatoid arthritis. Other groups tried to use human acceptor V regions that showed the closest similarity to their mouse donor V regions in an approach known as ''homology matching'' (also called ''best fit'' (Gorman et al.,

1991)). This was the approach taken by Queen et al. (1989) for the VH of the anti-TAC antibody, now marketed as Zenapax (Daclizumab) for the prophylaxis of acute organ rejection in patients receiving renal transplants. In this case, the VL was chosen to match the VH, that is, the same human antibody for both chains, while others have used the most similar VL and VH from different human antibodies (e.g., Daugherty et al., 1991). Variations on the best fit approach take into consideration the extent of sequence similarity (either the whole V region or the individual frameworks between the CDRs – chosen from either single or different human antibodies) and matching lengths of CDRs between the mouse and human V regions. Human V regions can also be chosen based on sequence similarity but with particular amino acid types fixed at positions deemed to be important for affinity, specificity, or stability. A subtle comparison of the fixed frameworks and best fit methods, in terms of the ease of producing a functional humanized antibody, can be found in the humanization of antibody M22 (Graziano et al., 1995). There the preferential choice appeared to be the latter, where the more sequence similar human KOL VH gave better binding than NEW. It has been argued that the advantage of the best fit approach might be outweighed by the wealth of experience that has been assembled using fixed frameworks (Hamilton et al., 1997). However, when the crystal structures of two humanized forms of antibody AF2 were determined, which differed in the sequence identity of the mouse VH to the humanized, the form with greater identity was significantly more structurally similar to the mouse antibody (Bourne et al., 2004). Since structure determines function, the more structurally similar humanized antibody would presumably reproduce the function of the mouse antibody more faithfully.

Both the fixed frameworks and best fit approaches to human V region selection can be limited to the processed V regions found in protein sequence databases, giving the advantage that the humanized molecule is more likely to be stable and expressed. However, this runs the risk of somatic mutations in these V regions creating immunogenic epitopes, even though human sequences are used. An alternative approach is to use the V regions from human consensus sequences where idiosyncratic somatic mutations will have been evened out (Shearman et al., 1991). It is still uncertain whether fixed frameworks, best fit, or consensus selection for humanized antibodies are best in terms of binding. Best fit and consensus selection were compared, in one case showing better binding with best fit (Sato et al., 1994) and in another case showing no difference (Kolbinger et al., 1993). Comparison of fixed frameworks and consensus selection (Maeda et al., 1991) showed loss of binding with the fixed frameworks. In several humanized antibodies, best fit V regions have been chosen from a protein sequence database, only to then exchange the residues in some positions for those of a consensus amino acid (e.g., Hakimi et al., 1993). Consensus sequences can also be selected in a fixed frameworks type of approach, regardless of sequence similarity to the mouse V region, using the knowledge that the most abundant human subgroups are VH subgroup III for the heavy chain and VL subgroup I for the kappa light chain.

Consensus sequences are artificial, having been created by taking the most frequent amino acid at a particular sequence position from a collection of sequences in a human V region subgroup. Although they have no unusual residues, they may contain unnatural sequence motifs that are immunogenic. An alternative approach is to use human germline sequences, originally suggested by Shearman et al. (1991), that do not contain the somatic hypermutations found in the protein- and cDNA-derived sequences in the databanks. Consensus and germline sequences can be selected in a best fit approach, with high sequence similarity to the mouse V region. The variations considered in the best fit approach are also possible with germline sequences – for instance, multiple individual germline frameworks corresponding to different segments of the V region can be used in an essentially mix-and-match procedure. So called "superhumanized" antibodies are humanized antibodies using germlines matched to the canonical templates (see section titled "Sequence Analysis" later in the chapter) of the mouse antibody (Tan et al., 2002).

Reshaped Antibodies

The first reported CDR-graft was performed using the donor VH CDRs of a murine anti-hapten antibody B1-8 grafted into acceptor VH frameworks from human antibody NEW (Jones et al., 1986) to determine whether the CDRs were independent of the framework. Although the binding of the hemi-CDR-grafted antibody was two-to-three-fold lower than the donor mouse antibody, the result was encouraging. This initial work was followed by a CDR graft using the VH CDRs of murine anti-lysozyme antibody D1.3 (Verhoeyen et al., 1988). The binding was 10-fold lower than the donor antibody and it was apparent that CDR loops were not stand-alone entities independent of the framework. The first humanized antibody of therapeutic interest using this approach took the six CDRs from rat antibody Campath-1R and grafted them into human VL from antibody REI and VH from NEW (Riechmann et al., 1988). For the first time, framework reversions (known as "backmutations") from human to rat were incorporated into the engineered antibody, now known as a "reshaped" antibody since the CDR-grafting was accompanied by backmutations to reshape the CDR loops (Figure 1.1: Reshaped). This was followed shortly after by the first reshaped mouse antibody, anti-TAC (Queen et al., 1989). In this case, the human VH framework was chosen based on similarity to the mouse VH, and the partner VL from the same human antibody was also used. Several backmutations were introduced based on a three-dimensional molecular model of the mouse variable regions. The authors proposed to call an antibody prepared in this manner "hyperchimeric" (Junghans et al., 1990) and certainly some reshaped antibodies contain so many framework backmutations that they might be considered almost chimeric. Later work (Schneider et al., 1993) showed the immunogenicity of the reshaped antibody was mainly caused by the CDRs rather than the modified human frameworks, supporting the validity of this approach. The backmutations are necessary to reproduce the affinity and specificity of the mouse antibody in the reshaped molecule. Sometimes they are also necessary to improve the expression yields, although these are rarely reported in the literature. In one case, an improvement in both the affinity and expression was accomplished by a single VL backmutation that improved not only the expression but also the affinity of the molecule (Saldanha et al., 1999). From the early humanizations, it was clear that any strategy for producing reshaped antibodies would require careful analysis of sequence and structure to determine the backmutations required in the final genetically engineered molecule.

Sequence Analysis

The CDRs are six highly variable sequence regions, three each in the VL and VH, of the donor antibody that structurally make up the antigen binding site (Figure 1.1: Mouse). The preponderance of backmutations reported in the literature at position 73 in VH suggests that the structural loop encompassing this residue may also be part of the antigen binding site in some antibodies. The CDRs contain the residues most likely to bind antigen and are defined by sequence according to Kabat (Wu & Kabat, 1970). The extents of the structural loops have also been defined by Chothia (Chothia et al., 1989) although this definition varies in the literature. The CDRs are grafted from the donor antibody into the acceptor human antibody. The Chothia structural loop extents are shorter than the Kabat sequence definition, thus resulting in less mouse sequence in the humanized antibody. However, the structural extent of the CDR-H1 loop encompasses residue positions 28–30 in VH, which are known to exacerbate the immunogenicity in humans (Tempest et al., 1995) whereas the Kabat sequence definition does not. The sequence definition of CDR-H1 often requires backmutations in the region covered by the structural extent of this loop, leading some to combine the definitions for CDR-H1 (e.g., Thomas et al., 1996). Conversely, the structural extent of the CDR-H2 loop usually requires several backmutations in the region covered by the sequence definition (e.g., Rodrigues et al., 1992).

Canonical residues are key residues in the CDR and/or framework that determine the conformation of the structural loop. Chothia and Lesk (1987) originally defined the canonical templates for each CDR conformation, which they later extended (Al-Lazikani et al., 1997). Canonical residues should be retained in the reshaped antibody if they are different from those in the chosen human frameworks. Note that particular CDRs or canonical residues might have no effect on the specificity or affinity of the reshaped antibody if that CDR does not contact the antigen, but there is no way of knowing this by consideration of the sequence alone.

Residues at the interface between VL and VH are also often analyzed in reshaped antibodies since they govern the packing of the variable domains, thus affecting the binding site. Their influence might also be functional since Nakamura et al. (2000) reported that although affinity was not affected, complement-dependent cytotoxicity (CDC), one of the effector functions of mAbs, was improved by a backmutation at the VL/VH interface. The interface residues were defined by Chothia et al. (1985) and have been improved by Vargas-Madrazo and Paz-García (2003).

Rare residues in the donor sequence can be determined by comparison with the Kabat subgroup (Kabat et al., 1987; 1991). Atypical residues near the antigen binding site, as determined from the crystal structure or molecular model (see section titled

"Structure Analysis" later in the chapter), may possibly contact the antigen and therefore should be backmutated. If they are not close to the binding site, then it is desirable to humanize them because they may represent immunogenic epitopes in the reshaped antibody. Sometimes unusual residues in the donor sequence are actually common residues in the human acceptor (Queen et al., 1989) and cause no such difficulties. Atypical residues in the human acceptor frameworks are not desirable because of the possibility of immunogenicity, unless of course they correspond to unusual residues in the donor and thus may be important functionally. Rarely occurring amino acids in the human frameworks have been mutated to human consensus residues (Co et al., 1991).

Potential N-glycosylation sites are specific to the consensus pattern asparagine-X-serine/threonine, where X can be any amino acid except proline, and most patterns on the surface of the protein are glycosylated. They may occur as part of the germline or arise through somatic hypermutation in the frameworks or CDRs. It was expected that addition or removal of N-glycosylation sites in reshaped antibodies might affect their binding or immunogenicity. Their removal has not destroyed the affinity thus far (Léger et al., 1997), even when they are found at canonical residues (Sato et al., 1996), and in some cases the affinity was even increased (Co et al., 1993). Any additional N-glycosylation sites introduced through the humanization procedure should be checked on a model to ensure that they do not interfere with the CDRs. O-glycosylation sites are usually found in helices and are therefore not common in the beta-sheet structure of antibodies.

Structure Analysis

Humanization using the fixed frameworks approach usually meant that the crystal structures of the human acceptor regions were available. These structures could be inspected to identify potential backmutations. Although some humanizations used only sequence analysis (e.g., Poul et al., 1995), other approaches to framework selection (best fit, consensus, germline) relied on a carefully built model of the mouse variable regions (e.g., Kettleborough et al., 1991) and in some cases the humanized variable regions, particularly when inspecting introduced N-glycosylation sites. Superposition of the mouse and humanized three-dimensional models and analysis of the size, charge, hydrophobicity, or hydrogen-bond potential between topologically equivalent residues allowed potential backmutations to be revealed. In some cases, a model of the antigen was also built (Nishihara et al., 2001). A model of the donor antibody docked to the antigen would be ideal for the design of a humanized antibody, in the absence of a crystal structure for the complex, and has been achieved by computer-guided docking (Zhang et al., 2005). The advantage is that CDRs not contacting antigen can be determined, and unnecessary grafting and backmutations avoided. Computer modeling can only be an interim measure on the way to determining the structure of the antibody or antibody-antigen complex by X-ray crystallography or nuclear magnetic resonance (NMR).

Antibody modeling is relatively simple compared to the modeling of other proteins, since the framework is so well conserved. This reduces the problem to modeling the CDRs, and the conformation of many of these CDRs can be inferred from the canonical templates (see section titled "Sequence Analysis" earlier in the chapter). It is rarely necessary to apply sophisticated loop modeling techniques to more than a couple of CDRs per antibody. Although there are no canonical templates available for CDR-H3, Shirai et al. (1996; 1999) showed that in many cases these loops exhibit "kinked" or "extended" C terminal regions predicted by sequence-based rules. These rules can be applied to determine additional features of CDR-H3 and aid its conformational prediction. It is possible to build a model completely automatically using programs such as Modeller (http://www.salilab.org/modeller/) and academic servers such as Swiss-Model (http://swissmodel.expasy.org/). However, the pitfall of allowing a computer to make all the decisions is highlighted in the humanization of antibody AT13/5 (Ellis et al., 1995), where the interaction between VH residues at positions 29 and 78 was not modeled correctly.

OTHER APPROACHES TO ANTIBODY HUMANIZATION

SDR-Transfer

CDR-grafting and reshaping do not necessarily eliminate the immunogenicity of the resultant molecule due to residual responses directed against the murine CDRs. An analysis of antibody structures determined that antigen binding usually involves only 20% to 33% of the CDR residues (Padlan, 1994) that have been given the label "specificity determining residues" (SDRs). Padlan et al. (1995) extended this work to determine the boundaries of the potential SDRs in different antigen-combining sites and called the segments thus found "abbreviated CDRs." The SDRs are commonly located at positions of high variability and are unique to each mAb. However, they can be identified by site-directed mutagenesis or determination of the 3D structure of the variable regions, or, in the absence of this information, the variability of positions within the abbreviated CDRs can be used to suggest which residues are SDRs. Transfer of SDRs only has been used successfully in the humanization of anticarcinoma mAb CC49, which specifically recognizes tumor-associated glycoprotein (TAG)-72 (Yoon et al., 2006). In that case, the lower affinity of the SDR-transferred antibody was improved by random mutagenesis of CDR-H3 (*in vitro* affinity maturation). SDR-transfer into human germline frameworks has been utilized in the humanization of murine mCOL-1, which specifically recognizes carcinoembryonic antigen (CEA). In this case, the SDR-transferred antibody had comparable binding activity to the reshaped equivalent and significantly higher activity compared with the abbreviated CDR-grafted antibody. It also showed decreased reactivity for anti-V region antibodies present in the sera of patients treated with mCOL-1 (Gonzales et al., 2004).

Veneering/Resurfacing

Another alternative to CDR-grafting/SDR transfer and reshaping is to replace only the surface residues of the murine variable regions with human residues while maintaining the murine core and CDRs (Figure 1.1: Veneered/Resurfaced). An early description of the differences in the pattern of surface residues on the three-dimensional structures of a small number of human and mouse antibody variable regions had already been published (Padlan, 1991); here the strategy of the replacement of solvent-exposed surface mouse with human residues found at equivalent positions was called "veneering." The analysis showed that the positions of surface residues were remarkably conserved between the two species. Also, the pattern of amino acid substitution was conserved within a species, but not between species – that is, no mouse variable region displayed the exact pattern of surface residues found in any human variable region. Thus, it was possible to convert a murine surface pattern to that of human with a small number of mutations. A later analysis of known three-dimensional protein structures to determine the relative solvent accessibility distributions of residues in human and mouse antibodies (Pedersen et al., 1994) resulted in the development of a similar surface replacement strategy known as "resurfacing." Staelens et al. (2006) modified this approach by comparing surface exposed residues on a molecular model of the murine variable domains with sequences of human antibodies with high identity and found some differences with the results of Pedersen et al. (1994). Thus molecular models are still required (as for reshaped antibodies) plus the choice of which solvent-exposed positions and types of residues to mutate to produce a characteristic human surface pattern without affecting the affinity or specificity of the parent antibody (e.g., Fontayne et al., 2006). Veneered/resurfaced antibodies are arguably easier to design and conceivably less immunogenic than reshaped antibodies, although this ignores the likelihood of T cell epitopes presented from the murine core of the antibody.

T Cell and B Cell Epitope Removal

The immunogenicity of antibodies (or other proteins) can be reduced by the identification and removal of potential helper T cell epitopes from the biopharmaceuticals and is usually combined with antibody veneering (based on Padlan's approach) to effectively humanize surface residues (thus removing B cell epitopes). This strategy is commonly known as DeImmunization™ (Hellendoorn et al., 2004). Helper T cell epitopes are short peptide sequences within proteins that bind to MHC class II molecules. These epitopes can be created by somatic mutations occurring naturally in human antibodies or by the CDR-grafting/SDR transfer, reshaping, veneering, or resurfacing process itself. The peptide-MHC class II complexes are recognized by T cells and trigger the activation and differentiation of helper T cells, thus stimulating a cellular immune response. Helper T cells initiate and maintain immunogenicity by interacting with B cells, resulting in the production of antibodies that bind specifically to the administered antibody. In DeImmunization, helper T cell epitopes are identified within the primary sequence of the antibody using prediction software, and these sequences are altered by amino acid substitution to avoid recognition by T cells. The computer software is principally based on modeling work with the crystal structures of MHC class II allotypes combined with a database search of known T cell epitopes. As a result, the modified antibody should no longer trigger T cell help. In this way immunogenicity may be eliminated or at least substantially reduced. However, particular peptides are not necessarily processed and presented by MHC class II, so some unnecessary epitope deletion is inevitable. Furthermore, there is the issue of tolerance of human antibodies, and this is handled by ignoring peptides present in human antibody sequences.

Another recent approach to removing T and B cell epitopes uses human string content (HSC) (Lazar et al., 2007). HSC is a metric of antibody "human-ness" computed by determining the peptide strings in a murine antibody that are also found within a set of human sequences. The computer program, through mouse to human substitutions in VH or VL, maximizes the HSC of the humanized molecule. To maintain the structural integrity, which might be disrupted by the substitutions, a sequence- and structure-based scoring method known as Analogous Contact Environments (ACE) is used. The method was applied to four antibodies of different antigen specificity and produced HSC humanized antibodies with comparable or higher affinity to the parent antibody and in some cases better expression levels. It was noted that the HSC scores of reshaped antibodies were close to, but not as good as, HSC humanized antibodies.

Phage Libraries

The relative importance of backmutations varies between different reshaped mAbs, and therefore the identification of important residue positions in the sequence and the determination of the optimal amino acid at those positions has proved challenging. With the advent of phage display of antibody fragments (Fvs, Fabs, etc.) (McCafferty et al., 1990) combined with efficient screening methods, large numbers of variants can be rapidly characterized for activity. This allows the properties of the humanized antibody to be optimized or even evolved *in vitro*, in contrast to iterative attempts at rational design. These combinatorial libraries have been used for the humanization of antibodies. Murine CDRs have been grafted into human frameworks from germline, consensus, or mature functional sources while selected buried positions in the frameworks were randomized with all possible combinations of murine/human amino acids in a phage library (Baca et al., 1997; Rosok et al., 1996). Thus the best binders were selected by screening many different reshaped Fabs differing only in their backmutations. The approach can also be used to optimize CDR residues (Wu et al., 1999) combining humanization and *in vitro* affinity maturation in the same procedure.

In the framework shuffling approach (Dall'Acqua et al., 2005), the CDRs are grafted into a pool of human germline frameworks, but residue positions in the frameworks are not combinatorially explored. The corresponding libraries are screened for binding to antigen. The process obviously does not require the building of a structural molecular model and the combinatorial power of this approach allows selection not only for binding and specificity but also expression yields (Damschroder et al., 2007).

A different strategy termed guided selection or chain shuffling has been used to isolate fully human mAbs from phage display libraries in a two-step process that does not require CDR-grafting. In the first stage, the source VH is paired with a repertoire of human VLs. The Fabs are displayed on filamentous phage and the selected human VL isolated from the screening process is paired in the second stage with a human VH repertoire. Therefore, the mouse variable domains are sequentially replaced by human variable domains (Jespers et al., 1994; Rader et al. 1998), although there is the risk of a drift in epitope recognition with this process (Ohlin et al., 1996). This was the approach taken in the development of the first fully human (Figure 1.1: Human) antibody approved by the FDA, Humira (adalimumab).

OUTLOOK

The predicted lowering of immunogenicity on moving from fully mouse to fully human antibodies via humanization has largely been proven (Hwang & Foote, 2005). The dominance of reshaped antibodies on the market (Table 1.1D) is testimony to the effectiveness of this approach. The author has participated in the design of nearly 50 successfully CDR-grafted and reshaped antibodies with several in clinical trials and two now on the market: Tysabri (Natalizumab) (Léger et al., 1997) for the treatment of multiple sclerosis and Crohn's disease, and Actemra (Tocilizumab) (Sato et al., 1993) licensed for Castleman's disease and rheumatoid arthritis in Japan. This success was in part due to the advances in protein sequence/structure analysis and modeling in the last 20 years. There are no FDA approved SDR-grafted, veneered/resurfaced, or T and B cell removed humanized antibodies at present – they may prove to be more effective than reshaped antibodies. There is only one CDR-grafted antibody (Table 1.1C): Eculizumab (Soliris) for the treatment of paroxysmal nocturnal hemoglobinuria (PNH). However, since this antibody uses a combination of Chothia's structural loops plus Kabat's sequence definition for CDR-H1, it is strictly speaking a reshaped antibody with two backmutations. Implicitly, CDR-grafting requires Kabat's sequence definition of CDRs for the grafting. Eleven such reshaped antibodies have received FDA approval, with many more in clinical trials. Undoubtedly, the couple of fully human antibodies on the market (Table 1.1E) are representative of only where we are at this time; undoubtedly, many more will receive approval, perhaps overtaking the number of reshaped antibodies, in the years to come.

REFERENCES

Al-Lazikani B, Lesk AM, Chothia C. (1997) Standard conformations for the canonical structure of immunoglobulins. *J. Mol. Biol.* **273**, 927–48.

Baca M, Presta LG, O'Connor SJ, Wells JA. (1997) Antibody humanization using monovalent phage display. *J. Biol. Chem.* **272**, 10678–84.

Boulianne GL, Hozumi N, Shulman MJ. (1984) Production of functional chimaeric mouse/human antibody. *Nature.* **312**, 643–6.

Bourne PC, Terzyan SS, Cloud G, Landolfi NF, Vasquez M, Edmundson AB. (2004) Three-dimensional structures of a humanized anti-IFN-gamma Fab (HuZAF) in two crystal forms. *Acta Crystallogr. D. Biol Crystallogr.* **60**, 1761–9.

Brüggemann M, Spicer C, Buluwela L, Rosewell I, Barton S, Surani MA, Rabbitts TH. (1991) Human antibody production in transgenic mice: expression from 100kb of the human IgH locus. *Eur. J. Immunol.* **21**, 1323–6.

Brüggemann M, Winter G, Waldmann H, Neuberger MS. (1989) The immunogenicity of chimeric antibodies. *J. Exp. Med.* **170**, 2153–7.

Chothia C, Lesk AM, Tramontano A, Levitt M, Smith-Gill SJ, Air G, Sheriff S, Padlan EA, Davies D, Tulip WR, Colman PM, Spinelli S, Alzari PM, Poljak RJ. (1989) Conformations of immunoglobulin hypervariable regions. *Nature* **342**, 877–83.

Chothia C, Lesk AM. (1987) Canonical structures for the hypervariable regions of immunoglobulins. *J. Mol. Biol.* **196**, 901–17.

Chothia C, Novotny J, Bruccoleri R, Karplus M. (1985) Domain association in immunoglobulin molecules. The packing of variable domains. *J. Mol. Biol.* **186**, 651–63.

Co MS, Deschamps M, Whitley RJ, Queen C. (1991) Humanized antibodies for antiviral therapy. *Proc. Natl. Acad. Sci. U.S.A.* **88**, 2869–73.

Co MS, Scheinberg DA, Avdalovic NM, McGraw K, Vasquez M, Caron PC, Queen C. (1993) Genetically engineered deglycosylation of the variable domain increases the affinity of an anti-CD33 monoclonal antibody. *Mol. Immunol.* **30**, 1361–7.

Dall'Acqua WF, Damschroder MM, Zhang J, Woods RM, Widjaja L, Yu J, Wu H. (2005) Antibody humanization by framework shuffling. *Methods* **36**, 43–60.

Damschroder MM, Widjaja L, Gill PS, Krasnoperov V, Jiang W, Dall'Acqua WF, Wu H. (2007) Framework shuffling of antibodies to reduce immunogenicity and manipulate functional and biophysical properties. *Mol. Immunol.* **44**, 3049–60.

Daugherty BL, DeMartino JA, Law MF, Kawka DW, Singer II, Mark GE. (1991) Polymerase chain reaction facilitates the cloning, CDR-grafting, and rapid expression of a murine monoclonal antibody directed against the CD18 component of leukocyte integrins. *Nucleic Acids Res.* **19**, 2471–6.

Ellis JH, Barber KA, Tutt A, Hale C, Lewis AP, Glennie MJ, Stevenson GT, Crowe JS. (1995) Engineered anti-CD38 monoclonal antibodies for immunotherapy of multiple myeloma. *J. Immunol.* **155**, 925–37.

Fontayne A, Vanhoorelbeke K, Pareyn I, Van Rompaey I, Meiring M, Lamprecht S, Roodt J, Desmet J, Deckmyn H. (2006) Rational humanization of the powerful antithrombotic anti-GPIbα antibody: 6B4. *Thromb. Haemost.* **96**, 671–84.

Gonzales NR, Padlan EA, De Pascalis R, Schuck P, Schlom J, Kashmiri SV. (2004) SDR grafting of a murine antibody using multiple human germline templates to minimize its immunogenicity. *Mol. Immunol.* **41**, 863–72.

Gorman SD, Clark MR, Routledge EG, Cobbold SP, Waldmann H. (1991) Reshaping a therapeutic CD4 antibody. *Proc. Natl. Acad. Sci. U.S.A.* **88**, 4181–5.

Graziano RF, Tempest PR, White P, Keler T, Deo Y, Ghebremariam H, Coleman K, Pfefferkorn LC, Fanger MW, Guyre PM. (1995) Construction and characterization of a humanized anti-gamma-Ig receptor type I (Fc gamma RI) monoclonal antibody. *J. Immunol.* **155**, 4996–5002.

Hakimi J, Ha VC, Lin P, Campbell E, Gately MK, Tsudo M, Payne PW, Waldmann TA, Grant AJ, Tsien WH, Schneider WP. (1993) Humanized Mik beta 1, a humanized antibody to the IL-2 receptor beta-chain that acts synergistically with humanized anti-TAC. *J. Immunol.* **151**, 1075–85.

Hamilton AA, Manuel DM, Grundy JE, Turner AJ, King SI, Adair JR, White P, Carr FJ, Harris WJ. (1997) A humanized antibody against human cytomegalovirus (CMV) gpUL75 (gH) for prophylaxis or treatment of CMV infections. *J. Infect. Dis.* **176**, 59–68.

Hellendoorn K, Jones T, Watkins J, Baker M, Hamilton A, Carr F. (2004) Limiting the risk of immunogenicity by identification and removal of T-cell epitopes (DeImmunisation™). *Cancer Cell Intl.* **4**, S20.

Hwang WY, Foote J. (2005) Immunogenicity of engineered antibodies. *Methods* **36**, 3–10.

Jaffers GJ, Fuller TC, Cosimi AB, Russell PS, Winn HJ, Colvin RB. (1986) Monoclonal antibody therapy. Anti-idiotypic and non-anti-idiotypic antibodies to OKT3 arising despite intense immunosuppression. *Transplantation* **41**, 572–8.

Jensen M, Klehr M, Bogel A, Schmitz S, Tawadros S, Mühlenhoff M, Plück A, Fischer T, Schomäcker K, Schultze, JL, Berthold F. (2007) One step generation of fully chimeric antibodies using Cγ1- and Cκ mutant mice. *J. Immunother.* **30**, 338–49.

Jespers LS, Roberts A, Mahler SM, Winter G, Hoogenboom HR. (1994) Guiding the selection of human antibodies from phage display repertoires to a single epitope of an antigen. *Biotechnology* **12**, 899–903.

Jones PT, Dear PH, Foote J, Neuberger MS, Winter G. (1986) Replacing the complementarity-determining regions in a human antibody with those from a mouse. *Nature* **321**, 522–5.

Junghans RP, Waldmann TA, Landolfi NF, Avdalovic NM, Schneider WP, Queen C. (1990) Anti-Tac-H, a humanized antibody to the interleukin 2 receptor with new features for immunotherapy in malignant and immune disorders. *Cancer Res.* **50**, 1495–502.

Kabat EA, Wu TT, Perry H, Gottesman K, Foeller C. (1991) *Sequences of Proteins of Immunological Interest*, 5th ed. NIH Publication No. 91–3242.

Kabat EA, Wu TT, Reid-Miller M, Perry H, Gottesman K. (1987) *Sequences of Proteins of Immunological Interest*, 4th ed. US Govt. Printing Office No. 165–492.

Kettleborough CA, Saldanha J, Heath VJ, Morrison CJ, Bendig MM. (1991) Humanization of a mouse monoclonal antibody by CDR-grafting: the importance of framework residues on loop conformation. *Protein Eng.* **4**, 773–83.

Köhler G, Milstein C. (1975) Continuous cultures of fused cells secreting antibody of predefined specificity. *Nature* **256**, 495–7.

Kolbinger F, Saldanha J, Hardman N, Bendig MM. (1993) Humanization of a mouse anti-human IgE antibody: a potential therapeutic for IgE-mediated allergies. *Protein Eng.* **6**, 971–80.

Lazar GA, Desjarlais JR, Jacinto J, Karki S, Hammond PW. (2007) A molecular immunology approach to antibody humanization and functional optimization. *Mol. Immunol.* **44**, 1986–1998.

Léger OJ, Yednock TA, Tanner L, Horner HC, Hines DK, Keen S, Saldanha J, Jones ST, Fritz LC, Bendig MM. (1997) Humanization of a mouse antibody against human alpha-4 integrin: a potential therapeutic for the treatment of multiple sclerosis. *Hum. Antibodies* **8**, 3–16.

Li J, Sai T, Berger M, Chao Q, Davidson D, et al. (2006) Human antibodies for immunotherapy development generated via a human B cell hybridoma technology. *Proc. Natl. Acad. Sci. U.S.A.* **103**, 3557–62.

Lv M, Li Y, Yu M, Sun Y, Lin Z, Qiao C, Luo Q, Gu X, Huang Y, Feng J, Shen B. (2007) Structured to reduce the mitogenicity of anti-CD3 antibody based on computer-guided molecular design. *Int. J. Biochem. Cell Biol.* **39**, 1142–55.

Maeda H, Matsushita S, Eda Y, Kimachi K, Tokiyoshi S, Bendig MM. (1991) Construction of reshaped human antibodies with HIV-neutralizing activity. *Hum. Antibodies Hybridomas.* **2**, 124–34.

McCafferty J, Griffiths AD, Winter G, Chiswell DJ. (1990) Phage antibodies: filamentous phage displaying antibody variable domains. *Nature* **348**, 552–4.

Morelock MM, Rothlein R, Bright SM, Robinson MK, Graham ET, Sabo JP, Owens R, King DJ, Norris SH, Scher DS, et al. (1994) Isotype choice for chimeric antibodies affects binding properties. *J. Biol. Chem.* **269**, 13048–55.

Morrison SL, Johnson MJ, Herzenberg LA, Oi VT. (1984) Chimeric human antibody molecules: mouse antigen-binding domains with human constant region domains. *Proc. Natl. Acad. Sci. U.S.A.* **81**, 6851–5.

Nakamura K, Tanaka Y, Fujino I, Hirayama N, Shitara K, Hanai N. (2000) Dissection and optimization of immune effector functions of humanized anti-ganglioside GM2 monoclonal antibody. *Mol. Immunol.* **37**, 1035–46.

Neuberger MS, Williams GT, Mitchell EB, Jouhal SS, Flanagan JG, Rabbitts TH. (1985) A hapten-specific chimaeric IgE antibody with human physiological effector function. *Nature* **314**, 268–70.

Nisihara T, Ushio Y, Higuchi H, Kayagaki N, Yamaguchi N, Soejima K, Matsuo S, Maeda H, Eda Y, Okumura K, Yagita H. (2001) Humanization and epitope mapping of neutralizing anti-human Fas ligand monoclonal antibodies: structural insights into Fas/Fas ligand interaction. *J. Immunol.* **167**, 3266–75.

Ohlin M, Owman H, Mach M, Borrebaeck CA. (1996) Light chain shuffling of a high affinity antibody results in a drift in epitope recognition. *Mol. Immunol.* **33**, 47–56.

Padlan EA, Abergel C, Tipper JP. (1995) Identification of specificity-determining residues in antibodies. *FASEB J.* **9**, 133–9.

Padlan EA. (1991) A possible procedure for reducing the immunogenicity of antibody variable domains while preserving their ligand-binding properties. *Mol. Immunol.* **28**, 489–98.

Padlan EA. (1994) Anatomy of the antibody molecule. *Mol. Immunol.* **31**, 169–217.

Pedersen JT, Henry AH, Searle SJ, Guild BC, Roguska M, Rees AR. (1994) Comparison of surface accessible residues in human and murine immunoglobulin Fv domains. Implication for humanization of murine antibodies. *J. Mol. Biol.* **235**, 959–73.

Poul MA, Ticchioni M, Bernard A, Lefranc MP. (1995) Inhibition of T cell activation with a humanized anti-beta 1 integrin chain mAb. *Mol. Immunol.* **32**, 101–16.

Queen C, Schneider WP, Selick HE, Payne PW, Landolfi NF, Duncan JF, Avdalovic NM, Levitt M, Junghans RP, Waldmann TA. (1989) A humanized antibody that binds to the interleukin 2 receptor. *Proc. Natl. Acad. Sci. U.S.A.* **86**, 10029–33.

Rader C, Cheresh DA, Barbas CF 3rd. (1998) A phage display approach for rapid antibody humanization: designed combinatorial V gene libraries. *Proc. Natl. Acad. Sci. U.S.A.* **95**, 8910–5.

Riechmann L, Clark M, Waldmann H, Winter G. (1988) Reshaping human antibodies for therapy. *Nature* **332**, 323–7.

Rodrigues ML, Shalaby MR, Werther W, Presta L, Carter P. (1992) Engineering a humanized bispecific F(ab')2 fragment for improved binding to T cells. *Int J Cancer* Suppl. 7, 45–50.

Rosok MJ, Yelton DE, Harris LJ, Bajorath J, Hellstrom KE, Hellstrom I, Cruz GA, Kristensson K, Lin H, Huse WD, Glaser SM. (1996) A combinatorial library strategy for the rapid humanization of anticarcinoma BR96 Fab. *J. Biol. Chem.* **271**, 22611–8.

Saldanha JW, Martin AC, Léger OJ. (1999) A single backmutation in the human kIV framework of a previously unsuccessfully humanized antibody restores the binding activity and increases the secretion in cos cells. *Mol. Immunol.* **36**, 709–19.

Sato K, Ohtomo T, Hirata Y, Saito H, Matsuura T, Akimoto T, Akamatsu K, Koishihara Y, Ohsugi Y, Tsuchiya M. (1996) Humanization of an anti-human IL-6 mouse monoclonal antibody glycosylated in its heavy chain variable region. *Hum. Antibodies. Hybridomas* **7**, 175–83.

Sato K, Tsuchiya M, Saldanha J, Koishihara Y, Ohsugi Y, Kishimoto T, Bendig MM. (1993) Reshaping a human antibody to inhibit the interleukin 6-dependent tumor cell growth. *Cancer Res.* **53**, 851–6.

Sato K, Tsuchiya M, Saldanha J, Koishihara Y, Ohsugi Y, Kishimoto T, Bendig MM. (1994) Humanization of a mouse anti-human interleukin-6 receptor antibody comparing two methods for selecting human framework regions. *Mol. Immunol.* **31**, 371–81.

Schneider WP, Glaser SM, Kondas JA, Hakimi J. (1993) The anti-idiotypic response by cynomolgus monkeys to humanized anti-Tac is primarily directed to complementarity-determining regions H1, H2, and L3. *J. Immunol.* **150**, 3086–90.

Schroff RW, Foon KA, Beatty SM, Oldham RK, Morgan AC Jr. (1985) Human anti-murine immunoglobulin responses in patients receiving monoclonal antibody therapy. *Cancer Res.* **45**, 879–85.

Shearman CW, Pollock D, White G, Hehir K, Moore GP, Kanzy EJ, Kurrle R. (1991) Construction, expression and characterization of humanized antibodies directed against the human alpha/beta T cell receptor. *J. Immunol.* **147**, 4366–73.

Shirai H, Kidera A, Nakamura H. (1996) Structural classification of CDR-H3 in antibodies. *FEBS Lett.* **399**, 1–8.

Shirai H, Kidera A, Nakamura H. (1999) H3-rules: identification of CDR-H3 structures in antibodies. *FEBS Lett.* **455**, 188–97.

Staelens S, Desmet J, Ngo TH, Vauterin S, Pareyn I, Barbeaux P, Van Rompaey I, Stassen JM, Deckmyn H, Vanhoorelbeke K. (2006) Humanization by variable domain resurfacing and grafting on a human IgG4, using a new approach for determination of non-human like surface accessible framework residues based on homology modeling of variable domains. *Mol. Immunol.* **43**, 1243–57.

Tan P, Mitchell DA, Buss TN, Holmes MA, Anasetti C, Foote J. (2002) ''Superhumanized'' antibodies: reduction of immunogenic potential by complementarity-determining region grafting with human germline sequences: application to an anti-CD28. *J. Immunol.* **169**, 1119–25.

Tempest PR, White P, Buttle M, Carr FJ, Harris WJ. (1995) Identification of framework residues required to restore antigen binding during reshaping of a monoclonal antibody against the glycoprotein gB of human cytomegalovirus. *Int. J. Biol. Macromol.* **17**, 37–42.

Thomas TC, Rollins SA, Rother RP, Giannoni MA, Hartman SL, Elliott EA, Nye SH, Matis LA, Squinto SP, Evans MJ. (1996) Inhibition of complement activity by humanized anti-C5 antibody and single-chain Fv. *Mol. Immunol.* **33**, 1389–401.

Vargas-Madrazo E, Paz-García E. (2003) An improved model of association for VH-VL immunoglobulin domains: asymmetries between VH and VL in the packing of some interface residues. *J. Mol. Recognit.* **16**, 113–20.

Verhoeyen M, Milstein C, Winter G. (1988) Reshaping human antibodies: grafting an antilysozyme activity. *Science* **239**, 1534–6.

Wu H, Nie Y, Huse WD, Watkins JD. (1999) Humanization of a murine monoclonal antibody by simultaneous optimization of framework and CDR residues. *J. Mol. Biol.* **294**, 151–62.

Wu TT, Kabat EA. (1970) An analysis of the sequences of the variable regions of Bence Jones proteins and myeloma light chains and their implications for antibody complementarity. *J. Exp. Med.* **132**, 211–50.

Yoon SO, Lee TS, Kim SJ, Jang MH, Kang YJ, Park JH, Kim KS, Lee HS, Ryu CJ, Gonzales NR, Kasmiri SV, Lim SM, Choi CW, Hong HJ. (2006) Construction, affinity maturation and biological characterization of an anti-tumor-associated glycoprotein-72 humanized antibody. *J. Biol. Chem.* **281**, 6985–92.

Zhang W, Feng J, Li Y, Guo N, Shen B. (2005) Humanization of an anti-human TNF-alpha antibody by variable region resurfacing with the aid of molecular modeling. *Mol. Immunol.* **42**, 1445–51.

CHAPTER TWO

Immunogenicity Assessment of Antibody Therapeutics

Philippe Stas, Jurgen Pletinckx, Yannick Gansemans, and Ignace Lasters

With over 20 therapeutic antibodies currently approved by the Food and Drug Administration (FDA) and close to 100 leads in clinical trials, therapeutic antibodies are responsible for a considerable part of the therapeutic proteins sales worldwide. The observation of immunogenicity with the early therapeutic antibodies did not come as a surprise, as many of them were murine antibodies or chimeric variants, consisting of murine variable parts in conjunction with a human constant domain. Over time, there has been a strong evolution toward the development of humanized and fully human antibodies, thereby reducing the observed immunogenicity to a significant extent. General side effects such as anaphylaxis and allergy against protein therapeutics are also less prevalent but this is due to better manufacturing processes giving more homogeneous products.

However, some of the currently available fully human antibodies have induced significant immunogenic responses over time. This has led to the regulatory instances in Europe and the United States supporting the development of guidelines to assess the likelihood of observing immunogenicity and its potential severity and side effects.

IMMUNOGENICITY DRIVERS

Several factors contribute to the potential immunogenicity of a protein therapeutic:

- Homology to human or endogenous proteins: The degree of "foreignness" of a protein to the host is one of the major contributors to an immune response. Indeed, the likelihood to observe immunogenicity related to a bacterium-derived protein therapeutic, such as staphylokinase, is higher than against proteins that show high homology to endogenous proteins, such as erythropoietin (EPO) and insulin. The overall immunogenicity of antibody therapeutics has been severely reduced by the development of fully human and humanized therapeutic antibodies as compared to the first-generation murine and chimeric antibodies (Hwang and Foote, 2005).

- Aggregates: Aggregates and immune-complexes are a second major driver in immune response and observed immunogenicity. They induce an immune response in two ways:

- The immune-complexes and aggregates can be more readily taken up by antigen presenting cells, leading to an increased humoral immune response (Rosenberg, 2006), and
- The aggregates can crosslink B cell receptors, thereby inducing B cell proliferation and activate an initial T cell independent immune response (Bachmann et al., 1993).

Aggregate formation can be caused by formulation, production processes, storage conditions, and/or the physicochemical characteristics of the protein drug itself. Even drug handling can impact the formation of (transient) aggregates, for instance, when using suboptimal dilution agents or upon fast dilution of the drug. When aggregates are formed in a repeated structure, such as present in viral-like particles, higher immunogenicity will be observed due to a T cell independent B cell response. In the characterization of this type of immune response, special care has to be taken to ensure that the antidrug antibodies (ADA) mounted against the latter type of aggregates are indeed cross-reactive with the free, nonaggregated drug.

- Dosing: Protein therapeutics used in a repeated or episodic dosing scheme, or with intermittent dosing scheme changes, have a higher likelihood to induce immunogenicity in patients as opposed to short dosing schemes to treat acute indications (Vermeire et al., 2007). It is expected that the observed ADA against antibody therapeutics will increase as patient groups are subjected to the drug over longer periods (Goldstein et al., 1986; Schroeder et al., 1989).
- Route of administration: Due to the different route of immunization, intravenous administration reduced the likelihood of an immune response as opposed to subcutaneous and intramuscular injection. (EMEA, 2007)
- Impurities, degradation products, and batch-to-batch variability: Contamination of the protein therapeutic with endotoxins, lipids, and production method–related DNA increase the risk for immunogenicity. However, anaphylactic shock or allergy due to the protein therapeutic is rare these days due to better quality control and optimized production processes, leading to less batch-to-batch variability. (EMEA, 2007)
- Immunomodulating conditions: Different immunomodulating factors will influence the observed immunogenicity of the protein drugs, such as the patient status, the immunostimulating or immunoreducing activity of the protein therapeutic and/or the concomitant use of immunomodulators. For example, the use of the disease modifying antirheumatic drug (DMARD) methotrexate (MTX) significantly reduces the observed immunogenicity both for adalimumab and infliximab (Baert et al. 2003).
- Protein structure: As protein drugs are high molecular weight molecules with complex chemical structures, often subject to posttranslational modification, there is subtle variability in the end product. Therefore, special attention must be given to glycosylation, deamidation, oxidation, and other factors (EMEA,

TABLE 2.1. Risk assessment for immunogenicity

In a risk assessment for immunogenicity of protein therapeutics, both the probability and the severity of immunogenicity should be estimated. To estimate the severity of observed immunogenicity, several aspects should be taken into account.

More severe	Less severe
Endogenous counterpart	Nonendogenous counterpart
Unique function/activity	Redundant activity
Sole therapy	Other therapies
Life-threatening disease	Non-life-threatening disease
Repetitive treatment chronic disease	Single-dose treatment end stage disease
Replacement therapy	Nonreplacement therapy
Nonreversible adverse effects	Reversible adverse effects

2007) as well as the presence of degradation products and alternative glycosylation patterns.

Table 2.1 gives an overview of some of the aspects to be taken into account in estimating the severity of the side effects related to immunogenicity of protein therapeutics.

OBSERVED IMMUNOGENICITY OF ANTIBODY THERAPEUTICS

While the current guidelines are developed for protein therapeutics in general, specific aspects should be taken into account in the development of antibody therapeutics.

The effect of ADA against therapeutic antibodies is generally restricted to altering the efficacy and pharmacokinetics of the drug by accelerating its rate of removal.

Special care should be taken regarding formulation, the avoidance of aggregates or degradation products, and controlling the development of immune-complexes. Recent developments focusing on Fc engineering increase the risk of immunogenicity due to amino acid substitutions in the antibody constant domains, thus raising the possibility of inducing cross-reactive antibodies against endogenous Fc. It seems unlikely however that Fc tolerance will be broken.

This situation is very different from the immunogenicity observed against non-antibody protein therapeutics. Indeed, the ADA response against humanlike protein therapeutics has the intrinsic risk of raising an immune response against endogenous counterparts of GM-CSF, EPO, and TPO. Immunogenicity has been measured against Factor-VIII and IFN-alpha. This ADA response may have severe medical consequences if the corresponding endogenous protein plays a key role in important biological processes (such as blood coagulation and haematopoesis). For example, anti-EPO ADA responses leading to prolonged red blood cell aplasia have been observed upon administration of recombinant EPO (Casadevall et al., 2002). Currently, the measurement and identification of ADA generated against therapeutic antibodies are a regulatory requirement. Moreover, new technologies to estimate the expected immunogenicity levels at a preclinical level are being developed.

STRATEGIES TO IDENTIFY ANTIDRUG ANTIBODIES

The measurement and characterization of antibodies formed against a therapeutic protein is not without technical challenges. A stratified approach has been suggested where different methods are combined to identify and characterize ADA upon administration of a drug (see Figure 2.1). In this approach, a screening assay is first developed to identify a potential ADA response in samples. Second, a confirmatory assay has to be developed to differentiate the positive from the false positive samples in the screening assay. Finally, assays should be established to further characterize the ADA response, by identifying the neutralizing character of the ADA and determining the specific isotypes of the ADA.

The assays in general rely on immunoreactivity such as direct, indirect, and bridging ELISA and are complemented with surface plasmon resonance, chemiluminescence, and/or radio-precipitation-based assays. In specific cases, cell-based assays are used in the characterization phase of the ADA response. Special care has to be taken to avoid "drug interference." ADA cannot be accurately measured in the presence of the therapeutic antibody so that a drug washout period is required. For antibodies with a long half-life, this may be an extensive period (Bearden et al., 2005; Mire-Sluis et al., 2004; Patton et al., 2005). The use of different assays and hence different sensitivities can lead to different readouts of immunogenicity. Therefore, the observed immunogenicity data cannot be easily compared throughout studies.

Table 2.2 presents a compilation of published data on antibody responses against therapeutic antibodies, including background data such as assay type and patient

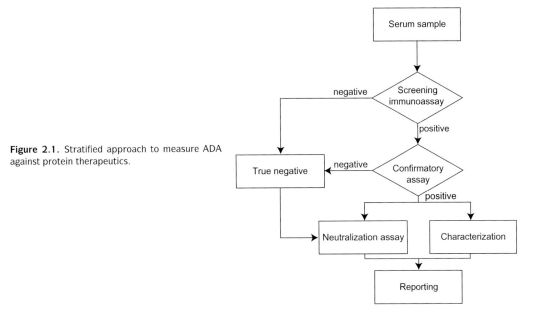

Figure 2.1. Stratified approach to measure ADA against protein therapeutics.

TABLE 2.2. Immunogenicity of therapeutic antibodies on the market or in clinical trials

Suppr: "+" (additional immunosuppressive drugs were used during treatment)

Name/% Antibody response	Population size	Type/Immunosuppression	Target/Dosage	Administration	Indication/Reference
HuBrE-3		Humanized	400 kDa breast epithelial mucin		Breast cancer
14	7	+	Single	iv	Kramer et al., 1998
hu-A33		Humanized	A33		Colorectal cancer (CRC)
73	11	.	Multiple	iv	Welt et al., 2003a
33	12	.	Multiple	iv	Scott et al., 2005
54	44	+	Multiple	iv	Ritter et al., 2001
59	13	+	Multiple	iv	Welt et al., 2003b
Tysabri/natalizumab		Humanized	a4 integrin		Crohn's disease
7	181	+	Multiple	iv	Ghosh et al., 2003
MLN02		Humanized	a4b7 integrin		Ulcerative colitis
44	118	.	Multiple	iv	Feagan et al., 2005
Eculizumab		Humanized	C5		Paroxysmal nocturnal hemoglobinuria (PNH)
0.2	43	+	Multiple	iv	Hillmen et al., 2006
Cantuzumab-mertansine		Humanized	Can		Colorectal cancer (CRC)
0	37	.	Multiple	iv	Tolcher et al., 2003
Hu23F2G		Humanized	CD11/CD18		Multiple sclerosis
0	24	.	Single	iv	Bowen et al., 1998
Raptiva/efalizumab		Humanized	CD11a		Psoriasis
2.3	501	.	Multiple	sc	Menter et al., 2005
4	292	+	Multiple	sc	Papp et al., 2006
6	1063	.	Multiple	sc	Package insert
B43-Genistein		Murine	CD19		Acute lymphoblastic leukemia (ALL)
33	9	+	Multiple	iv	Uckun et al., 1999
Bexxar/tositumomab		Murine	CD20		Non-Hodgkin's lymphoma (NHL)

Name/% Antibody response	Population size	Type/Immunosuppression	Target/Dosage	Administration	Indication/Reference
Rituxan/rituximab — 9	55	Chimeric — +	CD20 — Multiple	iv	Kaminski et al., 2001; Non-Hodgkin's lymphoma (NHL)
0	58	.	Multiple	iv	Davis et al., 2000
Rituxan/rituximab — 0	37	Chimeric — .	CD20 — Multiple	iv	Piro et al., 1999; Systemic lupus erythematosus
Rituxan/rituximab — 65	17	Chimeric — +	CD20 — Multiple	iv	Looney et al., 2004; Primary Sjögren's syndrome (PSS)
Zevalin/ibritumomab-tiuxetan — 27	15	Murine — +	CD20 — Multiple	iv	Pijpe et al., 2005; Non-Hodgkin's lymphoma (NHL)
Epratuzumab — 3	211	Humanized — .	CD22 — Multiple	iv	Package insert; Primary Sjögren's syndrome (PSS)
OKT3 — 19	16	Murine — .	CD3 — Multiple	iv	Steinfeld et al., 2006; Graft rejection
HuM291/vasilizumab — 54	82	Humanized — +	CD3 — Multiple	iv	McIntyre et al., 1996; Graft versus host disease (GVHD)
HuM195 — 0	13	Humanized — +	CD33 — Multiple	iv	Carpenter et al., 2002; Acute promyelocytic leukemia
Mylotarg/gemtuzumab-ozogamicin — 5	21	Humanized — +	CD33 — Multiple	iv	Jurcic et al., 2000; Acute myeloid leukemia
cM-T412 — 0	142	Chimeric — .	CD4 — Multiple	.	Package insert; Rheumatoid arthritis (RA)
hMAb BIWA 4/bivatuzumab — 75	12	Humanized — .	CD44v6 — Multiple	iv	Choy et al., 1998; Head and neck squamous cell carcinoma
10	20	+	Single	iv	Börjesson et al., 2003
0	10	.	Single	iv	Colnot et al., 2003

(continued)

TABLE 2.2 (continued)

Name/% Antibody response	Population size	Type/Immunosuppression	Target/Dosage	Administration	Indication/Reference
BIWI 1/bivatuzumab mertansine		Humanized	CD44v6		Squamous cell carcinoma
0	7		Multiple	iv	Tijink et al., 2006
0	31		Single/multiple	iv	Sauter et al., 2007
Mab BIWA 1		Murine	CD44v6		Head and neck squamous cell carcinoma
92	12		Single	iv	Stroomer et al., 2000
Campath-1H/alemtuzumab		Humanized	CD52		Rheumatoid arthritis (RA)
63	40		Multiple	iv	Weinblatt et al., 1995
10	10		Multiple	.	Reiff et al., 2005
75	4		Multiple	.	Reiff et al., 2005
29	31		Multiple	.	Reiff et al., 2005
53	30		Multiple	.	Reiff et al., 2005
0	5		Multiple	.	Reiff et al., 2005
Campath-1H/alemtuzumab		Humanized	CD52		B CLL
1.9	211			.	Package insert
Erbitux/cetuximab		Chimeric	EGFR		Cancer
5	1001		Multiple	iv	Package insert
ch14.18		Chimeric	Ganglioside GD2		Neuroblastoma
0	9		Multiple	iv	Handgretinger et al., 1995
Reopro/abciximab		Chimeric	GPIIb/IIIa		Coronary angioplasty
4	500		Single	iv	Tcheng et al., 2001
21	500		Multiple	iv	Tcheng et al., 2001
5	616		Single	iv	Package insert
7	616		Single	iv	Package insert
Herceptin/trastuzumab		Humanized	HER2		Breast cancer
0.1	903		Multiple	iv	Package insert
Xolair/omalizumab		Humanized	IgE		Asthma
0	22		Multiple	sc	Djukanović et al., 2005
0	268	+	Multiple	sc	Busse et al., 2001
Simulect/basiliximab		Chimeric	IL2R		Graft rejection

Name/% Antibody response	Population size	Type/Immunosuppression	Target/Dosage	Administration	Indication/Reference
0	30	+	Single	iv	Kovarik et al., 1997
1	339	+	Single	iv	Package insert
1	138	+	Single	iv	Package insert
Zenapax/HAT/daclizumab		Humanized	IL2R		Graft rejection
8	12	+	Multiple	iv	Vincenti et al., 1997
14	123	.	Multiple	iv	Package insert
34	61	.	Multiple	iv	Package insert
c-MOv18		Chimeric	Membrane folate receptor		Ovarian cancer
0	5	+	Multiple	iv	van Zanten-Przybysz et al., 2002
c-Nd2		Chimeric	Pancreatic mucin		Pancreatic cancer
0	10	.	Single	iv	Sawada et al., 1999
Denosumab		Humanized	RANKL		Osteoporosis/osteopenia
0.6	312	.	Multiple	sc	McClung et al., 2006
Synagis/palivizumab		Humanized	RSV		Hematopoietic stem cell transplants
0	6	.	Single	iv	Boeckh et al., 2001
Synagis/palivizumab		Humanized	RSV		Bronchopulmonary dysplasia
1	1002	.	Multiple	im	The Impact-RSV Study Group, 2006
Humicade/CDP571		Humanized	TNFa		Crohn's disease
7	111	+	Multiple	iv	Sandborn et al., 2001
Humira/adalimumab		Human	TNFa		Rheumatoid arthritis (RA)
12	434	+	Multiple	sc	van de Putte et al., 2004
1	209	+	Multiple	sc	Weinblatt et al., 2003
87	15	+	Multiple	sc	Bender et al., 2007
5	1062	+	Multiple	sc	Package insert
0.7	419	+	Multiple	sc	Keystone et al., 2004
Remicade/infliximab		Chimeric	TNFa		Rheumatoid arthritis (RA)
17.4	87	+/-	Multiple	iv	Maini et al., 1998
8	60	+	Multiple	iv	Lipsky et al., 2000

(continued)

TABLE 2.2 (continued)

Name/% Antibody response	Population size	Type/Immunosuppression	Target/Dosage	Administration	Indication/Reference
Remicade/infliximab		Chimeric	TNFa		Crohn's disease
6	50	+/−	Multiple	iv	Present et al., 1999
27	237	+/−	Multiple	iv	Hanauer et al., 2002
6	101	+/−	Multiple	iv	Targan et al., 1997
9	199	+	Multiple	iv	Hanauer, 1999
61	125	+	Multiple	iv	Baert et al., 2003
55	174	+/−	Multiple	iv	Vermeire et al., 2007
Certolizumab pegol		Humanized	TNFa		Crohn's disease
12	73	+/−	Multiple	sc	Schreiber et al., 2005
8	331	+/−	Multiple	sc	Sandborn et al., 2007
9	668	+/−	Multiple	sc	Schreiber et al., 2007
Avastin/bevacizumab		Humanized	VEGF		Solid tumors
0	25	+	Multiple	iv	Gordon et al., 2001
0	12	+	Multiple	iv	Margolin et al., 2001
Vitaxin		Humanized	avb3 integrin		Late stage cancer
0	17	.	Multiple	iv	Gutheil et al., 2000

population size. It should be noted that studies often comprise only a small number of patients, who are sometimes submitted to different treatment schemes based on their individual medical history and disease state. Therefore, care must be taken not to overinterpret immunogenicity data.

The variability of observed immunogenicity among similar clinical studies is illustrated with alemtuzumab, a lymphoid-cell-depleting humanized anti-CD52 antibody. The observed human antihuman antibody (HAHA) response varies from 0% to 75% in six clinical studies published between 1995 and 2005, for treatment of patients suffering from rheumatoid arthritis (RA) (Isaacs et al., 1992; Isaacs et al., 1996a, b; Reiff, 2005; Weinblatt et al., 1995). While the combined data of these six studies results in an immunogenicity of 45% for 120 patients, treatment of patients with B cell chronic lymphocytic leukemia (B-CLL) results in only 1.9% HAHA response for a group of 211 subjects, thus implicating the influence of the disease state on the antigenic response.

Similarly, rituximab, a chimeric antibody targeting the B cell differentiation antigen CD20, does not elicit a human antichimeric antibody (HACA) response in patients suffering from B-CLL (Piro et al., 1999; Davis et al., 2000). A possible explanation could be the loss of B cells and the concomitant use of immunosuppressive drugs and chemo treatment. However, the disease itself is probably a significant factor since patients treated with rituximab for the auto-immune diseases systemic lupus erythematosus and primary Sjögren's syndrome developed HACA in 65% and 27% of the cases, respectively, despite the concomitant use of immunosuppressive drugs (Looney et al., 2004; Pijpe et al., 2005).

PRECLINICAL IMMUNOGENICITY TESTING

The measurement and identification of ADA is mainly geared toward clinical phases and postmarketing monitoring. To date, no systems are available to estimate ADA in a preclinical or research setting, prior to the first dose in humans. While regulatory requirements include monitoring of the development of ADA during preclinical development in animal models, these data are difficult to map to the eventual immunogenicity measured in human subjects and is merely a covariate to take into account during the drug development. Indeed, ADA in animal models can interact with the drug and hence alter the toxicology and pharmacokinetics of the drug under investigation. One of the few cases when ADA observed in animal studies was predictive for the effect in humans related to the treatment of animals with autologous recombinant TPO inducing IgG-type ADA leading to thrombocytopenia (Koren, 2002). In the field of therapeutic antibodies, this predictivity has not been observed to date. Therefore, one has to rely on other methodologies to estimate the expected immunogenicity early in the development process.

T$_h$ EPITOPES

Mounting an ADA response through the T cell dependent immune-pathway generally involves three major types of cells: professional antigen presenting cells (APCs), T helper (T$_h$) cells, and B cells. Professional APCs include macrophages and dendritic cells, which can take up proteins such as the therapeutic antibody in a nonspecific manner through endocytosis. In the APC's endosome, the therapeutic antibody is digested into a mixture of peptides with lengths of up to 34 residues (Castellino et al., 1997). The endosome merges with the MIIC vesicle released from the Golgi apparatus containing membrane-bound human leucocyte antigen (HLA) Class II molecules. To bind to the HLA Class II receptor, the peptides have to displace the CLIP peptide bound to the HLA Class II. This process is mediated by HLA-DM, present in the MIIC vesicle (Kropshofer et al., 1999).

The HLA Class II molecule has the ability to bind a wide range of peptides, derived from the endocytosed protein. The peptides bind in an almost linearly outstretched conformation (Figure 2.2). The peptide-HLA Class II complex is transported to the APC's cell surface and can there be recognized by the T cell receptor (TCR) present on CD4+ T-helper-lymphocytes (T$_h$). The TCR is a highly variable immunoglobulin-like protein that recognizes the HLA-peptide complex in a clonotype specific manner (Davis & Bjorkman, 1988). Each peptide has a different affinity for the HLA Class II molecule because of its particular amino acid sequence. The peptides that bind are displayed on the surface of the APC until they dissociate after which the HLA becomes unstable and is internalized by the APC. As such, the concentration of a certain peptide presented is a function of the amount loaded and, crucially, of its affinity for HLA Class II.

The T$_h$ cell population as a whole has been selected not to respond to peptides that are derived from autologous proteins, that is, the self-peptides or self-epitopes. This selection process takes place in the thymus, where only developing T$_h$ cells that have a minimal affinity for HLA survive (Starr et al., 2003). T$_h$ cells with a TCR having a high affinity for HLA Class II displaying self-peptide are negatively selected. The activation of specific T$_h$ cells can be triggered by HLA Class II molecules displaying nonself-peptides, which will lead to proliferation and differentiation of the T$_h$ cell. The activated T$_h$ cell will produce the necessary cytokines to stimulate B cells

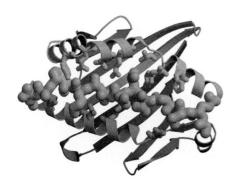

Figure 2.2. Top view of the HLA Class II DRB1*0101 binding groove, with α and β chains in blue and green, respectively, and the bound peptide in orange (PDB-code 1KLU). [See color plate.]

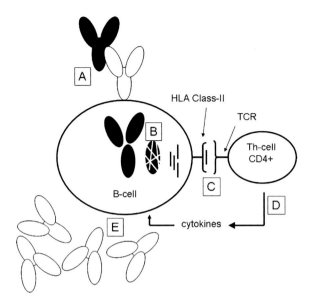

Figure 2.3. Schematic representation of antigen-specific activation of B cells by T$_h$ cells. (A) The B cell receptor (white) recognizes the therapeutic antibody or antigen (black). (B) The internalized antigen is digested in the endosomes. (C) The resulting peptides are mounted on HLA Class-II and presented on the surface of the B cell, where a selective T cell receptor (TCR) recognizes the expressed complex. (D) The activated T cell produces cytokines. E. The B cell is activated to produce antibodies against the antigen or therapeutic antibody.

producing antibodies against the protein. This specific stimulation is possible because the B cells themselves are also APCs, presenting peptides from the antigen they captured with their membrane-bound antibodies, and which the T$_h$ cell can recognize through its TCR (Figure 2.3).

In order to provide sufficient diversity in the response against potential antigens, the HLA Class II molecule is polymorphic and present in the population as different allotypes. The high degree of polymorphism of each HLA gene results in several different peptide-specificities within an individual and many more specificities within the human population. The polymorphisms are generally located at the level of the peptide binding site, illustrating the evolutionary benefit of having HLAs with different peptide specificities. Whereas the allotype determines the specific HLA Class II variant, the haplotype of a patient is the combination of the different HLA Class II alleles lying in the MHC locus. Differences exist in the frequencies of HLA allotypes (and hence haplotypes) among ethnicities around the world. The immunogenicity of a therapeutic protein should be assessed using a population representative for the patient population that is being targeted. The test population has to be large enough such that the HLAs prevalent in the patient population are present in representative amounts.

STRATEGIES FOR DETERMINING T CELL DRIVEN IMMUNOGENICITY

Binding of drug-derived peptides to HLA is a necessary step in T$_h$ cell activation. Therefore, determining the T cell epitopes in protein therapeutics allows us to estimate the potential immunogenicity. However, presentation of a peptide in the context of HLA does not necessarily lead to an immune response. Therefore, determining the T cell epitopes in a protein will be a worst case estimation of the true immunogenicity. T cell epitopes can be identified both with *in silico* and *in vitro* methods. Whereas the *in silico* methods focus on identifying the peptides presented in an HLA context, the *in vitro* tools measure T_h cell activation by the epitopes.

IN VITRO T CELL ACTIVATION ASSAYS

In vitro T cell activation and proliferation assays measure whether a therapeutic protein or peptide can elicit an immune response. This requires peptides bound to HLA that can be productively recognized by the TCR expressed on T cells. In order to measure T_h epitopes, a number of assays were optimized to characterize T cell responsiveness. Typically, the characterization is performed on peripheral blood mononuclear cells (PBMC) from patients or naïve donors. The PBMC are primed with whole antigen and after a number of days of culture, the cells are restimulated with autologous monocytes and whole antigen or fragments (peptides) of the antigen. For the identification of specific T cell epitopes of a given antigen, overlapping 15-amino acid synthetic peptides are used that span the whole sequence and overlap by 10 or 12 amino acids (Tangri et al., 2005). T cell proliferation can then be determined by pulsing the cells with 5-bromo-2'deoxyuridine and a subsequent detection by BrDU ELISA, or with tritiated thymidine followed by scintillation counting (Stickler et al., 2004; Warmerdam et al., 2002). Alternatively, ELISpot assays have been developed to count the number of activated antigen-specific T cells by measuring the secreted cytokines IFN-γ and/or IL2 after restimulation of the cells (Anthony & Lehmann, 2003).

An alternative method is the *i-mune*® approach, where dendritic cells are generated by differentiation from blood monocytes using appropriate cytokines (Anthony & Lehmann, 2003; Harding, 2003; Stickler et al., 2003; Stickler et al., 2004; Zhou & Tedder, 1996). The dendritic cells are co-cultured with purified T_h cells in the presence of peptide for 5 days followed by the assessment of T cell proliferation by tritiated thymidine incorporation or ELISpot analysis.

A drawback of the ELISpot and T cell proliferation assays is that the assays may be compromised by non-T cells contributing to the observed response. Therefore, alternative assays have been developed using flow cytometric approaches, where T cell-specific activation markers (such as CD25) can be measured in conjunction with intracellular or expressed cytokines, thereby optimally identifying the activated and proliferating T cell populations (Ostensen et al., 2005).

T cell activation assays are best used in the drug development phase in order to compare the potential immunogenicity of different formulations. Typically, T cell activation assays are performed on at least 50 donors for formulation testing and

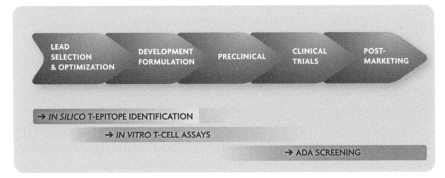

Figure 2.4. In the development process of therapeutic antibodies, the combination of *in silico* tools, *in vitro* T cell activation assays, and eventually ADA screening and characterization will allow a full assessment of the drug immunogenicity.

whole antigen assays. To identify specific T cell epitopes in a therapeutic protein, a multiple of this number of donors would be needed due to the high polymorphism in HLA and each patient expressing several HLA Class II molecules (Stickler et al., 2003). Therefore, the interpretation of T cell activation readouts for HLA preference of T cell epitopes should be supplemented with statistical as well as *in silico* T cell epitope analysis (Harding, 2003).

T CELL EPITOPE MAPPING TOOLS

Several methods have been developed to identify the binding affinity of peptides to HLA molecules and identify T cell epitopes. These include mass spectroscopy, binding assays, and T cell activation assays, each of which is described below. Tandem mass spectroscopy on elution profiles obtained from tissue samples allows sub-picomolar analysis of proteins and peptides (Chicz et al., 1992; Davenport et al., 1997; Eng et al., 1994; Falk et al., 1991; Hunt et al., 1992; Rudensky et al., 1991). Alternatively, direct binding assays determine the affinity of peptides for a given HLA Class II allotype using purified HLAs in solubilized or immobilized form (Rudolf et al., 2001; Sidney et al., 1998; Southwood et al., 1998; Tangri et al., 2005). Typically, the affinity of the peptides is determined in a competition assay with a labeled reference peptide yielding an IC50 value that can be converted into a dissociation constant Kd (Desmet et al., 2005). However, as peptides bind to HLA in a linearly outstretched conformation (Figure 2.4), the number of possible binding modes of any peptide is limited. This makes it possible to build *in silico* models that predict the affinity of peptides for a particular HLA allotype rather than obtaining the information through direct experimental measurement. The predictive computer methods for epitope prediction are of three different types: statistical (additive) methods based on inference, nonadditive methods based on inference, and structure-based methods. The earliest predictive models were entirely statistical (Sette et al., 1989). Given a number of peptides that are observed to be bound to a particular HLA allotype, the peptide sequences can be aligned and binding-motives are deduced. Initially, these methods were developed for HLA Class I molecules. For HLA Class II receptors, this alignment method is more complex as the peptide lengths can range from 9 to around 34 residues and extend outside the binding site (McFarland & Beeson, 2002). Nevertheless, given an alignment of binding peptides, a statistical profile, or substitution matrix can be constructed. The substitution matrix can be applied to a target sequence by performing an ungapped alignment to this matrix and adding up the relevant scores from each position of the peptide. The additive model works reasonably well for HLA Class I (Peters et al., 2003). For Class II, several ungapped alignments will be possible, and the one with the highest score is selected, estimating the peptide's true affinity. Examples of such statistical methods include Rankpep, Propred, Tepitope, Epimatrix, Bimas, and Syphpeiti (Borras-Cuesta et al., 2000; Hammer et al., 1994; Martin et al., 2003; Peters and Sette, 2005; Rammensee et al., 1999; Reche et al., 2004; Singh and Raghava, 2001; Sturniolo et al., 1999).

More elaborate predictive models based on inference have been developed, employing artificial neural networks (Gulukota et al., 1997; Milik et al., 1998), hidden Markov models (Mamitsuka, 1998), and support vector machines (SVMs) (Segal et al., 2001; Zhao et al., 2003).

More recently, structure-based methods have been successfully applied to both the Class I and the more difficult Class II system. These methods directly model the molecular interactions between peptide and molecule, using force fields or other structure-derived properties. As such, there is no need per se for experimental data to train the model. The methods also allow one to make accurate predictions for HLA Class II allotypes where little experimental data exist, as opposed to the methods by inference that suffer from data overfitting. Examples of structure-based methods are Epibase (Desmet et al., 2005) and the method of Davies et al. (2003).

The accuracy of predictive methods has evolved strongly over the past few years, and while the latest methods by inference work reasonably well compared to the first-generation tools, they do not attain the general accuracy level of the structure-based methods (Van Walle et al., 2007). *In silico* screening has the advantage of being relatively inexpensive and as such can be applied very early in the development cycle, during lead selection or as an integral part of the protein engineering cycle. As an example, upon the development of novel humanized therapeutic antibodies, one can apply structure-based prediction tools to ensure that CDR grafts or specific backmutations do not introduce potential T cell epitopes. Moreover, the tools can be used to rank the potential immunogenicity of different lead candidates binding to the same target. Differences in the number and HLA specificities of potential T cell epitopes in therapeutic antibodies provide a strong decision criterion for prioritizing the leads to be taken forward. For fully human therapeutic antibodies, screening for T cell epitopes allows a selection of leads with the lowest immunogenic CDRs. Indeed, as the constant domain and framework residues in the variable domain of fully human antibodies are in general self-peptides, as they are present in the germ line, the potential immunogenicity is driven by the CDR sequences, which are not germline encoded. In this case, re-engineering of the CDRs to remove the T cell epitopes will in general be difficult, as rational re-engineering of CDRs can lead to loss of affinity and efficacy of the therapeutic antibody.

CONCLUSIONS

As all therapeutic proteins and therapeutic antibodies will eventually show some level of immunogenicity, it is clear that the likelihood and the severity of ADA response should be evaluated throughout the development and lifetime of the drug. Whereas several guidelines and tools exist for the clinical and postmarketing assessment of immunogenicity, solutions are available to address potential immunogenicity risk during the research and development stage. As the ADA response against a therapeutic antibody will generally not lead to severe side effects and be merely deleterious for the drug, a suitable strategy has to be developed that addresses immunogenicity throughout the development process.

Techniques to assess immunogenicity at an early development stage, such as the monitoring of T cell driven immunogenicity and identification of T cell epitopes, have come of age in the past 5 years. They can be categorized into two largely complementary approaches. Structure based *in silico* epitope identification tools have the advantage of being very fast and accurate, and they can cope with the wide genetic variety of HLA Class II molecules. They are therefore ideal as a first screening tool, capable of pointing out which leads might show an increased immunogenicity and which part of their sequence can be the main driver. In general, CDRs of therapeutic antibody leads should be preferentially free from strong T cell epitopes.

When comparing formulations during development, particularly with respect to aggregate formation, one can extend the immunogenicity assessment with *in vitro* T cell activation assays. Indeed, by testing whole protein in a cell fluorometry–based system, specific T cell responses can be identified. The combination between the *in vitro* and the *in silico* tools facilitates the development of an HLA typing strategy during clinical trials, as their combined use leads to improved rationalization of the readouts, more accurate population risk assessments, and reduced costs. Eventually, when the drug enters clinical trials, ADA screening, confirmatory, neutralization, and characterization assays will be deployed to characterize the observed immunogenicity. Those assays are then further used during postmarketing surveillance.

Regulatory authorities are paying increased attention to the immunogenicity of therapeutic proteins. The current focus is on the monitoring and measurement of antibody responses against therapeutic antibodies as documented by several industry-backed white papers and on challenges associated with antibody assays such as the presence of circulating drugs and the formation of immune complexes (Bearden et al., 2005; Mire-Sluis et al., 2004; Patton et al., 2005). Whereas there are no formal requirements yet to measure T cell activation or provide T cell epitope data, the data are appreciated as supporting evidence of expected immunogenicity.

REFERENCES

Anthony DD and Lehmann PV. T-cell epitope mapping using the ELISPOT approach. *Methods* 2003; **29**:260–269.

Bachmann MF, Rohrer UH, Kundig TM, Burki K, Hengartner H, and Zinkernagel RM. The influence of antigen organization on B cell responsiveness. *Science* 1993; **262**:1448–1451.

Baert F, Noman M, Vermeire S, Van Assche G, D' Haens G, Carbonez A, and Rutgeerts P. Influence of immunogenicity on the long-term efficacy of infliximab in Crohn's disease. *N Engl J Med* 2003; **348**:601–608.

Bearden CM, Book BK, Sidner RA, and Pescovitz MD. Removal of therapeutic anti-lymphocyte antibodies from human sera prior to anti-human leukocyte antibody testing. *J Immunol Methods* 2005; **300**:192–199.

Bender NK, Heilig CE, Dröll B, Wohlgemuth J, Armbruster FP, and Heilig B. Immunogenicity, efficacy and adverse events of adalimumab in RA patients. *Rheumatol Int* 2007; **27**:269–274.

Boeckh M, Berrey MM, Bowden RA, Crawford SW, Balsley J, and Corey L. Phase 1 evaluation of the respiratory syncytial virus-specific monoclonal antibody palivizumab in recipients of hematopoietic stem cell transplants. *J Infect Dis* 2001; **184**:350–354.

Börjesson PK, Postema EJ, Roos JC, Colnot DR, Marres HA, van Schie MH, Stehle G, de Bree R, Snow GB, Oyen WJ, et al. Phase I therapy study with 186Re-labeled humanized monoclonal antibody BIWA 4 (bivatuzumab) in patients with head and neck squamous cell carcinoma. *Clin Cancer Res* 2003; **9**:3961s–3972s.

Borrás-Cuesta F, Golvano J, García-Granero M, Sarobe P, Riezu-Boj J, Huarte E, and Lasarte J. Specific and general HLA-DR binding motifs: comparison of algorithms. *Hum Immunol* 2000; **61**:266–278.

Bowen JD, Petersdorf SH, Richards TL, Maravilla KR, Dale DC, Price TH, St John TP, and Yu AS. Phase I study of a humanised anti-CD11/CD18 monoclonal antibody in multiple sclerosis. *Clin Pharmacol Ther* 1998; **64**:339–346.

Busse W, Corren J, Lanier BQ, McAlary M, Fowler-Taylor A, Cioppa GD, van As A, Gupta N. Omalizumab, anti-IgE recombinant humanized monoclonal antibody, for the treatment of severe allergic asthma. *J Allergy Clin Immunol* 2001; **108**:184–190.

Carpenter PA, Appelbaum FR, Corey L, Deeg HJ, Doney K, Gooley T, Krueger J, Martin P, Pavlovic S, Sanders J, et al. A humanised non-FcR-binding anti-CD3 antibody, visilizumab, for treatment of steroid-refractory acute graft-versus-host disease. *Blood* 2002; **99**:2712–2719.

Casadevall N, Nataf J, Viron B, Kolta A, Kiladjian JJ, Martin-Dupont P, Michaud P, Papo T, Ugo V, Teyssandier I, Varet B, and Mayeux P. Pure red-cell aplasia and antierythropoietin antibodies in patients treated with recombinant erythropoietin. *N Engl J Med* 2002; **346**(7):469–475.

Castellino F, Zhong G, and Germain RN. Antigen presentation by MHC class II molecules: invariant chain function, protein trafficking, and the molecular basis of diverse determinant capture. *Hum Immunol* 1997; **54**:159–169.

Chicz RM, Urban RG, Lane WS, Gorga JC, Stern LJ, Vignali DA, and Strominger JL. Predominant naturally processed peptides bound to HLA-DR1 are derived from MHC-related molecules and are heterogeneous in size. *Nature* 1992; **358**:764–768.

Choy EHS, Schantz A, Pitzalis C, Kingsley GH, and Panayi GS. The pharmacokinetics and human anti-mouse antibody response in rheumatoid arthritis patients treated with a chimeric anti-CD4 monoclonal antibody. *Br J Rheumatol* 1998; **37**:801–802.

Colnot DR, Roos JC, de Bree R, Wilhelm AJ, Kummer JA, Hanft G, Heider KH, Stehle G, Snow GB, and van Dongen GA. Safety, biodistribution, pharmacokinetics, and immunogenicity of 99mTc-labeled humanised monoclonal antibody BIWA 4 (bivatuzumab) in patients with squamous cell carcinoma of the head and neck. *Cancer Immunol Immunother* 2003; **52**:576–582.

Davenport MP, Smith KJ, Barouch D, Reid SW, Bodnar WM, Willis AC, Hunt DF, and Hill AV. HLA Class I binding motifs derived from random peptide libraries differ at the COOH terminus from those of eluted peptides. *J Exp Med* 1997; **185**:367–371.

Davies MN, Sansom CE, Beazley C, and Moss DS. A novel predictive technique for the MHC class II peptide-binding interaction. *Mol Med* 2003; **9**:220–225.

Davis MM and Bjorkman PJ. T-cell antigen receptor genes and T-cell recognition. *Nature* 1988; **334**:395–402.

Davis TA, Grillo-López AJ, White CA, McLaughlin P, Czuczman MS, Link BK, Maloney DG, Weaver RL, Rosenberg J, and Levy R. Rituximab anti-CD20 monoclonal antibody therapy in non-Hodgkin's lymphoma: safety and efficacy of re-treatment. *J Clin Oncol* 2000; **18**:3135–3143.

Desmet J, Meersseman G, Boutonnet N, Pletinckx J, De Clercq K, Debulpaep M, Braeckman T, and Lasters I. Anchor profiles of HLA-specific peptides: analysis by a novel affinity scoring method and experimental validation. *Proteins* 2005; **58**:53–69.

Djukanović R, Wilson SJ, Kraft M, Jarjour NN, Steel M, Chung KF, Bao W, Fowler-Taylor A, Matthews J, Busse WW, Holgate ST, and Fahy JV. Effects of treatment with anti-immunoglobulin E antibody omalizumab on airway inflammation in allergic asthma. *Am J Resp Crit Care Medicine*, 2005; **170**, 583–593.

European Agency for the Evaluation of Medicinal Products (EMEA) Guideline on immunogenicity assessment of biotechnology-derived therapeutic proteins. EMEA/CHMP/BMWP/14327/2006, draft 2007.

Eng JK, McCormack AL, and Yates JR III. An approach to correlate tandem mass spectral data of peptides with amino acid sequences in a protein database. *J Am Soc Mass Spectrom* 1994; **5**: 976–989.

Falk K, Roetzschke O, Stefanovic S, Jung G, and Rammensee HG. Allele-specific motifs revealed by sequencing of self-peptides eluted from MHC molecules. *Nature* 1991; **351**:290–296.

Feagan BG, Greenberg GR, Wild G, Fedorak RN, Paré P, McDonald JW, Dubé R, Cohen A, Steinhart AH, Landau S, et al. Treatment of ulcerative colitis with a humanised antibody to the alpha4beta7 integrin. *N Engl J Med* 2005; **352**:2499–2507.

Ghosh S, Goldin E, Gordon FH, Malchow HA, Rask-Madsen J, Rutgeerts P, Vyhnálek P, Zádorová Z, Palmer T, Donoghue S, et al. Natalizumab for active Crohn's disease. *N Engl J Med* 2003; **348**:24–32.

Goldstein G, Fuccello AJ, Norman DJ, Shield CF 3rd, Colvin RB, and Cosimi AB. OKT3 monoclonal antibody plasma levels during therapy and the subsequent development of host antibodies to OKT3. *Transplantation* 1986; **42**:507–511.

Gordon MS, Margolin K, Talpaz M, Sledge GW Jr, Holmgren E, Benjamin R, Stalter S, Shak S, and Adelman D. Phase I safety and pharmacokinetic study of recombinant human anti-vascular endothelial growth factor in patients with advanced cancer. *J Clin Oncol* 2001; **19**:843–850.

Gulukota K, Sidney J, Sette A, and DeLisi C. Two complementary methods for predicting peptides binding major histocompatibility complex molecules. *J Mol Biol* 1997; **267**:1258–1267.

Gutheil JC, Campbell TN, Pierce PR, Watkins JD, Huse WD, Bodkin DJ, and Cheresh DA. Targeted antiangiogenic therapy for cancer using Vitaxin: a humanized monoclonal antibody to the integrin alphavbeta3. *Clin Cancer Res* 2000; **6**:3056–3061.

Hammer J, Bono E, Gallazzi F, Belunis C, Nagy Z, and Sinigaglia F. Precise prediction of major histocompatibility complex class II-peptide interaction based on peptide side chain scanning. *J Exp Med* 1994; **180**:2353–2358.

Hanauer SB. Review article: safety of infliximab in clinical trials. *Aliment Pharmacol Ther* 1999; **13**:16–22.

Hanauer SB, Feagan BG, Lichtenstein GR, Mayer LF, Schreiber S, Colombel JF, Rachmilewitz D, Wolf DC, Olson A, Bao W, et al. Maintenance infliximab for Crohn's disease: the ACCENT I randomised trial. *Lancet* 2002; **359**:1541–1549.

Handgretinger R, Anderson K, Lang P, Dopfer R, Klingebiel T, Schrappe M, Reuland P, Gillies SD, Reisfeld RA, and Neithammer D. A phase I study of human/mouse chimeric antiganglioside GD2 antibody ch14.18 in patients with neuroblastoma. *Eur J Cancer* 1995; **31A**:261–267.

Harding F. CD4+ T cell epitope identification: applications to allergy. *Clin Exp Allergy* 2003; **33**: 557–565.

Hillmen P, Young NS, Schubert J, Brodsky RA, Socié G, Muus P, Röth A, Szer J, Elebute MO, Nakamura R, et al. The complement inhibitor eculizumab in paroxysmal nocturnal hemoglobinuria. *N Engl J Med* 2006; **355**; 1233–1243.

Hunt DF, Michel H, Dickinson TA, Shabanowitz J, Cox AL, Sakaguchi K, Appella E, Grey HM, and Sette A. Peptides presented to the immune system by the murine class II major histocompatibility complex molecule I-Ad. *Science* 1992; **256**:1817–1820.

Hwang W and Foote J. Immunogenicity of engineered antibodies. *Methods* 2005; **36**:3–10.

Isaacs JD, Manna VK, Rapson N, Bulpitt KJ, Hazleman BL, Matteson EL, St Clair EW, Schnitzer TJ, and Johnston JM. CAMPATH-1H in rheumatoid arthritis – an intravenous dose-ranging study. *Br J Rheumatol* 1996a; **35**:231–240.

Isaacs JD, Watts RA, Hazleman BL, Hale G, Keogan MT, Cobbold SP, and Waldmann H. Humanised monoclonal antibody therapy for rheumatoid arthritis. *Lancet* 1992; **340**:748–752.

Isaacs JD, Wing MG, Greenwood JD, Hazleman BL, Hale G, and Waldmann H. A therapeutic human IgG4 monoclonal antibody that depletes target cells in humans. *Clin Exp Immunol* 1996b; **106**:427–433.

Jurcic JG, DeBlasio T, Dumont L, Yao TJ, and Scheinberg DA. Molecular remission induction with retinoic acid and anti-CD33 monoclonal antibody HuM195 in acute promyelocytic leukemia. *Clin Cancer Res* 2000; **6**:372–380.

Kaminski MS, Zelenetz AD, Press OW, Saleh M, Leonard J, Fehrenbacher L, Lister TA, Stagg RJ, Tidmarsh GF, Kroll S, et al. Pivotal study of iodine I 131 tositumomab for chemotherapy-refractory low-grade or transformed low-grade B-cell non-Hodgkin's lymphomas. *J Clin Oncol* 2001; **19**:3918–3928.

Keystone EC, Kavanaugh AF, Sharp JT, Tannenbaum H, Hua Y, Teoh LS, Fischkoff SA, and Chartash EK. Radiographic, clinical, and functional outcomes of treatment with adalimumab (a human anti-tumor necrosis factor monoclonal antibody) in patients with active rheumatoid arthritis receiving concomitant methotrexate therapy: a randomized, placebo-controlled, 52-week trial. *Arthritis Rheum* 2004; **50**:1400–1411.

Koren, E. From characterization of antibodies to prediction of immunogenicity. *Dev Biol* 2002; **109**:87–95.

Kovarik J, Wolf P, Cisterne JM, Mourad G, Lebranchu Y, Lang P, Bourbigot B, Cantarovich D, Girault D, Gerbeau C, Schmidt AG, and Souillou JP. Disposition of basiliximab, an interleukin-2 receptor monoclonal antibody, in recipients of mismatched cadaver renal allografts. *Transplantation* 1997; **64**:1701–1705.

Kramer EL, Liebes L, Wasserheit C, Noz ME, Blank EW, Zabalegui A, Melamed J, Furmanski P, Peterson JA, and Ceriani RL. Initial clinical evaluation of radiolabeled MX-DTPA humanized BrE-3 antibody in patients with advanced breast cancer. *Clin Cancer Res* 1998; **4**:1679–1688.

Kropshofer H, Hämmerling GJ, and Vogt AB. The impact of the non-classical MHC proteins HLA-DM and HLA-DO on loading of MHC class II molecules. *Immunol Rev* 1999; **172**:267–278.

Lipsky PE, van der Heijde DM, St Clair EW, Furst DE, Breedveld FC, Kalden JR, Smolen JS, Weisman M, Emery P, Feldmann M, et al. Infliximab and methotrexate in the treatment of rheumatoid arthritis. Anti-Tumor Necrosis Factor Trial in Rheumatoid Arthritis with Concomitant Therapy Study Group. *N Engl J Med* 2000; **343**:1594–1602.

Looney RJ, Anolik JH, Campbell D, Felgar RE, Young F, Arend LJ, Sloand JA, Rosenblatt J, and Sanz I. B cell depletion as a novel treatment for systemic lupus erythematosus: a phase I/II dose-escalation trial of rituximab. *Arthritis Rheum* 2004; **50**:2580–2589.

Maini RN, Breedveld FC, Kalden JR, Smolen JS, Davis D, Macfarlane JD, Antoni C, Leeb B, Elliott MJ, Woody JN, et al. Therapeutic efficacy of multiple intravenous infusions of anti-tumor necrosis factor alpha monoclonal antibody combined with low-dose weekly methotrexate in rheumatoid arthritis. *Arthritis Rheum* 1998; **41**:1552–1563.

Mamitsuka H. Predicting peptides that bind to MHC molecules using supervised learning of Hidden Markov Models. *Proteins* 1998; **33**:460–474.

Margolin K, Gordon MS, Holmgren E, Gaudreault J, Novotny W, Fyfe G, Adelman D, Stalter S, and Breed J. Phase Ib trial of intravenous recombinant humanized monoclonal antibody to vascular endothelial growth factor in combination with chemotherapy in patients with advanced cancer: pharmacologic and long-term safety data. *J Clin Oncol* 2001; **19**:851–856.

Martin W, Sbai H, and De Groot AS. Bioinformatics tools for identifying class I-restricted epitopes. *Methods*, March 2003, **29**(3): 289–298.

McClung MR, Lewiecki EM, Cohen SB, Bolognese MA, Woodson GC, Moffett AH, Peacock M, Miller PD, Lederman SN, Chesnut CH, et al. Denosumab in postmenopausal women with low bone mineral density. *N Engl J Med* 2006; **354**:821–831.

McFarland BJ and Beeson C. Binding interactions between peptides and proteins of the class II major histocompatibility complex. *Med Res Rev* 2002; **22**:168–203.

McIntyre JA, Kincade M, and Higgins NG. Detection of IGA anti-OKT3 antibodies in OKT3-treated transplant recipients. *Transplantation* 1996; **61**:1465–1469.

Menter A, Gordon K, Carey W, Hamilton T, Glazer S, Caro I, Li N, and Gulliver W. Efficacy and safety observed during 24 weeks of efalizumab therapy in patients with moderate to severe plaque psoriasis. *Arch Dermatol* 2005; **141**:31–38.

Milik M, Sauer D, Brunmark AP, Yuan L, Vitiello A, Jackson MR, Peterson PA, Skolnick J, and Glass CA. Application of an artificial neural network to predict specific class I MHC binding peptide sequences. *Nat Biotechnol* 1998; **16**:753–756.

Mire-Sluis AR, Barrett YC, Devanarayan V, Koren E, Liu H, Maia M, Parish T, Scott G, Shankar G, Shores E, et al. Recommendations for the design and optimization of immunoassays used in the detection of host antibodies against biotechnology products. *J Immunol Methods* 2004; **289**:1–16.

Østensen M, Sicher P, Forger F, and Villiger PM. Activation markers of peripheral blood mononuclear cells in late pregnancy and after delivery: a pilot study. *Ann Rheum Dis* 2005; **64**:318–320.

Papp KA, Miller B, Gordon KB, Caro I, Kwon P, Compton PG, Leonardi CL, and Efalizumab Study Group. Efalizumab retreatment in patients with moderate to severe chronic plaque psoriasis. *J Am Acad Dermatol* 2006; **54**:S164–S170.

Patton A, Mullenix MC, Swanson SJ, and Koren E. An acid dissociation bridging ELISA for detection of antibodies directed against therapeutic proteins in the presence of antigen. *J Immunol Methods* 2005; **304**:189–195.

Peters B and Sette A: Generating quantitative models describing the sequence specificity of biological processes with the stabilized matrix method. BMC *Bioinformatics* 2005; **6**:132.

Peters B, Tong W, Sidney J, Sette A, and Weng Z. Examining the independent binding assumption for binding of peptide epitopes to MHC-I molecules. *Bioinformatics* 2003; **19**:1765–1772.

Pijpe J, van Imhoff GW, Spijkervet FK, Roodenburg JL, Wolbink GJ, Mansour K, Vissink A, Kallenberg CG, and Bootsma H. Rituximab treatment in patients with primary Sjögren's syndrome: an open-label phase II study. *Arthritis Rheum* 2005 **52**:2740–2750.

Piro LD, White CA, Grillo-López AJ, Janakiraman N, Saven A, Beck TM, Varns C, Shuey S, Czuczman M, Lynch JW, et al. Extended Rituximab (anti-CD20 monoclonal antibody) therapy for relapsed or refractory low-grade or follicular non-Hodgkin's lymphoma. *Ann Oncol* 1999; **10**:655–661.

Present DH, Rutgeerts P, Targan S, Hanauer SB, Mayer L, van Hogezand RA, Podolsky DK, Sands BE, Braakman T, DeWoody KL, et al. Infliximab for the treatment of fistulas in patients with Crohn's disease. *N Engl J Med* 1999; **340**:1398–1405.

Rammensee H, Bachmann J, Emmerich NP, Bachor OA, and Stevanovic S. SYFPEITHI: database for MHC ligands and peptide motifs. *Immunogenetics* 1999; **50**:213–219.

Reche PA, Glutting JP, Zhang H, and Reinherz EL. Enhancement to the RANKPEP resource for the prediction of peptide binding to MHC molecules using profiles. *Immunogenetics* 2004; **56**: 405–419.

Reiff A. A review of Campath in autoimmune disease: biologic therapy in the gray zone between immunosuppression and immunoablation. *Hematology* 2005; **10**:79–93.

Ritter G, Cohen LS, Williams C Jr, Richards EC, Old LJ, and Welt S. Serological analysis of human anti-human antibody responses in colon cancer patients treated with repeated doses of humanised monoclonal antibody A33. *Cancer Res* 2001; **61**:6851–6859.

Rosenberg AS. Effects of protein aggregates: an immunologic perspective. *AAPS J* 2006; **8**:E501–E507.

Rosenberg AS and Worobec A. A risk-based approach to immunogenicity concerns of therapeutic protein products – Part 1 – considering consequences of the immune response to a protein. *Biopharm Int* 2004a; **17**:22–26.

Rosenberg AS and Worobec A. A risk-based approach to immunogenicity concerns of therapeutic protein products – Part 2 – considering host-specific and product-specific factors impacting immunogenicity. *Biopharm Int* 2004b; **17**:34–42.

Rosenberg AS and Worobec A. A risk-based approach to immunogenicity concerns of therapeutic protein products – Part 3 – effects of manufacturing changes in immunogenicity and the utility of animal immunogenicity studies. *Biopharm Int* 2005; **18**:32–36.

Rudensky AY, Preston-Hurlburt P, Hong SC, Barlow A, and Janeway CA Jr. Sequence analysis of peptides bound to MHC class II molecules. *Nature* 1991; **353**:622–627.

Rudolf MP, Man S, Melief CJM, Sette A, and Kast WM. Human T-cell responses to HLA-A-restricted high binding affinity peptides of human papillomavirus type 18 proteins E6 and E7. *Clin Cancer Res* 2001; **7**:788s–795s.

Sandborn WJ, Feagan BG, Hanauer SB, Present DH, Sutherland LR, Kamm MA, Wolf DC, Baker JP, Hawkey C, Archambault A, et al. An engineered human antibody to TNF (CDP571) for active Crohn's disease: a randomized double-blind placebo-controlled trial. *Gastroenterology* 2001; **120**:1330–1338.

Sandborn WJ, Feagan BG, Stoinov S, Honiball PJ, Rutgeerts P, Mason D, Bloomfield R, Schreiber S, and PRECISE 1 Study Investigators. Certolizumab pegol for the treatment of Crohn's disease. *N Engl J Med* 2007; **357**:228–238.

Sauter A, Kloft C, Gronau S, Bogeschdorfer F, Erhardt T, Golze W, Schroen C, Staab A, Riechelmann H, and Hoermann K. Pharmacokinetics, immunogenicity and safety of bivatuzumab mertansine, a novel CD44v6-targeting immunoconjugate, in patients with squamous cell carcinoma of the head and neck. *Int J Oncol* 2007; **30**:927–935.

Sawada T, Nishihara T, Yamamoto A, Teraoka H, Yamashita Y, Okamura T, Ochi H, Ho JJ, Kim YS, and Hirakawa K. Preoperative clinical radioimmunodetection of pancreatic cancer by 111 In-labeled chimeric monoclonal antibody Nd2. *Jpn J Cancer Res* 1999; **90**:1179–1186.

Schreiber S, Rutgeerts P, Fedorak RN, Khaliq-Kareemi M, Kamm MA, Boivin M, Bernstein CN, Staun M, Thomsen OØ, Innes A, et al. A randomized, placebo-controlled trial of certolizumab pegol (CDP870) for treatment of Crohn's disease. *Gastroenterology* 2005; **129**:807–818.

Schreiber S, Khaliq-Kareemi M, Lawrance IC, Thomsen OØ, Hanauer SB, McColm J, Bloomfield R, Sandborn WJ, and PRECISE 2 Study Investigators. Maintenance therapy with certolizumab pegol for Crohn's disease. *N Engl J Med* 2007; **357**:239–250.

Schroeder TJ, First MR, Hurtubise PE, Marmer DJ, Martin DM, Mansour ME, and Melvin DB. Immunologic monitoring with Orthoclone OKT3 therapy. *J Heart Transplant* 1989; **8**:371–380.

Scott AM, Lee FT, Jones R, Hopkins W, MacGregor D, Cebon JS, Hannah A, Chong G, U P, Papenfuss A, et al. A phase I trial of humanized monoclonal antibody A33 in patients with colorectal carcinoma: biodistribution, pharmacokinetics, and quantitative tumor uptake. *Clin Cancer Res* 2005; **11**:4810–4817.

Segal MR, Cummings MP, and Hubbard AE. Relating amino acid sequence to phenotype: analysis of peptide-binding data. *Biometrics* 2001; **57**:632–642.

Sette A, Buus S, Appella E, Smith JA, Chesnut R, Miles C, Colon SM, and Grey HM. Prediction of major histocompatibility complex binding regions of protein antigens by sequence pattern analysis. *Proc Natl Acad Sci USA* 1989; **86**:3296–3300.

Sidney J, Southwood S, Oseroff C, del Guerico MF, Grey HM, and Sette A. Measurement of MHC/peptide interactions by gel filtration. In: *Current Protocols in Immunology*, Wiley, New York (1998):18.13.1–18.13.19.

Singh H and Raghava GP. ProPred: prediction of HLA-DR binding sites. *Bioinformatics* 2001; **17**:1236–1237.

Southwood S, Sidney J, Kondo A, del Guercio MF, Appella E, Hoffman S, Kubo RT, Chesnut RW, Grey HM, and Sette A. Several common HLA-DR types share largely overlapping peptide binding repertoires. *J Immunol* 1998; **160**:3363–3373.

Starr TK, Jameson SC, and Hogquist KA. Positive and negative selection of T cells. *Annu Rev Immunol* 2003; **21**:139–176.

Steinfeld SD, Tant L, Burmester GR, Teoh NK, Wegener WA, Goldenberg DM, and Pradier O. Epratuzumab (humanised anti-CD22 antibody) in primary Sjögren's syndrome: an open-label phase I/II study. *Arthritis Res Ther* 2006; **8**:R129.

Stickler M, Chin R, Faravashi N, Gebel W, Razo OJ, Rochanayon N, Power S, Valdes AM, Holmes S, and Harding FA. Human population-based identification of CD4+ T-cell peptide epitope determinants. *J Immunol Methods* 2003; **281**:95–108.

Stickler M, Rochanayon N, Razo OJ, Mucha J, Gebel W, Faravashi N, Chin R, Holmes S, and Harding FA. An in vitro human cell-based assay to rank the relative immunogenicity of proteins. *Toxicol Sci* 2004; **77**:280–289.

Stroomer JW, Roos JC, Sproll M, Quak JJ, Heider KH, Wilhelm BJ, Castelijns JA, Meyer R, Kwakkelstein MO, Snow GB, et al. Safety and biodistribution of ^{99m}Technetium-labeled anti-CD44v6 monoclonal antibody BIWA 1 in head and neck cancer patients. *Clin Cancer Res* 2000; **6**:3046–3055.

Sturniolo T, Bono E, Ding J, Raddrizzani L, Tuereci O, Sahin U, Braxenthaler M, Gallazzi F, Protti MP, Sinigaglia F, et al. Generation of tissue-specific and promiscuous HLA ligand databases using DNA microarrays and virtual HLA class II matrices. *Nat Biotechnol* 1999; **17**:555–561.

Tangri S, Mothé BR, Eisenbraun J, Sidney J, Southwood S, Briggs K, Zinckgraf J, Bilsel P, Newman M, Chesnut R, et al. Rationally engineered therapeutic proteins with reduced immunogenicity. *J Immunol* 2005; **174**:3187–3196.

Targan SR, Hanauer SB, van Deventer SJ, Mayer L, Present DH, Braakman T, DeWoody KL, Schaible TF, and Rutgeerts PJ. A short-term study of chimeric monoclonal antibody cA2 to tumor necrosis factor alpha for Crohn's disease. Crohn's Disease cA2 Study Group. *N Engl J Med* 1997; **337**: 1029–1035.

Tcheng JE, Kereiakes DJ, Lincoff AM, George BS, Kleiman NS, Sane DC, Cines DB, Jordan RE, Mascelli MA, Langrall MA, et al. Abciximab readministration: results of the ReoPro Readministration Registry. *Circulation* 2001; **104**:870–875.

The Impact-RSV Study Group. Palivizumab, a humanized respiratory syncytial virus monoclonal antibody, reduces hospitalization from respiratory syncytial virus infection in high-risk infants. *Pediatrics* 2006; 102:531–537.

Tijink BM, Buter J, de Bree R, Giaccone G, Lang MS, Staab A, Leemans CR, van Dongen GA. A phase I dose escalation study with anti-CD44v6 bivatuzumab mertansine in patients with incurable squamous cell carcinoma of the head and neck or esophagus. *Clin Cancer Res* 2006; **12**:6064–6072.

Tolcher AW, Ochoa L, Hammond LA, Patnaik A, Edwards T, Takimoto C, Smith L, de Bono J, Schwartz G, Mays T, et al. Cantuzumab mertansine, a maytansinoid immunoconjugate directed to the CanAg antigen: a phase I, pharmacokinetic, and biologic correlative study. *J Clin Oncol* 2003; **21**:211–222.

Uckun FM, Messinger Y, Chen CL, O'Neill K, Myers DE, Goldman F, Hurvitz C, Casper JT, and Levine A. Treatment of therapy-refractory B-lineage acute lymphoblastic leukemia with an apoptosis-inducing CD19-directed tyrosine kinase inhibitor. *Clin Cancer Res* 1999; **5**:3906–3913.

Van Walle I, Gansemans Y, Parren PW, Stas P, and Lasters I. Immunogenicity screening in protein drug development. *Expert Opin Biol Ther* 2007; **7**:405–418.

van de Putte LB, Atkins C, Malaise M, Sany J, Russell AS, van Riel PL, Settas L, Bijlsma JW, Todesco S, Dougados M, et al. Efficacy and safety of adalimumab as monotherapy in patients with rheumatoid arthritis for whom previous disease modifying antirheumatic drug treatment has failed. *Ann Rheum Dis* 2004; **63**:508–516.

van Zanten-Przybysz I, Molthoff C, Gebbinck JK, von Mensdorff-Pouilly S, Verstraeten R, Kenemans P, and Verheijen R. Cellular and humoral responses after multiple injections of unconjugated chimeric monoclonal antibody MOv18 in ovarian cancer patients: a pilot study. *J Cancer Res Clin Oncol* 2002; **128**:484–492.

Vermeire S, Noman M, Van Assche G, Baert F, D'Haens G, and Rutgeerts P. Effectiveness of concomitant immunosuppressive therapy in suppressing the formation of antibodies to infliximab in Crohn's disease. *Gut* 2007; **56**:1226–1231.

Vincenti F, Lantz M, Birnbaum J, Garovoy M, Mould D, Hakimi J, Nieforth K, and Light S. A phase I trial of humanized anti-interleukin 2 receptor antibody in renal transplantation. *Transplantation* 1997; **63**:33–38.

Warmerdam PA, Vanderlick K, Vandervoort P, De Smedt H, Plaisance S, De Maeyer M, and Collen D. Staphylokinase-specific cell-mediated immunity in humans. *J Immunol* 2002; **168**:155–161.

Weinblatt ME, Maddison PJ, Bulpitt KJ, Hazleman BL, Urowitz MB, Sturrock RD, Coblyn JS, Maier AL, Spreen WR, Manna VK, et al. CAMPATH-1H, a humanized monoclonal antibody, in refractory rheumatoid arthritis. An intravenous dose-escalation study. *Arthritis Rheum* 1995; **38**:1589–1594.

Weinblatt ME, Keystone EC, Furst DE, Moreland LW, Weisman MH, Birbara CA, Teoh LA, Fischkoff SA, and Chartash EK. Adalimumab, a fully human anti-tumor necrosis factor alpha monoclonal antibody, for the treatment of rheumatoid arthritis in patients taking concomitant methotrexate: the ARMADA trial. *Arthritis Rheum* 2003; **48**:35–45.

Welt S, Ritter G, Williams C Jr, Cohen LS, John M, Jungbluth A, Richards EA, Old LJ, and Kemeny NE. Phase I study of anticolon cancer humanized antibody A33. *Clin Cancer Res* 2003a; **9**:1338–1346.

Welt S, Ritter G, Williams C Jr, Cohen LS, Jungbluth A, Richards EA, Old LJ, and Kemeny NE. Preliminary report of a phase I study of combination chemotherapy and humanized A33 antibody immunotherapy in patients with advanced colorectal cancer. *Clin Cancer Res* 2003b; **9**:1347–1353.

Zhao Y, Pinilla C, Valmori D, Martin R, and Simon R. Application of support vector machines for T-cell epitopes prediction. *Bioinformatics* 2003; **19**:1978–1984.

Zhou LJ and Tedder TF. CD14+ blood monocytes can differentiate into functionally mature CD83+ dendritic cells. *Proc Natl Acad Sci USA* 1996; **93**:2588–2592.

In Vitro Screening for Antibody Immunogenicity

Frank J. Carr and Matthew P. Baker

A range of factors may contribute to the immunogenicity of therapeutic antibodies in patients but a major driver for immunogenicity is likely to be T cell help. Techniques have thus been developed that screen for MHC Class II restricted T cell epitopes in antibody variable region sequences to assess the potential for immunogenicity in therapeutic antibodies. Three such techniques are binding of peptides to human MHC Class II, binding of peptide-MHC complexes to T cell receptors, and *in vitro* human T cell assays. The most accurate measurement of T cell epitopes has been achieved using *in vitro* T cell assays, and these have demonstrated utility in testing antibodies as whole proteins as well as overlapping peptides from variable regions for the potency and location of T cell epitopes. Such *in vitro* T cell assays are now being used as a preclinical screen for antibody immunogenicity and for testing different formulations and manufacturing batches.

"NONSELF" ANTIBODIES

The evolution of a high affinity antibody response against an antigen *in vivo* is associated both with rearrangement of the variable and constant region genes as well as somatic hypermutation of the variable regions.[1] The resultant antibody secreted by a fully differentiated B cell (plasma cell) can be considered to be immunologically "nonself" by virtue of unique non-germline mutations introduced into the variable region sequences. However, such "nonself" antibodies are tolerated by the mammalian immune systems through various mechanisms of peripheral tolerance as well as by the fact that the effective concentration of any individual antibody present in the circulation at any given time is relatively low.

In contrast, treatment of humans with a therapeutic antibody presents them with an initially high concentration of an individual "nonself" antibody in the bloodstream or local tissue environment (if administering via the subcutaneous or intramuscular routes), typically exceeding the concentration of individual endogenous antibodies. Therefore it is not surprising that such therapeutic antibodies are often associated with immunogenicity in which antibodies are induced that bind to the

The authors would like to thank Laura Perry for critical reading of the review and Tim Jones for helpful discussions.

TABLE 3.1. Factors influencing the immunogenicity of antibody therapeutics

Intrinsic (antibody preparation)	Extrinsic (administration/patient status)
Aggregation	Dosage
Modification (e.g. glycosylation, deamidation)	Frequency of dose
Contaminants (adjuvants)	Route of administration (IV, SC,
Formulation	IM)
Sequence	Immunocompetence/patient
Helper T cell epitopes	disease status
B cell epitopes	MHC class II allotype
Size	Prior sensitization of patient/
Antigenic target(s)	cross-reactivity
Structure/disulphide bonding	Endogenous tolerance

therapeutic antibody (antitherapeutic antibodies) and can neutralize antigen binding (neutralizing antibodies).

The evolution of humanization and fully human antibody technologies has sought to create therapeutic antibodies that are immunologically "self" by providing variable regions as close to human germline as possible. In practice, due to the diversity of human frameworks expressed in the human population, identifying a common framework is not possible and some unique mutations are invariably required to create a high affinity antibody. Due to these factors, therapeutic antibodies are associated with a risk of immunogenicity in patients.[2] Techniques are being developed to quantify such risk at the preclinical stage in order to identify lead antibodies with reduced risk of immunogenicity and to prevent highly immunogenic antibodies from entering the clinic.

IMMUNOLOGICAL BASIS FOR ANTIBODY IMMUNOGENICITY

A range of factors has been proposed that potentially contributes to the immunogenicity of therapeutic antibodies and proteins as shown in Table 3.1. These are grouped into intrinsic factors that relate to the molecular properties of the therapeutic, extrinsic factors that relate to the administration of the therapeutic to patients, and the immune status of the patient.[25] While this is an extensive list of factors, it is likely that in all events where clinically significant immunogenicity is observed, T cell help (derived from CD4+ T cells) is a major influence in the production of antitherapeutic antibodies. The consequence of this T cell-dependent humoral response is the production of persistent high affinity antitherapeutic antibody responses and the generation of B cell memory. Indeed, experimental evidence in animal models has highlighted the link between T cell epitopes and high affinity

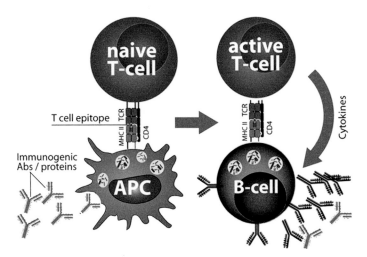

Figure 3.1. Stages in activation of helper T cell by therapeutic antibodies and subsequent induction of antibodies against the therapeutic.

anti-IFN-beta antibodies.[21] Furthermore there is a strong body of anecdotal evidence, for example relating to recombinant EPO (rEPO), that highlights the presence of T cell epitopes and the development of classic T cell dependent humoral responses in patients.[3,4,8]

Figure 3.1 outlines the stages in activation of T cells and the subsequent induction of a T cell dependent humoral response against a therapeutic protein. T cell epitopes are initially generated by the uptake and processing of protein antigens (including antibody therapeutics) by antigen-presenting cells (APCs) such as dendritic cells (DC). Peptides released by enzymatic cleavage in the endosomes are trafficked to vesicles containing MHC Class II molecules which, in turn, may bind these peptides and eventually display them at the cell surface. T cells recognize the peptide-MHC Class II complex by binding through the T cell receptor (TCR). Two signals are required for activation so that in addition to the signal through the TCR, T cells receive co-stimulation by interacting with molecules such as CD80 and CD86 on APCs, and CD28 on the T cells. Upon activation, T cells can differentiate and produce cytokines that support B cell activation/differentation and stimulate secondary B lymphopoeisis (somatic hypermutation and class switching of immunoglobulin genes). Furthermore, there is a cognate interaction between cell surface receptors expressed on activated B and T cells that provides additional stimulation for B cells. The specificity of this help is maintained because B cells are nonprofessional APCs that will take up and process the same antigen and present epitopes to specific T cell clones. Upon successful secondary B lymphopoiesis, B cells can differentiate into both plasma cells secreting antibody that binds to the original antigen, and into memory B cells.

It is clear that any of the intrinsic factors such as the presence of protein aggregates can, under certain circumstances, activate B cells independently of T cells and that these events can also facilitate a more effective T cell dependent humoral response.[5,23] Furthermore, enhanced antigen uptake and presentation of T cell epitopes can occur if the target antigen of the therapeutic antibody is present on APCs. Of the extrinsic factors, subcutaneous administration is associated with a higher risk of immunogenicity than intravenous or intramuscular administration,[6] probably because of a high local concentration of the injectable and high local level of specialized DC (Langerhans cells) in the skin. In spite of the risk factors, for any given therapeutic there is considerable heterogeneity in the frequency and magnitude of antitherapeutic antibody responses observed in patient populations. This is most likely due to a combination of risk factors relating to the patient and include MHC Class II haplotype, the degree of immunological tolerance that the patient exhibits toward the therapeutic antibody, the immunocompetence of the patient, and in certain cases, the severity of the disease, especially where inflammation is a factor.

IN VITRO SCREENING FOR IMMUNOGENICITY

Because T cell help is a key risk factor in the development of immunogenicity against therapeutic antibodies, there has been a major research initiative to develop preclinical *in vitro* screening tests to assess the potential for immunogenicity. Research in this area has centered on three types of *in vitro* test as follows: binding of peptides to MHC Class II, binding of peptide-MHC complex to TCRs, and *in vitro* human T cell assays.

Binding of Peptides to MHC Class II

The binding of peptides derived from therapeutic antibody variable region sequences to MHC Class II has been investigated as a potential screen for immunogenicity. Peptide binding to MHC Class II (Figure 3.1) is an essential molecular event in the activation of T cells. The established method for measuring the binding of peptides to MHC Class II uses test peptides in competition with standard high affinity MHC Class II binding peptides (normally radio- or biotin-labeled).[7] Typically, the solubilized MHC Class II molecule is immobilized after competition and the amount of bound standard peptide is measured. As such assays are technically laborious, many groups have developed *in silico* models for *in vitro* binding (reviewed by P. Stas in the previous chapter).

In vitro MHC Class II binding assays are limited because a majority of peptides bind a range of MHC Class II allotypes with some degree of affinity and because there are invariably many more medium and high affinity binders than actual T cell epitopes.[8] While the presence of peptides that bind a wide range of human MHC Class II allotypes with high affinity ("degenerate binders") provides some correlation with immunogenicity,[9] some moderate and low affinity peptides can also trigger T cell responses and some high affinity MHC Class II binders will not trigger a response.[10] The fact that *in vitro* MHC Class II binding assays tend to over-predict the number of actual immunogenic T cell epitopes has been known for some time and is largely ascribed to other factors that influence the formation of a T cell epitope, including binding affinity of peptide-MHC complex to TCRs, the need for co-stimulatory signals additional to peptide-MHC-TCR binding, and the requirement for a T cell to express a TCR specific for the peptide epitope. In addition, certain peptides may be destroyed or not effectively processed during antigen processing of therapeutic antibodies by APCs and therefore any *in vitro* MHC Class II binding analysis of such peptides will be irrelevant. However, an alternative method using mass spectrometry to detect processed peptides derived from proteins taken up by APC has recently been developed to account for antigen processing during the formation of a T cell epitope.[11]

Binding of Peptide-MHC Class II Complexes to T Cell Receptors

Tetramer technology[12] uses labeled complexes of peptides bound to isolated MHC Class II alleles which, in turn, bind to T cells with complementary T cell receptors. Tetramers have been used, for example, to detect and isolate T cells specific for HSV-2.[13] Similar to *in vitro* MHC Class II binding analysis, a major disadvantage of measuring the binding of peptide-MHC Class II complexes to T cells as described above is the level of over-prediction due to the inability to account for antigen processing. While this technology offers a more comprehensive assessment of T cell epitopes, it is still compounded by the difficulty in producing the peptide-MHC Class II complexes and the limited availability of variant MHC Class II alleles to allow for screening representative samples of the world population.

IN VITRO (EX VIVO) HUMAN T CELL ASSAYS

Three broad variations in the format of human T cell assays have been used to measure T cell activation as a model for immunogenicity of protein therapeutics: first, where T cells are expanded or cloned by repeated incubation with the antigen of interest;[8,15] second, where APCs are separated from T cells, differentiated *in vitro*, incubated with antigen, and then added back to autologous T cells;[14] and third, where antigen is added directly to unseparated peripheral blood mononuclear cells (PBMCs) that contain a physiological mixture of APCs and T cells.[15] For all formats, T cell responses can be detected to whole therapeutic antibodies or proteins using proliferation (e.g., tritiated thymidine incorporation) and cytokine release (e.g. ELIspot) assays. Furthermore an assessment of any associations between MHC Class II allotypes and T cell responses can be made given the known haplotypes of the individual donors in the study cohort.[22] *In vitro* T cell assays can also be used to determine the location of T cell epitopes by testing peptides derived from the protein sequence of interest. Peptides are normally designed to span the sequence (such as antibody variable region) and overlap the previous peptide to provide a high resolution T cell epitope map.[20] Typically, these assays require 50 or more donors normally selected for each assay to account for diversity in MHC Class II allotypes in the human population, and extensive assay development is required to differentiate signal from noise. A key step in the development of successful *in vitro* T cell assays is the ability to store frozen MHC Class II-typed PBMCs from donors so that cohorts representative of the world MHC Class II haplotype distribution can be selected at the time of a study.[15,24]

Of the three types of *in vitro* immunogenicity screen discussed above, *in vitro* human T cell assays theoretically provide the most accurate measurement of T cell responses since this assay format can assess antigen processing, peptide binding to MHC Class II, and T cell activation. Importantly, a correlation between T cell responses to protein therapeutics *in vitro* and clinical immunogenicity is emerging, thus confirming the importance of this type of assessment in preclinical screening for immunogenicity.[16]

PRACTICAL APPLICATIONS OF *IN VITRO* SCREENING

There are several stages of drug discovery and development where *in vitro* methods may be used to assess the immunogenicity of antibodies. At the research stage, *in vitro* screening has been used to analyze the potential immunogenicity of lead therapeutic antibodies prior to any decision on further development, including the testing of chimeric, humanized, and fully human antibodies, and also other antibody and antibody-like formats such as single-chain and single-domain antibodies. In the same manner, *in vitro* screening has been used to select between panels of lead antibodies for those with the lowest potential for immunogenicity. *In vitro* screening can also be used at the development stage to assess the potential immunogenicity of a therapeutic antibody in conjunction with immunogenicity testing in animals, as well as to assess the potential immunogenicity of different formulations. For example, new formulations of IFN-beta (Rebif®) in which human serum albumin had been removed were initially assessed using *in vitro* T cell assays. Selection of a lead formulation that exhibited fewer T cell responses in this *in vitro* study was corroborated by a later Phase IIIb clinical trial in which the same lead formulation was associated with a reduced risk of immunogenicity.[17,18] *In vitro* human T cell assays are also being used as a screen for manufacturing batches in order to detect effects on T cell responses related to physicochemical changes or impurities that might potentiate immunogenicity; this has important application in the *in vitro* screening for immunogenicity of biosimilars. Finally, *in vitro* human T cell assays are being used during clinical trials for analysis of T cell responses during therapy.

REMOVAL OF T CELL EPITOPES

A major application of *in vitro* screening for immunogenicity has been in the identification and removal of T cell epitopes from therapeutic antibodies and other proteins, a technique that is termed "deimmunization."[19] The screening of over-lapping peptides (typically 15mer peptides overlapping by 12 amino acids) derived from an antibody variable region sequence using *in vitro* human T cell assays can be used to locate T cell epitopes. Where the epitope is detected in one or more adjacent overlapping peptides, the location of the core 9mer that binds to MHC Class II can be defined using either *in vitro* or *in silico* techniques as described above. Removal of T cell epitopes typically involves substitution of amino acids within the MHC Class II binding core 9mer and testing of the deimmunized anti-body for retention of antigen binding. A disadvantage of the deimmunization technique is that some T cell epitopes are difficult to remove without loss of anti-body function. Since the risk of this occurring greatly depends upon the location of T cell epitopes in the starting antibody variable region sequences, an alternative approach developed in the authors' laboratory is to reconstruct the variable region sequences such that T cell epitopes are avoided. This is achieved by creating composite variable region sequences that involves joining together segments of sequences from other unrelated human antibody variable regions to create "com-posite human antibodies." The composite sequences are subject to assessment for T cell epitopes using data derived from *in vitro* human T cell assays as well as *in vitro/in silico* MHC Class II binding assays in order to avoid inclusion of T cell epitopes. Such antibodies can then be tested using *in vitro* human T cell assays to confirm the removal of T cell epitopes and are thus considered a low potential immunogenicity risk in patients.

CONCLUSIONS

In vitro screening for antibody immunogenicity is becoming an increasingly impor-tant factor in the discovery and development of new therapeutic antibodies. *In vitro* tests based on peptide binding to MHC Class II are being replaced by more accurate immunogenicity tests using *in vitro (ex vivo)* human T cell assays that can detect actual T cell recognition of epitopes rather than just the first MHC Class II binding step in a T cell response. There is an increasing body of evidence showing that T cell epitopes correlate with immunogenicity observed in patients. As a result, *in vitro* screening for antibody immunogenicity is now being actively used in the selection of lead therapeutic antibodies for clinical development and for the earlier screening of development-stage antibodies for potential immunogenicity. *In vitro* immunogenic-ity screening also has a role in testing different formulations and manufacturing batches of therapeutic antibodies. Finally, there is considerable utility in using *in vitro* human T cell assays to locate T cell epitopes in the variable regions of existing therapeutic antibodies that appear to be immunogenic in the clinic, thus enabling these epitopes to be specifically targeted for removal for improvement in the safety and efficacy of the antibodies.

REFERENCES

[1] Griffiths GM, Berek C, Kaartinen M, and Milstein C: Somatic mutation and the maturation of the immune response to 2-phenyl-oxazolone. *Nature* (1984) **312**: 271–274.

[2] Haraoui B, Cameron L, Ouellet M, and White B: Anti-infliximab antibodies in patients with rheumatoid arthritis who require higher doses of infliximab to achieve or maintain a clinical response. *J Rheumatol* (2006) **33**(1): 31–36.

[3] Schonholzer C, Keusch G, Nigg L, Robert D, and Wauters JP: High prevalence in Switzerland of pure red-cell aplasia due to anti-erythropoietin antibodies in chronic dialysis patients: report of five cases. *Nephrol Dial Transplant* (2004) **19**(8): 2121–2125.

[4] Bader F: Immunogenicity of Therapeutic Proteins: *A Case Report. Scientific Considerations Related to Developing Follow-On Protein Products FDA Public Workshop*, September 2004 (http://www.fda.gov/cder/meeting/followOn/Bader.ppt-**670**,3).

[5] Rosenberg AS: Effects of protein aggregates: an immunologic perspective. *AAPS J* (2006) **8**(3): E501–507.

[6] Howman R and Kulkarni H: Antibody-mediated acquired pure red cell aplasia (PRCA) after treatment with darbepoetin. *Nephrol Dial Transplant* (2007) **22**(5): 1462–1464.

[7] Sidney J, Southwood S, Oseroff C, del Guercio M-F, Grey HM, and Sette A: Measurement of peptide/MHC interactions by gel filtration. *Current Protocols in Immunology*, Wiley, New York (1988): 18.13.11.

[8] Tangri S, Mothé BF, Eisenbraun J, Sidney J, Southwood S, Briggs K, Zinckgraf J, Bilsel P, Newman M, Chesnut R, LiCalsi C, and Sette A: Rationally engineered therapeutic proteins with reduced immunogenicity. *J Immunol* (2005) **174**(6): 3187–3196.

[9] Southwood C, Sidney J, Kondo A, Chesnut RW, Grey HM, and Sette A: *J Immunol* (1998) **160**: 3363–3369.

[10] Barbosa MDFS and Celis E. Immunogenicity of protein therapeutics and the interplay between tolerance and antibody responses. *Drug Discov Today* (2007) **12**: 674–681.

[11] Röhn TA, Reitz A, Paschen A, Nguyen XD, Schadendorf D, Vogt AB, and Kropshofer H: A novel strategy for the discovery of MHC class II–restricted tumor antigens: identification of a melanotransferrin helper T-cell epitope. *Cancer Res* (2005) **65**: 10068–10078.

[12] Crawford F, Kozono H, White J, Marrack P, and Kappler J: Detection of antigen-specific T cells with multivalent soluble class II MHC covalent peptide complexes. *Immunity* (1998) **8**: 675–681.

[13] Novak EJ, Liu AW, Gebe JA, Falk BA, Nepom GT, Koelle DM, and Kwok WW: Tetramer-guided epitope mapping: rapid identification and characterization of immunodominant CD4+ T cell epitopes from complex antigens. *J Immunol* (2001) **166**: 6665–6670.

[14] Stickler M, Valdes AM, Gebel W, Razo OJ, Faravashi N, Chin R, Rochanayon N, and Harding FA: The HLA-DR2 haplotype is associated with an increased proliferative response to the immunodominant CD4(+) T-cell epitope in human interferon-beta. *Genes Immun* (2004) **5**(1): 1–7.

[15] Jones TD, Phillips WJ, Smith BJ, Bamford CA, Nayee PD, Baglin TP, Gaston JS, and Baker MP: Identification and removal of a promiscuous CD4+ T cell epitope from the C1 domain of factor VIII. *J Thromb Haemost* (2005) **3**(5): 991–1000.

[16] Baker MP and Jones TD: Identification and removal of immunogenicity in therapeutic proteins. *Curr Opin Drug Discov Devel* (2007) **18**(2): 219–227.

[17] Jaber A and Baker M: Assessment of the immunogenicity of different interferon beta-1a formulations using *ex vivo* T-cell assays. *J Pharm Biomed Anal* (2007) **43**(4): 1256–1261.

[18] Jaber A, Driebergen R, Giovannoni G, Schellekens H, Simsarian J, and Antonelli M: The Rebif® new formulation story. *Drugs R D* (2007) **8**(6): 335–348.

[19] Bander NH, Milowsky MI, Nanus DM, Kostakoglu L, Vallabhajosula S, and Goldsmith SJ: Phase I trial of 177lutetium-labeled J591, a monoclonal antibody to prostate-specific membrane antigen, in patients with androgen-independent prostate cancer. *J Clin Oncol* (2005) **23**(21): 4591–4601.

[20] Jones TD, Hanlon M, Smith BJ, Heise CT, Nayee PD, Sanders DA, Hamilton A, Sweet C, Unitt E, Alexander G, Lo K-M, Gillies SD, Carr FJ, and Baker MP: The development of a modified human IFN-α2b linked to the Fc portion of human IgG1 as a novel potential therapeutic for the treatment of hepatitis C virus infection. *J Interferon Cytokine Res* (2004) **24**: 560–572.

[21] Yeung VP, Chang J, Miller J, Barnett C, Stickler M, and Harding FA: Elimination of an immunodominant CD4 T cell epitope in human IFN-β does not result in an in vivo response directed at the subdominant epitope. *J Immunol* (2004), **172**: 6658–6665.

[22] Barbosa MDFS, Vielmetter J, Chu S, Smith DD, and Jacinto J: Clinical link between MHC class II haplotype and interferon-beta (IFN-β) immunogenicity. *Clinical Immunol* (2006) **118**(1): 42–50.

[23] Bachmann M and Zinkernagel R: Neutralizing antiviral B-cell responses. *Annu Rev Immunol* (1997) **15**: 235–270.

[24] Stickler M, Valdes AM, Gebel W, Razo OJ, Faravashi N, Chin R, Rochanayon N, and Harding FA: The HLA-DR2 haplotype is associated with an increased proliferative response to the immunodominant CD4(+) T-cell epitope in human interferon-beta. *Genes Immun* (2004) **5**(1): 1–7.

[25] Schellekens H and Casadevall N: Immunogenicity of recombinant human proteins: causes and consequences. *J Neurol* (2004) **251**(Suppl 2): II4–9.

PART II

GENERATION AND SCREENING OF ANTIBODY LIBRARIES

CHAPTER FOUR

Antibody Libraries from Naïve V Gene Sources

Gerald Beste and David Lowe

Recombinant human antibody repertoires are now used routinely for the identification of individual antibodies with defined specificities to any conceivable antigen. The generation of large libraries ($>10^{10}$) has been reported from many commercial and academic laboratories, along with a growing number of examples of isolated antibodies in clinical development for a range of therapeutic applications. Our laboratory has constructed nonimmunized libraries of human scFv antibody fragments with a combined size of $>10^{11}$ transformants that have been used for more than ten years to successfully isolate antibodies suitable for clinical development.

LIBRARY DESIGN CONSIDERATIONS

Natural Antibody Diversity

The common aim of all nonimmunized recombinant antibody libraries is to mirror the immune system's ability to provide binding specificity to any antigen. For naïve human antibody libraries this is achieved by capturing the full spectrum of antibody sequences available from the human B cell repertoire.

The primary repertoire of variable heavy and light chain DNA sequences is generated by the recombination of V, J, and in case of the heavy chain, also D gene segments, which can recombine to give 7,650 (16,218 considering the use of multiple reading frames for the D segments) different V_H and 324 different V_L sequences (Corbett et al., 1997; Nossal, 2003). Imprecise joining of these gene segments and addition of nucleotides at splice sites introduce further variation giving an estimated primary repertoire in excess of 10^9 different antibody sequences. It is worth noting that the diversity of this repertoire is concentrated in the CDR3 regions where the gene recombination occurs. To clone the primary repertoire, mRNA from the naïve B cell population – that is, from B cells that have not yet encountered antigen – is used. These naïve cells are predominantly found in bone marrow and peripheral blood where they constitute approximately 60% of the B cell total (Klein et al., 1998).

The secondary repertoire of antibody DNA sequences is generated from B cells that undergo somatic hypermutation upon antigen stimulation to differentiate into memory and plasma B cells. Hypermutation results from stepwise incorporation of single nucleotide substitutions into the antibody variable gene (Di Noia & Neuberger, 2007) followed by selection of B cells producing antibodies with improved affinity for the antigen. The average mutation frequency found in the resulting antibody genes away from the germline sequence is between 2% and 6%, equivalent to 15–45 mutations per variable region (Goossens et al., 1998). Beneficial mutations are found more frequently within CDR regions than in framework regions. To capture the natural antibody gene diversity generated by somatic hypermutation, mRNA from tissues containing high levels of plasma and memory B cells is used for library generation. Tissues include secondary lymphoid organs such as spleen and tonsils as well as peripheral blood lymphocytes (PBL) with memory B cells and plasma cells constituting approximately 40% and 1% of total PBL, respectively (Klein et al., 1998).

For the construction of an antibody library, it is important to consider that the ratio of antibody genes representative of the primary and secondary repertoires is also determined by the level of Ig mRNA found in the different types of B cells. Memory B cells have 5- to 10-fold (Klein et al., 1997), and active, antibody-secreting plasma cells have 100- to 180-fold (Kelley & Perry, 1986; Matthes et al., 1994) increased Ig mRNA levels over resting naïve B cells.

Tissues should be sourced from multiple donors to ensure that V gene diversity is maximized and the effects of biases in any given individual's immune repertoire are minimized. The libraries that have been generated in our laboratory have been derived from B lymphocytes from over 100 healthy human donors.

Library Diversity

Following the isolation of mRNA from B cells and its reverse transcription into cDNA, V_H and V_L regions are amplified separately and recombined in a random fashion to create the antibody library. This chain-shuffling procedure introduces non-native diversity into the antibody repertoire, which is believed to be crucial for the isolation of antibodies with high specificity for human self-antigens from naïve antibody libraries by creating antigen-binding sites *de novo* (Griffiths et al., 1993; Hoet et al., 2005). Further non-natural diversity is usually introduced by PCR errors during the library construction process and antibody variable genes may have undergone several PCR amplifications for V_H and V_L amplification and assembly. The most commonly used Taq polymerase has an error rate of $\sim 10^{-4}$/bp, resulting in approximately 8 mutations on average over 100 PCR cycles for a scFv gene.

Regarding the isolation of human anti-self antibodies, it is worth noting that despite immunological tolerance mechanisms that prevent the antigen-driven expansion of B cells with self-specificities (Nossal, 1989), a considerable fraction of B lymphocytes in healthy individuals carry polyreactive and to a lesser degree monoreactive receptors with auto-antigen-binding capacity, which seem to play a role in general homeostasis (Avrameas et al., 2007). As a result of chain shuffling and the introduction of PCR errors, techniques that have been used extensively for *in vitro* antibody affinity maturation (Marks et al., 1992), some of these low affinity antibodies are presumably converted to monospecific binders with higher affinity during library construction.

Library Size and Quality

Based on theoretical considerations, an antibody repertoire of 10^7 different molecules has been estimated to recognize 99% of epitopes, with an average affinity of 10^{-5} M proportionally increasing with library size (Perelson, 1989; Perelson & Oster, 1979). The first libraries of human antibody fragments were 10^7–10^8 in size and generally produced micromolar to nanomolar affinity clones. Such low affinities render antibodies impractical for most applications and are not compatible with the requirement for testing them in cell-based functional assays in the context of therapeutic antibody generation. Antibodies from larger repertoires generated by increasing the numbers of transformations (Vaughan et al., 1996), by employing more efficient cloning techniques (de Haard et al., 1999), or by exploiting *in vivo* bacterial recombination of the V genes (Griffiths et al., 1994; Sblattero & Bradbury, 2000) have been shown to be of higher affinity, with even sub-nanomolar affinity constants being measured for certain clones (Vaughan et al., 1996). To date, the repertoire sizes of the most commonly used phage displayed antibody libraries have reached a ceiling of ~10^{11} transformants, given the practical limitations on bacterial transformation.

In addition to the generally quoted total number of transformants produced, it is also important to assess and monitor the percentage of functional antibodies to describe the size of an antibody fragment library. Important parameters to determine the functional library size include the proportion of truncated clones and clones with frameshifts or stop codons, the overrepresentation of clones, the proportion of clones that can be expressed in the expression system of choice as well as the display level for the display format used. For phage displayed antibody libraries it seems that despite concerns that as few as 1% to 10% of transformants express full-length antibody fragments (McCafferty, 1996) over 50% of transformants, in both scFv and Fab libraries, express full-length protein (de Haard et al., 1999; Vaughan et al., 1996).

The ultimate test for a naïve antibody library, however, is whether it can be used to isolate diverse panels of specific high affinity antibodies to any given antigen. The antibody libraries constructed in our laboratory containing >10^{11} transformants have been used to successfully isolate antibodies against a large number of targets from different target classes. Panels of more than 1,000 antibodies different in amino acid sequence have been generated against some targets (Edwards et al., 2003) and antibodies with therapeutical potential have been isolated straight from the library without the need for further affinity maturation (Dobson et al., 2002; Edwards, 2003).

Combination of Naïve and Synthetic Repertoires

The combination of naïve and synthetic repertoires for the generation of antibody libraries has a long-standing history. More recent examples include the isolation of heavy and light chain CDR from human lymphoid tissue, and subsequent transplantation into synthetically constructed V_H (3–23) and V_L (1-g) frameworks chosen for improved bacterial expression and folding (Söderlind et al., 2000) or the use of a single synthetic V_H framework (3–23), containing targeted mutations to the antigen-binding CDR1 and 2 regions, paired with a repertoire of CDR3 sequences and entire V_L genes isolated from human donors (Hoet et al., 2005).

These semisynthetic approaches to antibody repertoire generation have several attractive features. Unique restriction enzyme recognition sites can be incorporated into the chosen framework sequence to facilitate further engineering of antibody fragments through CDR loop or framework shuffling. Improved bacterial expression can be achieved by designing a library around a framework that is known to express and fold efficiently in *E. coli*. Particular frameworks such as V_H3 and κ chains enable the use of protein A or L for detection/purification and as an indicator of proper folding.

This has to be balanced against potential disadvantages of semisynthetic antibody repertoires in comparison to fully naïve V gene sources. Synthetic repertoire moieties may introduce features selected against in natural repertoires such as protease cleavage sites, glycosylation sites, or an increased tendency for aggregation. If a repertoire is restricted to a particular set of V genes, antibody paratopes formed by other V genes may be missed. When one constructs synthetic CDR sequences, care should be taken to avoid the introduction of T cell epitopes that could result in a higher risk of immunogenicity. A semisynthetic library can be constructed using codons optimized for bacterial expression. The codon usage, however, may not be compatible with the eukaryotic expression of the antibody in IgG format, resulting in reduced expression yields.

Display of Naïve Antibody Repertoires Using Ribosome Display

Since its inception in 1990 (McCafferty et al., 1990), phage display of antibody fragments has been the method of choice for the screening of large naïve antibody repertoires despite the development of alternative display formats, such as ribosome display (Hanes & Plückthun, 1997) and cell surface display (Chen et al., 2001; Feldhaus et al., 2003). To a large degree, this is because phage display has proven to be a very robust technique that allows for the efficient enrichment of rare antibodies from nonimmune repertoires during the critical initial selection rounds.

As one of the alternative display technologies, ribosome display has so far been mainly applied in the context of antibody optimization, where it offers some unique advantages over phage display. Such advantages include the ability to manipulate mRNA: ribosome ratios to give monovalent display using excess mRNA to prevent polysome formation, affinity-independent elution through complex destabilization, ease of sequence diversification via DNA manipulation between selection rounds, and tailored folding conditions for stability screening (Groves & Osbourn, 2005).

The use of ribosome display for the screening of naïve antibody libraries, however, has shown to be technically more challenging than for an already enriched population due to the difficulty in recovering sufficient amounts of cDNA following the initial selection rounds (Groves et al., 2006; Villemagne et al., 2006) and only a few successful applications using nonimmune antibody libraries have been reported (Hanes et al., 2000; Yan et al., 2005; Yau et al., 2003). Markedly improved cDNA yields that can facilitate naïve library selections have recently been achieved by using reconstituted translation systems that do not suffer from the rapid energy depletion and mRNA degradation associated with the conventional *E. coli* S30 cell extract (Villemagne et al., 2006).

These more robust systems enable the use of the intrinsic features that make ribosome display a valuable complementary technology to phage display viable for the screening of naïve antibody libraries. Since the repertoire size using ribosome display is not limited by transformation efficiency, larger libraries with up to 10^{14} members can be realized, with the upper limit depending primarily on the scale of the *in vitro* translation performed. This has implications for the average affinity that can be isolated from a library as discussed before. In addition to antibody affinity, expression levels are crucial for the successful enrichment of binders over several selection cycles. For individual antibody fragments these will be different for the *E. coli*-based phage display system compared to the *in vitro* transcription/translation systems used with ribosome display. This can lead to the preferential enrichment of a different set of clones when both technologies are used in parallel, providing greater choice from a more diverse panel of antibodies as has been shown for enriched repertoires during affinity maturation (Groves et al., 2006). In contrast to phage display where mutations occur rarely, ribosome display is a more dynamic system where the introduction of PCR errors in each cycle increases the sequence space screened. This could result in the isolation of higher affinity binders from the same initial repertoire (Hanes et al., 2000). An advantage of phage display over ribosome display is that it is more tolerant toward the use of unpurified target antigens for selection, which pose technical challenges when used with ribosome display due to the labile nature of the ternary ribosome-antibody-mRNA complex.

Taken together, both technologies are complementary and can be used in parallel to yield more diverse panels of antibodies from naïve repertoires than can be achieved with one technology alone.

LIBRARY CONSTRUCTION

The following paragraphs describe the generation of a large naïve phage display library of human scFv antibody fragments as performed in our laboratory. An overview of the process is shown in Figure 4.1.

Sourcing of mRNA and Reverse Transcription

The source tissues of the B cell–derived antibody V genes include spleen, bone marrow, tonsil, and peripheral blood mononuclear cells (PBMC). These tissue sources have been chosen to represent as wide a diversity of V genes as possible and to include both primary and secondary immune sources. B lymphocyte cDNA template can either be purchased from manufacturers (e.g., Clontech Quick-Clone cDNA) or prepared directly from appropriate tissue. For PBMC, 50 ml of whole blood yield

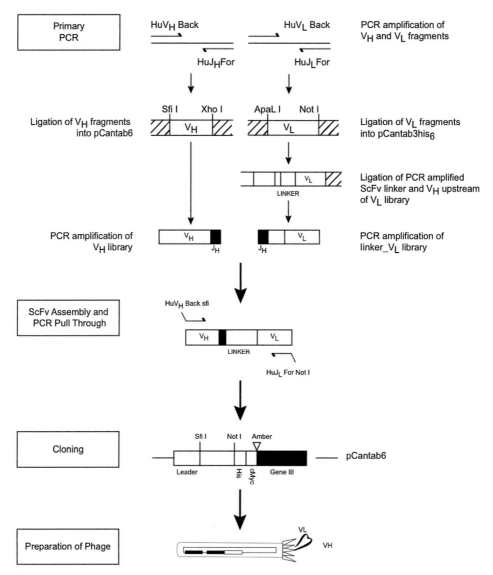

Figure 4.1. Overview for construction of the scFv phagemid library.

approximately 10^7 cells, following Ficoll gradient centrifugation as detailed by Marks et al. (1991). The mRNA is immediately isolated using an oligo(dT)-purification system. First-strand cDNA from the mRNA template is synthesized using random hexamer primers. This allows all five antibody classes (IgM, IgG, IgA, IgD, and IgE) to be represented and increases library diversity. From each tissue source approximately 15ng cDNA are required for the initial PCR amplification of V_H and V_L repertoires.

Amplification of V_H and V_L Repertoires

The primers used to amplify the V_H and V_L genes are designed to anneal to all heavy and light chain gene families and are based on those originally described by Marks

TABLE 4.1. Distribution of functional V genes on Ig locus

V_H family	$V_H1/7$	V_H2	V_H3	V_H4	V_H5	V_H6			
Proportion of pool	12/49	3/49	21/49	10/49	2/49	1/49			
V_κ family	$V_\kappa1$	$V_\kappa2$	$V_\kappa3$	$V_\kappa4$	$V_\kappa5$	$V_\kappa6$			
Proportion of pool	17/35	7/35	7/35	1/35	1/35	2/35			
V_λ family	$V_\lambda1$	$V_\lambda2$	$V_\lambda3$	$V_\lambda4$	$V_\lambda5$	$V_\lambda6$	$V_\lambda7/8$	$V_\lambda9$	$V_\lambda10$
Proportion of pool	5/31	5/31	9/31	3/31	3/31	1/31	3/31	1/31	1/31

Source: V-BASE directory, MRC Centre for Protein Engineering, Cambridge UK; http://vbase.mrc-cpe.cam.ac.uk.

et al. (1991), including additional gene families that have since been discovered (Tomlinson et al., 1992; Vaughan et al., 1996). To capture maximum diversity and to avoid a bias in V gene representation (Sheets et al., 1998) separate PCR reactions for each V_H, V_λ and V_κ exon are performed – that is, each V gene–specific 5′ primer is paired with a pool of J region–specific 3′ primers.

To facilitate cloning, 5′ and 3′ primers contain *Sfi*I and *Xho*I restriction sites (V_H) or *Apa*L1 and *Not*I sites (V_L), respectively. For each PCR, 0.5 ng of first-strand cDNA are used. Following amplification, the different PCR products are quantified and pooled in a normalized fashion based on the relative size of each V_H and V_L family as determined by the number of functional V segments on the relevant Ig locus (Table 4.1). The pooled products are digested with the appropriate restriction enzymes and inserted into separate vectors. The V_H pool is inserted into pCANTAB6 (McCafferty et al., 1994). Electroporation of the ligation product should yield a library size of 10^8. The V_κ and V_λ pools can either be kept separate to generate individual κ and λ libraries or can be pooled. The separate or combined V_L pools are cloned into pCANTAB3his_6 (McCafferty et al., 1994) to generate V_κ and V_λ repertoire sizes of 10^5 to 10^6.

scFv Assembly and Cloning

As a first step to facilitate scFv assembly, a $(Gly_4Ser)_3$ scFv-linker is attached to the V_L repertoire. This is achieved by amplifying the linker together with an irrelevant V_H from an existing scFv via PCR and inserting this fragment into the V_L repertoire upstream of the V_L gene segments as a *Hin*dIII-*Apa*LI digested fragment. This should generate a V_L repertoire with an upstream scFv linker of between 10^6 and 10^7 recombinants.

The V_H and linker-V_L DNA fragments are then amplified separately from each of the cloned repertoires (V_H in pCANTAB6 and linker-V_L in pCANTAB3his_6). To facilitate assembly of the two repertoires, the 3′ primer set for the V_H amplification and the 5′ primer set for the linker-V_L amplification overlap on the J_H region with the latter set introducing the necessary mutations into the monoclonal J_H derived from the dummy V_H sequence to sample all different J_H gene families. V_H and linker-V_L PCR products are subsequently mixed in equal amounts and assembled via PCR. Following the assembly step, individual pull-through PCR reactions for each V_H-gene specific 5′ primer paired with each pool of J_λ and J_κ 3′ primers are performed.

The resulting PCR products are pooled, digested with *Sfi*I and *Not*I, and inserted into the phagemid vector pCANTAB6. To generate a library of 10^{10} transformants, at least 100 electroporations are performed and spread onto 243mm x 243mm agar plates. The scFv antibody library is stored as bacterial suspension in aliquots at $-70°C$.

Phage Preparation

To generate the phage library for use in selections, the phagemid particles are rescued with the helper phage M13K07 (New England Biolabs). The resultant library phages are PEG precipitated and caesium-banded, allowing storage at 4°C for long periods.

Assessment of Diversity

To assess the diversity of the antibody libraries generated in our laboratory, DNA sequence analysis was performed. Approximately 500 random scFv antibody clones were taken directly from the unselected libraries (i.e., clones that have not been isolated by panning against a particular antigen) and analyzed. More than 80% of the sequences were found to encode full-length antibody genes without frameshifts or stop codons. Within the pool of functional genes, the vast majority of V_H germline gene segments (44/49) was observed. The different germline gene segments were represented in 0.2% to 11% of antibodies isolated, demonstrating a broad spread of germline gene usage, with no one particular family dominating. V_L usage in the sample was also extensive with a total of 22/31 V_λ and 16/35 V_κ germline segments observed. Despite the small sample size, approximately 300 different V_H-V_L combinations were identified; and with only two combinations appearing more than 10 times, no strong bias toward one particular pairing was observed.

The extensive sampling of the possible V gene repertoire by such libraries is potentially advantageous over libraries designed around single synthetic frameworks, as the range of structurally different antibodies will more closely match that of the natural immune response and could represent a more diverse coverage of possible paratopes. It has been proposed that different germline V gene families evolved to exploit the diversity created by somatic hypermutation, which, in contrast to the primary repertoire, is more focused at the periphery of the binding site rather than the center (Tomlinson et al., 1996). For example, we have previously reported the isolation of over 1,000 different antibodies to a single protein antigen (Edwards et al., 2003) from our naïve human scFv antibody libraries. This diverse panel was made up of 42/49 different V_H genes, coupled with light chains representing 19/31 and 13/35 of the possible V_λ and V_κ genes and covered both biologically functional and nonfunctional epitopes.

SUMMARY

The development of naïve repertoires of human antibodies allows the rapid isolation of antibodies to every conceivable immunogen, including toxic antigens and those that are highly conserved among mammalian species, which have traditionally been difficult to isolate via conventional immunization strategies. Moreover, such libraries typically yield panels of unique antibodies in the range of hundreds to thousands. Combining such diverse repertoires with automated antibody selection and screening advances has led to the industrialization of the humoral antibody response. This provides researchers and developers with a range of options when considering the optimum desired profile for a new therapeutic, or a set of bespoke tools with exquisite specificity for supporting clinical research.

REFERENCES

Avrameas, S., Ternynck, T., Tsonis, I.A., Lymberi, P., 2007. Naturally occurring B-cell autoreactivity: A critical overview. *J. Autoimmun.* **29**, 213–218.

Chen, G., Hayhurst, A., Thomas, J.G., Harvey, B.R., Iversen, B.L., Georgiou, G., 2001. Isolation of high-affinity ligand-binding proteins by periplasmic expression with cytometric screening (PECS). *Nat. Biotechnol.* **19**, 537–542.

Corbett, S.J., Tomlinson, I.M., Sonnhammer, E.L.L., Buck, D., Winter, G., 1997. Sequence of the human immunoglobulin diversity (D) segment locus: a systematic analysis provides no evidence for the use of DIR segments, inverted D segments, ''minor'' D segments or D-D recombination. *J. Mol. Biol.* **270**, 587–597.

de Haard, H.J., van Neer, N., Reurs, A., Hufton, S.E., Roovers, R.C., Henderikx, P., de Bruine, A.P., Arends, J.W., Hoogenboom, H.R., 1999. A large non-immunized human Fab fragment phage library that permits rapid isolation and kinetic analysis of high affinity antibodies. *J. Biol. Chem.* **274**, 18218–18230.

Di Noia, J.M., Neuberger, M.S., 2007. Molecular mechanisms of antibody somatic hypermutation. *Annu. Rev. Biochem.* **76**, 1–22.

Dobson, C.L., Edwards, B.M., Main, S.H., Minter R., Williams, E., Salcedo, T., Choi, G.H., Albert, V.R., Vaughan, T.J., 2002. Generation of human therapeutic anti-TRAIL-R1 agonistic antibodies by phage display. 93rd Annual Meeting AACR, San Francisco, CA, USA.

Edwards, B.M., Barash, S.C., Main, S.H., Choi, G.H., Minter, R., Ullrich, S., Williams, E., Du Fou, L., Wilton, J., Albert, V.R., Ruben, S.M., Vaughan, T.J., 2003. The remarkable flexibility of the human antibody repertoire; isolation of over one thousand different antibodies to a single protein, BLys. *J. Mol. Biol.* **334**, 103–118.

Edwards, B.M., 2003. Isolation of agonistic human monoclonal antibodies to TRAIL-R2 that display potent *in vitro* and *in vivo* anti-tumour activities. *Antibody-based Therapeutics for Cancer*, Banff, Alberta, Canada.

Feldhaus, M.J., Siegel, R.W., Opresko, L.K., Coleman, J.R., Weaver Feldhaus, J.M., Yeung, Y.A., Cochran, J.R., Heinzelman, P., Colby, D., Swers, J., Graff, C., Wiley, H.S., Wittrup, K.D., 2003. Flow-cytometric isolation of human antibodies from a nonimmune *Saccharomyces cerevisiae* surface display library. *Nat. Biotechnol.* **21**, 163–170.

Goossens, T., Klein, U., Küppers, R., 1998. Frequent occurrence of deletions and duplications during somatic hypermutation: Implications for oncogene translocations and heavy chain disease. *Proc. Natl. Acad. Sci. USA* **95**, 2463–2468.

Griffiths, A.D., Malmqvist, M., Marks, J.D., Bye, J.M., Embleton, M.J., McCafferty, J., Baier, M., Holliger, K.P., Gorick, B.D., Hughes-Jones, N.C., Hoogenboom, H.R., Winter, G., 1993. Human anti-self antibodies with high specificity from phage display libraries. *EMBO J.* **12**, 725–734.

Griffiths, A.D., Williams, S.C., Hartley, O., Tomlinson, I.M., Waterhouse, P., Crosby, W.L., Kontermann, R.E., Jones, P.T., Low, N.M., Allison, T.J., Prospero, T.D., Hoogenboom, H.R., Nissim, A., Cox, J.P.L., Harrison, J.L., Zaccolo, M., Gherardi, E., Winter, G., 1994. Isolation of high affinity human antibodies directly from large synthetic repertoires. *EMBO J.* **13**, 3245–3260.

Groves, M.A.T., Osbourn, J.K., 2005. Applications of ribosome display to antibody drug discovery. *Expert Opin. Biol. Ther.* **5**, 125–135.

Groves, M., Lane, S., Douthwaite, J., Lowne, D., Rees, D.G., Edwards, B., Jackson, R.H., 2006. Affinity maturation of phage display antibody populations using ribosome display. *J. Immunol. Meth.* **313**, 129–139.

Hanes, J., Plückthun, A., 1997. *In vitro* selection and evolution of functional proteins by using ribosome display. *Proc. Natl. Acad. Sci. USA* **94**, 4937–4942.

Hanes, J., Schaffitzel, C., Knappik, A., Plückthun, A., 2000. Picomolar affinity antibodies from a fully synthetic naïve library selected and evolved by ribosome display. *Nat. Biotechnol.* **18**, 1287–1292.

Hoet, R.M., Cohen, E.H., Kent, R.B., Rookey, K., Schoonbroodt, S., Hogan, S., Rem, L., Frans, N., Daukandt, M., Pieters, H., van Hegelsom, R., Neer, N.C., Nastri, H.G., Rondon, I.J., Leeds, J.A., Hufton, S.E., Huang, L., Kashin, I., Devlin, M., Kuang, G., Steukers, M., Viswanathan, M., Nixon, A.E., Sexton, D.J., Hoogenboom, H.R., Ladner, R.C., 2005. Generation of high-affinity human antibodies by combining donor-derived and synthetic complementarity-determining-region diversity. *Nat. Biotechnol.* **23**, 344–348.

Kelley, D.E., Perry, R.P., 1986. Transcriptional and posttranscriptional control of immunoglobulin mRNA production during B lymphocyte development. *Nucleic Acids Res.* (Online) **14**, 5431–5447.

Klein, U., Küppers, R., Rajewsky, K., 1997. Evidence for a large compartment of IgM-expressing memory B cells in humans. *Blood* **89**, 1288–1298.

Klein, U., Rajewsky, K., Küppers, R., 1998. Human immunoglobulin (Ig)M+IgD+ peripheral blood B cells expressing the CD27 cell surface antigen carry somatically mutated variable region genes: CD27 as a general marker for somatically mutated (memory) B cells. *J. Exp. Med.* **188**, 1679–1689.

Marks, J.D., Hoogenboom, H.R., Bonnert, T.P., McCafferty, J., Griffiths, A.D., Winter, G., 1991. By-passing immunization. Human antibodies from V-gene libraries displayed on phage. *J. Mol. Biol.* **222**, 581–597.

Marks, J.D., Tristem, M., Karpas, A., Winter, G., 1991. Oligonucleotide primers for polymerase chain reaction amplification of human immunoglobulin variable genes and design of family-specific oligonucleotide probes. *Eur. J. Immunol.* **21**, 985–991.

Marks, J.D., Griffiths, A.D., Malmqvist, M., Clackson, T., Bye, J.M., Winter, G., 1992. By-passing immunization: building high affinity human antibodies by chain shuffling. *Biotechnology* **10**, 779–783.

Matthes, T., Kindler, V., Zubler, R.H., 1994. Semiquantitative, nonradioactive RT-PCR detection of immunoglobulin mRNA in human B cells and plasma cells. *DNA Cell. Biol.* **13**, 429–436.

McCafferty, J., 1996. Phage display: factors affecting panning efficiency. In Kay, B., Winter, L., McCafferty, J., eds. *Display of Peptides and Proteins.* San Diego, 261–276.

McCafferty, J., Fitzgerald, K.J., Earnshaw, J., Chiswell, D.J., Link, J., Smith, R., Kenten, J., 1994. Selection and rapid purification of murine antibody fragments that bind a transition-state analog by phage display. *Appl. Biochem. Biotechn.* **47**, 157–173.

McCafferty, J., Griffiths, A.D., Winter, G., Chiswell, D.J., 1990. Phage antibodies: filamentous phage displaying antibody variable domains. *Nature* **348**, 552–554.

Nossal, G.J., 1989. Immunologic tolerance: collaboration between antigen and lymphokines. *Science* **245**, 147–153.

Nossal, G.J.V., 2003. The double helix and immunology. *Nature* **421**, 440–444.

Perelson, A.S., Oster, G.F., 1979. Theoretical studies of clonal selection: minimal antibody repertoire size and reliability of self-non-self discrimination. *J. Theor. Biol.* **81**, 645–670.

Perelson, A.S. 1989. Immune network theory. *Immunol. Rev.* **110**, 5–33.

Sblattero, D., Bradbury, A., 2000. Exploiting recombination in single bacteria to make large phage antibody libraries. *Nat. Biotechnol.* **18**, 75–80.

Sheets, M.D., Amersdorfer, P., Finnern, R., Sargent, P., Lindquist, E., Schier, R., Hemingsen, G., Wong, C., Gerhart, J.C., Marks, J.D., 1998. Efficient construction of a large nonimmune phage antibody library: the production of high-affinity human single-chain antibodies to protein antigens. *Proc. Natl. Acad. Sci. USA* **95**, 6157–6162.

Söderlind, E., Strandberg, L., Jirholt, P., Kobayashi, N., Alexeiva, V., Aberg, A.M., Nilsson, A., Jansson, B., Ohlin, M., Wingren, C., Danielsson, L., Carlsson, R., Borrebaeck, C.A., 2000. Recombining germline-derived CDR sequences for creating diverse single-framework antibody libraries. *Nat. Biotechnol.* **18**, 852–856.

Tomlinson, I.M., Walter, G., Marks, J.D., Llewelyn, M.B., Winter, G., 1992. The repertoire of human germline VH sequences reveals about fifty groups of VH segments with different hypervariable loops. *J. Mol. Biol.* **227**, 776–798.

Tomlinson, I.M., Walter, G., Jones, P.T., Dear, P.H., Sonnhammer, E.L., Winter, G., 1996. The imprint of somatic hypermutation on the repertoire of human germline V genes. *J. Mol. Biol.* **256**, 813–817.

Vaughan, T.J., Williams, A.J., Pritchard, K., Osbourn, J.K., Pope, A.R., Earnshaw, J.C., McCafferty, J., Hodits, R.A., Wilton, J., Johnson, K.S. 1996. Human antibodies with sub-nanomolar affinities isolated from a large non-immunized phage display library. *Nat. Biotechnol.* **14**, 309–314.

Villemagne, D., Jackson, R., Douthwaite, J.A., 2006. Highly efficient ribosome display selection by use of purified components for *in vitro* translation. *J. Immunol. Meth.* **313**, 140–148.

Yan, X.H., Xu, Z.R., 2005. Production of human single-chain variable fragment (scFv) antibody specific for digoxin by ribosome display. *Indian J. Biochem. Biophys.* **42**, 350–357.

Yau, K.Y.F., Groves, M.A.T., Li, S., Sheedy, C., Lee, H., Tanha, J., MacKenzie, C.R., Jermutus, L., Hall, J.C., 2003. Selection of hapten-specific single-domain antibodies from a non-immunized llama ribosome display library. *J. Immunol. Meth.* **281**, 161–175.

CHAPTER FIVE

Antibodies from IgM Libraries

Stefan Knackmuss and Vera Molkenthin

IgM antibodies exist both in a pentameric soluble form and as membrane-bound monomers mainly on the surface of naïve B cells, where they are part of the antigen receptor complex. Naïve B cells, constituting 75% of the peripheral blood B cell repertoire in humans (Klein et al., 1997), contain the largest diversity of an individual's rearranged immunoglobulin genes. The naturally occurring antibody repertoire contains specific antibodies against various antigens. In a primary immune response, B cells expressing antigen-specific IgM molecules are activated and differentiate into antibody-producing and -secreting plasma cells. Secreted antigen-specific IgM molecules are the first immunoglobulins occurring during a primary immune response. On the other hand, so-called natural antibodies exist independently of antigenic stimulation and are thought to contribute to the first line of defense against infections (Carsetti et al., 2004; Ochsenbein & Zinkernagel, 2000) as well as malignancy (Brändlein et al., 2003).

In addition to antibody-secreting plasma cells, memory B cells are generated during a primary immune response, a process that includes somatic hypermutation in the germinal centers. Most of the memory B cells have undergone a class switch and do not express IgM. In humans, however, IgM molecules with somatic mutations have been identified (Van Es et al., 1992). These somatically mutated IgM molecules contribute to an individual's immunological memory and constitute about 10% of the total peripheral blood B cell repertoire (Klein et al., 1997). IgM-expressing memory B cells protect against infections by encapsulated bacteria, and develop during the first year of life (Kruetzmann et al., 2003).

IgM Specificities

B cells expressing autoreactive antibodies are counterselected at two checkpoints – in the bone marrow and in the periphery – but 20% of the mature naïve B cells still appear to express anti-self antibodies (Wardemann et al., 2003). An enormous number of completely new specificities can be created from this basic IgM repertoire by randomly combining the variable heavy and light chains, thus significantly increasing the chances of isolating antibodies against any human antigen (for examples, see Bobrzynski et al., 2005; De Haard et al., 1999; Griffiths et al., 1993; Knackmuss et al., 2007; Schwarz et al., 2004; Sheets et al., 1998; Zuber et al., 2008).

Affinities of antibody fragments isolated from the IgM repertoire of unimmunized donors are likely to be lower than the ones isolated from immune IgG libraries (Burton et al., 1991; Finnern et al., 1997; Kausmally et al., 2004; Kramer et al., 2005), as the latter repertoire includes the somatically mutated sequences selected during the *in vivo* process of affinity maturation. These immune libraries will, however, only allow the isolation of high-affinity antibodies against the immunizing antigen. For ethical reasons, immunizations of human beings are restricted to approved vaccines or naturally occurring infections.

Antibody fragments with affinities in the nanomolar and sub-nanomolar range have been isolated from a large nonimmunized library (Vaughan et al., 1996), suggesting that affinities of isolated antibody fragments are dependent on the library size and diversity (De Haard et al., 1999; Hoogenboom et al., 1998; Sheets et al., 1998). Affinity maturation by chain shuffling can substitute for size limitations of a library and will increase the affinity of isolated antibodies if the optimal VH-VL combination has not been selected from the original library. Shuffling of both light chain and heavy chain segments has been successfully carried out to increase the affinity of isolated antibodies (Marks et al., 1992; Schier et al., 1996a). Furthermore, single mutations introduced at key positions in the CDRs as well as in the framework sequences can increase the affinity (Barbas et al., 1994; Boder et al., 2000; Chames et al., 1998; Daugherty et al., 2000; De Pascalis et al., 2003; Glaser et al., 1992; Gram et al., 1992; Pavoni et al., 2006; Pini et al., 1998; Rajpal et al., 2005; Riaño-Umbarila et al., 2005; Schier et al., 1996b; Tachibana et al., 2004; Wu et al., 1998; Yelton et al., 1995).

GENERATION OF IgM LIBRARIES

Source of Rearranged Immunoglobulin Sequences

B cells that have left the bone marrow express IgM molecules with individual variable sequences on their surface. For the generation of *in vitro* phage display antibody libraries, RNA from B cells is first reversely transcribed into cDNA followed by the PCR amplification of VH and VL sequences, which are then cloned and recombined in phage display vectors. Peripheral blood lymphocytes and spleen biopsy material are frequently used as a source of material for nonimmunized libraries (De Haard et al., 1999; Griffiths et al., 1993; Marks et al., 1991; Schwarz et al., 2004). To prevent a bias of the library by overexpressed individual immunoglobulins, the amplification of IgG sequences is avoided and care is taken to use material from healthy donors who are not generating an excess of disease-related antibodies. To ensure the isotype-specific amplification of VH sequences, primers specifically annealing to the different constant domains of IgA, IgD, IgE, IgG, and IgM have to be used either for reverse transcription or in the amplification step. Amplification of the VL chains is, however, independent of the isotype of the immunoglobulin molecule of which they had originally been a part, thus emphasizing the importance of using healthy donors to avoid biased libraries.

Besides comprising the most diverse repertoire of rearranged immunoglobulin sequences, there are indications for a participation of IgM-expressing B cells in the defense against malignant cells, suggesting that IgM libraries are a potential source of tumor-specific antibodies. Tumor-specific IgM molecules with unmutated, germ-line-like sequences have been isolated from tumor patients as well as from healthy donors, pointing to an antigen-independent presence of tumor-specific IgM anti-bodies (Brändlein et al., 2003). Some autoantibodies appear to be present from birth throughout life; anti-FcεRIα antibodies were isolated from IgM libraries derived from healthy donors, from patients with chronic urticaria, and from human cord blood (Bobrzynski et al., 2005). On the other hand, the somatically mutated IgM memory B cell pool develops during the first years of life. For example, antibodies with partic-ular specificities that bind to encapsulated bacteria appear to be restricted to this special B cell pool (Kruetzmann et al., 2003). IgM libraries derived from healthy adult human donors contain the variable sequences of the so-called natural antibodies (Bobrzynski et al., 2005; Brändlein et al., 2003; Carsetti et al., 2004; Ochsenbein & Zinkernagel, 2000) that occur without antigenic stimulation, as well as the somati-cally mutated IgM memory B cell repertoire. They therefore appear to represent the most diverse and useful antibody repertoires for isolating antibodies against a large variety of antigens.

Amplification of Rearranged Immunoglobulin Sequences

For cloning into the phage display vector, an amplification of the immunoglobulin sequences by PCR is required. On the cDNA level, priming in the variable sequences cannot be avoided, and a set of various primers has to be used to cover the whole repertoire of VH and VL sequences. The literature describes several primer sets (De Haard et al., 1999; Little et al., 1999; Marks et al., 1991; Sblattero et al., 1998; Welschof et al., 1995) that were designed to cover most if not all occurring sequences and to avoid errors by cross-priming. Restriction sites for cloning the amplified fragments into the phage display vector can easily be introduced via the PCR primers during the amplification step. The choice of restriction sites is of considerable importance, since the variable immunoglobulin sequences contain recognition sites for a number of restriction enzymes with varying frequencies. A table with percentages of recognized Ig sequences for several restriction enzymes is given in Welschof et al. (1995).

Cloning of a Phage Display Library

The amplified VH and VL sequences are randomly combined with one another in a phage display vector. In the case of a scFv library, at least two different principal strategies exist to combine the VH and VL domains. In a two-step cloning procedure, either VH or VL fragments are cloned into the phage display vector, and the second variable domain is cloned in a second step (Little et al., 1999). In an alternative strategy, the VH and VL domains are combined in an assembly PCR, and the entire scFv coding sequence is cloned into the phage display vector (Marks et al., 1991;

Sheets et al., 1998; Vaughan et al., 1996). The vectors are usually introduced into bacterial cells by electroporation, the number of transformants reflecting the complexity of the library. To demonstrate the quality of the library, a large number of individual, randomly picked clones from the library has to be sequenced. These data provide information on sequence diversity, percentage of correctly expressed full-length clones, and frequency of germline family usage.

EXAMPLES OF ANTIBODIES FROM IgM LIBRARIES

Large naïve repertoires facilitate the isolation of highly specific antibodies having sufficient affinity to meet the requirements of particular therapeutic applications. The following examples outline the isolation of several highly selective antibodies from a naïve library made by the firm Affimed Therapeutics.

High Affinity Antibodies from Naïve Repertoires

The affinity of antibodies selected from naïve libraries is correlated with the size of the library, ranging from 10^{-6} to 10^{-7} M for a small library with 10^7 individual clones (Griffiths et al., 1993; Marks et al., 1991), and from 10^{-8} to 10^{-10} M for very large repertoires with 10^{10} clones (Hoogenboom et al., 1998; Vaughan et al., 1996). Vaughan et al. (1996) describe the isolation of scFv with nanomolar and sub-nanomolar affinities against various targets. From an IgM library with a complexity of 1.7×10^9 described in Schwarz et al. (2004), scFv with affinities in the range of 10^{-8} M were raised against antigens such as EpCAM and CD30.

Isolation of an Anti IL-13-receptor Antibody Blocking IL-13-driven Cell Proliferation

IL-13 is a critical mediator of allergic inflammation. The functional IL-13 receptor is formed by a heterodimer composed of the IL-4Rα and IL-13Rα1 subunits. Pharmaceuticals targeting specifically the cytokine-receptor interaction might be beneficial for the treatment of allergic disorders (Hershey, 2003). Selection of a naïve library (Schwarz et al., 2004) against the recombinant IL-13Rα1, a subunit of the IL-13 receptor complex, led to the isolation of a set of scFv clones binding to the receptor on the surface of transiently transfected cells (Knackmuss et al., 2007). Measurements of IL-13-dependent proliferation of TF-1 cells, IL-13-dependent gene transcription, as well as inhibition of IL-13-induced STAT6 tyrosine phosphorylation in human blood monocytes in the presences of various scFv clones identified one clone that specifically inhibited IL-13 signaling (Knackmuss et al., 2007). Figure 5.1A/B shows the effect of this IL-13Rα1 blocking scFv on IL-13- and IL-4-driven cell proliferation. While an irrelevant anti-estradiol scFv as well as two IL-13Rα1 binding clones (14IIIN, 37VIS) had no effect on the proliferation of TF-1 cells, increasing amounts of clone 6IN resulted in a dose-dependent inhibition on IL-13 stimulation. In contrast, no inhibition of IL-4-stimulated cells was observed.

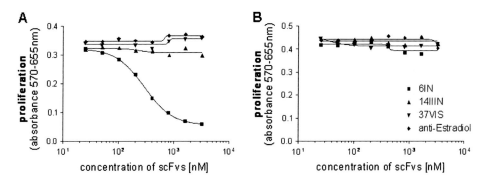

Figure 5.1. A/B Test for inhibition of IL-13 dependent cell proliferation by IL-13Rα1 binding scFvs. Proliferation was determined by means of an MTT assay (CellTiter 96 Non-radioactive Cell Proliferation Assay; Promega, Mannheim, Germany). Starved samples of TF-1 cells were incubated with human IL-13 (A) and for control purposes with human IL-4 (B).

Isolation of an Anti-CD16 Antibody Highly Specific for the A Isoform

CD16A (also known as FcγRIIIA), a low-affinity receptor for the Fc portion of IgGs, is known to be involved in antibody-dependent cellular cytotoxicity (ADCC). It is expressed on macrophages, mast cells, and NK cells as a transmembrane receptor. FcγRIIIB is present on polymorphonuclear granulocytes (PMN) as a glycosyl-phosphatidylinositol (GPI)-anchored receptor (FcγRIIIB isoform), which cannot trigger tumor cell killing (van de Winkel & Capel, 1993). Considering all known allelic variants of the two isoforms, they consistently differ in only two amino acid positions. Three rounds of selection on a CD16A-Fc fusion molecule identified a single chain molecule highly specific for the A-isoform of the receptor.

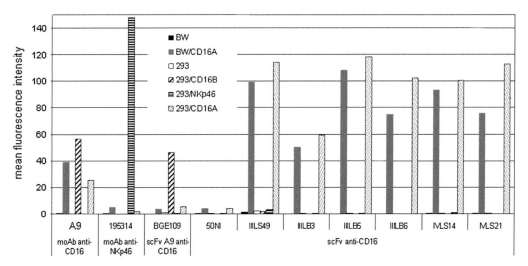

Figure 5.2. Anti-CD16 scFv bind to cell transfectants expressing CD16A but not to cells expressing CD16B in flow cytometry. Murine BW cells and BW cells stably transfected with CD16A (BW/CD16A), HEK-293 cells and HEK-293 cells transiently transfected with CD16B (293/CD16B), CD16A (293/CD16A), or NKp46 (293/NKp46) were used for flow cytometric analysis. Cells were stained with the MAb A9 (anti-CD16) or MAb 195314 (anti-NKp46) followed by a FITC-conjugated goat anti-mouse IgG. The anti-CD16 scFv were detected with MAb 13/45/31-2 (anti-Hexa His) followed by FITC-conjugated goat anti-mouse IgG.

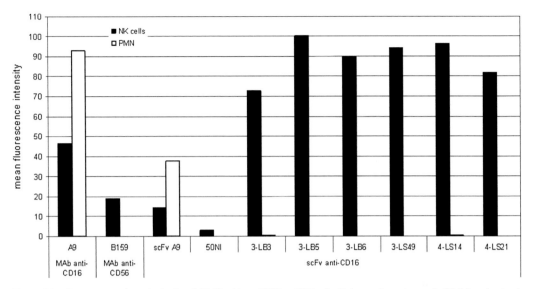

Figure 5.3. Flow cytometric analysis of anti-CD16 scFv on PMN and NK cells. Polymorphonuclear cells (PMN) and natural killer (NK) cells were isolated from peripheral blood from a healthy donor and used for flow cytometric analysis. The cells were stained with the anti-CD16 MAb A9 and the anti-CD56 MAb B159 followed by a FITC-conjugated goat anti-mouse IgG. All scFv were detected with MAb 13/45/31-2 (anti-Hexa His) followed by a FITC-conjugated goat anti-mouse IgG.

Subsequent affinity maturation led to several variants ranging in affinity between 10^{-7} and 10^{-8} M. Figure 5.2 outlines the binding of different clones to 293 cells transiently transfected with either the A or B isoform in flow cytometry. A stably transfected CD16A expressing cell line (BWCD16A) was included as an additional control. While the monoclonal anti-CD16 antibody A9 (Kipriyanov et al., 2002) and its scFv derivative (BGE 109) recognized both isoforms, all scFv variants revealed exclusive binding to the A form. The difference in binding of the anti-CD16 scFv to the two isoforms was clearly demonstrated by staining freshly isolated NK cells expressing CD16A on their surface in comparison to CD16B-expressing granulocytes (Figure 5.3).

CONCLUSION

It is possible to isolate highly specific antibody clones with relatively high affinities from IgM-based libraries. A crucial factor for successful screening is the diversity and quality of the library, particularly regarding the percentage of full-length functional clones. Although the library is of human origin, we have succeeded in isolating highly specific antibodies to a large number of human target molecules. In one particular case, the isolated antibody was able to sharply distinguish between two isoforms that differed by only three amino acids. Current improvements to this library are expected to result in even higher yields of high-quality specific antibodies.

REFERENCES

Barbas III, C.F., Hu, D., Dunlop, N., Sawyer, L., Cababa, D., Hendry, R.M., Nara, P.L., and Burton, D.R. (1994). *In vitro* evolution of a neutralizing human antibody to human immunodeficiency virus type 1 to enhance affinity and broaden strain cross-reactivity. *Proc. Natl. Acad. Sci. USA*, **91**, 3809–3813.

Bobrzynski, T., Fux, M., Vogel, M., Stadler, M.B., Stadler, B.M., and Miescher, S.M. (2005). A high-affinity natural autoantibody from human cord blood defines a physiologically relevant epitope on the FcepsilonRIalpha. *J. Immunol.*, **175**, 6589–6596.

Boder, E.T., Midelfort, K.S., and Wittrup, K.D. (2000). Directed evolution of antibody fragments with monovalent femtomolar antigen-binding affinity. *Proc. Natl. Acad. Sci. USA*, **97**(20), 10701–10705.

Brändlein, S., Pohle, T., Ruoff, N., Wozniak, E., Müller-Hermelink, H.-K., and Vollmers, H.P. (2003). Natural IgM antibodies and immunosurveillance mechanisms against epithelial cancer cells in humans. *Cancer Res*, **63**, 7995–8005.

Burton, D.R., Barbas III, C.F., Persson, M.A.A., Koenig, S., Channock, R.M., and Lerner, R.A. (1991). A large array of human monoclonal antibodies to type 1 human immunodeficiency virus from combinatorial libraries of asymptomatic seropositive individuals. *Proc. Natl. Acad. Sci. USA*, **88**, 10134–10137.

Carsetti, R., Rosado, M.M., and Wardemann, H. (2004). Peripheral development of B cells in mouse and man. *Immunol. Rev.*, **197**, 179–191.

Chames, P., Coulon, S., and Baty, D. (1998). Improving the affinity and the fine specificity of an anti-cortisol antibody by parsimonious mutagenesis and phage display. *J. Immunol.*, **161**, 5421–5429.

Daugherty, P.S., Chen, G., Iverson, B.L., and Georgiou, G. (2000). Quantitative analysis of the effect of the mutation frequency on the affinity maturation of single chain Fv antibodies. *Proc. Natl. Acad. Sci. USA*, **97**(5), 2029–2034.

De Haard, H.J., Van Neer, N., Reurs, A., Hufton, S.E., Roovers, R.C., Henderikx, P., de Bruïne, A.P., Arends, J.-W., and Hoogenboom, H.R. (1999). A large non-immunized human Fab fragment phage library that permits rapid isolation and kinetic analysis of high affinity antibodies. *J. Biol. Chem.*, **274**(26), 18218–18230.

De Pascalis, R., Gonzales, N.R., Padlan, E.A., Schuck, P., Batra, S.K., Schlom, J., and Kashmiri, S.V.S. (2003). *In vitro* affinity maturation of a specificity-determining region-grafted humanized anti-carcinoma antibody: Isolation and characterization of minimally immunogenic high-affinity variants. *Clin. Cancer Res.*, **9**, 5521–5531.

Finnern, R., Pedrollo, E., Fisch, I., Wieslander, J., Marks, J.D., Lockwood, C.M., and Ouwehand, W.H. (1997). Human autoimmune anti-proteinase 3 scFv from a phage display library. *Clin. Exp. Immunol.*, **107**, 269–281.

Glaser, S.M., Yelton, D.E., and Huse, W.D. (1992). Antibody engineering by codon-based mutagenesis in a filamentous phage vector system. *J. Immunol.*, **149**(12), 3903–3913.

Gram, H., Marconi, L.-A., Barbas III, C.F., Collet, T.A., Lerner, R.A., and Kang, A.S. (1992). *In vitro* selection and affinity maturation of antibodies from a naive combinatorial immunoglobulin library. *Proc. Natl. Acad. Sci. USA*, **89**, 3576–3580.

Griffiths, A.D., Malmqvist, M., Marks, J.D., Bye, J.M., Embleton, M.J., McCafferty, J., Baier, M., Holliger, K.P., Gorick, B.D. Hughes-Jones, N.C., Hoogenboom, H.R., and Winter, G. (1993). Human anti-self antibodies with high specificity from phage display libraries. *EMBO J.*, **12**(2), 725–734.

Hershey, G.K.H. (2003). IL-13 receptors and signaling pathways: An evolving web. *J. Allergy Clin. Immunol.*, **111**, 677–690.

Hoogenboom, H.R., de Bruïne, A.P., Hufton, S.E., Hoet, R.M., Arens, J.-W., and Roovers, R.C. (1998). Review article: Antibody phage display technology and its applications. *Immunotechnology*, **4**, 1–20.

Kausmally, L., Waalen, K., Løbersli, I., Hvattum, E., Berntsen, G., Michaelsen, T.E., and Brekke, O.H. (2004). Neutralizing human antibodies to varicella-zoster virus (VZV) derived from a VZV patient recombinant antibody library. *J. Gen. Virol.*, **85**, 3493–3500.

Kipriyanov, S., Cochlovius, B., Schäfer, H.J., Moldenhauer, G., Bähre, A., LeGall, F., Knackmuss, S., and Little, M. (2002). Synergistic antitumor effect of bispecific CD19xCD3 and CD19xCD16 diabodies in a preclinical model of non-Hodgkin's lymphoma. *J. Immunol.*, **169**, 137–144.

Klein, U., Küppers, R., and Rajewsky, K. (1997). Evidence for a large compartment of IgM-expressing memory B cells in humans. *Blood*, **89**, 1288–1298.

Knackmuss, S., Krause, S., Engel, K., Reusch, U., Virchow, J.C., Mueller, T., Kraich, M., Little, M., Luttmann, W., and Friedrich, K. (2007). Specific inhibition of interleukin-13 activity by a recombinant human single-chain immunoglobulin domain directed against the IL-13 receptor alpha1 chain. *Biol. Chem.*, **388**(3), 325–330.

Kramer, R.A., Marissen, W.E., Goudsmit, J., Visser, T.J., Clijsters-Van der Horst, M., Bakker, A.Q., de Jong, M., Jongeneelen, M., Thijsse, S., Backus, H.H.J., Rice, A.B., Weldon, W.C., Rupprecht, C.E., Dietzschold, B., Bakker, A.B.H., and de Kruif, J. (2005). The human antibody repertoire specific for rabies virus glycoprotein as selected from immune libraries. *Eur. J. Immunol.*, **35**, 2131–2145.

Kruetzmann, S., Rosado, M.M., Weber, H., Germing, U., Tournilhac, O., Peter, H.-H., Berner, R., Peters, A., Boehm, T., Plebani, A., Qzinit, I., and Carsetti, R. (2003). Human immunoglobulin M memory B cells controlling *Streptococcus pneumoniae* infections are generated in the spleen. *J. Exp. Med.*, **197**(7), 939–945.

Little, M., Welschof, M., Bruanagel, M., Hermes, I., Christ, C., Keller, A., Rohrbach, P., Kürschner, T., Schmidt, S., Kleist, C., and Terness, P. (1999). Generation of a large complex antibody library from multiple donors. *J. Immunol. Meth.*, **231**, 3–9.

Marks, J.D., Hoogenboom, H.R., Bonnert, T.P., McCafferty, J., Griffiths, A.D., and Winter, G. (1991). By-passing immunization. Human antibodies from V-gene libraries displayed on phage. *J. Mol. Biol*, **222**, 581–597.

Marks, J.D., Griffiths, A.D., Malmqvist, M., Clackson, T.P., Bye, J.M., and Winter, G. (1992). By-passing immunization: Building high affinity human antibodies by chain shuffling. *Bio/Technology*, **10**, 779–783.

Ochsenbein, A.F., and Zinkernagel, R.M. (2000). Natural antibodies and complement link innate and acquired immunity. *Immunol. Today*, **21**(12), 624–630.

Pavoni, E., Flego, M., Dupuis, M.L., Barca, S., Petronzelli, F., Anastasi, A.M., D'Alessio, V., Pelliccia, A., Vaccaro, P., Monteriù, G., Ascione, A., De Santis, R., Felici, F., Cianfriglia, M., and Minenkova, O. (2006). Selection, affinity maturation, and characterization of a human scFv antibody against CEA protein. *BMC Cancer*, **6**, 41.

Pini, A., Viti, F., Santucci, A., Carnemolla, B., Zardi, L., Neri, P., and Neri, D. (1998). Design and use of a phage display library. *J. Biol. Chem.*, **273**(34), 21769–21776.

Rajpal, A., Beyaz N., Haber, L., Cappuccilli, G., Yee, H., Bhatt, R.R., Takeuchi, T., Lerner, R.A., and Crea, R. (2005). A general method for greatly improving the affinity of antibodies by using combinatorial libraries. *Proc. Natl. Acad. Sci. USA*, **102**(24), 8466–8471.

Riaño-Umbarila, L., Juárez-González, V.R., Olamendi-Portugal, T., Ortíz-León, M., Possani, L.D., and Becerril, B. (2005). A strategy for the generation of specific human antibodies by directed evolution and phage display. An example of a single-chain antibody fragment that neutralizes a major component of scorpion venom. *FEBS J.*, **272**(10), 2591–2601.

Sblattero, D., and Bradbury, A. (1998). A definitive set of oligonucleotide primers for amplifying human V regions. *Immunotechnology*, **3**, 271–278.

Schier, R., Bye, J., Apell, G., McCall, A., Adams, G.P., Malmqvist, M., Weiner, L.M. and Marks, J.D. (1996a). Isolation of high-affinity monomeric human anti-c-erbB-2 single chain Fv using affinity-driven selection. *J. Mol. Biol.*, **255**, 28–43.

Schier, R., McCall, A., Adams, G.P., Marshall, K.W., Merritt, H., Yim, M., Crawford, R.S., Weiner, L.M., Marks, C., and Marks, J.D. (1996b). Isolation of picomolar affinity anti-c-erbB-2 single-chain Fv by molecular evolution of the complementarity determining regions in the center of the antibody binding site. *J. Mol. Biol.*, **263**, 551–567.

Schwarz, M., Röttgen, P., Takada, Y., Le Gall, F., Knackmuss, S., Bassler, N., Büttner, C., Little, M., Bode, C., and Peter, K. (2004). Single-chain antibodies for the conformation-specific blockade of activated platelet integrin alphaIIbbeta3 designed by subtractive selection from naïve human phage libraries. *FASEB J.*, **18**, 1704–1706.

Sheets, M.D., Amersdorfer, P., Finnern, R., Sargent, P., Lindqvist, E., Schier, R., Hemingsen, G., Wong, C., Gerhart, J.C., and Marks, J.D. (1998). Efficient construction of a large nonimmune phage antibody library: The production of high-affinity human single-chain antibodies to protein antigens. *Proc. Natl. Acad. Sci. USA*, **95**, 6157–6162.

Tachibana, H., Matsumoto, N., Cheng, X.-J., Tsukamoto, H., and Yoshihara, E. (2004). Improved affinity of a human anti-*Entamoeba histolytica* Gal/GalNAc lectin Fab fragment by a single amino acid modification of the light chain. *Clin. Diagn. Lab. Immunol.*, **11**(6), 1085–1088.

Van de Winkel, J.G., and Capel P.J. (1993). Human IgG Fc receptor heterogeneity: molecular aspects and clinical implications. *Immunol. Today*, **14**(5), 215–221.

Van Es, J.H., Meyling, F.H., and Logtenberg, T. (1992). High frequency of somatically mutated IgM molecules in the human adult blood B cell repertoire. *Eur. J. Immunol.*, **22**, 2761–2764.

Vaughan, T.J., Williams, A.J., Pritchard, K., Osbourn, J.K., Pope, A.R., Earnshaw, J.C., McCafferty, J., Hodits, R.A., Wilton, J., and Johnson, K.S. (1996). Human antibodies with sub-nanomolar affinities isolated from a large non-immunized phage display library. *Nat. Biotechnol.*, **14**, 309–314.

Wardemann, H., Yurasov, S., Schaefer, A., Young, J.W., Meffre, E., and Nussenzweig, M.C. (2003). Predominant autoantibody production by early human B cell precursors. *Science*, **301**, 1374–1377.

Welschof, M., Terness, P., Kolbinger, F., Zewe, M., Dübel, S., Dörsam, H., Hain, C., Finger, M., Jung, M., Moldenhauer, G., Hayashi, N., Little, M., and Opelz, G. (1995). Amino acid sequence based PCR primers for amplification of rearranged human heavy and light chain immunoglobulin variable region genes. *J. Immunol. Meth.*, **179**, 203–214.

Wu, H., Beuerlein, G., Nie, Y., Smith, H., Lee, B.A., Hensler, M., Huse, W.D., and Watkins, J.D. (1998). Stepwise *in vitro* affinity maturation of Vitaxin, an alphav beta3-specific humanized mAb. *Proc. Natl. Acad. Sci. USA*, **95**(11), 6037–6042.

Yelton, D.E., Rosok, M.J., Cruz, G., Cosand, W.L., Bajorath, J., Hellström, I., Hellström, K.E., Huse, W.D., and Glaser, S.M. (1995). Affinity maturation of the BR96 anti-carcinoma antibody by codon-based mutagenesis. *J. Immunol.*, **155**, 1994–2004.

Zuber, C., Knackmuss, S., Rey, C., Reusch, U., Röttgen, P., Fröhlich, T., Arnold, G.J., Pace, C., Mitteregger, G., Kretzschmar, H.A., Little, M., and Weiss, S. (2008). Single chain Fv antibodies directed against the 37 kDa/67 kDa laminin receptor as therapeutic tools in prion diseases. *Mol. Immunol.*, **45**(1), 144–151.

CHAPTER SIX

Generation and Screening of the Synthetic Human Combinatorial Antibody Library HuCAL GOLD

Ingo M. Klagge

Nowadays, monoclonal antibodies are the fastest growing class of biopharmaceuticals. By the end of 2007, the U.S. Food and Drug Administration (FDA) had approved 21 therapeutic antibodies. Since 1975, with the seminal work of Köhler and Milstein (Köhler & Milstein, 1975) describing the use of hybridoma technology for monoclonal antibody generation, major advances in the field allowed for the development of antibody libraries using recombinant technologies (reviewed by Hoogenboom, 2005, and Sergeeva et al., 2006). Various display technologies and the integration of automated screening methods now enable researchers to quickly identify multiple target specific antibodies for later development as biopharmaceuticals.

This chapter will look at MorphoSys's latest fully human antibody library, the Human Combinatorial Antibody Library HuCAL GOLD based on phage display of Fab antibody fragments. Besides a comprehensive introduction of the design and generation of the library, the chapter will describe the HuCAL-specific CysDisplay technology, explore the use of MorphoSys's proprietary AgX technology, and give some examples on the use of HuCAL-based antibody optimization by using standard affinity maturation approaches or the recently developed RapMAT technology.

HuCAL CONCEPT

The HuCAL technology is a unique and innovative concept for the *in vitro* generation of highly diverse fully human antibodies. The structural basis for the HuCAL libraries is provided by seven heavy chain and seven light chain variable region genes (Knappik et al., 2000). These consensus framework sequences encompass the sequence information of each frequently used heavy chain variable domain (VH) and light chain variable domain (VL) germline family leading to 49 combinations of HuCAL master genes. This broad coverage of the structural diversity of the human antibody repertoire is considered to be quite important, since framework residues can influence the folding of complementarity determining region (CDR)

HuCAL, HuCAL GOLD, RapMAT, AutoCAL, AutoPan, AutoScreen, AgX are registered trademarks of the MorphoSys AG. Abbreviations used: CDR, complementarity determining region; ELISA, enzyme-linked immunosorbent assay; HuCAL, Human Combinatorial Antibody Library; IHC, immunohistochemistry; K_D, affinity constant; SET, solution equilibrium titration; TRIM, trinucleotide mutagenesis; VH, variable region of the heavy chain; VL, variable region of the light chain.

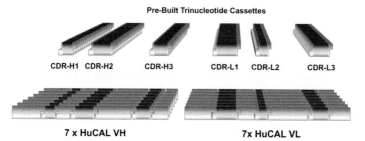

Figure 6.1. The HuCAL concept. Seven HuCAL framework mastergenes for each variable domain of the heavy chain (VH) and light chain (VL) cover the naturally occurring structural diversity of human antibodies resulting in up to 49 framework combinations. In HuCAL GOLD, every CDR in each VH and VL is diversified. The modular nature of the library, because of unique restriction sites flanking the CDRs and the framework regions, allows for rapid conversion into alternative antibody formats and for easy antibody optimization using prebuilt CDR libraries.

stretches and can also participate in the interaction with the antigen (Ewert et al., 2004). By superimposing highly variable DNA cassettes on these frameworks, the CDRs as occurring in the human antibody repertoire are mimicked (Figure 6.1).

During the design of HuCAL, the focus was on obtaining a high number of correct antibody fragments, thus emphasizing the functional and not the apparent library size. In line with this approach, all genes and CDR cassettes were prepared and assembled by chemical synthesis avoiding the use of error-prone polymerase chain reaction (PCR)-based approaches. In addition, the genes were optimized for expression and folding in *E. coli*. To ensure a high-quality library with a large number of functional gene products, the diversity of the CDR cassettes was achieved by employing MorphoSys's proprietary trinucleotide mutagenesis (TRIM) technology (Virnekäs et al., 1994). The use of precoupled trinucleotides specially selected for codon usage in *E. coli* leads to improved expression rates in the bacterial expression strains, avoids the insertion of stop codons, and allows the expression of recombinant Fabs with defined amino acid compositions.

To generate optimal libraries of CDR cassettes for each framework, an in-depth analysis of databases of rearranged naturally occurring human antibody molecules was made. The information on CDR length and amino acid composition for any given position within each CDR was used to design templates for the generation of framework-specific CDR cassettes. Employing TRIM technology, the three CDRs for each individual framework were synthesized to mimic the length of each CDR and the amino acid composition for every individual position within this CDR. Therefore, each of the six HuCAL CDRs in every one of the 14 frameworks reflects the natural composition of CDRs in terms of length and amino acid distribution in its natural framework context as found in human antibodies.

Another important feature of HuCAL is its modular gene structure. Each CDR and framework region is flanked by unique restriction sites. The availability of compatible vector modules allows for the easy conversion of selected Fab fragments into different antibody formats, for the addition of effector functions, and for further antibody optimization by exchanging CDR regions of selected binders with prebuilt CDR cassette libraries of high diversity.

The first HuCAL library utilized the scFv antibody format and only CDR-L3 and CDR-H3 were diversified (Knappik et al., 2000). In the HuCAL-Fab1 library, all characteristic features of the HuCAL concept were combined with the superior characteristics of the Fab antibody formats (Rauchenberger et al., 2003).

HuCAL GOLD AND CysDISPLAY

The latest and most powerful antibody library developed by MorphoSys so far, the HuCAL GOLD library, maintains the display of Fab fragments, but in contrast to HuCAL Fab-1, all six CDRs are simultaneously diversified using TRIM technology (Rothe et al., 2008). The library harbors 1.6×10^{10} different Fab-fragment coding phage particles of which as many as 77% were estimated to represent functional antibody genes. Additionally, HuCAL GOLD employs MorphoSys's proprietary CysDisplay technology (Löhning, 2001). For the design of frameworks and CDR composition in HuCAL GOLD, the different germline families were analyzed separately, which better facilitated the design of libraries comprising several canonical conformations (for details, see Rothe et al., 2008).

Pannings carried out with the HuCAL GOLD library yielded Fab antibodies from each subfamily reflecting the structural repertoire and distribution found in humans (Figure 6.2). However, for the VH4 germline family and for Vλ3 antibodies we observed a deviation from this pattern, with VH4 being underrepresented and Vλ3 being more frequently selected from the HuCAL GOLD library compared to the naturally occurring frequency of these two antibody subfamilies. The reasons for these findings are unclear.

Overall, the HuCAL GOLD library allows for the selection of specific Fab antibodies which, correlating well with natural antibodies, are distributed over all consensus framework families. As a result, and also owing to its large size and high quality, the HuCAL GOLD library facilitates the selection of antibodies against proteinacious and non-proteinacious targets presented as purified molecules immobilized to various surfaces, in solution, or presented on cell surfaces.

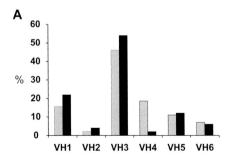 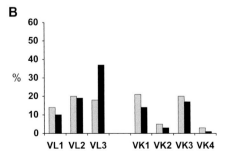

Figure 6.2. VH and VL distribution. The VH (A) and VL (B) subfamily usage of HuCAL GOLD antibodies (black bars) compared to the family distribution of rearranged human antibodies used for CDR library design reflecting the usage in humans (gray bars). More than 5,000 HuCAL VH domains and more than 1,000 HuCAL VL domains were used for analysis. Adapted from Rothe et al., 2008.

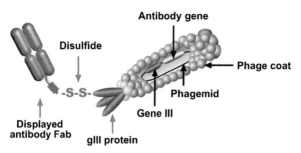

Figure 6.3. The CysDisplay. The schematical drawing shows one incorporated engineered gIII protein at the tip of the phage particle. The Fab fragment is displayed on the phage via a disulfide bond between an unpaired N-terminal cysteine of the engineered pIII and an unpaired cysteine of the Fab C_H1 domain, and couples the phenotype to the genotype encoded by the packaged phagemid.

With CysDisplay, HuCAL GOLD uses a novel and efficient display technology for selecting high-affinity binders from antibody libraries using filamentous phage. Unlike conventional phage display, the antibody Fab fragment is not genetically fused to the phage coat protein but linked to an engineered pIII phage coat protein by forming a disulfide linkage between the two molecules (Figure 6.3). The Fab fragment with its genetically introduced unpaired cysteine residue at the C-terminus of the C_H1 domain is translocated across the periplasmic membrane into the periplasmic space. The engineered gene III protein is inserted into the inner membrane with another unpaired N-terminal cysteine residue oriented toward the periplasm. This simultaneous periplasmic exposure results in the disulfide bond formation between both partners. The subsequent incorporation of this protein complex into the phage particle during phage morphogenesis couples the genotype to the phenotype.

Besides Fab-pIII complexes, Fab-Fab as well as pIII-pIII complexes form, making up the major products. Although being a minor species, the heterodimeric Fab-pIII complexes are incorporated into the phage coat and, as a side effect, result in a strictly monovalent display on the phage surface, thus supporting the selection of high-affinity antibodies. Since the disulfide linkage between the antibody fragment and the engineered pIII protein is sensitive to reducing agents, an efficient elution procedure for phage recovery can be carried out irrespective of the affinity of the displayed Fab fragment. As this procedure can furthermore be applied to any type of antigen and any type of panning conditions, the CysDisplay technology is ideally suited for high-throughput applications as well as for the recovery of affinity-improved antibodies.

AutoCAL AND HuCAL AgX

Right from the beginning, the design of the HuCAL libraries aimed at a high modularity to ease the manipulation of selected binders and to facilitate the automation of the whole panning and screening process. With AutoCAL, MorphoSys developed procedures for automated panning (AutoPan) and screening (AutoScreen). The very high expression rates in *E. coli* due to the Fab format, the applied *E. coli* codon usage, and the selection of well-expressing frameworks allowed massive miniaturization of expression and screening systems. As a consequence, standard selection and screening processes were simplified and miniaturized for adaptation to a system of specialized workstations for antibody selections in 384 well plate formats (Krebs et al., 2001). The AutoCAL process is modular and expendable and allows for the generation of high-quality, validated, and sequenced antibodies in a high-throughput fashion against hundreds of different antigens. These features make AutoCAL extremely suitable for identification of promising antibody candidates in target research or target validation programs (Sun et al., 2003).

HuCAL AgX was developed by MorphoSys as a generally applicable method for the high-throughput generation of antibodies to protein antigen domains (Frisch et al., 2003). Using proprietary expression plasmids, protein domains (length 100 to 300 amino acids) are expressed as polypeptides fused to the N1-domain of the gIII-protein of filamentous phage M13 in *E. coli* as inclusion bodies. After a standardized purification and efficient refolding procedure, these AgX polypeptides can enter the AutoCAL process. The identification of protein domains within target proteins of interest and their expression employing the HuCAL AgX technology facilitates three-dimensional structures to be retained and formed after refolding. This allows for the fast generation of antibodies binding to conformational epitopes present in the full-length protein of interest achieving higher success rates than approaches using short linear peptide antigens.

Antibodies identified by this technique are suitable for use in various biochemical methods like Western blotting, ELISA, immunoprecipitation, IHC, or flow cytometry. For *in situ* protein expression profiling, staining of tissues with antibodies is a powerful method in the area of target identification and validation. Ideally suited for applications in IHC are bivalent Fab formats like MorphoSys's Fab-dHLX mimicking full-length immunoglobulin proteins (Pack & Plückthun, 1992). HuCAL GOLD-derived antibodies working in IHC could be identified by various approaches using, for example, proteins or protein fragments (Ohara et al., 2006). Jarutat and colleagues reported the selection of specific Fab-dHLX antibodies employing a subtractive panning approach on formalin-fixed paraffin-embedded tissue (Jarutat et al., 2007).

Due to their fully human nature and modular design, HuCAL-derived antibodies identified during target identification and validation processes may then immediately be developed as lead candidates for drug development; this can be done, for example, by changing the final antibody format from a Fab molecule into a full-length IgG antibody or by improving the affinity using HuCAL's sophisticated *in vitro* affinity maturation processes.

HuCAL ANTIBODY OPTIMIZATION

Antibodies can be isolated directly from HuCAL libraries showing affinities in the low nanomolar to even sub-nanomolar range without any further engineering step. Nevertheless, for certain therapeutic applications of monoclonal antibodies it may be desirable to improve antibody affinities to achieve increased drug potency, thereby lowering the effective therapeutic dose needed. With HuCAL, a targeted approach exploiting again the modularity of the library and relying on the use of prebuilt CDR cassettes using TRIM (Knappik et al., 2000; Virnekäs et al., 1994) is possible. Figure 6.4 illustrates this principal approach schematically: without touching the consensus framework sequences, by using the unique restriction sites flanking the CDR chosen for exchange the respective prebuilt CDR cassettes are introduced into the selected constructs. Again, by the use of the TRIM technology, with complete control over the amino acid composition thereby avoiding stop codons and with the optimized codon usage for prokaryotic expression, the resulting CDR libraries are of substantially higher quality than can be obtained using, for example, conventional mutagenesis approaches. After thorough analyses of the naturally occurring human CDR sequences, the constructed CDR libraries mimic the CDRs of the natural human antibody repertoire, just as the six CDRs of HuCAL GOLD do, but in addition providing very high sequence variability.

MorphoSys employs two individual approaches to optimize antibody affinity; one is a standard affinity maturation process that involves grafting the prebuilt and highly diverse CDR cassettes into selected HuCAL antibodies. The other approach, RapMAT, employs affinity maturation within the process of antibody selection. Both technologies are schematically illustrated in Figure 6.5. With both technologies, significant affinity improvements can be achieved that made the development of a reliable and reproducible high-throughput affinity determination method necessary. With MorphoSys's own solution equilibrium titration (SET) method, these demands are perfectly covered, thus facilitating a fast kinetic analysis of selected binders. Especially with the determination of extremely high-affinity binders in the low or even sub-picomolar range, SET is superior over other technologies relying, for example, on surface plasmon resonance (Haenel et al., 2005).

HuCAL ANTIBODY OPTIMIZATION BY STANDARD AFFINITY MATURATION

Preselected HuCAL antibody candidates identified after a first set of screening and antibody characterization are affinity optimized by a simple "mix and match" process as schematically shown in Figures 6.4 and 6.5. Figure 6.6 illustrates the power of HuCAL's standard optimization process listing the affinities determined for antibody candidates of therapeutic antibody projects using the HuCAL GOLD library.

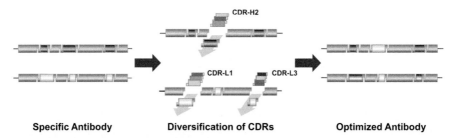

    Specific Antibody   Diversification of CDRs   Optimized Antibody

Figure 6.4. Principle of antibody optimization using HuCAL libraries. The HuCAL technology dramatically simplifies the optimization of antibodies. The modular design of HuCAL with its unique restriction sites flanking each of the six CDRs allows easy exchange with prebuilt CDR cassettes in one cloning step without touching the consensus frameworks of the HuCAL antibodies.

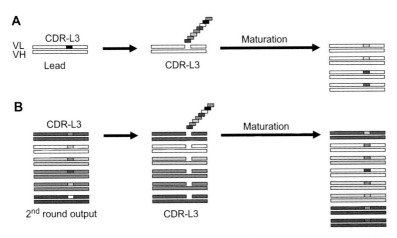

Figure 6.5. HuCAL antibody optimization by standard affinity maturation or RapMAT. Standard optimization as shown in A starts with a preselected characterized HuCAL binder, which, during a lead or pool optimization, undergoes targeted exchange of the selected CDR. In contrast, as shown in B, the RapMAT process is integrated into an ongoing antibody selection process.

The exchange of CDRs by TRIM-derived cassettes permits for a directed affinity maturation of single antibodies ("lead optimization") or even antibody pools ("pool maturation"). Each of the six CDRs can be chosen for introduction of sequence diversity. Even a maturation process involving an iterative exchange of more than one CDR, termed "CDR walking" (Barbas et al., 1994; Yang et al., 1995), can easily be performed with HuCAL libraries. For example, for the generation of HLA-DR specific Fab fragments, first the CDR-L3 of the corresponding Fab antibody fragments were exchanged with TRIM-based CDR-L3 cassettes. After selection of improved Fab derivatives, these binders were then further diversified by replacing the CDR-L1 in the same way to achieve additional affinity optimization (Nagy et al., 2002).

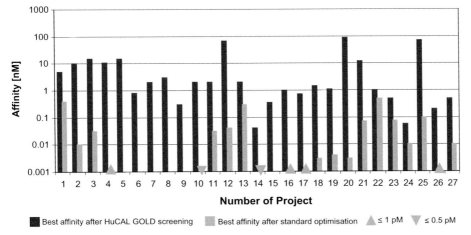

Figure 6.6. Affinity distribution in therapeutic antibody projects before/after affinity maturation using HuCAL GOLD. After affinity maturation, 18 of 21 antibody candidates show affinities below 100 pM with 10 antibody candidates in the single-digit picomolar or even sub-picomolar affinity range.

Brocks and colleagues improved the affinity of TIMP-1-specific HuCAL antibodies by performing CDR walking on lead candidates (Brocks et al., 2006). Antibodies selected directly out of the HuCAL library were characterized for functional inhibition of TIMP-1 and the best candidates subjected to affinity improvement. Working with the HuCAL Fab-1 library, with only the CDR-H3 and CDR-L3 being diversified, additional affinity maturation was carried out by replacing CDR-H1 and CDR-H2 simultaneously with respective diversified CDR cassettes followed by exchange of the CDR-L3. This extensive CDR walking approach led to the identification of binders having affinities and activities in the sub-nanomolar range.

Besides standard proteinacious antigens, HuCAL also allows the identification of antibodies specific to small molecules. A valid application of such antibodies might be their use as smart probes for diagnostic imaging. Hillig and colleagues describe the identification of a HuCAL antibody, MOR03268, which is specific for tetrasulfocyanine (TSC), a near-infrared *in vivo* imaging agent (Hillig et al., 2007; Hillig et al., 2008). Specific Fabs, upon binding to TSC, caused a significant alteration of the photophysical properties. Again, the employment of a standard optimization strategy by a stepwise exchange of the CDR-L3 regions followed by CDR-H2 maturation led to the identification of antibodies with affinities in the low and sub-picomolar range. These Fabs provide the basis for the development of bispecific antibodies that might direct the fluorescent probe *in vivo* specifically to cellular targets of choice.

A recently published very successful example of the use of HuCAL's optimization strategy led to the identification of MorphoSys's lead candidate MOR04357, specific for human GM-CSF, which is currently being tested in a Phase I clinical trial for the treatment of rheumatoid arthritis (Steidl et al., in press). In this particular project, antibody candidates selected directly from the HuCAL GOLD library by standard pannings were improved by a parallel CDR-L3 and CDR-H2 standard maturation. For each selected parental antibody candidate, several affinity-improved CDR-L3 or CDR-H2 variants were identified. In a process called cross-cloning, the CDR-H2 and CDR-L3 of improved derivatives of one parental antibody were combined to test whether it is possible to yield antibodies with even better affinities. By exploiting maturation in two CDR regions and using cross-cloning, the lead antibody MOR04357 showed a 5,000-fold lower K_D compared to the parental antibody (Table 6.1).

HuCAL ANTIBODY OPTIMIZATION BY RapMAT

The introduction of RapMAT illustrates again the flexibility of the HuCAL technology. RapMAT extends the possibilities for isolating high-affinity and functional potent antibodies directly from the HuCAL GOLD library at early stages of antibody selection. Compared to a standard antibody maturation process where already characterized antibody candidates are optimized, RapMAT is easily included in our standard antibody selection process and adds roughly only two additional weeks to an ongoing antibody selection program. Figure 6.7 compares the antibody selection strategies that can be performed with the HuCAL technology and shows the affinity ranges expected for these strategies.

TABLE 6.1. Affinities of Fab antibodies to recombinant human GM-CSF determined by surface plasmon resonance (Biacore) and solution equilibrium titration (SET)

		Biacore	SET
MOR0#	Origin	K_D (pM)	K_D (pM)
3929	Parent	4260	2000
4302	CDR-L3 optimization	174	63.5
4287	CDR-H2 optimization	Nd[a]	17.9
4252	CDR-H2 optimization	55	6.0
4290	CDR-H2 optimization	122	11.1
4350	Cross-cloning: 4302x4287	19	1.1
4354	Cross-cloning: 4302x4290	21	2.8
4357	Cross-cloning: 4302x4252	7	0.4

[a] Nd = not done.

An exemplary RapMAT process starts with the polyclonal phage output after two rounds of standard antibody selection. Without further characterization, this pool of antibodies, preenriched for binders with a desired specificity, is further diversified by the displacement of a selected CDR with TRIM-based maturation cassettes whereby CDR-H3 is left untouched. In principle, a preselected binder out of the polyclonal pool after round two thereby gives rise to a plethora of derivatives diversified in the chosen CDR. Two further selection rounds on this diversified binder pool, applying high stringency conditions, allow for the identification of derivatives with improved affinities.

With MorphoSys's standard optimization process, antibodies can be generated with affinities and potencies in the low to sub-picomolar range. Using RapMAT, one can achieve early on in an antibody project a repertoire of highly diverse fully human antibodies having affinities in the mid-picomolar range. Figure 6.8 exemplifies the

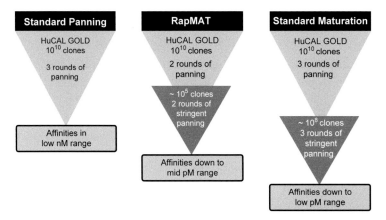

Figure 6.7. Comparison of standard panning with standard affinity optimization and RapMAT. Standard pannings result in the selection of specific binders with affinities in the low nanomolar range directly from HuCAL libraries. Such antibody candidates can be further improved if necessary by standard maturation leading to low picomolar affinity antibodies. With RapMAT, an affinity improvement already within the selection process takes place by diversifying a binder pool enriched for antigen-specific antibodies. With only a minor additional effort, compared to standard pannings, monoclonal antibodies with mid-picomolar affinities can easily be identified.

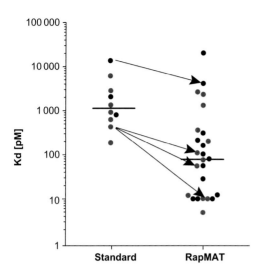

Figure 6.8. Affinity range RapMAT versus standard panning. β-galactosidase was used as a model antigen in standard or RapMAT pannings. Antibodies sharing identical VH are found in standard as well as in RapMAT pannings (indicated by identical shading). Exemplified by two arrows, parental antibodies identified in the standard pannings are coupled to their respective derivatives in the RapMAT pannings.

affinity improvements observed by employing RapMAT within a standard antibody selection using the model antigen β-galactosidase.

RapMAT pannings on β-galactosidase resulted in multiple derivatives of parental binders found in standard pannings. This diversification of the already specific antibody led to the selection of binders with generally improved affinities. In this example, comparing the best antibodies, an overall affinity improvement by 37-fold was achieved, with the highest affinity antibody found by RapMAT showing an affinity of 5 pM. RapMAT therefore is an excellent alternative to standard maturation with several outstanding characteristics. This in-process maturation delivers antibodies in the range of mid-picomolar affinities by adding only minor additional time on the selection procedure. The identified antibodies can be characterized in functional assays much better because of their high affinity and thus improved activity. And finally, a family of antibodies differing only in one CDR can be generated that most likely possess similar affinities and potencies in functional assays. Out of this family, the best candidate can be selected having the optimal characteristics regarding, for example, production and later development.

SUMMARY

This chapter describes the Human Combinatorial Antibody Library (HuCAL) technology. It shows that HuCAL is highly versatile for target research processes and therapeutic applications. Examples given underline the power and the success of this *in vitro* technology. Selections can be done on purified molecules immobilized to various surfaces, held in solution, or presented on cell surfaces. The ease in utilizing the HuCAL libraries is based on the fully automated approach AutoCAL provides. Its modular structure and sophisticated methods for optimization of lead candidates by standard optimization or by in-process optimization using RapMAT pannings permit the identification of antibodies with extremely high affinities and high potency. These fully human antibodies with a reduced risk of inducing immunogenicity can be easily converted into various formats and antibody isotypes without changing the parental antibody sequence. Therefore, HuCAL technology allows for the identification and optimization of antibodies ideally suited for target research and especially for therapeutic use.

REFERENCES

Barbas, C.F., III, Hu, D., Dunlop, N., Sawyer, L., Cababa, D., Hendry, R.M., Nara., P.L., Burton, D.R. (1994). *In vitro* evolution of a neutralizing human antibody to human immunodeficiency virus type 1 to enhance affinity and broaden strain cross-reactivity. *Proceedings of the National Academy of Sciences USA*, **91**, 3809–18.

Brocks, B., Kraft, S., Zahn, S., Noll, S., Pan, C., Schauer, M., Krebs, B. (2006). Generation and optimization of human antagonistic antibodies against TIMP-1 as potential therapeutic agents in fibrotic diseases. *Human Antibodies*, **15**, 115–24.

Ewert, S., Honegger, A., Plückthun, A. (2004). Stability improvement of antibodies for extracellular and intracellular applications: CDR grafting to stable frameworks and structure-based framework engineering. *Methods*, **34**, 184–99.

Frisch, C., Brocks, B., Ostendorp, R., Hoess, A., von Rüden, T., Kretzschmar, T. (2003). From EST to ICH: human antibody pipeline for target research. *Journal of Immunological Methods*, **75**, 203–12.

Haenel, C., Satzger, M., Della Ducata, D., Ostendorp, R., Brocks, B. (2005). Characterization of high-affinity antibodies by electrochemiluminescence-based equilibrium titration. *Analytical Biochemistry*, **339**, 182–4.

Hillig, R.C., Urlinger, S., Fanghänel, J., Brocks, B., Haenel, C., Stark, Y., Sülzle, D., Svergun, D.I., Baesler, S., Malawski, G., Moosmayer, D., Menrad, A., Schirner, M., Licha, K. (2008). Fab MOR03268 triggers absorption shift of a diagnostic dye via packaging in a solvent-shielded Fab dimer interface. *Journal of Molecular Biology*, **377**, 206–19.

Hillig, R.C., Baesler, S., Urlinger, S., Stark, Y., Bauer, S., Badock, V., Huber, M., Bahr, I., Schirner, M., Licha, K. (2007). Crystallization and molecular-replacement solution of a diagnostic fluorescent dye in complex with a specific Fab fragment. *Acta Crystallographica Section F*, **63**, 217–23.

Hoogenboom, H.R. (2005). Selecting and screening recombinant antibody libraries. *Nature Biotechnology*, **23**, 1105–16.

Jarutat, T., Nickels, C., Frisch, C., Stellmacher, F., Hofig, K.P., Knappik, A., Merz, H. (2007). Selection of vimentin-specific antibodies from the HuCAL phage display library by subtractive panning on formalin-fixed, paraffin-embedded tissue. *Biological Chemistry*, **388**, 651–8.

Knappik, A., Ge, L., Honegger, A., Pack, P., Fischer, M., Wellnhofer, G., Hoess, A., Wölle, J., Plückthun, A., Virnekäs, B. (2000). Fully synthetic human combinatorial antibody libraries (HuCAL) based on modular consensus frameworks and CDRs randomized with trinucleotides. *Journal of Molecular Biology*, **296**, 57–86.

Köhler, G. and Milstein, C. (1975). Continuous cultures of fused cells secreting antibody of predefined specificity. *Nature*, **256**, 495–7.

Krebs, B., Rauchenberger, R., Reiffert, S., Rothe, C., Tesar, M., Thomassen, E., Cao, M., Dreier, T., Fischer, D., Höß, A., Landon, I., Knappik, A., Marget, M., Pack., P., Meng., X.-Q., Schier, R., Söhlemann, P., Winter, J., Wölle, J., Kretzschmar, T. (2001). High-throughput generation and engineering of recombinant human antibodies. *Journal of Immunological Methods*, **254**, 67–84.

Löhning, C. (2001). Novel methods for displaying (poly)peptides/proteins on bacteriophage particles via disulfide bonds. WO 01/05950.

Nagy, Z.A., Hubner, B., Löhning, C., Rauchenberger, R., Reiffert, S., Thomassen-Wolf, E., Zahn, S., Leyer, S., Schier, E.M., Zahradnik, A., Brunner, C., Lobenwein, K., Rattel, B., Stanglmaier, M., Hallek, M., Wing, M., Anderson, S., Dunn, M., Kretzschmar, T., Tesar, M. (2002). Fully human,

HLA-DR-specific monoclonal antibodies efficiently induce programmed death of malignant lymphoid cells. *Nature Medicine*, **8**, 801–7.

Ohara, R., Knappik, A., Shimada, K., Frisch, C., Ylera, F., Koga, H. (2006). Antibodies for proteomic research: comparison of traditional immunization with recombinant antibody technology. *Proteomics*, **6**, 2638–46.

Pack, P. and Plückthun, A. (1992). Miniantibodies: use of amphipathic helices to produce functional, flexibly linked dimeric FV fragments with high avidity in *Escherichia coli*. *Biochemistry*, **31**, 1579–84.

Rauchenberger, R., Borges, E., Thomassen-Wolf, E., Rom, E., Adar, R., Yaniv, Y., Malka, M., Chumakov, I., Kotzer, S., Resnitzky, D., Knappik, A., Reiffert, S., Prassler, J., Jury, K., Waldherr, D., Bauer, S., Kretzschmar, T., Yayon, A., Rothe, C. (2003). Human combinatorial Fab library yielding specific and functional antibodies against the human fibroblast growth factor receptor 3. *Journal of Biological Chemistry*, **278**, 38194–205.

Rothe, C., Urlinger, S., Löhning, C., Prassler, J., Stark, Y., Jäger, U., Hubner, B., Bardroff, M., Pradel, I., Boss, M., Bittlingmaier, R., Bataa, T., Frisch, C., Brocks, B., Honegger, A., Urban, M. (2008). The Human Combinatorial Antibody Library HuCAL GOLD combines diversification of all six CDRs according to the natural immune system with a novel display method for efficient selection of high-affinity antibodies. *Journal of Molecular Biology*, **376**, 1182–200.

Sergeeva, A., Kolonin, M.G., Molldrem, J.J., Pasqualini, R., Arap, W. (2006). Display technologies: application for the discovery of drug and gene delivery agents. *Advanced drug Delivery Reviews*, **58**, 1622–54.

Steidl, S., Ratsch, O., Brocks, B., Dürr, M., Thomassen-Wolf, E. (in press). *In vitro* affinity maturation of human GM-CSF antibodies by targeted CDR-diversification. *Molecular Immunology*.

Sun, C., Kilburn, D., Lukashin, A., Crowell, T., Gardner, H., Brundiers, R., Diefenbach, B., Carulli, J.P. (2003). Kirrel2, a novel immunoglobulin superfamily gene expressed primarily in β cells of the pancreatic islets. *Genomics*, **82**, 130–42.

Virnekäs, B., Ge, L., Plückthun, A., Schneider, K.C., Wellnhofer, G. Moroney, S.E. (1994). Trinucleotide phosphoramidites: ideal reagents for the synthesis of mixed oligonucleotides for random mutagenesis. *Nucleic Acids Research*, **22**, 5600–7.

Yang, W.P., Green, K., Pinz-Sweeney, S., Briones, A.T., Burton, D.R., Barbas, C.F., III. (1995). CDR walking mutagenesis for the affinity maturation of a potent human anti-HIV-1 antibody into the picomolar range. *Journal of Molecular Biology*, **254**, 392–403.

PART III

TRANSGENIC HUMAN ANTIBODY REPERTOIRES

CHAPTER SEVEN

Therapeutic Antibodies from XenoMouse Transgenic Mice

Aya Jakobovits

For close to two decades, realization of the promise of monoclonal antibody (mAb) technology for the generation of therapeutic "magic bullets" has been challenged primarily by limited efficacy and safety related to immunogenicity of mouse antibodies in human patients. Among the technologies developed to overcome these hurdles were transgenic mice genetically engineered with a "humanized" humoral immune system. One such transgenic technology, the XenoMouse, has succeeded in recapitulating the human antibody response in mice by introducing nearly the entire human immunoglobulin (Ig) loci into the germline of mice with inactivated mouse antibody machinery. XenoMouse strains have been used to generate a large array of high-affinity, potent, fully human antibodies directed to targets in multiple disease indications, many of which are advancing in clinical development. Full validation of the technology has been achieved with the recent regulatory approval of panitumumab, a fully human antibody directed against epidermal growth factor receptor, for the treatment of advanced colorectal cancer. The successful development of panitumumab, as the first antibody derived from human antibody transgenic mice, signifies an important milestone for XenoMouse and other human antibody transgenic technologies and points to their potential contributions for future therapeutics.

RATIONALE FOR DEVELOPING HUMAN ANTIBODY-PRODUCING TRANSGENIC MICE

The discovery of hybridoma technology in 1975 for the isolation of high-specificity and high-affinity mouse monoclonal antibodies (mAbs)[1] opened the door to a new class of therapeutics with a potential to substantially impact both therapy and diagnosis of many human diseases. However, the path for realization of the therapeutic potential of mAbs took more than a quarter of a century, with the majority of the 21 commercialized mAbs achieving regulatory approval by the U.S. Federal Drug Administration (FDA) during the last 12 years.

The primary challenge for the development of therapeutic antibodies stemmed from the limited efficacy and safety related to immunogenicity of mouse antibodies in human patients. Therefore, the predominant contribution to the successful development of therapeutic mAbs during the last decade derived from the technical progress in humanizing monoclonal antibodies, thus making them safer, more stable, and more efficacious. Until the early 1990s, most product candidates in development were mouse mAbs that elicited production of human anti-mouse antibodies (HAMA) in humans, resulting in rapid clearance, limited efficacy, and safety risks, such as immunogenicity and allergic reactions.[2] The limitations of mouse mAbs were especially problematic in the treatment of chronic and recurring human diseases that require repeated antibody administration. These issues became the driving force for the development of numerous approaches to generate partially or fully human mAbs. Application of the hybridoma methodology to generate human mAbs from human B cells was limited by the scarcity of human B cells expressing antibodies of the desired antigen specificity and affinity and by difficulty in achieving immortalization.[3] The replacement of parts of the mouse mAbs with human sequences to generate chimeric[4] or humanized antibodies [5] with reduced immunogenicity requires case-by-case molecular modeling and engineering. Furthermore, these mAbs still retain some mouse sequences. The generation of large human immunoglobulin (Ig) gene combinatorial libraries has opened an avenue for the cloning of antigen-specific fully human antibodies.[6,7] However, in many cases, derivation of high-affinity human antibodies by this technology, particularly to human antigens, requires extensive *in vitro* manipulation that can affect the authenticity of the human antibody sequences.[8] The limitations associated with in vitro production of partially or fully human therapeutic mAbs redirected attention to the mouse machinery as a simple but robust tool for generation and selection of authentic human mAbs. Mice engineered with the human humoral immune system could harness the natural recombination and affinity maturation processes to generate a large and diverse repertoire of high-affinity antibodies to any target, including human antigens. Furthermore, the well-established mouse hybridoma technology provides an efficient and accessible process to derive and select the desired mAbs.

This rationale was the basis for generating XenoMouse strains, in which the inactivated mouse antibody machinery was "humanized" with megabase (Mb)-sized human Ig loci to substantially reproduce the human humoral immune system in mice and to produce a wide diversity of high-affinity human mAbs.

GENERATION OF XENOMOUSE STRAINS

The strategy for the creation of XenoMouse aimed at recapitulation of the human humoral immune system in mice. It required two major genetic manipulations of the mouse genome: (1) inactivation of mouse antibody production machinery, and (2) stable cloning and introduction of human Ig heavy and light chain loci. Both genetic modifications were carried out in mouse embryonic stem (ES) cells, which provided an effective tool for transmission of defined and selected genetic modifications into the mouse germline. The mouse heavy and kappa (κ) light chain genes were inactivated in ES cells by gene-targeted-deletion of crucial cis-acting sequences involved in the process of mouse Ig gene rearrangement and expression.[9] Deletion of the mouse J_H region completely inhibited the heavy chain recombination machinery and thus abolished mouse Ig production. Deletion of the mouse Cκ region inactivated the mouse Igκ locus. Successive crosses of J_H and Cκ homozygous mice led to a double inactivated (DI) strain, in which production of antibodies and, therefore, B cell development were completely arrested.[10,11] These mice, however, maintained the necessary trans-acting factors for antibody rearrangement and expression and therefore provided the proper genetic background for introduction of unrearranged human Ig loci.

Recapitulation of the human antibody repertoire in mice emphasized the need for cloning and transferring large portions of the human Ig loci in order to preserve the large variable gene diversity and proper regulation of antibody maturation and expression. The genes encoding human Ig heavy and Ig κ light chains each span over 1.5 Mb on chromosome 14 and 2, respectively, containing hundreds of gene segments that encode and control the expression of the huge diversity of the humoral immune response. In their germline configuration, these loci consist of the variable segments encoding the variable (95 V_H, 76 Vκ genes), diversity (30 D_H genes) and joining (6 J_H and 5 Jκ genes) domains, the segments that encode the constant (C) domains, and the interspersed cis-regulatory elements that control antibody expression, allelic exclusion, class switching, and affinity maturation.[12–14] Therefore, reproduction of the human antibody response in mice demanded the ability to clone and reconstruct large portions of the human Ig heavy and light chain loci in their germline configuration, and their introduction in intact form into ES cells. Cloning of the large human heavy and light chain loci was facilitated by the yeast artificial chromosome (YAC) technology, which permitted the stable isolation and efficient genetic manipulation of Mb-sized DNA fragments.[15] By cloning and recombining DNA fragments in yeast, we reconstructed a 970 kb human heavy chain YAC, encompassing in germline configuration 66 different consecutive V_H genes (80% of the human V_H gene repertoire), all 30 D_H and 6 J_H genes, and the Cμ and Cδ constant regions.[16] The Cδ region was retrofitted with human γ1, γ2, or γ4 constant region, in conjunction with the mouse 3′ enhancer, to generate three different yH2 YACs, each equipped with a different heavy chain isotype (IgG_1, IgG_2, and IgG_4). A similar cloning strategy was applied for reconstruction of an 800 kb yK2 YAC containing, in germline configuration, the human κ chain proximal locus, including 32 Vκ genes, 5 Jκ genes, Cκ region, κ deleting element (Kde), and Igκ intronic and 3′ enhancers.[16] Inasmuch as the κ chain distal locus mainly duplicates the proximal region and the proximal Vκ genes are the ones most commonly used in human, yK2 captures 80% of the human Vκ chain gene repertoire.[17]

The large human yH2 and yκ2 YACs were introduced into the mouse genome by the fusion of YAC-containing yeast spheroplasts and ES cells. This methodology yielded a high frequency of ES cells in which the large DNA fragments are integrated in the mouse genome in intact and unrearranged form and are transmitted faithfully through the mouse germline.[18] ES cells, containing intact yH2 or yK2 YACs, were utilized to transmit these human Ig fragments into the mouse germline with no apparent deletions or rearrangements and to generate yH2-and yK2-bearing transgenic mice expressing human heavy or κ chain protein, respectively.[11,16] The crossbreeding of these mouse strains yielded mouse strain expressing fully human antibodies in the presence of mouse antibodies. The crossbreeding of these mice with DI mice yielded XenoMouse strains that produce fully human antibodies.[16] Our strategy yielded three different XenoMouse strains, each producing fully human antibodies with only one of the three isotypes (IgG$_1$κ, IgG$_2$κ, IgG$_4$κ) allowing the generation of antigen-specific mAbs with the desired effector function for specific disease indications. Subsequently, the entire human Igλ chain locus on YAC was also introduced into XenoMouse strains to generate three mouse strains, XMG1-KL, XMG2-KL, and XMG3-KL, each producing both human IgGκ and IgGλ antibodies (at 60:40 ratio) with the corresponding isotype.[19]

RECAPITULATION OF HUMAN HUMORAL IMMUNE SYSTEM IN XENOMOUSE STRAINS

Analysis of XenoMouse lymphoid organs and serum demonstrated that the human Ig YACs were fully compatible with the mouse machinery to restore proper B cell development and antibody production.[10,16] Characterization of the mouse humoral immune system confirmed faithful reconstitution of human antibody response from a broad primary immune response that utilizes the wide range of variable gene repertoire to proper secondary response, including class switching and affinity maturation, leading to a large and diverse repertoire of authentic human antibodies.[16,20] Sequence analysis of XenoMouse-derived antibody transcripts revealed a broad and diverse utilization of the different V, D, and J genes across the entire length of the YACs that is reminiscent of their utilization in humans.[19,20] The critical role of the large and diverse V gene repertoire in the recapitulation of human humoral response was validated when XenoMouse strains were compared to mice engineered with smaller V gene repertoires, whether contained on YACs[11] or on minigene constructs.[21,22] In addition to more efficient B cell development and higher levels of circulating antibodies, the utilization at high frequency of V genes, which are rarely used in the overall repertoire, in sequences of mAbs with selected specificity and function, underscores the need for a large V gene array to support generation of antibodies to specific epitopes.

GENERATION OF HIGH-AFFINITY, POTENT, FULLY HUMAN mABs

Utilization of the large human repertoire in XenoMouse for generation of a diverse human antibody response was manifested by the production of antigen-specific, high-affinity human antibodies to numerous antigens, including interleukin-8 (IL-8), epidermal growth factor (EGFR), tumor necrosis factor-α (TNF-α), interleukin-6 (IL-6), L-selectin, GROα, and CD147,[16,19,23] MUC18,[24] platelet-derived growth factor-D (PDGFR-D),[25] insulin growth factor receptor-1 (IGF-1R),[26] cytotoxic

T lymphocyte associated antigen 4 (CTLA-4),[27] CD40,[28,29] hepatocyte growth factor (HGF),[30] receptor activator of nuclear factor Kappa B (RANK) Ligand,[31] and prostate stem cell antigen (PSCA).[32] XenoMouse animals consistently produced mAbs of high affinity between 10^{-9} and 10^{-11} M,[16,19] with some mAbs, such as mAb to RANK ligand (AMG 162, denosumab), exhibiting a very high affinity of 10^{-12} M[31]. These findings reflect the broad and diverse utilization of the variable genes and the efficient affinity maturation processes in XenoMouse strains. The selected antibodies also demonstrated high potency in blocking the *in vitro* and *in vivo* biological effects of their respective antigens on human cells indicating their therapeutic potential,[23–32] and providing the rationale for their clinical development. The mAb pharmacokinetics is influenced by the nature of its target and the related biology, such that a mAb targeting a circulating antigen may have a different pharmacokinetics profile from that of a mAb targeting a cell surface receptor that can mediate internalization of the receptor-mAb complex. For example, XenoMouse-derived mAbs directed to IL-8 (ABX-IL8)[33] and CTLA-4 (ticilimumab),[34] exhibited in patients pharmacokinetics similar to that of an endogenous human IgG, which has a half-life of 21 days. The mAb to RANK ligand, denosumab, exhibited a very long half-life supporting dosing as infrequently as every 3 or 6 months.[31] Data from clinical trials with XenoMouse-derived mAbs have indicated no or a very low rate of immunogenicity, including subjects who received up to 3 months of treatment with ABX-IL8 or denosumab.[31,33,35,36]

PANITUMUMAB – THE FIRST APPROVED ANTIBODY FROM HUMAN ANTIBODY TRANSGENIC MICE

Panitumumab is a fully human IgG$_2$κ mAb that binds specifically to EGFR with very high affinity (Kd~0.05 nM), allowing it to compete effectively with EGFR ligands, including EGF and transforming growth factor-alpha.[37] The IgG$_2$ isotype was chosen to minimize potential toxicity to EGFR-expressing normal tissues, such as skin, liver, kidney, and lung, from recruitment of antibody-dependent cell-mediated cytotoxicity (ADCC) and complement-dependent cytotoxicity (CDC). EGFR has been considered to play a critical role in the development and progression of solid tumors due to its overexpression in many human epithelial cancers often associated with poor clinical prognosis, and increased production of ligands by the tumor cells, suggesting an autocrine regulatory loop for EGFR stimulation.[38,39] Ligand binding to EGFR leads to receptor dimerization and autophosphorylation, which triggers a cascade of signaling pathways that regulate cell proliferation, survival, motility, transformation, and angiogenesis.[38,39] Panitumumab binding to EGFR blocked ligand binding, inhibited receptor autophosphorylation and activation of EGFR-mediated signal transduction pathways, and induced receptor down regulation. As a result, the antibody inhibited tumor cell proliferation and production of angiogenic factors by tumor cells, and induced cell apoptosis.[37,40] In various xenograft mouse models, representing human tumors expressing different levels of EGFR, panitumumab has demonstrated significant antitumor activity, including eradication of large established tumors, with enhanced activity when combined with chemotherapy.[37,40,41]

Early clinical development of panitumumab included a series of Phase I studies, which evaluated the antibody pharmacokinetics and safety in EGFR-expressing tumors.[41,42] In dose escalation studies, panitumumab exhibited nonlinear pharmacokinetics, with longer antibody half-life associated with increasing dose.[43] This pharmacokinetic profile indicates antibody clearance by EGFR-expressing tissues. Upon saturation of this elimination pathway, pharmacokinetics was linear. The antibody clearance decreased with increasing dose and approached the clearance value for endogenous IgG, suggesting EGFR saturation at weekly doses >2 mg/kg. Comparison of different dosing schedules of 2.5 mg/kg weekly, 6 mg/kg every 2, or 9 mg/kg every 3 weeks have shown that steady-state panitumumab concentrations were obtained after 6 weeks of treatment with mean half-life values of 8.5, 7.5, and 8.4 days for these three regimens, respectively.[42] The antibody was generally well tolerated and skin toxicity (acneiform skin rash) was the most common dose-related adverse event.

Phase II studies focused largely on patients with metastatic colorectal cancer whose disease had progressed during or after one or more prior chemotherapy regimens.[41] Evaluating panitumumab as monotherapy in this patient population, detected an overall response rate of 9%, and overall stable disease rate was 29%, for an overall disease control rate of 38%.[44] No differences in response rate were observed between patients with tumors with low and high EGFR-staining intensity. Panitumumab was well tolerated. Over 90% of patients experienced skin-related toxicities (most were grade 1 or 2 in severity). No anti-panitumumab antibodies were detected.

Panitumumab (Vectibix) was approved by the Food and Drug Administration in the United States in September 2006 based on a randomized, Phase III, multicenter, open-label trial comparing panitumumab (at 6 mg/kg every other week) plus best supportive care (BSC) with BSC alone in patients with metastatic colorectal cancer who had disease progression after fluoropyrimidine-, irinotecan-, and oxaliplatin-containing chemotherapy regimens.[45] Panitumumab plus BSC significantly improved progression-free survival compared with BSC alone by approximately 46% (hazard ratio = 0.54, 95% CI: 0.44–0.66; p<0.0001). In subset analyses, progression-free survival favored panitumumab over BSC for all subsets studied based on gender, age, Eastern Cooperative Oncology Group (ECOG) status, primary tumor type, prior number of regimens, and EGFR staining categories. Objective responses favored panitumumab over BSC (10% vs. 0%, respectively, p<0.001). No differences in overall survival were observed between treatment groups (hazard ratio = 1.00, 95% CI: 0.82–1.22). Overall survival could have been confounded by the fact that about 75% of patients in the BSC arm crossed over to receive panitumumab at a median time of 7 weeks, as similar activity of panitumumab was observed in the crossover study as in the Phase III study. Panitumumab was generally well tolerated, with main toxicities including skin rash, hypomagnesemia, and diarrhea. No grade 3/4 infusion reactions were observed. As seen with other EGFR inhibitors, response rate, progression-free survival, and overall survival were associated with skin toxicity. In both the pivotal trial and in the pooled safety summary of panitumumab, the incidence of antibody formation against panitumumab was low with no discernible effect on pharmacokinetics or the safety profile. The rate of immunogenicity and infusion reactions differentiate between panitumumab and cetuximab (Erbitux), a chimeric IgG$_1$ antibody (Kd = 0.39 nM) that was the first therapeutic mAb directed to EGFR approved for the treatment of colorectal cancer and squamous cell carcinoma of the head and neck.[38,46,47] Published evidence indicates a severe infusion reaction rate of 3% with cetuximab and a total infusion reaction rate of approximately 20%,[46] and immunogenicity rate of 5% (Erbitux prescribing information, 2006). The two antibodies also differ in their half-life and dosing requirements, which may reflect the differences between the fully human nature of panitumumab, its higher affinity, and lower immunogenicity, which contribute to slower clearance, more avid binding, and lower dose requirement for EGFR saturation. Both antibodies demonstrated overall similar clinical efficacy and similar skin toxicity, a pattern that is now considered a class effect.[41]

XENOMOUSE-DERIVED HUMAN ANTIBODIES IN CLINICAL DEVELOPMENT

At present, eleven antibodies are progressing in clinical development for treatment of different indications, including cancer, inflammation, and bone loss (Table 7.1). Two of these antibodies, denosumab and ticilimumab, are in advanced Phase III studies.

Denosumab (AMG 162) is an IgG$_2\kappa$ mAb with very high affinity (Kd~10^{-12} M) directed to RANK ligand, a TNF family member that stimulates the maturation and activation of osteoclasts, cells that mediate bone resorption.[31] The IgG$_2$ isotype was chosen to avoid an undesirable potential toxic profile caused by RANK ligand-producing stromal, osteoblasts, and T cells.[48] The antibody is being tested in multiple Phase III clinical trials for treatment of patients with a variety of metabolic and inflammatory bone disorders, including postmenopausal women and cancer patients with metastatic lytic bone metastases. Phase I studies evaluating the pharmacokinetics and effect of a subcutaneous injection of single dose showed a rapid onset (within 12 hours) of antibody effect in blocking bone resorption that was sustained for up to 6 months, with no reported serious adverse effect.[49] In another study, administration of 3-month and 6-month repeat dosing of denosumab in postmenopausal women showed increased bone density even in patients given only 60 mg every 6 months. A single-dose study in patients with multiple myeloma or breast cancer patients with bone metastases showed decreased bone metabolism that persisted for the 84-day study follow-up period.[36] A terminal half-life between 32 and 46 days was detected at the 3mg/kg dose. Very low incidence of anti-denosumab antibodies has been detected. These favorable pharmcokinetic parameters allow for infrequent dosing, which makes this antibody very attractive for the chronic treatment of these patient populations. In the current Phase III

TABLE 7.1. XenoMouse-derived mAbs in Clinical Development

mAb	Target	Indication	Company (developer)	Clinical trial stage
Panitumumab (Vectibix)	EGFR	Cancer – solid tumors	Amgen	approved; 2, 3
Denosumab (AMG 162)	RANK ligand	Osteoporosis, treatment induced bone loss, bone metastases, multiple myeloma	Amgen	2,3
AMG 102	HGF	Cancer – solid tumors	Amgen	1
AMG 655	Trail receptor 2	Cancer – solid tumors	Amgen	1,2
Ticilimumab (CP-675,206)	CTLA-4	Cancer – solid tumors	Pfizer	3
CP-870,893	CD40 agonist	Cancer – solid tumors	Pfizer	1
CP-751,871	IGF-IR	Cancer – solid tumors	Pfizer	2
HCD122	CD40 antagonist	Cancer – hematologic tumors	Novartis/Xoma	1
CROO2	PDGFR	Kidney inflammation	CuraGen	1b
CRO11-vcMMAE	GPNMB	Cancer – melanoma	CuraGen	1
HGS004	CC chemokine receptor 5 (CCR5)	HIV	Human Genome Sciences	2
AGS-1C4D4	PSCA	Cancer – solid tumors	Agensys(Astellas)	2
AGS-16M18	AGS-16	Cancer – solid tumors	Agensys(Astellas)	1
AGS-8M4	AGS-8	Cancer – solid tumors	Agensys(Astellas)	1
PSMA-vcMMAE	PSMA	Cancer – solid tumors	Progenics	1

trials with postmenopausal women, the effect of denosumab (administered subcutaneously at 60 mg every 6 months) on bone mineral density is compared to alendronate. In trials with pre-metastatic prostate and breast cancer patients, denosumab is being administered subcutaneously at 120 mg monthly to analyze the antibody effect on bone loss related to androgen deprivation or aromatase inhibitor therapy, respectively.

Ticilimumab (CP-675206) is an $IgG_2\kappa$ mAb directed to CTLA-4,[27] a negative T cell signaling molecule that binds to the two ligands CD80 and CD86, which are also recognized by the positive T cell signaling molecule CD28.[50] The binding of antibodies to CTLA-4 results in blocking of ligand binding leading to activation of T cell response and thus enhanced immune responses and inhibition of tumor growth in xenograft mouse models.[50] Clinical trials with ticilimumab have demonstrated objective and durable antitumor responses in patients with metastatic melanoma.[34,51,52] In a Phase I single dose monotherapy, dose escalation in metastatic melanoma, with patients receiving up to 15 mg/kg, a 10% overall response rate was reported. A terminal half-life of 22 days was measured, with no measurable anti-ticilimumab antibody response.[34] The reported serious adverse effects of ticilimumab are immune-related inflammatory responses including rash, enterocolitis, and hypophystis.[34] They are regarded as target-related toxicities and have been correlated with clinical responses.[52] Although this mechanism of action involves a potent up-modulation of patient immune response, denosumab does not appear to induce immunogenicity in treated patients or accelerated clearance.

CONCLUSIONS

The regulatory approval of panitumumab marked the commercial validation of XenoMouse technology and signifies an important milestone for the development of therapeutic antibodies from human antibody transgenic mouse platform technologies. The path from initiation of XenoMouse technology development to regulatory approval took approximately 15 years, including 6 years for the mouse strains derivation and mAb development and 6.5 years of clinical development. The numerous XenoMouse-derived antibody products selected for clinical development prove the technology as a reliable source for generation and selection of mAbs with the desired isotype, affinity, specificity, and therapeutic potency. The clinical experience with XenoMouse–derived mAbs in human patients demonstrate their behavior as authentic fully human antibodies with long terminal half-life and very low rate of immunogenicity. In addition, some of these antibody products already demonstrate good safety profile and promising efficacy. These findings suggest that XenoMouse-derived mAbs are likely to develop into products that will benefit patients in different disease indications.

REFERENCES

[1]   G. Kohler & C. Milstein. Continuous cultures of fused cells secreting antibody of predefined specificity. *Nature*, **256** (1975), 495–497.

[2]   C. Pendley, A. Schantz, & C. Wagner. Immunogenicity of therapeutic monoclonal antibodies. *Curr Opin Mol Ther*, **5** (2003), 172–179.

[3]   G. Winter & C. Milstein. Man-made antibodies. *Nature*, **349** (1991), 293–299.

[4]   S.L. Morrison & V.T. Oi. Chimeric immunoglobulin genes, in *Immunoglobulin genes* (London, UK: Academic Press, 1975), pp. 260–274.

[5]   L. Riechmann, M. Clark, H. Waldmann, & G. Winter. Reshaping human antibodies for therapy. *Nature*, **332** (1988), 323–327.

[6]   D.R. Burton & C.F. Barbas. Human antibodies from combinatorial libraries, in *Protein engineering of antibody molecules for prophylactic and therapeutic antibodies in man* (ed. M. Clark) (Nottingham, UK: Nottingham Academic Titles, 1993), pp. 65–82.

[7]   H.R. Hoogenboom. Selecting and screening recombinant antibody libraries. *Nat Biotechnol*, **23** (2005), 1105–1116.

[8]   N. Lonberg. Human antibodies from transgenic animals. *Nat Biotechnol*, **23** (2005), 1117–1125.

[9]   A. Jakobovits, et al. Analysis of homozygous mutant chimeric mice: deletion of the immunoglobulin heavy-chain joining region blocks B-cell development and antibody production. *Proc Natl Acad Sci USA*, **90** (1993), 2551–2555.

[10] L.L. Green & A. Jakobovits. Regulation of B cell development by variable gene complexity in mice reconstituted with human immunoglobulin yeast artificial chromosomes. *J Exp Med*, **188** (1998), 483–495.

[11]   L.L. Green, et al. Antigen-specific human monoclonal antibodies from mice engineered with human Ig heavy and light chain YACs. *Nat Genet*, **7** (1994), 13–21.

[12]   F. Matsuda & T. Honjo. Organization of the human immunoglobulin heavy-chain locus. *Adv Immunol*, **62** (1996), 1–29.

[13]   G.P. Cook & I.M. Tomlinson. The human immunoglobulin VH repertoire. *Immunol Today*, **16** (1995), 237–242.

[14]   E. Max. Immunoglobulins: molecular genetics, in *Fundamental immunology* (ed. W.E. Paul), (New York: Raven Press, 1993), pp. 315–382.

[15]   M.J. Mendez, et al. Analysis of the structural integrity of YACs comprising human immuno-globulin genes in yeast and in embryonic stem cells. *Genomics*, **26** (1995), 294–307.

[16]   M.J. Mendez, et al. Functional transplant of megabase human immunoglobulin loci recapit-ulates human antibody response in mice. *Nat Genet*, **15** (1997), 146–156.

[17]   G.M. Weichhold, R. Ohnheiser, & H.G. Zachau. The human immunoglobulin kappa locus consists of two copies that are organized in opposite polarity. *Genomics*, **16** (1993), 503–511.

[18]   A. Jakobovits, et al. Germ-line transmission and expression of a human-derived yeast artificial chromosome. *Nature*, **362** (1993), 255–258.

[19]   S.A. Kellermann & L.L. Green. Antibody discovery: the use of transgenic mice to generate human monoclonal antibodies for therapeutics. *Curr Opin Biotechnol*, **13** (2002), 593–597.

[20]   M.L. Gallo, V.E. Ivanov, A. Jakobovits, & C.G. Davis. The human immunoglobulin loci intro-duced into mice: V (D) and J gene segment usage similar to that of adult humans. *Eur J Immunol*, **30** (2000), 534–540.

[21]   D.M. Fishwild, et al. High-avidity human IgG kappa monoclonal antibodies from a novel strain of minilocus transgenic mice. *Nat Biotechnol*, **14** (1996), 845–851.

[22]   N. Lonberg, et al. Antigen-specific human antibodies from mice comprising four distinct genetic modifications. *Nature*, **368** (1994), 856–859.

[23]   S. Huang, et al. Fully humanized neutralizing antibodies to interleukin-8 (ABX-IL8) inhibit angiogenesis, tumor growth, and metastasis of human melanoma. *Am J Pathol*, **161** (2002), 125–134.

[24]   E.C. McGary, et al. A fully human antimelanoma cellular adhesion molecule/MUC18 anti-body inhibits spontaneous pulmonary metastasis of osteosarcoma cells in vivo. *Clin Cancer Res*, **9** (2003), 6560–6566.

[25]   T. Ostendorf, et al. A fully human monoclonal antibody (CR002) identifies PDGF-D as a novel mediator of mesangioproliferative glomerulonephritis. *J Am Soc Nephrol*, **14** (2003), 2237–2247.

[26]   B.D. Cohen, et al. Combination therapy enhances the inhibition of tumor growth with the fully human anti-type 1 insulin-like growth factor receptor monoclonal antibody CP-751,871. *Clin Cancer Res*, **11** (2005), 2063–2073.

[27]   D.C. Hanson. Preclinical in vitro characterization of anti-CTLA4 therapeutic antibody CP-675-206. *Proc Am Assoc Cancer Res*, **45** (2004), 877.

[28]   R.P. Gladue & V. Bedian. Identification and characterization of a human CD40 agonist anti-body with efficacy against human tumors SCID mice. *Proc Am Assoc Cancer Res*, **47** (2006), Abstract #1355.

[29]   L. Long, et al. Antagonist anti-CD40 monoclonal antibody, CHIR-12.12, inhibits growth of a rituximab-resistant NHL xenograft model and achieves synergistic activity when combined with ineffective rituximab. *Blood*, **104** (2004), Abstract #3281.

[30]   T. Burgess, et al. Fully human monoclonal antibodies to hepatocyte growth factor with ther-apeutic potential against hepatocyte growth factor/c-Met-dependent human tumors. *Cancer Res*, **66** (2006), 1721–1729.

[31]   P.J. Bekker, et al. A single-dose placebo-controlled study of AMG 162, a fully human monoclonal antibody to RANKL, in postmenopausal women. *J Bone Miner Res*, **19** (2004), 1059–1066.

[32]   A. Jakobovits, et al. A fully human monoclonal antibody to prostate stem cell antigen (PSCA) for the treatment prostate pancreatic cancers. *J Clin Oncol*, **23**(16s) (2005), Abstract #4722.

[33]   D.A. Mahler, S. Huang, M. Tabrizi, & G.M. Bell. Efficacy and safety of a monoclonal antibody recognizing interleukin-8 in COPD: a pilot study. *Chest*, **126** (2004), 926–934.

[34] A. Ribas, L.H. Camacho, & G. Lopez-Berestein, et al. Antitumor activity in melanoma and anti-self responses in a phase I trial with the anti-cytotocix T lymphocyte-associated antigen 4 monoclonal antibody. *J. Clin Oncol*, **23** (2005), 8968–8977.

[35] M.R. McClung, et al. Denosumab in postmenopausal women with low bone mineral density. *N Engl J Med*, **354** (2006), 821–831.

[36] J.J. Body, et al. A study of the biological receptor activator of nuclear factor-kappaB ligand inhibitor, denosumab, in patients with multiple myeloma or bone metastases from breast cancer. *Clin Cancer Res*, **12** (2006), 1221–1228.

[37] X.D. Yang, et al. Eradication of established tumors by a fully human monoclonal antibody to the epidermal growth factor receptor without concomitant chemotherapy. *Cancer Res*, **59** (1999), 1236–1243.

[38] J. Mendelsohn & J. Baselga. Epidermal growth factor receptor targeting in cancer. *Semin Oncol*, **33** (2006), 369–385.

[39] Y. Yarden & M.X. Sliwkowski. Untangling the ErbB signalling network. *Nat Rev Mol Cell Biol*, **2**, (2001), 127–137.

[40] X.D. Yang, L.K. Roskos, C.G. Davis, & G. Schwab. From XenoMouse® technology to panitu-mumab, in *Cancer drug discovery and development, the oncogenomics handbook* (eds. W.J. LaRochelle & R.A. Shimkets) (Totowa, NJ: Humana Press, 2005), 647–657.

[41] A. Jakobovits, R.G. Amado, & X. Yang, et al. From XenoMouse technology to panitumumab, the first fully human antibody product from transgenic mice. *Nat Biotechnol*, **25** (2007), 1134–1143.

[42] L.M. Weiner, et al. Updated results from a dose and schedule study of Panitumumab (ABX-EGF) monotherapy, in patients with advanced solid malignancies. *J Clin Oncol*, **23** (suppl 16) (2005), Abstract #3059.

[43] E.K. Rowinsky, et al. Safety, pharmacokinetics, and activity of ABX-EGF, a fully human anti-epidermal growth factor receptor monoclonal antibody in patients with metastatic renal cell cancer. *J Clin Oncol*, **22** (2004), 3003–3015.

[44] J.R. Hecht, et al. Panitumumab monotherapy in patients with previously treated metastatic colorectal cancer. *Cancer*, **110** (2007), 980–987.

[45] E. Van Cutsem, et al. An open-label, randomized, phase 3 clinical trial of panitumumab plus best supportive care versus best supportive care in patients with chemotherapy-refractory metastatic colorectal cancer. *J Clin Oncol*, **25** (2007), 1658–1664.

[46] D. Cunningham, et al. Cetuximab monotherapy and cetuximab plus irinotecan in irinotecan-refractory metastatic colorectal cancer. *N Engl J Med*, **351** (2004), 337–345.

[47] B. Burtness, M.A. Goldwasser, W. Flood, B. Mattar, & A.A. Forastiere. Phase III randomized trial of cisplatin plus placebo compared with cisplatin plus cetuximab in metastatic/recurrent head and neck cancer: an Eastern Cooperative Oncology Group study. *J Clin Oncol*, **23** (2005), 8646–8654.

[48] E.M. Schwarz & C.T. Ritchlin. Clinical development of anti-RANKL therapy. *Arthritis Res Ther*, **9** (2007), S:7.

[49] P.J. Bekker, D. Holloway, & S. Ramussen, et al. A single-dose placebo-controlled study of AMG 162, a fully human monoclonal antibody to RANKL, in postmenopausal women. *J Bone Miner Res*, **19** (2004), 1059–1066.

[50] A.J. Korman, K.S. Peggs, & J.P. Allison. Checkpoint blockade in cancer immunotherapy. *Adv Immunol*, **90** (2006), 297–339.

[51] A. Ribas, J.A. Glaspy, & Y. Lee, et al. Role of dendritic cell phenotype, determinant spreading, and negative costimulatory blockade in dendritic cell-based melanoma immunotherapy. *J Immunother*, **27** (2004), 354–367.

[52] J.M. Reuben, B.N. Lee, & C. Li, et al. Biologic and immunomodulatory events after CTLA-4 blockade with ticilimumab in patients with advanced malignant melanoma. *Cancer*, **106** (2006), 2437–2444.

PART IV

ANTIBODY EFFECTOR FUNCTION

CHAPTER EIGHT

VelocImmune: Immunoglobulin Variable Region Humanized Mice

Andrew Murphy

The study of immunology is inexorably linked to the practice of animal husbandry. For example, the word "vaccinate" is derived from the Latin *vaccinus* meaning "of or from cows." The name stems from the practice of protecting people from the deadly smallpox virus by inoculating them with an extract derived from sores of cow udders infected with the innocuous cowpox virus.[1] Later, the serum of animals that had been repeatedly exposed to sublethal doses of diptheria toxin was shown to protect humans against diphtheria, a discovery that eventually led to the discovery of antibodies.[2] Eventually the study of antibody-producing cells in mice led to the invention of monoclonal antibody technology by Kohler and Milstein in 1975.[3] Thus, it is no surprise that germline engineering of the mouse was put to immunological use soon after this powerful technology was developed.[4] Here I describe the VelocImmune® mouse[5,6] created several years ago by megabase-scale humanization of the variable portion of mouse immunoglobulin (Ig) loci, by far the largest such precision genome-engineering project to date, and compare it with other methods for the generation of humanized or fully human monoclonal antibody therapeutics.

ANTIBODY THERAPEUTICS

Monoclonal antibodies have numerous advantages as drugs. They possess the qualities of (1) high affinity and exquisite specificity leading to few off-target effects and generally superb safety profiles, (2) long half-life leading to infrequent dosing, and (3) reproducible physical characteristics leading to routine production and shortened development time lines. However, because typical monoclonal antibodies are mouse proteins, they are highly immunogenic, and upon repeated administration to humans, humans develop natural antibodies that bind and neutralize the activity of mouse monoclonal antibody therapeutics. This neutralization response, termed HAMA for human anti-mouse antibodies, rendered the first attempts at using monoclonal antibodies as therapeutics largely ineffective. Of additional concern, the HAMA response can be so severe as to generate a toxic anaphylactic reaction. Much work has been done over the past 20 years to create therapeutic monoclonal antibodies that more closely resemble natural human antibodies and would thus be seen as self by the patient's immune system, avoiding an immune response.

The first and most straightforward approach toward reducing HAMA response was the creation of chimeric antibodies[7,8] in which the antigen-binding variable domains of a mouse monoclonal antibody were fused to constant domains of a human antibody by simple cDNA engineering and expression in a cell-culture system. The engineering of chimeric antibodies is uniformly successful in producing well-expressed and well-behaved antibodies that retain the affinity and selectivity of the parent mouse antibody, perhaps because the junction between variable and constant domains of an antibody has been selected by evolution to be very promiscuous in order to generate a large diversity of antigen specificities (many different variable domains created by differential rearrangement) and effector functions (several different constant domains can be added to the same variable domain during class switching). Several chimeric antibodies have gained regulatory approval and have become important therapeutics.[9–12] However, chimeric antibodies still retain a significant amount of mouse-derived sequence and immunogenicity (termed HACA for human antichimeric antibody response). Administration of chimeric antibody therapeutics is often accompanied by premedication with anti-inflammatory agents like antihistamines, glucocorticoids, or NSAIDs, and many of the approved chimeric antibodies themselves possess anti-inflammatory or antibody-suppressing properties.

Most therapeutic antibodies are currently being generated using a set of techniques (Table 8.1) that produce monoclonal antibodies with a higher degree of similarity to natural human antibodies than that of the chimeric antibodies. Most of these methods are extensively described within this volume or elsewhere, so they will be only minimally described here in order to compare them to the VelocImmune system.

The first two methods listed in Table 8.1 were the first to be developed and to come under widespread use. Neither method takes full advantage of the immune system's natural ability to select for not only high-affinity binding but also a number of other characteristics that make an antibody maximally effective in an *in vivo* mammalian setting. Many of these same characteristics are highly desirable in the therapeutic setting as outlined in Table 8.2. In contrast, researchers isolating antibody variable regions using phage display, for example, may be unwittingly selecting for properties that are irrelevant to the desired therapeutic uses. First, a process of "natural" selection occurs to bias for antibody sequences most compatible with rapid growth of phage in *E. coli* and with most efficient display on phage virions.

TABLE 8.1. Methods for generation of human or humanized mABs

Methods for generation of human or humanized mAbs	References
• Display technologies	[13,14]
• Humanization of mouse mAbs	[15,16]
• Transgenic mice with human Ig loci	[17,18]
• Trans-chromosome mice with human Ig minichromosomes	[19]
• VelocImmune mice with humanized variable loci	[5,6]
• Immunization of human subjects	[20]

TABLE 8.2. Advantages of in vivo selected antibodies for therapeutic use

In vivo selected Ab characteristic	Advantage in therapeutic setting
• High affinity	• High efficacy at low dose
• High-level production	• Feasibility of large scale production
• Long *in vivo* half life	• Infrequent dosing
• Stability	• Long shelf life and convenient storage
• Solubility (lack of a tendency to form aggregates at high concentrations)	• Convenient subcutaneous dosing and low immunogenicity
• Specificity	• Lack of off-target side effects
• Low intrinsic immunogenicity	• Safety and efficacy (due to lack of neutralizing antibody response)

Second, a somewhat "unnatural" *in vitro* selection process of panning to an immobilized target is employed to isolate binding antibodies. Finally, because initial "hits" are almost always suboptimal, additional rounds of mutagenesis and "unnatural" selection (often given fanciful names like "molecular evolution" or "directed evolution") are required to fix them. Likewise, humanization of antibodies is a labor-intensive process that transplants naturally selected, antigen-binding residues from a mouse antibody onto a human antibody scaffold. In the process, antibody engineers may unwittingly lose many of the attractive antibody attributes that were selected in the mouse. Thus, humanized antibodies also often need to undergo additional rounds of mutagenesis and *in vitro* selection, subjecting them to the same potential pitfalls as antibodies isolated from display libraries.

On the other hand, most display technologies do not suffer as dramatically from the issues of tolerance that affect the other methods listed in Table 8.1 that rely on immunization. Tolerance means that self-antigens (antigens identical or very similar to an endogenous protein, sugar, etc.) do not produce as robust an antibody response in animals as do foreign antigens. The immune system suppresses responses to self-antigens by failing to provide T cell help, by inhibiting B cells that express auto-antibodies, and possibly by removing V, D, or J chain segments with a propensity for self-recognition during the course of evolution, although little evidence of the last exists. Since antibody display libraries are derived from human variable gene sequences, they would also be subject to any evolutionary depletion of self-reactivity, but most would not be subject to the other mechanisms of auto-antibody suppression that affect the immunization strategies. Of course, most human antigens are dissimilar enough from their mouse orthologues for them to generate robust immune responses in mice. In addition, there are immunization methods that enhance antibody responses against self-antigens in mice. For instance, there are many mouse models of autoimmune disease that are initiated by immunization with a self-antigen expressed in the target tissue, like collagen to induce a response similar to rheumatoid arthritis or myelin components to induce a response similar to multiple sclerosis. Finally, mice that are genetically prone to autoimmunity or deficient in the gene encoding the auto-antigen can be immunized.

Transgenic (TGx) and trans-chromosome (TC) human Ig mice have been used to generate many high-affinity, fully human antibodies possessing all of the attributes expected of *in vivo* selection.[21] Antibodies isolated from these mice are most often immediately ready for clinical development upon expression in high-yield mammalian production systems. These mice were created by inactivating the endogenous mouse Ig heavy and kappa light chain loci using small targeted deletions in mouse embryonic stem (ES) cells, for example, by deleting the J-region of the heavy chain locus (Figure 8.1A), and then breeding the resulting mice to distinct strains in which functional human Ig loci have been inserted using one of three methods: pronuclear injection with engineered Ig "mini-loci,"[17,22] introduction of human Ig-loci-bearing yeast artificial chromosomes (YACs) into mouse ES cells by spheroplast fusion,[18,23] and mini-cell fusion to introduce Ig-loci-bearing self-replicating human chromosome fragments into ES cells.[19] Each of these TGx and TC hIg mouse strains have produced high-quality fully human antibodies to specific antigens upon immunization, and many of these antibodies are either approved drugs[24] or are in clinical development.[25–28] However, these mice have exhibited a quantitative deficit in either serum Ig levels and/or numbers of mature B cells in the spleen when compared to wild-type mice. This indicates that the TGx or TC human Ig loci in these mice, while functional, do not appear to be functioning at the same efficiency as the endogenous mouse Ig loci. VelocImmune mice were created to overcome this apparent inefficiency.

THE VELOCIMMUNE MOUSE

The construction of the VelocImmune mouse, described in detail elsewhere,[5] involved the precise replacement of approximately 3 Mb (megabases, 1 Mb = 1,000,000 base pairs) of mouse chromosome 12, containing all of the Ig heavy chain

A. Human Ig Transgene Mice

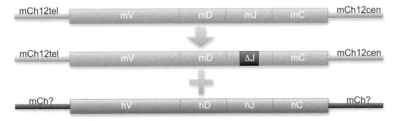

B. VelocImmune Ig Variable Humanized Mice

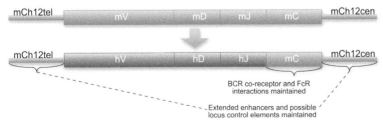

Figure 8.1. Schematic representation of the engineering of immunoglobulin heavy chain loci of human Ig transgene mice versus VelocImmune mice.

variable (V), diversity (D), and joining (J) gene segments, in ES cells with the orthologous 1 Mb region of human chromosome 14, containing essentially all human V, D, and J gene segments, using the VelociGene method.[29] Similarly, the variable region of the mouse Ig kappa light chain locus was humanized in ES cells by the replacement of 3 Mb of mouse chromosome 2, containing all of the V kappa and J kappa gene segments, with about 500 kb (kilobases, 1 kb = 1,000 base pairs) of human chromosome 2, containing the proximal V repeat and J region of the kappa light chain locus. Most, but not all human, genomes contain a second, distal repeat of V kappa gene segments that sits about 800 kb upstream of the proximal repeat in an inverted orientation. Many of the V gene segments in the distal repeat are identical to their counterparts in the proximal repeat and the rest show an extreme degree of similarity. Therefore, little diversity would be gained by including the distal repeat, and it was not included in the final VelocImmune mouse. The VelocImmune heavy chain locus was constructed by nine sequential ES cell modification steps and the light chain locus was constructed in eight sequential steps in a separate ES cell lineage. The final modified ES cells were used to generate mouse lines[30] that were bred to each other to generate the final VelocImmune mice. The antibodies produced by VelocImmune mice contain fully human variable domains and mouse constant domains. The fully human variable domains are cloned onto human constant domains to make fully human antibodies in a manner analogous to the construction of chimeric antibodies.

Extensive analysis of VelocImmune mice[6] revealed that they are quantitatively identical to wild-type mice in every measure of efficiency that has been investigated (see Table 8.3). These include the aforementioned serum Ig concentrations and numbers of mature B cells, as well as the ratio of human kappa light chains to mouse lambda light chains expressed from the endogenous mouse lambda locus. Between 5% and 10% of mouse Igs contain lambda light chains. In contrast, a higher proportion of antibodies containing lambda light chains have been reported for transgenic Ig mice,[19,23,31] indicating that the kappa light chain loci in these mice are operating at lower efficiencies than the mouse kappa locus. In addition, head-to-head comparisons were performed to test the immune response of VelocImmune mice to target antigens. VelocImmune mice and their wild-type littermates were immunized in parallel with a variety of antigens. Although there is animal-to-animal variation,

---

TABLE 8.3. Attributes of VelocImmune mice that are quantitatively indistinguishable from wild-type littermates

- Numbers and distribution of B cells in spleen and lymph node
- B cell differentiation in bone marrow
- Allelic exclusion
- Variable region usage and junctional diversity
- Somatic hypermutation
- Serum levels for all Ig isotypes (IgM, IgG1, IgG2a, IgG2b, IgG3, IgE, IgA)
- Kappa:lambda light chain ratios (human kappa to mouse lambda)
- Immune responses to target antigens
- Ability to generate hybridomas

the distributions and average antigen-specific antibody titers to each antigen were the same between cohorts of VelocImmune mice and cohorts of their littermates. Such a head-to-head comparison has not been reported for human Ig transgenic or trans-chromosome mice.

The apparent enhanced efficiency of the VelocImmune Ig loci over the human Ig TGx or TC mice could occur at either the protein or DNA levels (Table 8.4). At the protein level, the mouse heavy chain constant domains of VelocImmune antibodies may interact more efficiently with the numerous mouse Fc receptors than do human constant domains. In addition, the heavy chain constant domain of every isotype of both mouse and human antibodies is expressed in two forms through alternate splicing: a secreted soluble form and a membrane-bound form that is part of a B cell receptor. The mouse heavy chain constant domains in these B cell receptors may interact more efficiently with their mouse co-receptors than do human constant domains. At the DNA level, either the endogenous mouse intronic enhancers that reside in the J-C introns of both heavy and kappa light chain loci, or the powerful 3′ enhancers located downstream of the constant genes may function at a higher level in mice than do their human counterparts. It is also possible that as yet unidentified locus control elements located upstream, or far downstream, of the Ig loci, and absent from the Ig TGx and TC mice, contribute to the transcriptional or recombinational efficiency of the loci. While not affecting the efficiency of antibody production, VelocImmune mice have the additional advantage of having only two genetically modified and well-behaved alleles as opposed to the four alleles (heavy and light chain knockout alleles and separate heavy and light chain transgene alleles) of the human Ig transgene mice. This dramatically simplifies crossing these mice to additional mutant alleles or backcrossing them to the genetic background of different inbred strains.

The last method mentioned in Table 8.1 is the immunization of human subjects. In theory, the best human antibodies would be those produced by humans responding to an antigen challenge. In practice, immunization of humans with most self-antigens would be dangerous, and in cases where immunization is practical – for instance, by vaccination against infectious diseases or toxins – the ability to isolate high-affinity antibodies has been hampered by the inaccessibility of the B cells that produce them and the inability to immortalize human B cells by hybridoma formation. Recently, the isolation of high-affinity human antibodies by cloning antibody genes from single human B cells in circulation following influenza vaccination

---

TABLE 8.4. Possible advantages of variable region humanization versus Ig loci transgenics

- Functionality equivalent to mouse loci
  - More faithful interactions between transmembrane Ig and B cell receptor co-receptors
  - More faithful interactions between Fc region of Igs and FcRs
  - Transcriptional control by endogenous mouse flanking locus control elements
- Two vs. four modified alleles simplifies breeding
  - Backcrossing to different strain backgrounds
  - Crossing to other mutations

was demonstrated.[20] It remains to be seen how useful this method will be for generating therapeutic monoclonal antibodies.

REFERENCES

[1]   Waldmann, T.A., Immunotherapy: past, present and future. *Nat Med*, 2003. **9**(3): pp. 269–77.

[2]   Llewelyn, M.B., R.E. Hawkins, and S.J. Russell, Discovery of antibodies. *BMJ*, 1992. **305**(6864): pp. 1269–72.

[3]   Kohler, G. and C. Milstein, Continuous cultures of fused cells secreting antibody of predefined specificity. *Nature*, 1975. **256**(5517): pp. 495–7.

[4]   Kitamura, D., et al., A B cell-deficient mouse by targeted disruption of the membrane exon of the immunoglobulin mu chain gene. *Nature*, 1991. **350**(6317): pp. 423–6.

[5]   Macdonald, L.E., S. Stevens, et al., Humanization of several megabases of mouse immunoglobulin variable gene loci. *Manuscript in preparation*.

[6]   Stevens, S., L.E. Macdonald, et al., Mouse immunoglobulin gene loci with megabase humanization of only the variable region function with as efficiently as normal mouse immunoglobulin loci. *Manuscript in preparation*.

[7]   Morrison, S.L., et al., Chimeric human antibody molecules: mouse antigen-binding domains with human constant region domains. *Proc Natl Acad Sci USA*, 1984. **81**(21): pp. 6851–5.

[8]   Boulianne, G.L., N. Hozumi, and M.J. Shulman, Production of functional chimaeric mouse/human antibody. *Nature*, 1984. **312**(5995): pp. 643–6.

[9]   Elliott, M.J., et al., Randomised double-blind comparison of chimeric monoclonal antibody to tumour necrosis factor alpha (cA2) versus placebo in rheumatoid arthritis. *Lancet*, 1994. **344**(8930): pp. 1105–10.

[10] Popma, J.J. and L.F. Satler, Early and late clinical outcome following coronary angioplasty performed with platelet glycoprotein IIb/IIIa receptor inhibition: the EPIC Trial results. *J Invasive Cardiol*, 1994. 6 Suppl A: pp. 19A–28A; discussion 45A–50A.

[11] Nashan, B., et al., Randomised trial of basiliximab versus placebo for control of acute cellular rejection in renal allograft recipients. CHIB 201 International Study Group. *Lancet*, 1997. **350**(9086): pp. 1193–8.

[12] Maloney, D.G., et al., IDEC-C2B8 (Rituximab) anti-CD20 monoclonal antibody therapy in patients with relapsed low-grade non-Hodgkin's lymphoma. *Blood*, 1997. **90**(6): pp. 2188–95.

[13] McCafferty, J., et al., Phage antibodies: filamentous phage displaying antibody variable domains. *Nature*, 1990. **348**(6301): pp. 552–4.

[14] Machold, K.P. and J.S. Smolen, Adalimumab – a new TNF-alpha antibody for treatment of inflammatory joint disease. *Expert Opin Biol Ther*, 2003. **3**(2): pp. 351–60.

[15] Queen, C., et al., A humanized antibody that binds to the interleukin 2 receptor. *Proc Natl Acad Sci USA*, 1989. **86**(24): pp. 10029–33.

[16] Carter, P., et al., Humanization of an anti-p185HER2 antibody for human cancer therapy. *Proc Natl Acad Sci USA*, 1992. **89**(10): pp. 4285–9.

[17] Lonberg, N., et al., Antigen-specific human antibodies from mice comprising four distinct genetic modifications. *Nature*, 1994. **368**(6474): pp. 856–9.

[18] Green, L.L., et al., Antigen-specific human monoclonal antibodies from mice engineered with human Ig heavy and light chain YACs. *Nat Genet*, 1994. **7**(1): pp. 13–21.

[19] Tomizuka, K., et al., Double trans-chromosomic mice: maintenance of two individual human chromosome fragments containing Ig heavy and kappa loci and expression of fully human antibodies. *Proc Natl Acad Sci USA*, 2000. **97**(2): pp. 722–7.

[20] Wrammert, J., et al., Rapid cloning of high-affinity human monoclonal antibodies against influenza virus. *Nature*, 2008. **453**(7195): pp. 667–71.

[21] Lonberg, N., Human antibodies from transgenic animals. *Nat Biotechnol*, 2005. **23**(9): pp. 1117–25.

[22] Fishwild, D.M., et al., High-avidity human IgG kappa monoclonal antibodies from a novel strain of minilocus transgenic mice. *Nat Biotechnol*, 1996. **14**(7): pp. 845–51.

[23] Mendez, M.J., et al., Functional transplant of megabase human immunoglobulin loci recapitulates human antibody response in mice. *Nat Genet*, 1997. **15**(2): pp. 146–56.

[24] Giusti, R.M., et al., FDA drug approval summary: panitumumab (Vectibix). *Oncologist*, 2007. **12**(5): pp. 577–83.

[25] Leonardi, C.L., et al., Efficacy and safety of ustekinumab, a human interleukin-12/23 monoclonal antibody, in patients with psoriasis: 76-week results from a randomised, double-blind, placebo-controlled trial (PHOENIX 1). *Lancet*, 2008. **371**(9625): pp. 1665–74.

[26] Miller, P.D., et al., Effect of denosumab on bone density and turnover in postmenopausal women with low bone mass after long-term continued, discontinued, and restarting of therapy: A randomized blinded phase 2 clinical trial. *Bone*, 2008. **43**(2): pp. 222–29.

[27] Hagenbeek, A., et al., First clinical use of ofatumumab, a novel fully human anti-CD20 monoclonal antibody in relapsed or refractory follicular lymphoma: results of a phase 1/2 trial. *Blood*, 2008. **111**(12): pp. 5486–95.

[28] Kay, J., et al., Golimumab in patients with active rheumatoid arthritis despite treatment with methotrexate: a randomized, double-blind, placebo-controlled, dose-ranging study. *Arthritis Rheum*, 2008. **58**(4): pp. 964–75.

[29] Valenzuela, D.M., et al., High-throughput engineering of the mouse genome coupled with high-resolution expression analysis. *Nat Biotechnol*, 2003. **21**(6): pp. 652–9.

[30] Poueymirou, W.T., et al., F0 generation mice fully derived from gene-targeted embryonic stem cells allowing immediate phenotypic analyses. *Nat Biotechnol*, 2007. **25**(1): pp. 91–9.

[31] Jakobovits, A., Production and selection of antigen-specific fully human monoclonal antibodies from mice engineered with human Ig loci. *Adv Drug Deliv Rev*, 1998. **31**(1–2): pp. 33–42.

CHAPTER NINE

Mechanisms of Tumor Cell Killing by Therapeutic Antibodies

Ross Stewart and Carl Webster

Since its reemergence following the discovery of monoclonal antibodies in the early 1980s, the field of antibody therapy in cancer has progressed in leaps and bounds. From murine to chimeric, through humanized to fully human, we are now in a situation where, with over 200 antibodies having passed through some kind of clinical testing (Reichert & Valge-Archer, 2007), the monoclonal is now an accepted form of treatment for malignancy. In fact, for some malignancies, most notably non-Hodgkin's lymphoma, monoclonals are routinely used as frontline therapy. As such, we are past the point of asking whether monoclonal therapy works and into the more expansive territory of asking how it works and how we can make it work better.

While antibodies can function to combat a tumor in a number of ways – for example, sequestration of factors essential to survival or growth and stimulation of the immune response – one of the best-studied mechanisms of action is direct tumor cell killing. Here we will begin by looking in detail at the mechanisms by which antibodies can mediate cell killing, and which of these mechanisms is likely to be most important. Subsequently, we will review briefly the possible ways that this cell killing can be increased through the process of protein engineering, several of which will be expanded upon by the authors of subsequent chapters.

ANTIBODY STRUCTURE AND MECHANISMS OF CELL KILLING

All therapeutic antibodies to date have been of the immunoglobulin G (IgG) isotype, which is formed from four polypeptide chains, one pair of heavy chains, and one pair of light chains. Heavy chains are composed of four domains: three constant domains that do not vary between antibodies and one variable domain; the light chains are composed of a single constant and single variable domain. The four chains interact through covalent and noncovalent interactions to form three separate binding domains, which are linked together by a flexible hinge. Two of these domains, each formed by association of one light chain with the variable and first constant domain of one heavy chain, are termed Fab domains. They are identical to each other and are responsible for binding of antibody to target antigen. The remaining binding domain is generated by interaction of the four remaining heavy chain constant regions – two from each heavy chain – and is termed the Fc domain. The Fc domain is responsible for interactions with other parts of the immune system, including interaction with the C1q complement component and the various Fc gamma receptors (FcγRs). This multifunctional, multidomain nature of antibodies means that they can mediate tumor cell killing by a variety of mechanisms that can work in isolation or in concert; studies conducted over the last 10 years are only now beginning to pull apart these mechanisms.

Broadly speaking, there are two main routes by which unconjugated antibodies can directly trigger death of a target cell. The first is by delivery of an apoptotic signal to the cell, and a good example of this is the agonistic anti-TRAIL-R1 (TNF-related apoptosis-inducing ligand receptor 1) antibody, HGS-ETR1, which mimics the receptor's natural ligand in order to deliver apoptotic signals to a number of tumor cell types (Pukac et al., 2005). Such effects are mediated by binding of Fab to a surface antigen and are usually independent of the Fc domain of the antibody; in fact, many such signals can be generated using only Fab or $F(ab')^2$ molecules rather than the whole antibody. The second route is by recruiting components of the patient immune system to attack tumor cells. Such recruitment occurs via interaction of the Fc domain of a therapeutic antibody with the C1q protein, which is part of the complement cascade, or with Fcγ receptors (FcγRs) expressed on the surface of immune effector cells. Interaction with C1q results in recruitment of further complement components and, ultimately, lysis of the target cell in a process termed complement-dependent cytotoxicity (CDC). Interaction with FcγRs can recruit a number of different cell types, including neutrophils, macrophages, and natural killer (NK) cells, which are capable of killing a target cell by a variety of mechanisms, such as phagocytosis and antibody-dependent cell-mediated cytotoxicity (ADCC). It is also possible for antibodies to trigger cell death in an indirect manner – for example, the monoclonal therapeutic Cetuximab acts by blocking survival signals through the epidermal growth factor receptor (EGFR) (Wong, 2005), which in turn leads to tumor cell death. Given the multifunctional nature of antibodies, these mechanisms are by no means mutually exclusive and the extent to which each one acts will depend upon the particular antibody therapy in question.

CELL KILLING BY DIRECT INDUCTION OF APOPTOSIS

Many cell surface receptors are capable of delivering pro-apoptotic signals when engaged by their cognate ligands, and it is often possible to use antibodies to mimic those ligands and elicit an apoptotic response in a target cell. By targeting surface receptors that trigger their apoptotic effects preferentially in tumor cells, therapeutic antibodies can be used to deliver an apoptotic signal to tumors. The best examples of this approach are the anti-TRAIL receptor antibodies currently being developed or in clinical trials by a number of companies, including Human Genome Sciences (HGS-ETR1, HGS-ETR2 and HGS-TR2J), Genentech (Apomab), Amgen (AMG 655), Novartis (LBY135), and Daiichi Sankyo (CS-1008). These antibodies bind agonistically to members of the TRAIL receptor family expressed on the surface of a number of tumor cell types and deliver lethal apoptotic signals (Takeda et al., 2007). These signals are largely Fab-domain driven and can, under some circumstances, be recapitulated using antibody fragments such as scFv rather than whole IgG, although whole antibody is generally more effective since greater cross linking occurs via FcγR binding and because of the molecule's bivalent nature.

Several other monoclonal antibodies are also believed to act predominantly through induction of apoptosis, including Seattle Genetics' anti-CD30 (SGN-30) (Wahl et al., 2002), the anti-CD23 lumuliximab (Biogen) (Pathan et al., 2007), and the anti-HLA-DR antibody 1D093C (GPC Biotech) (Carlo-Stella et al., 2006), while both Cetuximab and some anti-HER2 monoclonals are believed to act at least partially via this mechanism (Bianco et al., 2005; Hinoda et al., 2004). More controversially, a number of studies have demonstrated the potential for anti-CD20 to deliver cell death signals direct to B cells, although there has been some disagreement over whether this death is classical, caspase-dependent apoptosis (Deans et al., 2002; Hofmeister et al., 2000; Shan et al., 2000) or some alternative form of cell death (Chan et al., 2003; van der Kolk et al., 2002). In addition, anti-CD20 induced apoptosis is far from being universal among B cell lines (Golay et al., 2000), and since all such apoptotic studies have been conducted *in vitro*, it is difficult to extrapolate from them to an *in vivo* mechanism of action, and the role apoptotic signaling plays in the therapeutic activity of anti-CD20 remains questionable.

Fc DOMAIN-DEPENDENT TUMOR CELL KILLING

The Fc domain of an IgG antibody can interact with a number of different receptors in humans. Together with soluble C1q, there are four main cell surface-expressed FcγRs: the high-affinity FcγRI and the two low-affinity receptors FcγRIIa and FcγRIIIa, which deliver activating signals, and a low-affinity inhibitory receptor FcγRIIb. Each of these cellular receptors shows a limited expression pattern, with the exception of FcγRIIb, which is expressed relatively widely (Siberil et al., 2007), and debate continues over which receptors and effector cell populations are key to the anti-tumor response. Anti-CD20 monoclonals have been utilized extensively as a model in studies attempting to address this question, in part because the use of anti-CD20 clinically, in the form of Rituximab, is well established, but also because the action of anti-CD20 is specific to B cells, which are a discrete and easily studied population. What follows is a brief summary of this research, followed by consideration of how well anti-CD20 might model the action of other therapeutic antibodies.

Cellular Effector Function

The conclusive evidence for the role of cellular effector function in the action of anti-CD20 comes from mouse xenograft models in which the efficacy of Rituximab, and other therapeutic antibodies, was significantly reduced following deletion of the common gamma chain, a central component in the signaling of the activating FcγRs (Clynes et al., 2000). Subsequent to these initial findings, the majority of attention

has focused upon the action of FcγRIIIa, whose expression is limited to the natural
killer (NK) cell population. This initial interest in the role of FcγRIIIa stemmed from
work that linked polymorphisms in this receptor to clinical response to Rituximab
(Cartron et al., 2002). This work showed that individuals carrying a phenylalanine at
position 158 in FcγRIIIa have a receptor with reduced affinity for the Fc of IgG1, and
that this correlated with a reduced response to treatment with Rituximab. This was,
and remains, some of the only evidence from human studies for the role of Fc gamma
receptors in the action of therapeutic antibodies and clearly points to a central role
for the NK cell population. This role has subsequently been supported by studies in
patients that show increases in NK cell activity following treatment with Rituximab
(Fischer et al., 2006), by *in vitro* studies that implicate NK cells as the primary cells
responsible for ADCC directed against tumor cells (Golay et al., 2003), and by *in vivo*
xenograft models that show the activity of Rituximab can be enhanced by expanding
the NK cell population with interleukin-2 (Lopes de Menezes et al., 2007).

In opposition to this, a number of subsequent clinical studies have shown no link
between FcγRIIIa polymorphisms and response to Rituximab treatment (Carlotti
et al., 2007; Farag et al., 2004; Galimberti et al., 2007; Mitrovic et al., 2007), suggesting
that NK cells may not be as dominant as initially thought. In support of this, work in
Jeffrey Ravetch's group, using mouse models, has indicated that the key factor in
determining antibody efficacy *in vivo* is strength of binding to the activating FcγRs
relative to inhibitory FcγRIIb – what they term the activating/inhibitory (A/I) ratio
(Clynes et al., 2000; Nimmerjahn & Ravetch, 2005). They show that antibodies with a
high A/I ratio perform better with respect to tumor cell clearance, and since NK cells
express no FcγRIIb, their contribution was not dominant. It is, however, quite difficult to translate these findings to humans, since mice have a family of FcγRs with
different affinities, specificities, and expression patterns to those found in humans
and additionally have a set of IgG subclasses that is also different.

The second low-affinity activating receptor, FcγRIIa, has also been implicated in
the action of anti-CD20. In humans, FcγRIIa is found, together with FcγRI, on the
surface of neutrophils and on cells of the monocytic lineage (Nuutila et al., 2007),
such as macrophages (Nuutila et al., 2007). Both these cell types are capable of
mediating ADCC of tumor cells (Lefebvre et al. 2006; van der Kolk et al. 2002), and
one study has indicated that polymorphisms in FcγRIIa can influence antibody
efficacy in the clinic (Weng & Levy, 2003). Neutrophils can account for up to 70%
of circulating leukocytes, and as such they present an attractive candidate effector
cell in antitumor responses. However, while studies in mice have shown that depletion of neutrophils can reduce efficacy of Rituximab (Hernandez-Ilizaliturri et al.,
2003), there is little evidence for their *in vivo* role in humans. Additionally, most
ADCC activity of neutrophils appears to be due to the action of FcγRI (van der Kolk
et al., 2002), and it has been postulated that FcγRI is saturated *in vivo* by nonspecific
antibody in sera due to its high affinity for monomeric IgG (van de Winkel & Capel,
1993) and is unavailable to take part in any antitumor response. Recently, there has
been an increased interest in the monocytic phagocyte network as a potential effector cell population, with two recent papers demonstrating that clodronate-mediated
depletion of macrophages prevented depletion of circulating B cells in mice, while

removal of other effector populations such as NK cells had little effect (Gong et al., 2005; Uchida et al., 2004). It is important, however, to note that these studies focus on the depletion of normal B cells, the majority of which recirculate to some degree, thus allowing them access to various parts of the monocytic phagocyte network – the Kupffer cells of the liver, for example. Malignant B cells are in general part of a solid tumor mass and do not recirculate in the same way. It is therefore difficult to directly transfer these observations of normal B cell depletion to that of their malignant counterparts.

The mixed messages presented by these various studies can be partially reconciled if we accept that all the FcγRs have a role to play, and indeed this is the message that work in knockout mice delivers, where removal of any one individual FcγR has little effect on the ability of anti-CD20 to deplete B cells, but removal of all three results in a dramatic loss of depletion (Gong et al. 2005; Uchida et al. 2004). It is likely that the exact contribution each receptor makes to the activity of anti-CD20 will be dependent on the specific model used or lymphoid malignancy being treated.

C1q and Complement-Dependent Cytotoxicity (CDC)

The role of complement in the action of anti-CD20 has been a point of greater discussion than that of the cellular FcγRs. The *in vivo* animal data regarding complement is contradictory, with some mouse models demonstrating dependence on complement for anti-CD20 activity (Di Gaetano et al., 2003; Golay et al., 2006) and others showing no such requirement (Hamaguchi et al., 2006; Nimmerjahn & Ravetch, 2005; Uchida et al., 2004), while *in vitro* studies supporting a dominant role for CDC are scarce (Harjunpaa et al., 2000). Recent studies have indicated that the extent to which anti-CD20 triggers complement activation may be linked to the expression level of CD20 on the target cell (van Meerten et al., 2006), the ability of the antibody in question to translocate CD20 into lipid rafts (Cragg & Glennie, 2004), and the specific epitope it binds (Teeling et al., 2006). Since often the models used to study anti-CD20 function utilize different antibodies and cell lines with different CD20 expression levels, this may go some way to explaining the discrepancies seen between studies.

Tumor cells, like many cells of the body, are protected from CDC by surface-expressed complement defense molecules such as CD55 and CD59. In support of a role for complement in the action of anti-CD20, there is evidence that inhibiting the action of these molecules *in vitro* with a blocking antibody can increase the sensitivity of cell lines and tumor samples to Rituximab-mediated killing (Golay et al., 2000; Golay et al., 2001; Harjunpaa et al., 2000; Treon et al., 2001). Additionally, the expression levels of these defense molecules are generally lower on samples taken from those types of lymphoma more sensitive to Rituximab – for example, follicular lymphoma – when compared to those more resistant to treatment, such as chronic lymphocytic leukaemia (Manches et al., 2003), although this finding does not seem to apply within tumors of the same type (Weng & Levy, 2001). Whatever its involvement in cell killing complement is definitely activated and consumed following dosing of patients with Rituximab (Kennedy et al., 2004; van der Kolk et al., 2001), and it is worth bearing in mind that complement has many roles aside from CDC (inflammation, opsonization, chemotaxis), all of which may feed into a larger anti-tumor immune response.

Other Monoclonal Therapeutics

While anti-CD20 antibodies have provided a wealth of information with respect to the role of effector functions in tumor killing by antibodies, it is not to be assumed that these findings will translate directly to antibodies against other targets. CD20 is quite an unusual antigen that lends itself to targeting by antibodies that utilize immune effector functions for a number of reasons. First, it is expressed at relatively high levels, and the extent of ADCC against target cells *in vitro* can be dependent on antigen-expression level (Golay et al., 2001). Second, it undergoes very little internalization upon antibody binding (Press et al., 1989; Sieber et al., 2003), which allows for retention of antibody at the surface, increasing the exposure to effector cells. Third, it has no essential, or even notable, function in normal tissue. The extent to which antibodies directed against other targets utilize immune effector mechanisms and how much value there might be in increasing this response through protein engineering will likely be different according to the antigen being targeted.

The closest correlates to anti-CD20 are likely to be antibodies targeting other lymphoid or myeloid surface markers, but even here there are clear differences in the contribution that direct cell killing makes to the mechanism of each antibody. For example, antibodies directed against CD22 do not notably trigger CDC or ADCC, presumably because CD22 is rapidly internalized when bound by antibody (Carnahan et al., 2007); similarly, anti-CD33 has little ADCC activity (Caron et al., 1995). Both, however, have been employed in forms that lack effector triggering capabilities but rely on internalization to deliver a toxic payload to the cell (Fenton & Perry, 2006; Kreitman & Pastan, 2006). In contrast, antibodies directed against both CD19, which internalizes at a more moderate rate (Press et al. 1989), and CD30 are capable of mediating B cell depletion both *in vivo* and *in vitro* (Borchmann et al., 2003; Yazawa et al., 2005; Zhukovsky, 2007), and while neither is as potent as anti-CD20 in this respect, it is possible to improve the killing potential of both antibodies by engineering them for greater interaction with Fc receptors (Hammond et al., 2005; Zhukovsky, 2007). Anti-CD40 antibodies are also capable of mediating ADCC against both multiple myeloma (MM) and chronic lymphocytic leukaemia (CLL) cell lines (Tai et al., 2005a; Tai et al., 2005b; Xia Tong, 2004), although the value of engineering greater killing into such antibodies may be less than for CD19 or CD20. First, because anti-CD40 also acts by blocking survival signals to target cells and second, because the wider expression of CD40 throughout the immune system and elsewhere may make increasing killing detrimental to therapy; for example, CD40 is highly expressed on macrophages and antigen-presenting cells, and removal of such populations may hinder the immune system's ability to contribute to the antitumor response.

Where CD20 may be less useful as a model antitumor monoclonal is in predicting the mechanisms of an antibody directed against solid tumors, since the morphology of such tumors and their accessibility to the immune system is likely to be very different to that of lymphomas and myelomas. Currently, there are two such antibodies in clinical use: Trastuzumab (Herceptin), which targets human EGF receptor 2 (HER2) and is used in the treatment of metastatic breast cancer, and Cetuximab (Erbitux), which targets EGF receptor and is used in the treatment of metastatic colorectal cancer. Both of these antibodies are capable of mediating ADCC against tumor cells *in vitro* (Cooley et al., 1999; Kimura et al., 2007), as are monoclonals directed against other cell surface molecules such as epithelial cell adhesion molecule (Ep-CAM) (Prang et al., 2005) and mucin-1 (Danielczyk et al. 2006), and there is additional evidence that this activity also plays a role *in vivo*. In the case of Trastuzumab, mouse xenograft models have shown that much of the therapeutic effect of the antibody is dependent on FcγR expression (Clynes et al., 2000) and on use of full-length IgG rather than F(ab′) (Barok et al., 2007). Studies in the clinic have indicated that treatment with Trastuzumab can result in increased tumor infiltration by lymphocytes and NK cells (Arnould et al., 2006) and that the extent of infiltration together with the ability to mediate ADCC may correlate with response (Gennari et al., 2004). In the case of Cetuximab, a recent study has shown a correlation between the FcγR polymorphisms carried by patients and response to treatment, although for FcγRIIIa this correlation was the inverse of that seen with Rituximab (Zhang et al., 2007). Importantly, unlike anti-CD20, both Trastuzumab and Cetuximab are directed against targets with obvious cellular functions, and as such they have numerous potential mechanisms of action that aren't open to anti-CD20 – for example, blocking of survival signals, induction of cell cycle arrest, inhibition of angiogenesis, and receptor down-regulation (Marshall, 2006; Valabrega et al., 2007). In the context of such complex biology, it is very difficult to estimate what contribution immune-mediated killing may play in the action of these antibodies. It is likely, however, that it plays a role and as such increasing effector function triggering by antibody engineering could be beneficial to the action of these antibodies. With this in mind, an engineered form of Trastuzumab, with increased binding to FcγRIIIa, has been generated and shows increased activity *in vitro* (Suzuki et al., 2007). It will be interesting to see how this antibody performs clinically, as this could reveal much about the contribution ADCC makes to the action of antibodies directed against solid tumors.

PROTEIN ENGINEERING FOR IMPROVED TUMOR CELL KILLING

To date, the majority of antibodies that bind tumor-expressed surface antigens seem to utilize Fc-driven effector functions, or apoptosis, to some degree to mediate tumor cell killing. As such, engineering antibodies to trigger increased effector function or apoptosis would be expected to be positive or neutral with respect to their therapeutic efficacy. With this in mind, even as research is ongoing to unravel the mechanisms of antibody therapy, a closely related effort is being applied to increasing the ability of antibodies to drive cell killing.

It has been suggested that the level of cell death triggered by different anti-CD20 antibodies depends upon which cell death pathway they trigger, on their ability to generate higher order clustering of target antigen, and on whether they translocate CD20 into lipid rafts (Glennie et al., 2007), and it is possible that such clustering, or lipid raft effects, may also influence the ability of antibodies against other targets to trigger apoptosis. Additionally, choice of epitope, affinity for target antigen, and the on/off rate of an antibody are all likely to determine the extent of apoptosis induced upon cell binding. These properties can all be biased favorably during the initial selection from antibody libraries and in the subsequent screening of antibody panels, using the techniques detailed in earlier sections of this book and elsewhere (Hoogenboom, 2005). Subsequently, it may be possible to gain further improvements in the properties of a specific monoclonal by employing one of a number of antibody optimization strategies (Dufner et al., 2006).

The level of Fc-driven effector function triggered by an antibody can also be strongly influenced by the affinity and epitope specificity of its Fab domain (Teeling et al., 2006; Tang et al., 2007), and as such, it would be possible to use similar methods to those referenced earlier in order to identify antibodies with optimized effector function–triggering properties. More intriguing though is the possibility of engineering the Fc domain of antibodies for improved effector function. The region of the Fc domain involved in FcγR binding was initially mapped, using IgG mutagenesis and binding studies (Canfield & Morrison, 1991; Duncan et al., 1988; Lund et al., 1992; Woof et al., 1986), to the CH2 domain and the lower hinge region, and subsequent crystal structures for the interaction of IgG with FcγRIIIa have largely borne out the conclusions of these studies (Radaev et al., 2001; Sondermann et al., 2000). While crystal structures are unavailable for the interaction between IgG and the other FcγRs, conservations in structure and mode of binding between family members have been used in order to model the interaction of IgG with FcγRI and FcγRII (Sondermann et al., 2001). Binding of IgG to C1q is more complex than FcγR binding due to the size and multivalent nature of C1q. In studies similar to those for the FcγRs, the binding site for the head of C1q was mapped on mouse IgG2b to the CH2 domain of the heavy chain (Duncan & Winter, 1988), and while further studies have indicated that the specific residues involved may vary between species, and indeed between isotypes of IgG in the same species, in all cases the CH2 domain is maintained as the site of C1q binding (Brekke et al., 1994; Duncan & Winter, 1988; Idusogie et al., 2000; Morgan et al., 1995; Sensel et al., 1997; Tao et al., 1991; Tao et al., 1993; Thommesen et al., 2000; Xu et al., 1994).

An initial attempt at protein engineering an Fc domain with improved effector function was made by Genentech, who used an alanine scanning methodology in order to identify surface residues on IgG1 important for the interaction with FcγRs (Shields et al., 2001). Subsequent to this initial proof of principle, a number of different methodologies have been attempted to improve IgG effector function further (Dall'Acqua et al., 2006; Stavenhagen et al., 2007), the most exhaustive, arguably, being Xencor's use of intelligent and computational driven protein design (Lazar et al., 2006). In addition to these protein engineering efforts, it has also been possible to use modification of the IgG carbohydrate side chains, which are essential to FcγR binding (Jefferis, 2007), with the most prominent examples being Biowa's Potelligent™ antibody technology (Niwa et al., 2005). At present, all of these technologies have been utilized only *in vitro* and for *in vivo* animal models; however, both Xencor and Medarex (in collaboration with Biowa) have Fc engineered anti-CD30 antibodies entering Phase I clinical trials imminently, and further trials of engineered antibodies against other targets will inevitably follow, allowing a more complete assessment of what benefits they might provide to patients.

CONCLUSIONS

The reality is that while well established in clinical use, the mechanisms for most antibody therapeutics in oncology remain theoretical and difficult to prove conclusively. The studies performed to date indicate that the role played by complement, FcγR-driven effector function and more direct induction of apoptosis in driving efficacy of therapeutic antibodies varies between targets, between antibodies against the same target, and even across indications for the same antibody. Given this variability, it seems likely that while one mechanism may take priority in driving the therapeutic effects of a given antibody, alternative mechanisms may be able to complement or augment those effects. It may be that as the marketplace expands to take in antibodies against new targets – and more particularly, antibodies engineered with particular mechanisms of action in mind – our understanding of the way in which these drugs mediate their therapeutic effects will become more complete. The hope is that with that understanding there will come further opportunities for increases in efficacy and safety, which can translate directly to patient benefit.

REFERENCES

Arnould, L., M. Gelly, et al. (2006). "Trastuzumab-based treatment of HER2-positive breast cancer: an antibody-dependent cellular cytotoxicity mechanism?" *Br J Cancer* **94**(2): 259–67.

Barok, M., J. Isola, et al. (2007). "Trastuzumab causes antibody-dependent cellular cytotoxicity-mediated growth inhibition of submacroscopic JIMT-1 breast cancer xenografts despite intrinsic drug resistance." *Mol Cancer Ther* **6**(7): 2065–72.

Bianco, R., G. Daniele, et al. (2005). "Monoclonal antibodies targeting the epidermal growth factor receptor." *Curr Drug Targets* **6**(3): 275–87.

Borchmann, P., J.F. Treml, et al. (2003). "The human anti-CD30 antibody 5F11 shows in vitro and in vivo activity against malignant lymphoma." *Blood* **102**(10): 3737–42.

Brekke, O.H., T.E. Michaelsen, et al. (1994)."Human IgG isotype-specific amino acid residues affecting complement-mediated cell lysis and phagocytosis." *Eur J Immunol* **24**(10): 2542–7.

Canfield, S.M. and S.L. Morrison (1991). "The binding affinity of human IgG for its high affinity Fc receptor is determined by multiple amino acids in the CH2 domain and is modulated by the hinge region." *J Exp Med* **173**(6): 1483–91.

Carlo-Stella, C., M. Di Nicola, et al. (2006). "The anti-human leukocyte antigen-DR monoclonal antibody 1D09C3 activates the mitochondrial cell death pathway and exerts a potent antitumor activity in lymphoma-bearing nonobese diabetic/severe combined immunodeficient mice." *Cancer Res* **66**(3): 1799–808.

Carlotti, E., G.A. Palumbo, et al. (2007). "FcgammaRIIIA and FcgammaRIIA polymorphisms do not predict clinical outcome of follicular non-Hodgkin's lymphoma patients treated with sequential CHOP and rituximab." *Haematologica* **92**(8): 1127–30.

Carnahan, J., R. Stein, et al. (2007). "Epratuzumab, a CD22-targeting recombinant humanized antibody with a different mode of action from rituximab." *Mol Immunol* **44**(6): 1331–41.

Caron, P.C., L.T. Lai, et al. (1995). "Interleukin-2 enhancement of cytotoxicity by humanized monoclonal antibody M195 (anti-CD33) in myelogenous leukemia." *Clin Cancer Res* **1**(1): 63–70.

Cartron, G., L. Dacheux, et al. (2002). "Therapeutic activity of humanized anti-CD20 monoclonal antibody and polymorphism in IgG Fc receptor FcgammaRIIIa gene." *Blood* **99**(3): 754–8.

Chan, H.T., D. Hughes, et al. (2003). "CD20-induced lymphoma cell death is independent of both caspases and its redistribution into triton X-100 insoluble membrane rafts." *Cancer Res* **63**(17): 5480–9.

Clynes, R.A., T.L. Towers, et al. (2000). "Inhibitory Fc receptors modulate in vivo cytoxicity against tumor targets." *Nat Med* **6**(4): 443–6.

Cooley, S., L.J. Burns, et al. (1999). "Natural killer cell cytotoxicity of breast cancer targets is enhanced by two distinct mechanisms of antibody-dependent cellular cytotoxicity against LFA-3 and HER2/neu." *Exp Hematol* **27**(10): 1533–41.

Cragg, M.S. and M.J. Glennie (2004). "Antibody specificity controls in vivo effector mechanisms of anti-CD20 reagents." *Blood* **103**(7): 2738–43.

Dall'Acqua, W.F., K.E. Cook, et al. (2006). "Modulation of the effector functions of a human IgG1 through engineering of its hinge region." *J Immunol* **177**(2): 1129–38.

Danielczyk, A., R. Stahn, et al. (2006). "PankoMab: a potent new generation anti-tumour MUC1 antibody." *Cancer Immunol Immunother* **55**(11): 1337–47.

Deans, J.P., H. Li, et al. (2002). "CD20-mediated apoptosis: signalling through lipid rafts." *Immunology* **107**(2): 176–82.

Di Gaetano, N., E. Cittera, et al. (2003). "Complement activation determines the therapeutic activity of rituximab in vivo." *J Immunol* **171**(3): 1581–7.

Dufner, P., L. Jermutus, et al. (2006). "Harnessing phage and ribosome display for antibody optimisation." *Trends Biotechnol* **24**(11): 523–9.

Duncan, A.R. and G. Winter (1988). "The binding site for C1q on IgG." *Nature* **332**(6166): 738–40.

Duncan, A.R., J.M. Woof, et al. (1988). "Localization of the binding site for the human high-affinity Fc receptor on IgG." *Nature* **332**(6164): 563–4.

Farag, S.S., I.W. Flinn, et al. (2004). "Fc gamma RIIIa and Fc gamma RIIa polymorphisms do not predict response to rituximab in B-cell chronic lymphocytic leukemia." *Blood* **103**(4): 1472–4.

Fenton, C. and C.M. Perry (2006). "Spotlight on gemtuzumab ozogamicin in acute myeloid leukaemia." *BioDrugs* **20**(2): 137–9.

Fischer, L., O. Penack, et al. (2006). "The anti-lymphoma effect of antibody-mediated immunotherapy is based on an increased degranulation of peripheral blood natural killer (NK) cells." *Exp Hematol* **34**(6): 753–9.

Galimberti, S., G.A. Palumbo, et al. (2007). "The efficacy of rituximab plus Hyper-CVAD regimen in mantle cell lymphoma is independent of FCgammaRIIIa and FCgammaRIIa polymorphisms." *J Chemother* **19**(3): 315–21.

Gennari, R., S. Menard, et al. (2004). "Pilot study of the mechanism of action of preoperative trastuzumab in patients with primary operable breast tumors overexpressing HER2." *Clin Cancer Res* **10**(17): 5650–5.

Glennie, M.J., R.R. French, et al. (2007). "Mechanisms of killing by anti-CD20 monoclonal antibodies." *Mol Immunol* **44**(16): 3823–37.

Golay, J., E. Cittera, et al. (2006). "The role of complement in the therapeutic activity of rituximab in a murine B lymphoma model homing in lymph nodes." *Haematologica* **91**(2): 176–83.

Golay, J., M. Lazzari, et al. (2001). "CD20 levels determine the in vitro susceptibility to rituximab and complement of B-cell chronic lymphocytic leukemia: further regulation by CD55 and CD59." *Blood* **98**(12): 3383–9.

Golay, J., M. Manganini, et al. (2003). "Rituximab-mediated antibody-dependent cellular cytotoxicity against neoplastic B cells is stimulated strongly by interleukin-2." *Haematologica* **88**(9): 1002–12.

Golay, J., L. Zaffaroni, et al. (2000). "Biologic response of B lymphoma cells to anti-CD20 monoclonal antibody rituximab in vitro: CD55 and CD59 regulate complement-mediated cell lysis." *Blood* **95**(12): 3900–8.

Gong, Q., Q. Ou, et al. (2005). "Importance of cellular microenvironment and circulatory dynamics in B cell immunotherapy." *J Immunol* **174**(2): 817–26.

Hamaguchi, Y., Y. Xiu, et al. (2006). "Antibody isotype-specific engagement of Fcgamma receptors regulates B lymphocyte depletion during CD20 immunotherapy." *J Exp Med* **203**(3): 743–53.

Hammond, P.W., O. Vafa, et al. (2005). "A humanized anti-CD30 monoclonal antibody, XmAbTM2513, with enhanced in vitro potency against CD30-positive lymphomas mediated by high affinity Fc-receptor binding." *The American Society of Hematology 47th Annual Meeting and Exposition.*

Harjunpaa, A., S. Junnikkala, et al. (2000). "Rituximab (anti-CD20) therapy of B-cell lymphomas: direct complement killing is superior to cellular effector mechanisms." *Scand J Immunol* **51**(6): 634–41.

Hernandez-Ilizaliturri, F.J., V. Jupudy, et al. (2003). "Neutrophils contribute to the biological anti-tumor activity of rituximab in a non-Hodgkin's lymphoma severe combined immunodeficiency mouse model." *Clin Cancer Res* **9**(16 Pt 1): 5866–73.

Hinoda, Y., S. Sasaki, et al. (2004). "Monoclonal antibodies as effective therapeutic agents for solid tumors." *Cancer Sci* **95**(8): 621–5.

Hofmeister, J.K., D. Cooney, et al. (2000). "Clustered CD20 induced apoptosis: src-family kinase, the proximal regulator of tyrosine phosphorylation, calcium influx, and caspase 3-dependent apoptosis." *Blood Cells Mol Dis* **26**(2): 133–43.

Hoogenboom, H.R. (2005). "Selecting and screening recombinant antibody libraries." *Nat Biotechnol* **23**(9): 1105–16.

Idusogie, E.E., L.G. Presta, et al. (2000). "Mapping of the C1q binding site on rituxan, a chimeric antibody with a human IgG1 Fc." *J Immunol* **164**(8): 4178–84.

Jefferis, R. (2007). "Antibody therapeutics: isotype and glycoform selection." *Expert Opin Biol Ther* **7**(9): 1401–13.

Kennedy, A.D., P.V. Beum, et al. (2004). "Rituximab infusion promotes rapid complement depletion and acute CD20 loss in chronic lymphocytic leukemia." *J Immunol* **172**(5): 3280–8.

Kimura, H., K. Sakai, et al. (2007). "Antibody-dependent cellular cytotoxicity of cetuximab against tumor cells with wild-type or mutant epidermal growth factor receptor." *Cancer Sci* **98**(8): 1275–80.

Kreitman, R.J. and I. Pastan (2006). "BL22 and lymphoid malignancies." *Best Pract Res Clin Haematol* **19**(4): 685–99.

Lazar, G.A., W. Dang, et al. (2006). "Engineered antibody Fc variants with enhanced effector function." *Proc Natl Acad Sci USA* **103**(11): 4005–10.

Lefebvre, M.L., S.W. Krause, et al. (2006). "Ex vivo-activated human macrophages kill chronic lymphocytic leukemia cells in the presence of rituximab: mechanism of antibody-dependent cellular cytotoxicity and impact of human serum." *J Immunother (1997)* **29**(4): 388–97.

Lopes de Menezes, D.E., K. Denis-Mize, et al. (2007). "Recombinant interleukin-2 significantly augments activity of rituximab in human tumor xenograft models of B-cell non-Hodgkin lymphoma." *J Immunother (1997)* **30**(1): 64–74.

Lund, J., J.D. Pound, et al. (1992). "Multiple binding sites on the CH2 domain of IgG for mouse Fc gamma R11." *Mol Immunol* **29**(1): 53–9.

Manches, O., G. Lui, et al. (2003). "In vitro mechanisms of action of rituximab on primary non-Hodgkin lymphomas." *Blood* **101**(3): 949–54.

Marshall, J. (2006). "Clinical implications of the mechanism of epidermal growth factor receptor inhibitors." *Cancer* **107**(6): 1207–18.

Mitrovic, Z., I. Aurer, et al. (2007). "FCgammaRIIIA and FCgammaRIIA polymorphisms are not associated with response to rituximab and CHOP in patients with diffuse large B-cell lymphoma." *Haematologica* **92**(7): 998–9.

Morgan, A., N.D. Jones, et al. (1995). "The N-terminal end of the CH2 domain of chimeric human IgG1 anti-HLA-DR is necessary for C1q, Fc gamma RI and Fc gamma RIII binding." *Immunology* **86**(2): 319–24.

Nimmerjahn, F. and J.V. Ravetch (2005). "Divergent immunoglobulin g subclass activity through selective Fc receptor binding." *Science* **310**(5753): 1510–2.

Niwa, R., A. Natsume, et al. (2005). "IgG subclass-independent improvement of antibody-dependent cellular cytotoxicity by fucose removal from Asn297-linked oligosaccharides." *J Immunol Methods* **306**(1–2): 151–60.

Nuutila, J., U. Hohenthal, et al. (2007). "Simultaneous quantitative analysis of FcgammaRI (CD64) expression on neutrophils and monocytes: A new, improved way to detect infections." *J Immunol Methods* **228**(1–2): 189–200.

Pathan, N.I., P. Chu, et al. (2007). "Mediation of apoptosis by and anti-tumor activity of lumiliximab in chronic lymphocytic leukemia cells and CD23+ lymphoma cell lines." *Blood* **111**(3): 1594–1602.

Prang, N., S. Preithner, et al. (2005). "Cellular and complement-dependent cytotoxicity of Ep-CAM-specific monoclonal antibody MT201 against breast cancer cell lines." *Br J Cancer* **92**(2): 342–9.

Press, O.W., A.G. Farr, et al. (1989). "Endocytosis and degradation of monoclonal antibodies targeting human B-cell malignancies." *Cancer Res* **49**(17): 4906–12.

Pukac, L., P. Kanakaraj, et al. (2005). "HGS-ETR1, a fully human TRAIL-receptor 1 monoclonal antibody, induces cell death in multiple tumour types in vitro and in vivo." *Br J Cancer* **92**(8): 1430–41.

Radaev, S., S. Motyka, et al. (2001). "The structure of a human type III Fcgamma receptor in complex with Fc." *J Biol Chem* **276**(19): 16469–77.

Reichert, J.M. and V.E. Valge-Archer (2007). "Development trends for monoclonal antibody cancer therapeutics." *Nat Rev Drug Discov* **6**(5): 349–56.

Sensel, M.G., L.M. Kane, et al. (1997). "Amino acid differences in the N-terminus of C(H)2 influence the relative abilities of IgG2 and IgG3 to activate complement." *Mol Immunol* **34**(14): 1019–29.

Shan, D., J.A. Ledbetter, et al. (2000). "Signaling events involved in anti-CD20-induced apoptosis of malignant human B cells." *Cancer Immunol Immunother* **48**(12): 673–83.

Shields, R.L., A.K. Namenuk, et al. (2001). "High resolution mapping of the binding site on human IgG1 for Fc gamma RI, Fc gamma RII, Fc gamma RIII, and FcRn and design of IgG1 variants with improved binding to the Fc gamma R." *J Biol Chem* **276**(9): 6591–604.

Siberil, S., C.A. Dutertre, et al. (2007). "FcgammaR: The key to optimize therapeutic antibodies?" *Crit Rev Oncol Hematol* **62**(1): 26–33.

Sieber, T., D. Schoeler, et al. (2003). "Selective internalization of monoclonal antibodies by B-cell chronic lymphocytic leukaemia cells." *Br J Haematol* **121**(3): 458–61.

Sondermann, P., R. Huber, et al. (2000). "The 3.2-A crystal structure of the human IgG1 Fc fragment-Fc gammaRIII complex." *Nature* **406**(6793): 267–73.

Sondermann, P., J. Kaiser, et al. (2001). "Molecular basis for immune complex recognition: a comparison of Fc-receptor structures." *J Mol Biol* **309**(3): 737–49.

Stavenhagen, J.B., S. Gorlatov, et al. (2007). "Fc optimization of therapeutic antibodies enhances their ability to kill tumor cells in vitro and controls tumor expansion in vivo via low-affinity activating Fcgamma receptors." *Cancer Res* **67**(18): 8882–90.

Suzuki, E., R. Niwa, et al. (2007). "A nonfucosylated anti-HER2 antibody augments antibody-dependent cellular cytotoxicity in breast cancer patients." *Clin Cancer Res* **13**(6): 1875–82.

Tai, Y.T., X. Li, et al. (2005). "Human anti-CD40 antagonist antibody triggers significant antitumor activity against human multiple myeloma." *Cancer Res* **65**(13): 5898–906.

Tai, Y.T., X.F. Li, et al. (2005). "Immunomodulatory drug lenalidomide (CC-5013, IMiD3) augments anti-CD40 SGN-40-induced cytotoxicity in human multiple myeloma: clinical implications." *Cancer Res* **65**(24): 11712–20.

Takeda, K., J. Stagg, et al. (2007). "Targeting death-inducing receptors in cancer therapy." *Oncogene* **26**(25): 3745–57.

Tang, Y., J. Lou, et al. (2007). "Regulation of antibody-dependent cellular cytotoxicity by IgG intrinsic and apparent affinity for target antigen." *J Immunol* **179**(5): 2815–23.

Tao, M.H., S.M. Canfield, et al. (1991). "The differential ability of human IgG1 and IgG4 to activate complement is determined by the COOH-terminal sequence of the CH2 domain." *J Exp Med* **173**(4): 1025–8.

Tao, M.H., R.I. Smith, et al. (1993). "Structural features of human immunoglobulin G that determine isotype-specific differences in complement activation." *J Exp Med* **178**(2): 661–7.

Teeling, J.L., W.J. Mackus, et al. (2006). "The biological activity of human CD20 monoclonal anti-bodies is linked to unique epitopes on CD20." *J Immunol* **177**(1): 362–71.

Thommesen, J.E., T.E. Michaelsen, et al. (2000). "Lysine 322 in the human IgG3 C(H)2 domain is crucial for antibody dependent complement activation." *Mol Immunol* **37**(16): 995–1004.

Treon, S.P., C. Mitsiades, et al. (2001). "Tumor Cell Expression of CD59 Is Associated With Resistance to CD20 Serotherapy in Patients With B-Cell Malignancies." *J Immunother* **24**(3): 263–271.

Uchida, J., Y. Hamaguchi, et al. (2004). "The innate mononuclear phagocyte network depletes B lymphocytes through Fc receptor-dependent mechanisms during anti-CD20 antibody immuno-therapy." *J Exp Med* **199**(12): 1659–69.

Valabrega, G., F. Montemurro, et al. (2007). "Trastuzumab: mechanism of action, resistance and future perspectives in HER2-overexpressing breast cancer." *Ann Oncol* **18**(6): 977–84.

van de Winkel, J.G. and P.J. Capel (1993). "Human IgG Fc receptor heterogeneity: molecular aspects and clinical implications." *Immunol Today* **14**(5): 215–21.

van der Kolk, L.E., M. de Haas, et al. (2002). "Analysis of CD20-dependent cellular cytotoxicity by G-CSF-stimulated neutrophils." *Leukemia* **16**(4): 693–9.

van der Kolk, L.E., L.M. Evers, et al. (2002). "CD20-induced B cell death can bypass mitochondria and caspase activation." *Leukemia* **16**(9): 1735–44.

van der Kolk, L.E., A.J. Grillo-Lopez, et al. (2001). "Complement activation plays a key role in the side-effects of rituximab treatment." *Br J Haematol* **115**(4): 807–11.

van Meerten, T., R.S. van Rijn, et al. (2006). "Complement-induced cell death by rituximab depends on CD20 expression level and acts complementary to antibody-dependent cellular cytotoxicity." *Clin Cancer Res* **12**(13): 4027–35.

Wahl, A.F., K. Klussman, et al. (2002). "The anti-CD30 monoclonal antibody SGN-30 promotes growth arrest and DNA fragmentation in vitro and affects antitumor activity in models of Hodg-kin's disease." *Cancer Res* **62**(13): 3736–42.

Weng, W.K. and R. Levy (2001). "Expression of complement inhibitors CD46, CD55, and CD59 on tumor cells does not predict clinical outcome after rituximab treatment in follicular non-Hodgkin lymphoma." *Blood* **98**(5): 1352–7.

Weng, W.K. and R. Levy (2003). "Two immunoglobulin G fragment C receptor polymorphisms independently predict response to rituximab in patients with follicular lymphoma." *J Clin Oncol* **21**(21): 3940–7.

Wong, S.F. (2005). "Cetuximab: an epidermal growth factor receptor monoclonal antibody for the treatment of colorectal cancer." *Clin Ther* **27**(6): 684–94.

Woof, J.M., L.J. Partridge, et al. (1986). "Localisation of the monocyte-binding region on human immunoglobulin G." *Mol Immunol* **23**(3): 319–30.

Xia Tong, G.V.G., Li Long, Susan O'Brien, Anas Younes, Mohammad Luqman(2004). "In Vitro Activ-ity of a Novel Fully Human Anti-CD40 Antibody CHIR-12.12 in Chronic Lymphocytic Leukemia: Blockade of CD40 Activation and Induction of ADCC." *46th ASH Annual Meeting.*

Xu, Y., R. Oomen, et al. (1994). "Residue at position 331 in the IgG1 and IgG4 CH2 domains contributes to their differential ability to bind and activate complement." *J Biol Chem* **269**(5): 3469–74.

Yazawa, N., Y. Hamaguchi, et al. (2005). "Immunotherapy using unconjugated CD19 monoclonal antibodies in animal models for B lymphocyte malignancies and autoimmune disease." *Proc Natl Acad Sci USA* **102**(42): 15178–83.

Zhang, W., M. Gordon, et al. (2007). "FCGR2A and FCGR3A polymorphisms associated with clinical outcome of epidermal growth factor receptor expressing metastatic colorectal cancer patients treated with single-agent cetuximab." *J Clin Oncol* **25**(24): 3712–8.

Zhukovsky, E., S.Chu, M. Bernett, S. Karki, W. Dang, P. Hammond, C. Edler, N. Polder, C. Chan, J. Jacinto, J. Desjarlais (2007). "XmAb Fc engineered anti-CD19 monoclonal antibodies with enhanced in vitro efficacy against multiple lymphoma cell lines." *Journal of Clinical Oncology,* 2007 ASCO Annual Meeting Proceedings Part I **25**(18S) (June 20 Supplement): 3021.

CHAPTER TEN

Optimization of Fc Domains to Enhance Antibody Therapeutics

Greg A. Lazar and Aaron K. Chamberlain

The Fc region of an antibody is the central link between the targeted antigen and the immune system. It is responsible for mediating a spectrum of effector functions that monoclonal antibodies (mAbs) use against tumors and pathogens. Whereas historically drug developers have kept the Fc region fixed, over the past decade there has been substantial effort to engineer it for improved effector function activity. This new direction has grown from a more mature understanding of the role of immune receptors in antibody therapy and the development of Fc modifications to control antibody/receptor interactions. In this chapter, we discuss how Fc engineering is being used to enhance antibody therapeutics for cellular effector functions, complement-mediated activities, and pharmacokinetic properties.

SITES FOR ENGINEERING AND OPTIMIZABLE PROPERTIES

The Fc region mediates binding of the antibody to all endogenous receptors other than target antigen. Although vaguely defined, an antibody's Fc region typically refers to the C-terminal portion of the hinge and the CH2 and CH3 domains, approximately residues 226 to the C-terminus using the EU numbering scheme.[1] The human effector ligands that bind Fc can be divided into three groups (Figure 10.1): FcγRs, complement protein C1q, and the neonatal Fc receptor FcRn. The FcγRs all bind to essentially the same site on Fc, specifically the lower hinge and proximal CH2 region.[2] Interaction with these receptors can elicit a variety of cellular effector functions that destroy target cells and regulate the immune system. C1q binds to a region in CH2 and the hinge overlapping with the binding site for FcγRs. Interaction with this protein mediates the classical (antibody-dependent) complement pathway that includes both noncellular and cellular cytotoxic mechanisms. Finally, FcRn binds Fc in the interfacial region of the CH2 and CH3 domains, enabling endosomal recycling that determines in part the long serum half-life of antibodies. The principal strategy of all Fc engineering efforts is to optimize the affinity for these effector ligands, and thus the activities that they mediate, to improve the clinical performance of therapeutic mAbs.

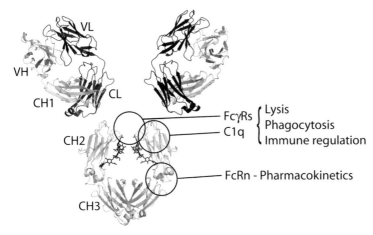

VL

VH

CH1

CL

CH2

FcγRs — Lysis
C1q — Phagocytosis
Immune regulation

FcRn - Pharmacokinetics

CH3

Figure 10.1. Fc sites for engineering. A ribbon diagram of the full-length antibody structure is shown, with light chains shown in black and heavy chains shown in gray. The flexible hinge that links CH1 and CH2 is not shown. Black lines represent the attached carbohydrate at N297. Sites for binding to FcγRs, complement protein C1q, and FcRn are shown, along with the properties that may be optimized by engineering Fc to improve their interaction. FcγRs bind monomerically and asymetrically to the Fc homodimer. In contrast, C1q and FcRn bind to each side of the Fc homodimer (only one side is illustrated), and thus can bind as dimers.

OPTIMIZING FcγR-MEDIATED EFFECTOR FUNCTIONS

FcγR Biology and Links to Therapeutic Relevance

The family of human FcγRs consists of six known members in three subgroups: FcγRI (CD64); FcγRIIa,b,c (CD32a,b,c); and FcγRIIIa,b (CD16a,b). The differences between the receptors in expression, signaling, and affinities for the IgG isotypes make this biological system versatile and highly regulated. Four of the receptors are activating due to their possession of a cytoplasmic immunoreceptor tyrosine-based activation motif (ITAM), which is either part of the receptor polypeptide chain (FcγRIIa,c) or gained by the association of the receptor subunit with a common ITAM γ-chain (FcγRI and FcγRIIIa). In contrast, FcγRIIb possesses an inhibitory motif (ITIM) in its cytoplasmic domain that generates negative intracellular signals that down-regulate effector functions. FcγRIIIb does not signal because it is linked to the membrane with a glycosyl phosphatidyl inositol (GPI) anchor. In the generally accepted mechanism, clustering of receptors by bound immune complexes initiates activating (ITAM) or inhibitory (ITIM) intracellular signaling. Monomeric IgG, in contrast, is unable to initiate signaling of the FcγRII and FcγRIII receptors due to its low affinity (10^{-5} – 10^{-7} M). FcγRI uniquely binds with high affinity (10^{-10} M) to monomeric IgG, and therefore is poor at distinguishing between monomeric IgG and immune complexed antigen.

Allelic variants of the receptors exist that interact differentially with IgG, which can thereby bring about differences in the magnitude of immune response.[3] Two notable polymorphisms with respect to Fc optimization are an H/R variation at position 131 of FcγRIIa and a V/F variation at position 158 of FcγRIIIa. Only the H131 form of FcγRIIa binds IgG2 and is able to carry out IgG2-mediated neutrophil and monocyte phagocytosis.[4–6] For FcγRIIIa, the presence of a valine at position 158 provides the receptor with a higher affinity for IgG1 and IgG3 relative to the phenylalanine form.[7] Many studies have characterized the relationship between these polymorphisms and susceptibility to autoimmune and infectious diseases.[3,8] Correlations between polymorphisms and clinical response to antibody antitumor therapy have also been established.[9]

The differences in receptor expression on various immune cells enable versatility in cellular responses to immune challenge. The cell types that are likely most relevant for therapeutic antibodies are natural killer (NK) cells, monocytes/macrophages, dendritic cells (DCs), and neutrophils (Figure 10.2). Although other cell types such as basophils, eosinophils, mast cells, B cells, and γδ T cells are presumed less relevant for antibody drugs, awareness of their FcγR expression is nonetheless important for the development of antibodies with altered Fc regions. The presence of neutrophils,[10,11] macrophages,[12] DCs,[13] and in some cases NK cells[14] in the tumor microenvironment suggests that they do play a role in fighting tumors. The highly coordinated response by these cell types against infectious pathogens and the role of antibody-mediated immunity in microbial clearance[15,16] are well established. Natural killer cells are unique in that they typically express only the activating receptor FcγRIIIa, although due to allelic variation, some individuals express NK cell FcγRIIc.[17] Cells of the myeloid lineage, including monocytes, macrophages, DCs, and neutrophils, have more complex FcγR expression profiles.[18–21] All express FcγRIIa and the inhibitory receptor FcγRIIb. Macrophages and DCs also express FcγRI and FcγRIIIa depending on their source and activation state. Neutrophils express FcγRI when activated by granulocyte macrophage colony–stimulating factor (GM-CSF) and FcγRIIIb rather than FcγRIIIa. Although FcγRIIIb has no intrinsic signaling capacity, some studies have shown that it can mediate neutrophil effector functions through cooperation or colocalization with other receptors such as FcγRIIa or complement receptor CR3.[22–24]

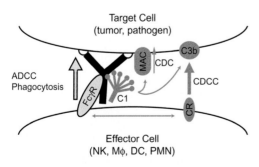

Figure 10.2. FcγR- and complement-mediated effector functions of antibodies. Interaction of antibody (shown in black) with FcγRs expressed on effector cells such as NK cells (NK), macrophages (MΦ), dendritic cells (DC), and neutrophils (PMN) can mediate effector functions such as ADCC and phagocytosis against target tumor or microbial cells. Interaction of antibody with complement protein C1 deposits a variety of complement proteins on the target cell membrane that can mediate noncellular and cellular activities. CDC is a noncellular effector function carried out by the MAC protein complex. In contrast, cellular pathways (CDCC) are mediated by interaction between complement receptors (CR) and opsonic C3b (as well as iC3b and C4b, not shown). Complement receptors also synergize with FcγRs to enhance FcγR-mediated effector functions.

Engagement of FcγRs on these cells by immune-complexed antibody can mediate an array of effector functions including cytolysis, phagocytosis, cytokine and chemokine release, as well as major histocompatibility complex (MHC) presentation and T cell activation (Figure 10.2). Three general sets of results suggest that FcγRs are relevant to clinical efficacy, and thus that optimizing their interactions with Fc is a good strategy for improving therapeutic antibodies. First is the relationship between receptor affinity and *in vitro* effector function. Early mutagenesis work showed not only that the affinity of an IgG for Fc receptors affects antibody-dependent cell-mediated cytotoxicity (ADCC) in cell-based assays, but further that affinity improvements could be used to enhance activity.[25] Second, the dependence of *in vivo* activity on Fc receptors has been well established using animal models. Experiments with genetic knockout mice showed that the common γ-chain, utilized by all murine activating FcγRs, is essential to the antitumor activity for the anti-Her2 antibody trastuzumab (Herceptin®) and the anti-CD20 antibody rituximab (Rituxan®).[26, 27] Later studies also showed that depletion of normal B cells by murine anti-CD20 antibodies is dependent on the common γ-chain and the antibody isotype.[28, 29] Finally, perhaps the most compelling motivation for improving FcγR interactions comes from the greater clinical benefit observed in patients with the higher affinity alleles for activating FcγRs. FcγR polymorphism associations have been studied as predictors of autoimmune disease incidence and susceptibility to microbial infections,[3, 8, 30] and more recently, clinical response to anticancer antibody drugs.[9] The high-affinity (V158) allele of FcγRIIIa is correlated with significantly greater therapeutic benefit from rituximab for treatment of B cell malignancies,[31–35] and trastuzumab for treatment of metastatic breast cancer.[36] Although a number of these studies also documented significant associations with the H131 allele of FcγRIIa, these results appear to be due to linkage disequilibrium between FcγRIIa and FcγRIIIa,[37] consistent with the lack of affinity preference of IgG1 for either FcγRIIa allele. The strongest direct support for FcγRIIa-mediated antitumor effects is the greater progression-free survival observed in neuroblastoma patients with the homozygous R131 genotype when treated with an anti-GD2 murine IgG3 antibody,[38] which binds with greater affinity to the R131 allele relative to the H131 form. Altogether, *in vitro* data, results from animal models, and clinical associations with receptor polymorphisms have firmly established the link between FcγRs and mAb therapeutic activity.

Amino Acid Engineering to Improve FcγR-mediated Effector Functions

Amino acid modification provides a versatile approach for optimizing binding to FcγRs. From the standpoint of protein engineering, controlling FcγR affinity is challenging due to the 1:1 asymmetric binding of the Fc homodimer to monomeric receptor (Figure 10.1) and the virtually identical Fc binding site of the different Fc receptors. Engineering efforts have been aided by the crystal structures of the Fc/FcγRIIIb complex[39,40] and aggressive screening approaches that include alanine scanning and site-directed mutagenesis,[41] computational structure-based design,[42,43] and selection-based methods.[44] Receptor binding has consistently been the primary screen or selection criterion, with subsequent evaluation of selected hits in cell-based effector function assays, typically ADCC. The most well-characterized variants include substitutions at positions 298, 333, and 334;[41] 239, 332, 330, and 236;[42,43] and 243, 292, 300, 305, and 396.[44] However, a much larger number of variants, on the order of thousands, are described in patents, and the Fc region at the FcγR binding interface has been virtually saturated with all possible mutations.

An early goal of engineering efforts was to improve affinity to FcγRIIIa, based primarily on its clinical relevance inferred from polymorphism data and the dominance of NK cells among other peripheral blood mononuclear cell (PBMC) components in ADCC assays. A small number of mutations can create greater affinity for this receptor of between one and two orders of magnitude, providing substantial enhancements in ADCC.[41,42,44] Increased FcγRIIa affinity is another target receptor profile, specifically for the goal of enhancing the effector functions of macrophages, DCs, and neutrophils. Variants with up to 70-fold greater affinity to FcγRIIa relative to native IgG1 have been generated that provide substantial enhancements to macrophage phagocytosis.[43] More challenging goals are selective affinity enhancement to activating receptors relative to the inhibitory receptor FcγRIIb. Variants that improve Fc affinity for FcγRIIIa relative to FcγRIIb have been generated,[41,42,44] although as of yet no clear effector function benefit has been conclusively attributed to this selectivity. Variants have also been engineered that provide selective enhancement to FcγRIIa relative to FcγRIIb,[43] a particularly formidable selectivity to achieve given their near identical extracellular domains (93%). Interestingly, the greater macrophage phagocytosis of these variants depended primarily on their absolute affinity for FcγRIIa, with no impact from FcγRIIb binding, a result that is counter to the perceived role of FcγRIIb for this cell type. This result underscores the value of variants with diverse FcγR affinities for not only improving antibody drugs but also for better understanding FcγR biology.

A major obstacle to exploring which FcγR affinities and selectivities are optimal for improving antibody efficacy is the asymmetry between mouse and human Fc receptor biology. Substantial differences in sequence homology, isotype affinities, and receptor expression patterns[9,45] limit the utility of standard mouse models to study the *in vivo* activity of variants that are engineered for improved interaction with human receptors. Nonetheless, improvements in activity have been demonstrated in standard SCID xenograft models.[46] Animal models that more accurately represent human FcγR biology include mice engrafted transiently with human immune cells, mice engineered transgenically with human receptors, and cynomolgus monkeys. Experiments exploring the impact of Fc variants in mice transgenic for human FcγRIIIa[44] and in monkey B cell depletion models[42,47] have confirmed that the affinity/activity relationship observed *in vitro* does indeed translate to greater antibody activity *in vivo*. Antibody drug candidates with some of these variants, which represent the first generation of therapeutic mAbs Fc-engineered for enhanced cytotoxicity, are just beginning to make their entry into clinical trials.[9]

Glycoengineering to Improve FcγR-mediated Effector Functions

The development of glycoform engineering as a strategy for improving effector function was motivated by the observation that ADCC is affected by different Asn297 carbohydrate compositions, produced by varying cell line and culture conditions.[48] The earliest attempts to control Fc glycosylation involved overexpression of β(1,4)-*N*-acetylglucosaminyltransferase III (GnTIII), which causes both a lack of fucose and a bisecting *N*-acetylglucosamine (GlcNAc). Originally it was not clear which modifications were responsible for the improved ADCC activity.[49,50] Later work, however, showed that the absence of fucose is the sole determinant of enhanced FcγR affinity,[51,52] suggesting that the impact of GnTIII was due not to bisecting GlcNAc directly but rather its preclusion of subsequent modification by α1,6-fucosyltransferase.

Much of the work studying the impact of glycoforms on antibody activity has been carried out with the Chinese hamster ovary (CHO) cell line Lec13 and the rat hybridoma cell line YB2/0, which naturally generate fucose-deficient antibodies. These cells, however, are impractical for large scale mAb manufacturing because they are poor at antibody expression and produce mixtures of fucosylated and afucosylated antibodies. Engineered CHO cell lines that more robustly and efficiently produce afucosylated antibodies inducibly express GnTIII[49] or are deleted for the enzyme α-1,6-fucosyltransferase (FUT8).[53] Non-mammalian expression systems lacking fucosylation enzymes have been also been engineered in yeast, plants, and moss.[54–56] Afucosylated antibodies produced by these methods, in general, provide one to two orders of magnitude greater affinity for both iosoforms of FcγRIIIa.[57,58] The same challenges of characterization in mouse models apply equally to glycoengineered antibodies. Notably, improved antitumor activity has been demonstrated for an afucosylated antibody using mice engrafted with human PBMCs.[59] Clinical candidates based on some of these glycoengineering technologies are currently being developed, the most advanced of which is an anti-GD3 antibody being tested for metastatic melanoma.[60]

There has been some incertitude regarding the mechanism by which afucosylation increases FcγR affinity and ADCC. Structural work has suggested that absence of fucose causes subtle conformational changes that result in improved FcγR binding.[61] In contrast, other studies have indicated that removal of Fc fucose relieves a steric interaction between Fc and a receptor carbohydrate at Asn162.[57] The latter model is supported by the lack of enhancement by afucosylation when receptor carbohydrate is removed enzymatically,[57] and the binding improvement to only human FcγRIIIa/b and mouse FcγRIV,[57,62] which are the only receptors in these organisms that possess an asparagine at the 162 position. The affinity increase by glycoengineering to only FcγRIIIa/b among the human receptors highlights a key distinction from amino acid modifications, which can create a more diverse range of effects. The receptor carbohydrate mechanism has several ramifications. First, it suggests that variability in FcγRIIIa glycosylation, known to occur for some effector cell types,[63,64] could impact *in vivo* benefit. Second, it reaffirms that lack of fucose is the most important if not the sole factor for enhancement, and accordingly, that afucosylation is afucosylation irrespective of the method used to generate it. Thus the only difference between the various expression systems with respect to receptor enhancement should be percentage of afucosylated antibody and commercial viability. A cautionary note is that although lack of fucose appears to be the only modification that improves FcγRIIIa affinity, other sugar structures can adversely affect antibody Fc properties.[65,66]

Target FcγR Profiles for Improving Therapeutic mAb Activity

A current gap for Fc engineering efforts is the lack of clarity regarding the optimal FcγR profile(s) for a given indication, antigen, and antibody. There is an incomplete understanding of the roles of different immune cell types in destroying tumor or pathogenic target cells *in vivo*, and the specific FcγR-dependencies of each cell type are poorly defined. Natural killer cells have developed a prominent reputation as target cell killers due to their efficient ADCC of antibody-opsonized tumor cells lines *in vitro*.[67] Moreover, the correlations observed between clinical response to rituximab and FcγRIIIa polymorphism have foremost been attributed to the involvement of NK cells, a plausible hypothesis given that they express only this receptor among the FcγRs. However, despite the recent observation of NK cells in breast cancer tissue after treatment with trastuzumab,[14] the capacity of NK cells to infiltrate solid tumors is generally considered poor.[68] FcγR-positive effector populations with stronger reputations for infiltrating tumors are the monocytic phagocytes, including macrophages[12] and DCs[13] as well as neutrophils.[10,11] The importance of monocytes in antibody-mediated tumor reduction is supported by data from mouse models.[28,29] Macrophages and DCs express FcγRIIIa, and the correlations observed between polymorphism of this receptor and clinical outcome apply equally to these cell types as they do to NK cells. Recent data have indicated that FcγRIIa in particular is a key receptor for macrophages, with smaller contributions from FcγRI and FcγRIIIa, and no impact from FcγRIIb.[43] Dendritic cells have also been shown to be dependent on FcγRIIa for immune-complex stimulated maturation,[18] an important step in cross-presentation of target cell–derived antigens to antitumor cytotoxic T cells (CTLs).[69] Neutrophil ADCC is also known to be strongly dependent on FcγRIIa, with a cooperative role for FcγRIIIb.[22,23,70] Given the strong involvement of FcγRIIa in their effector functions and their capacity to infiltrate tumors, the observed correlations between FcγRIIa polymorphism and clinical outcome[38] would seem to support a role for macrophages, DCs, and/or neutrophils in antibody efficacy.

Overall, the current data support the greatest roles for FcγRIIa, FcγRIIb, and FcγRIIIa,[9] and thus far the emphasis of Fc engineering has been on optimizing interaction profiles with these receptors. At first glance, the ideal FcγR selectivity profile of an engineered antibody would be high affinity for FcγRIIa and FcγRIIIa but low affinity for the inhibitory FcγRIIb. A significant obstacle to such specificity is the high homology between these receptors, particularly FcγRIIa and FcγRIIb. Whether a single optimal FcγR selectivity profile exists for cytotoxic mAbs or whether practically the best set of receptor affinities is a compromise remains to be determined. Addressing this question will no doubt become more feasible as the toolkit of Fc variants becomes more diverse.

OPTIMIZING COMPLEMENT-MEDIATED EFFECTOR FUNCTIONS

Complement Biology and Links to Therapeutic Relevance

The classical, or antibody-dependent, complement pathway is initiated by binding of complement protein C1q to the antibody Fc region. A series of reactions results that ultimately leads to deposition on the target cell of complement proteins that mediate both noncellular and cellular cytotoxic mechanisms (Figure 10.2). The most widely recognized mechanism of target cell destruction is noncellular, referred to as complement-dependent cytotoxicity (CDC), and is mediated by the membrane attack complex (MAC or C5b-9). Cellular mechanisms are mediated by interaction between opsonic C3 and C4 components (specifically C3b, iC3b, and C4b) and complement receptors (CR1, CR3, and CR4) expressed on effector cells. One of these mechanisms is mediated by direct binding of CR to opsonin and is referred to as complement-dependent cell-mediated cytotoxicity (CDCC), or CR-dependent cellular cytotoxicity (CR-DCC). This activity is activated by cell wall β-glucan and thus is thought to be relevant against pathogenic target cells but not tumors. The other cellular mechanism involves enhancement of FcγR-mediated effector functions by the CR/opsonin interaction. This activity does not require micro-organism danger signals, making it a potential cytotoxic mechanism for both antitumor and anti-infectious disease antibodies. CR-enhancement of FcγR-mediated effector functions is activated by opsonic complement protein C5a, which is chemotactic for effector cells and also selectively increases expression of activating FcγRs relative to FcγRIIb on macrophages.[71,72] Thus, there is significant synergy between complement and FcγR effector pathways (Figure 10.2).

In vitro and *in vivo* data support the role of complement in the antimicrobial activity of mAbs.[73–76] Indeed, infectious diseases are the most intuitive applications for complement-enhanced mAbs, given the activation of complement pathways by microbial surfaces. However, little clinical support is available due to the low number of antipathogen antibody drugs that have progressed through clinical trials.[77] For anticancer applications, the role of complement is generally not well established. Doubts arise particularly because tumors overexpress complement regulatory proteins (CRPs) that protect them from complement-mediated injury.[78,79] However, *in vivo* work with an anti-GD2 antibody demonstrated complement mechanisms against tumor cells even when they expressed high levels of complement inhibitors.[80] For anti-CD20, the most well studied system for complement activity, some experiments in animal models have demonstrated a dependence of activity on complement,[81–83] whereas others have not.[29,84] Similarly, although expression of CRPs in lymphoma patients correlates with a lower response to rituximab,[85,86] no differences in complement-mediated cytotoxicity *in vitro* were observed using tumor cells from the different response groups.[87] A strong argument for a role for complement is that complement is consumed in chronic lymphocytic leukemia (CLL) patients as a result of rituximab treatment.[88] In addition, recent work has investigated the relationship between complement polymorphisms and clinical response, similar to the FcγR studies, and has found an association between C1q polymorphism and breast cancer metastasis.[89]

Amino Acid Engineering to Improve Complement-mediated Effector Functions

Although a structure of the Fc/C1q complex is unavailable, mutagenesis data have aided engineering by elucidating the role of the hinge and Fc positions 234, 235, 270, 322, 326, 329, 331, and 333 in binding.[90–96] An important consideration for Fc engineering is that this site overlaps with the binding site for FcγRs (Figure 10.1). Several groups have successfully engineered mutations that improve mAb/complement interactions and *in vitro* complement-dependent cytotoxicity (CDC), including substitutions at 326 and 333,[97] hinge modifications,[98] and IgG1/IgG3 isotype switch variants.[99] Some work has been aimed at increasing the valency of antibody and target antigen, a critical parameter for complement activity. Generation of covalent dimers by engineering C-terminal disulfide bonds resulted in up to 200-fold greater CDC activity.[100]

Recent data showing improved B cell depletion in a monkey model by an engineered anti-CD20 with improved C1q affinity and CDC has provided important *in vivo* validation for the strategy.[99] Because of the early stage, as of yet there are no antibodies in clinical development with modifications that improve complement activity. Obviously, the first such antibody drug will be an important test for this area of Fc engineering. Given the overlapping biochemistry, it will be particularly exciting to see how enhanced complement activity may synergize with enhanced FcγR-mediated effects.

REMOVING Fc-MEDIATED EFFECTOR FUNCTIONS

The removal of FcγR- and/or complement-mediated effector functions may also be a means for improving the clinical properties of antibodies. "Knockout" or "silent" Fc regions can be valuable when FcγR and/or complement interactions result in off-mechanism toxicity, when the goal is to block a surface antigen but not deplete the target cell, or when the primary application of a non-cytotoxic antibody is co-therapy with one that is – for example, an anti-angiogenic or immunomodulatory mAb with one that targets a tumor. Additionally, FcγRs and complement provide mechanisms of elimination, and thus reducing antibody interactions with them can potentially result in improved pharmacokinetic properties.[101,102] A critical criterion for engineering a therapeutic candidate with silent Fc regions, and often a difficult one to meet, is the knowledge that FcγR- and/or complement-mediated effects are definitively not part of a mAb's mechanism of action.

Use of IgG Isotypes to Reduce Fc-mediated Activities

The use of weaker effector function isotypes, specifically human IgG2 and IgG4, is one approach to reducing Fc-mediated effects. However, although the Fc's of these isotypes are typically not as potent as IgG1 and IgG3, the view that they are absent FcγR binding and effector function is inaccurate. IgG2 binds with significant affinity to FcγRIIa, particularly the H131 allele, allowing it to promote phagocytic capacity by neutrophils and monocytes.[5,6] IgG4 binds with high affinity to FcγRI and weak but significant affinity to FcγRIIa/b and is capable of Fc-mediated effects.[103] The engagement of Fc receptors by IgG4 has been suggested as a possible explanation for the disastrous clinical outcome of TGN1412,[104] an anti-CD28 antibody that caused a dangerous cytokine storm in six Phase I patients. The superior bactericidal activity of IgG2 and IgG4 relative to the IgG1 and IgG3 in a fungal infection model[105] further supports the notion that the natural immunology is more complex than high- and low-effector function isotypes. Another important consideration for drug development is that the IgG2 and IgG4 isotypes can exhibit problematic solution properties. In particular, IgG4 heavy chains readily exchange with one another. This process occurs regardless of antigen specificity, and thus exchange can create heterogenous mixtures of homodimeric and heterodimeric antibodies.[106] There is also some indication that IgG2 can form covalent dimers, a property apparently related to its disulfide pairing.[107] Overall, the differences between the IgG isotypes are not simplistic, and selection of which isotype best suits a clinical candidate requires careful consideration.[108]

Amino Acid Engineering to Reduce Fc-mediated Activities

The residual Fc interactions of IgG2 and IgG4 and their suboptimal solution properties have motivated efforts to engineer silent Fc's. The generation of knockout variants with minimal creation of new epitopes has been accomplished using inter-sequence variants of the IgG1, IgG2, and IgG4 isotypes.[109,110] Reduction of the unfavorable exchange behavior of IgG4 has also been achieved using amino acid modifications.[111] Much of the engineering work in this area has been carried in the context of anti-CD3 and anti-CD4 mAbs, the most well-characterized cases for which Fc interactions are undesirable.[112,113] Muromonab-CD3 (Orthoclone OKT3) is a murine anti-CD3 antibody used for transplant rejection, whose beneficial Fv-mediated activity is corrupted by off-mechanism Fc-mediated effects, specifically the rapid induction of a cytokine storm upon administration.[112,114,115] Variant Fc domains created to address this problem include an N297A IgG1 variant that lacks Fc carbohydrate,[116] L234A/L235A variants of IgG1 and IgG4 isotypes,[117] and a V234A/G237A variant of IgG2.[118] Successfully, Phase I clinical trials of these variant mAbs demonstrated that they maintain Fv-mediated immunosuppressive activity yet elicit minimal acute side effects.[119–121] In the case of an anti-CD4 antibody, the IgG4 isotype was mutated with L235E to reduce residual FcγRI binding and with S228P to stabilize the hinge disulfides and reduce heavy chain exchange.[113,122] This antibody, referred to as IgG4-PE, retained the Fv-mediated capacity to inhibit CD4 interaction with MHC II, but did not deplete CD4+ T cells in a chimpanzee model.[113,122] The successful preclinical and clinical results with these modified anti-CD3 and -CD4 antibodies illustrate how simple but well-designed modifications can dramatically improve the *in vivo* properties of therapeutic mAbs.

OPTIMIZING INTERACTION WITH FcRn

FcRn Biology and IgG Homeostasis

The role of the neonatal Fc receptor, FcRn, in IgG homeostasis and transport across epithelial barriers provides the foundation for Fc engineering efforts aimed at improving the pharmacokinetic (PK) properties of antibodies and Fc fusions. FcRn is a heterodimer of a 50kD alpha chain and an 18kD beta chain known as beta-2-microglobulin. FcRn has also been called the IgG protection receptor or the Brambell receptor after Brambell's hypothesis that an Fc receptor mediates IgG catabolism and transport from the mother to neonate.[123,124] It has also been referred to as the MHC-class I-related receptor because of its structural similarity to MHC-I. For more detail on FcRn biology and function, the reader is referred to a number of useful reviews and to the chapter by Andersen and Sandlie in this book.[125–127]

FcRn protects IgG from degradation and is therefore responsible in part for the long half-lives (~21 days) of antibodies in circulation. The first indication of this function was the observation that IgG of mice lacking beta-2-microglobulin have a much shorter half-life and lower serum concentrations than IgG of normal mice.[128] More recently, this result was demonstrated in mice lacking the FcRn heavy chain.[129] Mechanistically, FcRn protects IgG from degradation by binding IgG in endosomes and recycling it to the cell surface (Figure 10.3). Central to this mechanism is the pH-dependent binding of the IgG/FcRn interaction. Due to several histidines at the interface, FcRn binds IgG at the low pH of the endosome (pH 6–6.5), but not at the higher pH of blood (pH 7.4). Endosomal IgG/FcRn binding salvages IgG from lysosomal degradation,[130] as evidenced by the rapid turnover of antibodies lacking an Fc domain or antibodies with a point mutant (H435A) that disrupts receptor binding.[131] The transport of IgG back to the membrane can occur in small vesicles moving from the endosome to the membrane or through tubular structures linking the endosome to a fairly distant portion of the membrane.[132] Variation is also seen in the exocytic vesicle fusion with the membrane, which can be a complete fusion event or can involve only partial mixing of membrane components and a slower release of vesicle contents.[133] Interestingly, in some of the slower releasing vesicles, the IgG does not appear to dissociate completely from FcRn, which may indicate that the local pH does not fully raise to the external pH or that the IgG remains

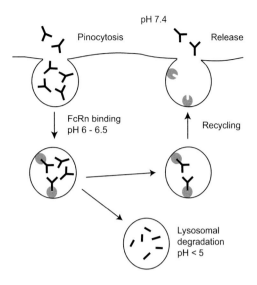

Figure 10.3. Mechanism of FcRn-mediated endosomal recycling of antibodies. Antibodies (black) are pinocytosed from circulation by endothelial (and other) cells. FcRn (gray) binds antibody at pH 6–6.5. Unbound antibodies are sorted to the lysosome where they are degraded at lower pH. In contrast, bound antibodies are recycled to the cell membrane where they are released back into circulation due to lack of binding at physiological pH.

bound at the higher pH. These complexities, and the incomplete understanding of the process by which FcRn traffics antibodies, present obstacles to engineering efforts aimed at controlling antibody PK. Nonetheless, the well-established role of FcRn in IgG serum turnover and the importance of pH to the interaction provide the opportunity to control antibody half-lives.

Engineering Optimized Interaction with FcRn to Improve PK

FcRn binds to IgG in the interface between the CH2 and CH3 domains (Figure 10.1),[134,135] allowing one Fc domain to bind two FcRn molecules.[136] This site also mediates binding to microbial proteins A and G, an important consideration for engineering work given the use of these reagents for large-scale manufacturing. Early mutagenesis studies with mouse IgG1 provided important structural characterization of the Fc binding site, demonstrating the particular importance of I253 and histidines at positions 310 and 435.[137,138] To date, literally hundreds of mutations to human IgG have been made in the interface region to study the contribution of each residue and to select mutations that improve FcRn binding.[41,139–144]

An early obstacle to establishing improved PK *in vivo* was the irregular binding of human IgG to mouse FcRn, specifically the binding of human IgG to mouse FcRn with 10-fold greater affinity than to human FcRn. The first engineered antibodies tested in mice, including most notably a M252Y/S254T/T256E variant, resulted in reduced antibody serum concentrations relative to native IgG1 and no discernible changes in half-life.[139] This result was attributed to the inability of recycled variant antibodies to release from FcRn even at the higher pH of the extracellular environment. Experiments in cynomolgus monkeys, whose FcRn is more similar to that of human, have shown increased half-life by antibody variants engineered by several different groups. A T250Q/M428L variant of an anti-hepatitis B virus antibody increased the terminal half-life to 27.2 days (IgG2 antibody) or 34 days (IgG1 antibody) compared to 14 days for the WT (IgG1 or IgG2).[140,145] The M252Y/S254T/T256E variant, which reduced serum concentration in mice, showed a 21 day half-life in monkeys compared to 6 days for native IgG1 in the context of an antirespiratory sincytial virus (RSV) antibody.[146] Finally, an N434A variant increased the half-life of an anti-BR3 antibody from 9.0 days to 14.1 days.[141]

Importantly, variants with increased FcRn binding have not always improved antibody serum half-life in cynomolgus monkeys. In one study, the T250Q/M428L variant and a P257I/Q311I variant with similarly improved FcRn affinity had wild-type pharmacokinetics.[147] These variants were constructed in an anti-TNF antibody and injected at a low dose of 0.5 or 0.75 mg/kg. The reason for the negative results with these variants is not clear, though it may be that lack of antigen saturation due to the low dose precluded FcRn binding. Moreover, although increased half-life can clearly be achieved with improved FcRn binding, correlations between FcRn affinity and half-life have been shown to be poor.[148] The measurements of binding affinity are also complicated by the 2:1 binding ratio of FcRn to IgG and possibly other factors that require more sophisticated modeling to interpret.[149] Finally, antigen binding, effector functions, immunogenicity, stability, and protease sensitivity may all affect antibody pharmacokinetics in ways that are little understood at the present moment. Predicting which FcRn variants will improve and what other parameters impact serum half-life remains a challenging task for the field.

Fortunately, mice containing human FcRn and lacking endogenous murine FcRn have been created and used successfully to study the half-lives of variant antibodies.[150] In these transgenic mice, the N434A variant, which demonstrated improved PK in monkeys, resulted in a half-life of 3.9 days compared to 1.7 days for the native IgG1. The half-life shortened to only 1 day using either FcRn$^{-/-}$ mice or a knockout variant, I253A, further confirming the FcRn dependence. In our own work with these mice, engineered variants with improved FcRn affinity increase half-life from 2.6 days to over 9 days (unpublished results). These human FcRn mice greatly facilitate *in vivo* studies relative to the more laborious and costly cynomolgus studies and will help researchers develop a better understanding of the relationship between FcRn affinity and half-life.

Biologics with increased half-lives may allow less frequent dosing schedules, enabling lower cost and greater convenience to patients and medical staff. This advantage is the principal aim of the extended half-life version of the anti-RSV antibody palivizumab (Synagis®), which is to our knowledge the only antibody engineered for greater FcRn affinity under development.[146] An additional and intriguing application of variants with improved FcRn binding is their potential to reduce the concentration of endogenous autoantibodies for treatment of autoimmune diseases.[151,152] As the PK benefit of Fc variants engineered for FcRn binding becomes more established clinically, we will no doubt see their expanded use in therapeutic agents.

SUMMARY

Fc engineering exploits the relationship between the affinity of an antibody for Fc effector ligands and the activities that they mediate. A growing variety of amino acid and glycoform modifications provide drug developers with the capacity to control antibody interactions with FcγRs, complement, and FcRn in order to tune them for optimized immunological and pharmacokinetic properties. Though challenges remain, particularly with respect to understanding the precise mechanisms by which Fc mediates its various effects, the potential of these modifications to improve the performance of antibody drugs is enormous. The current clinical development of a number of Fc-engineered antibodies based on these optimizations is both a sign of progress, and a harbinger of greater improvements to come.

REFERENCES

[1] Edelman, G.M. et al. (1969) The covalent structure of an entire gammaG immunoglobulin molecule. *Proc Natl Acad Sci USA* **63**(1), 78–85.

[2] Sondermann, P. et al. (2001) Molecular basis for immune complex recognition: a comparison of Fc-receptor structures. *J Mol Biol* **309**(3), 737–749.

[3] van Sorge, N.M. et al. (2003) FcgammaR polymorphisms: Implications for function, disease susceptibility and immunotherapy. *Tissue Antigens* **61**(3), 189–202.

[4] Parren, P.W. et al. (1992) On the interaction of IgG subclasses with the low affinity Fc gamma RIIa (CD32) on human monocytes, neutrophils, and platelets. Analysis of a functional polymorphism to human IgG2. *J Clin Invest* **90**(4), 1537–1546.

[5] Salmon, J.E. et al. (1992) Allelic polymorphisms of human Fc gamma receptor IIA and Fc gamma receptor IIIB. Independent mechanisms for differences in human phagocyte function. *J Clin Invest* **89**(4), 1274–1281.

[6] Sanders, L.A. et al. (1995) Human immunoglobulin G (IgG) Fc receptor IIA (CD32) polymorphism and IgG2-mediated bacterial phagocytosis by neutrophils. *Infect Immun* **63**(1), 73–81.

[7] Koene, H.R. et al. (1997) Fc gammaRIIIa-158V/F polymorphism influences the binding of IgG by natural killer cell Fc gammaRIIIa, independently of the Fc gammaRIIIa-48L/R/H phenotype. *Blood* **90**(3), 1109–1114.

[8] Lehrnbecher, T. et al. (1999) Variant genotypes of the low-affinity Fcgamma receptors in two control populations and a review of low-affinity Fcgamma receptor polymorphisms in control and disease populations. *Blood* **94**(12), 4220–4232.

[9] Desjarlais, J.R. et al. (2007) Optimizing engagement of the immune system by anti-tumor antibodies: an engineer's perspective. *Drug Discov. Today* **12**(21–22), 898–910.

[10] van Egmond, M. (2008) Neutrophils in antibody-based immunotherapy of cancer. *Expert Opin Biol Ther* **8**(1), 83–94.

[11] Di Carlo, E. et al. (2001) The intriguing role of polymorphonuclear neutrophils in antitumor reactions. *Blood* **97**(2), 339–345.

[12] Mantovani, A. et al. (2002) Macrophage polarization: tumor-associated macrophages as a paradigm for polarized M2 mononuclear phagocytes. *Trends Immunol* **23**(11), 549–555.

[13] Guiducci, C. et al. (2005) Redirecting in vivo elicited tumor infiltrating macrophages and dendritic cells towards tumor rejection. *Cancer Res* **65**(8), 3437–3446.

[14] Arnould, L. et al. (2006) Trastuzumab-based treatment of HER2-positive breast cancer: an antibody-dependent cellular cytotoxicity mechanism? *Br J Cancer* **94**(2), 259–267.

[15] Casadevall, A. and Pirofski, L.A. (2004) New concepts in antibody-mediated immunity. *Infect. Immun.* **72**(11), 6191–6196.

[16] Keller, M.A. and Stiehm, E.R. (2000) Passive immunity in prevention and treatment of infectious diseases. *Clin. Microbiol. Rev.* **13**(4), 602–614.

[17] Ernst, L.K. et al. (2002) Allelic polymorphisms in the FcgammaRIIC gene can influence its function on normal human natural killer cells. *J Mol Med* **80**(4), 248–257.

[18] Boruchov, A.M. et al. (2005) Activating and inhibitory IgG Fc receptors on human DCs mediate opposing functions. *J Clin Invest* **115**(10), 2914–2923.

[19] Michon, J.M. et al. (1998) In vivo induction of functional Fc gammaRI (CD64) on neutrophils and modulation of blood cytokine mRNA levels in cancer patients treated with G-CSF (rMetHuG-CSF). *Br J Haematol* **100**(3), 550–556.

[20] Pricop, L. et al. (2001) Differential modulation of stimulatory and inhibitory Fc gamma receptors on human monocytes by Th1 and Th2 cytokines. *J Immunol* **166**(1), 531–537.

[21] Schakel, K. et al. (1998) A novel dendritic cell population in human blood: one-step immunomagnetic isolation by a specific mAb (M-DC8) and *in vitro* priming of cytotoxic T lymphocytes. *Eur J Immunol* **28**(12), 4084–4093.

[22] Edberg, J.C. et al. (1998) Differential regulation of human neutrophil FcgammaRIIa (CD32) and FcgammaRIIIb (CD16)-induced Ca2+ transients. *J Biol Chem* **273**(14), 8071–8079.

[23] Fernandes, M.J. et al. (2006) CD16b associates with high-density, detergent-resistant membranes in human neutrophils. *Biochem J* **393**(Pt 1), 351–359.

[24] Stockinger, H. (1997) Interaction of GPI-anchored cell surface proteins and complement receptor type 3. *Exp Clin Immunogenet* **14**(1), 5–10.

[25] Clark, M.R. (1997) IgG effector mechanisms. *Chem Immunol* **65**, 88–110.

[26] Clynes, R. et al. (1998) Fc receptors are required in passive and active immunity to melanoma. *Proc Natl Acad Sci USA* **95**(2), 652–656.

[27] Clynes, R.A. et al. (2000) Inhibitory Fc receptors modulate in vivo cytoxicity against tumor targets. *Nat Med* **6**(4), 443–446.

[28] Hamaguchi, Y. et al. (2006) Antibody isotype-specific engagement of Fcgamma receptors regulates B lymphocyte depletion during CD20 immunotherapy. *J Exp Med* **203**(3), 743–753.

[29] Uchida, J. et al. (2004) The innate mononuclear phagocyte network depletes B lymphocytes through Fc receptor-dependent mechanisms during anti-CD20 antibody immunotherapy. *J Exp Med* **199**(12), 1659–1669.

[30] Karassa, F.B. et al. (2004) The role of FcgammaRIIA and IIIA polymorphisms in autoimmune diseases. *Biomed Pharmacother* **58**(5), 286–291.

[31] Cartron, G. et al. (2002) Therapeutic activity of humanized anti-CD20 monoclonal antibody and polymorphism in IgG Fc receptor FcgammaRIIIa gene. *Blood* **99**(3), 754–758.

[32] Kim, D.H. et al. (2006) FCGR3A gene polymorphisms may correlate with response to frontline R-CHOP therapy for diffuse large B-cell lymphoma. *Blood* **108**(8), 2720–2725.

[33] Weng, W.K. and Levy, R. (2003) Two immunoglobulin G fragment C receptor polymorphisms independently predict response to rituximab in patients with follicular lymphoma. *J Clin Oncol* **21**(21), 3940–3947.

[34] Weng, W.K. and Levy, R. (2005) Genetic polymorphism of the inhibitory IgG Fc receptor Fc gamma RIIb is not associated with clinical outcome of rituximab treated follicular lymphoma patients. ASH Annual Meeting, Abstract 2430.

[35] Treon, S.P. et al. (2005) Polymorphisms in FcgammaRIIIA (CD16) receptor expression are associated with clinical response to rituximab in Waldenstrom's macroglobulinemia. *J Clin Oncol* **23**(3), 474–481.

[36] Musolino, A. et al. (2007) Immunoglobulin G fragment C receptor polymorphisms and response to trastuzumab-based treatment in patients with HER-2/neu-positive metastatic breast cancer. AACR Annual Meeting, Abstract 4188.

[37] Hatjiharissi, E. et al. (2007) Genetic linkage of Fc gamma RIIa and Fc gamma RIIIa and implications for their use in predicting clinical responses to CD20-directed monoclonal antibody therapy. *Clin Lymphoma Myeloma* **7**(4), 286–290.

[38] Cheung, N.K. et al. (2006) FCGR2A polymorphism is correlated with clinical outcome after immunotherapy of neuroblastoma with anti-GD2 antibody and granulocyte macrophage colony-stimulating factor. *J Clin Oncol* **24**(18), 2885–2890.

[39] Radaev, S. et al. (2001) The structure of a human type III Fcγ receptor in complex with Fc. *J Biol Chem* **276**(19), 16469–16477.

[40] Sondermann, P. et al. (2000) The 3.2-A crystal structure of the human IgG1 Fc fragment-FcγRIII complex. *Nature* **406**(6793), 267–273.

[41] Shields, R.L. et al. (2001) High resolution mapping of the binding site on human IgG1 for Fc gamma RI, Fc gamma RII, Fc gamma RIII, and FcRn and design of IgG1 variants with improved binding to the Fc gamma R. *J Biol Chem* **276**(9), 6591–6604.

[42] Lazar, G.A. et al. (2006) Engineered antibody Fc variants with enhanced effector function. *Proc Natl Acad Sci USA* **103**(11), 4005–4010.

[43] Richards, J.O. et al. (2008) Optimization of antibody binding to FcγRIIa enhances macrophage phagocytosis of tumor cells. *Molecular Cancer Therapeutics*, **7**(8), 2517–2527.

[44] Stavenhagen, J.B. et al. (2007) Fc optimization of therapeutic antibodies enhances their ability to kill tumor cells in vitro and controls tumor expansion *in vivo* via low-affinity activating Fcgamma receptors. *Cancer Res* **67**(18), 8882–8890.

[45] Clynes, R. (2006) Antitumor antibodies in the treatment of cancer: Fc receptors link opsonic antibody with cellular immunity. *Hematol Oncol Clin North Am* **20**(3), 585–612.

[46] Horton et al. (2008) Potent in vitro and in vivo activity of an Fc-engineered anti-CD19 monoclonal antibody against lymphoma and leukemia. *Cancer Res* **68**(19), 8049–8057.

[47] Zalevsky et al. (2009) The impact of Fc engineering on an anti-CD19 antibody: increased Fc gamma receptor affinity enhances B-cell clearing in nonhuman primates. *Blood*, in press.

[48] Lifely, M.R. et al. (1995) Glycosylation and biological activity of CAMPATH-1H expressed in different cell lines and grown under different culture conditions. *Glycobiology* **5**(8), 813–822.

[49] Umana, P. et al. (1999) Engineered glycoforms of an antineuroblastoma IgG1 with optimized antibody-dependent cellular cytotoxic activity. *Nat Biotechnol* **17**(2), 176–180.

[50] Davies, J. et al. (2001) Expression of GnTIII in a recombinant anti-CD20 CHO production cell line: Expression of antibodies with altered glycoforms leads to an increase in ADCC through higher affinity for FC gamma RIII. *Biotechnol Bioeng* **74**(4), 288–294.

[51] Shinkawa, T. et al. (2003) The absence of fucose but not the presence of galactose or bisecting N-acetylglucosamine of human IgG1 complex-type oligosaccharides shows the critical role of enhancing antibody-dependent cellular cytotoxicity. *J Biol Chem* **278**(5), 3466–3473.

[52] Shields, R.L. et al. (2002) Lack of fucose on human IgG1 N-linked oligosaccharide improves binding to human Fcgamma RIII and antibody-dependent cellular toxicity. *J Biol Chem* **277**(30), 26733–26740.

[53] Yamane-Ohnuki, N. et al. (2004) Establishment of FUT8 knockout Chinese hamster ovary cells: an ideal host cell line for producing completely defucosylated antibodies with enhanced antibody-dependent cellular cytotoxicity. *Biotechnol Bioeng* **87**(5), 614–622.

[54] Cox, K.M. et al. (2006) Glycan optimization of a human monoclonal antibody in the aquatic plant Lemna minor. *Nat Biotechnol* **24**(12), 1591–1597.

[55] Li, H. et al. (2006) Optimization of humanized IgGs in glycoengineered Pichia pastoris. *Nat Biotechnol* **24**(2), 210–215.

[56] Nechansky, A. et al. (2007) Compensation of endogenous IgG mediated inhibition of antibody-dependent cellular cytotoxicity by glyco-engineering of therapeutic antibodies. *Mol Immunol* **44**(7), 1815–1817.

[57] Ferrara, C. et al. (2006) The carbohydrate at FcgammaRIIIa Asn-162. An element required for high affinity binding to non-fucosylated IgG glycoforms. *J Biol Chem* **281**(8), 5032–5036.

[58] Okazaki, A. et al. (2004) Fucose depletion from human IgG1 oligosaccharide enhances binding enthalpy and association rate between IgG1 and FcgammaRIIIa. *J Mol Biol* **336**(5), 1239–1249.

[59] Niwa, R. et al. (2004) Defucosylated chimeric anti-CC chemokine receptor 4 IgG1 with enhanced antibody-dependent cellular cytotoxicity shows potent therapeutic activity to T-cell leukemia and lymphoma. *Cancer Res* **64**(6), 2127–2133.

[60] Forero, A. et al. (2006) A phase I study of an anti-GD3 monoclonal antibody, KW-2871, in patients with metastatic melanoma. *Cancer Biother Radiopharm* **21**(6), 561–568.

[61] Matsumiya, S. et al. (2007) Structural comparison of fucosylated and nonfucosylated Fc fragments of human immunoglobulin G1. *J Mol Biol* **368**(3), 767–779.

[62] Masuda, K. et al. (2007) Enhanced binding affinity for FcgammaRIIIa of fucose-negative antibody is sufficient to induce maximal antibody-dependent cellular cytotoxicity. *Mol Immunol.*

[63] Drescher, B. et al. (2003) Glycosylation of FcgammaRIII in N163 as mechanism of regulating receptor affinity. *Immunology* **110**(3), 335–340.

[64] Edberg, J.C. and Kimberly, R.P. (1997) Cell type-specific glycoforms of Fc gamma RIIIa (CD16): differential ligand binding. *J Immunol* **159**(8), 3849–3857.

[65] Kanda, Y. et al. (2007) Comparison of biological activity among nonfucosylated therapeutic IgG1 antibodies with three different N-linked Fc oligosaccharides: the high-mannose, hybrid, and complex types. *Glycobiology* **17**(1), 104–118.

[66] Scallon, B.J. et al. (2007) Higher levels of sialylated Fc glycans in immunoglobulin G molecules can adversely impact functionality. *Mol Immunol* **44**(7), 1524–1534.

[67] Abdullah, N. et al. (1999) The role of monocytes and natural killer cells in mediating antibody-dependent lysis of colorectal tumour cells. *Cancer Immunol Immunother* **48**(9), 517–524.

[68] Albertsson, P.A. et al. (2003) NK cells and the tumour microenvironment: implications for NK-cell function and anti-tumour activity. *Trends Immunol* **24**(11), 603–609.

[69] Dhodapkar, K.M. et al. (2005) Selective blockade of inhibitory Fcgamma receptor enables human dendritic cell maturation with IL-12p70 production and immunity to antibody-coated tumor cells. *Proc Natl Acad Sci USA* **102**(8), 2910–2915.

[70] Nagarajan, S. et al. (2000) Cell-specific, activation-dependent regulation of neutrophil CD32A ligand-binding function. *Blood* **95**(3), 1069–1077.

[71] Godau, J. et al. (2004) C5a initiates the inflammatory cascade in immune complex peritonitis. *J Immunol* **173**(5), 3437–3445.

[72] Konrad, S. et al. (2006) Intravenous immunoglobulin (IVIG)-mediated neutralisation of C5a: a direct mechanism of IVIG in the maintenance of a high Fc gammaRIIB to Fc gammaRIII expression ratio on macrophages. *Br J Haematol* **134**(3), 345–347.

[73] Kelly-Quintos, C. et al. (2006) Characterization of the opsonic and protective activity against Staphylococcus aureus of fully human monoclonal antibodies specific for the bacterial surface polysaccharide poly-N-acetylglucosamine. *Infect Immun* **74**(5), 2742–2750.

[74] Preston, M.J. et al. (1998) Production and characterization of a set of mouse-human chimeric immunoglobulin G (IgG) subclass and IgA monoclonal antibodies with identical variable regions specific for Pseudomonas aeruginosa serogroup O6 lipopolysaccharide. *Infect Immun* **66**(9), 4137–4142.

[75] Wells, J. et al. (2006) Complement and Fc function are required for optimal antibody prophylaxis against Pneumocystis carinii pneumonia. *Infect Immun* **74**(1), 390–393.

[76] Han, Y. et al. (2001) Complement is essential for protection by an IgM and an IgG3 monoclonal antibody against experimental, hematogenously disseminated candidiasis. *J Immunol* **167**(3), 1550–1557.

[77] Baker, M. (2006) Anti-infective antibodies: finding the path forward. *Nat Biotechnol* **24**(12), 1491–1493.

[78] Gelderman, K.A. et al. (2004) Complement function in mAb-mediated cancer immunotherapy. *Trends Immunol* **25**(3), 158–164.

[79] Li, L. et al. (2001) CD55 is over-expressed in the tumour environment. *Br J Cancer* **84**(1), 80–86.

[80] Imai, M. et al. (2005) Complement-mediated mechanisms in anti-GD2 monoclonal antibody therapy of murine metastatic cancer. *Cancer Res* **65**(22), 10562–10568.

[81] Cragg, M.S. and Glennie, M.J. (2004) Antibody specificity controls in vivo effector mechanisms of anti-CD20 reagents. *Blood* **103**(7), 2738–2743.

[82] Di Gaetano, N. et al. (2003) Complement activation determines the therapeutic activity of rituximab in vivo. *J Immunol* **171**(3), 1581–1587.

[83] Golay, J. et al. (2006) The role of complement in the therapeutic activity of rituximab in a murine B lymphoma model homing in lymph nodes. *Haematologica* **91**(2), 176–183.

[84] Hamaguchi, Y. et al. (2005) The peritoneal cavity provides a protective niche for B1 and conventional B lymphocytes during anti-CD20 immunotherapy in mice. *J Immunol* **174**(7), 4389–4399.

[85] Bannerji, R. et al. (2003) Apoptotic-regulatory and complement-protecting protein expression in chronic lymphocytic leukemia: relationship to in vivo rituximab resistance. *J Clin Oncol* **21**(8), 1466–1471.

[86] Treon, S.P. et al. (2001) Tumor cell expression of CD59 is associated with resistance to CD20 serotherapy in patients with B-cell malignancies. *J Immunother* **24**(3), 263–271.

[87] Weng, W.K. and Levy, R. (2001) Expression of complement inhibitors CD46, CD55, and CD59 on tumor cells does not predict clinical outcome after rituximab treatment in follicular non-Hodgkin lymphoma. *Blood* **98**(5), 1352–1357.

[88] Kennedy, A.D. et al. (2004) Rituximab infusion promotes rapid complement depletion and acute CD20 loss in chronic lymphocytic leukemia. *J Immunol* **172**(5), 3280–3288.

[89] Racila, E. et al. (2006) The pattern of clinical breast cancer metastasis correlates with a single nucleotide polymorphism in the C1qA component of complement. *Immunogenetics* **58**(1), 1–8.

[90] Hezareh, M. et al. (2001) Effector function activities of a panel of mutants of a broadly neutralizing antibody against human immunodeficiency virus type 1. *J Virol* **75**(24), 12161–12168.

[91] Idusogie, E.E. et al. (2000) Mapping of the C1q binding site on rituxan, a chimeric antibody with a human IgG1 Fc. *J Immunol* **164**(8), 4178–4184.

[92] Thommesen, J.E. et al. (2000) Lysine 322 in the human IgG3 C(H)2 domain is crucial for antibody dependent complement activation. *Mol Immunol* **37**(16), 995–1004.

[93] Redpath, S. et al. (1998) Activation of complement by human IgG1 and human IgG3 antibodies against the human leucocyte antigen CD52. *Immunology* **93**(4), 595–600.

[94] Sensel, M.G. et al. (1997) Amino acid differences in the N-terminus of C(H)2 influence the relative abilities of IgG2 and IgG3 to activate complement. *Mol Immunol* **34**(14), 1019–1029.

[95] Tao, M.H. et al. (1991) The differential ability of human IgG1 and IgG4 to activate complement is determined by the COOH-terminal sequence of the CH2 domain. *J Exp Med* **173**(4), 1025–1028.

[96] Tao, M.H. et al. (1993) Structural features of human immunoglobulin G that determine isotype-specific differences in complement activation. *J Exp Med* **178**(2), 661–667.

[97] Idusogie, E.E. et al. (2001) Engineered antibodies with increased activity to recruit complement. *J Immunol* **166**(4), 2571–2575.

[98] Dall'Acqua, W.F. et al. (2006) Modulation of the effector functions of a human IgG1 through engineering of its hinge region. *J Immunol* **177**(2), 1129–1138.

[99] Natsume, A. et al. (2008) Engineered antibodies of IgG1/IgG3 mixed isotype with enhanced cytotoxic activities. *Cancer Res* (in press).

[100] Shopes, B. (1992) A genetically engineered human IgG mutant with enhanced cytolytic activity. *J Immunol* **148**(9), 2918–2922.

[101] Gillies, S.D. et al. (1999) Improving the efficacy of antibody-interleukin 2 fusion proteins by reducing their interaction with Fc receptors. *Cancer Res* **59**(9), 2159–2166.

[102] Hutchins, J.T. et al. (1995) Improved biodistribution, tumor targeting, and reduced immunogenicity in mice with a gamma 4 variant of Campath-1H. *Proc Natl Acad Sci USA* **92**(26), 11980–11984.

[103] Isaacs, J.D. et al. (1996) A therapeutic human IgG4 monoclonal antibody that depletes target cells in humans. *Clin Exp Immunol* **106**(3), 427–433.

[104] Wise, M.P. et al. (2006) T-cell costimulation. *N Engl J Med* **355**(24), 2594–2595; author reply 2595.

[105] Beenhouwer, D.O. et al. (2007) Human immunoglobulin G2 (IgG2) and IgG4, but not IgG1 or IgG3, protect mice against Cryptococcus neoformans infection. *Infect Immun* **75**(3), 1424–1435.

[106] van der Neut Kolfschoten, M. et al. (2007) Anti-inflammatory activity of human IgG4 antibodies by dynamic Fab arm exchange. *Science* **317**(5844), 1554–1557.

[107] Yoo, E.M. et al. (2003) Human IgG2 can form covalent dimers. *J Immunol* **170**(6), 3134–3138.

[108] Salfeld, J.G. (2007) Isotype selection in antibody engineering. *Nat Biotechnol* **25**(12), 1369–1372.

[109] Armour, K.L. et al. (1999) Recombinant human IgG molecules lacking Fcgamma receptor I binding and monocyte triggering activities. *Eur J Immunol* **29**(8), 2613–2624.

[110] Strohl, W.R. Merck. Non-immunostimulatory antibody and compositions containing the same, USSN 11/581,931.

[111] Angal, S. et al. (1993) A single amino acid substitution abolishes the heterogeneity of chimeric mouse/human (IgG4) antibody. *Mol Immunol* **30**(1), 105–108.

[112] Chatenoud, L. (2004) Anti-CD3 antibodies: towards clinical antigen-specific immunomodulation. *Curr Opin Pharmacol* **4**(4), 403–407.

[113] Newman, R. et al. (2001) Modification of the Fc region of a primatized IgG antibody to human CD4 retains its ability to modulate CD4 receptors but does not deplete CD4(+) T cells in chimpanzees. *Clin Immunol* **98**(2), 164–174.

[114] Raasveld, M.H. et al. (1993) Complement activation during OKT3 treatment: a possible explanation for respiratory side effects. *Kidney Int* **43**(5), 1140–1149.

[115] Vallhonrat, H. et al. (1999) In vivo generation of C4d, Bb, iC3b, and SC5b-9 after OKT3 administration in kidney and lung transplant recipients. *Transplantation* **67**(2), 253–258.

[116] Bolt, S. et al. (1993) The generation of a humanized, non-mitogenic CD3 monoclonal antibody which retains in vitro immunosuppressive properties. *Eur J Immunol* **23**(2), 403–411.

[117] Xu, D. et al. (2000) *In vitro* characterization of five humanized OKT3 effector function variant antibodies. *Cell Immunol* **200**(1), 16–26.

[118] Cole, M.S. et al. (1997) Human IgG2 variants of chimeric anti-CD3 are nonmitogenic to T cells. *J Immunol* **159**(7), 3613–3621.

[119] Friend, P.J. et al. (1999) Phase I study of an engineered aglycosylated humanized CD3 antibody in renal transplant rejection. *Transplantation* **68**(11), 1632–1637.

[120] Norman, D.J. et al. (2000) Phase I trial of HuM291, a humanized anti-CD3 antibody, in patients receiving renal allografts from living donors. *Transplantation* **70**(12), 1707–1712.

[121] Woodle, E.S. et al. (1999) Phase I trial of a humanized, Fc receptor nonbinding OKT3 antibody, huOKT3gamma1(Ala-Ala) in the treatment of acute renal allograft rejection. *Transplantation* **68**(5), 608–616.

[122] Reddy, M.P. et al. (2000) Elimination of Fc receptor-dependent effector functions of a modified IgG4 monoclonal antibody to human CD4. *J Immunol* **164**(4), 1925–1933.

[123] Brambell, F.W. (1966) The transmission of immunity from mother to young and the catabolism of immunoglobulins. *Lancet* **2**(7473), 1087–1093.

[124] Brambell, F.W. et al. (1964) A theoretical model of gGamma-globulin catabolism. *Nature* **203**, 1352–1354.

[125] Ghetie, V. and Ward, E.S. (2000) Multiple roles for the major histocompatibility complex class I- related receptor FcRn. *Annu Rev Immunol* **18**, 739–766.

[126] Lencer, W.I. and Blumberg, R.S. (2005) A passionate kiss, then run: exocytosis and recycling of IgG by FcRn. *Trends Cell Biol* **15**(1), 5–9.

[127] Yoshida, M. et al. (2006) IgG transport across mucosal barriers by neonatal Fc receptor for IgG and mucosal immunity. *Springer Semin Immunopathol* **28**(4), 397–403.

[128] Junghans, R.P. and Anderson, C.L. (1996) The protection receptor for IgG catabolism is the beta2-microglobulin-containing neonatal intestinal transport receptor. *Proc Natl Acad Sci USA* **93**(11), 5512–5516.

[129] Roopenian, D.C. et al. (2003) The MHC class I-like IgG receptor controls perinatal IgG transport, IgG homeostasis, and fate of IgG-Fc-coupled drugs. *J Immunol* **170**(7), 3528–3533.

[130] Ober, R.J. et al. (2004) Visualizing the site and dynamics of IgG salvage by the MHC class I-related receptor, FcRn. *J Immunol* **172**(4), 2021–2029.

[131] Ward, E.S. et al. (2003) Evidence to support the cellular mechanism involved in serum IgG homeostasis in humans. *Int Immunol* **15**(2), 187–195.

[132] Prabhat, P. et al. (2007) Elucidation of intracellular recycling pathways leading to exocytosis of the Fc receptor, FcRn, by using multifocal plane microscopy. *Proc Natl Acad Sci USA* **104**(14), 5889–5894.

[133] Ober, R.J. et al. (2004) Exocytosis of IgG as mediated by the receptor, FcRn: an analysis at the single-molecule level. *Proc Natl Acad Sci USA* **101**(30), 11076–11081.

[134] Burmeister, W.P. et al. (1994) Crystal structure of the complex of rat neonatal Fc receptor with Fc. *Nature* **372**(6504), 379–383.

[135] Martin, W.L. et al. (2001) Crystal structure at 2.8 A of an FcRn/heterodimeric Fc complex: mechanism of pH-dependent binding. *Mol Cell* **7**(4), 867–877.

[136] Martin, W.L. and Bjorkman, P.J. (1999) Characterization of the 2:1 complex between the class I MHC-related Fc receptor and its Fc ligand in solution. *Biochemistry* **38**(39), 12639–12647.

[137] Kim, J.K. et al. (1999) Mapping the site on human IgG for binding of the MHC class I-related receptor, FcRn. *Eur J Immunol* **29**(9), 2819–2825.

[138] Medesan, C. et al. (1997) Delineation of the amino acid residues involved in transcytosis and catabolism of mouse IgG1. *J Immunol* **158**(5), 2211–2217.

[139] Dall'Acqua, W.F. et al. (2002) Increasing the affinity of a human IgG1 for the neonatal Fc receptor: biological consequences. *J Immunol* **169**(9), 5171–5180.

[140] Hinton, P.R. et al. (2004) Engineered human IgG antibodies with longer serum half-lives in primates. *J Biol Chem* **279**(8), 6213–6216.

[141] Adams, C.W. et al. Genentech. Polypeptide variants with altered effector function, USSN 11/208,422.

[142] Allan, B. et al. Eli Lilly. Variant Fc regions, USSN 11/572,634.

[143] Chamberlain, A.K. et al. Xencor. Fc variants with altered binding to FcRn, USSN 11/436,266.

[144] Farrington, G.K. et al. Biogen Idec. Neonatal Fc receptor (FcRn)-binding polypeptide variants, dimeric Fc binding proteins and methods related thereto, USSN 11/432,872.

[145] Hinton, P.R. et al. (2006) An engineered human IgG1 antibody with longer serum half-life. *J Immunol* **176**(1), 346–356.

[146] Dall'Acqua, W.F. et al. (2006) Properties of human IgG1s engineered for enhanced binding to the neonatal Fc receptor (FcRn). *J Biol Chem* **281**(33), 23514–23524.

[147] Datta-Mannan, A. et al. (2007) Monoclonal antibody clearance. Impact of modulating the interaction of IgG with the neonatal Fc receptor. *J Biol Chem* **282**(3), 1709–1717.

[148] Gurbaxani, B. et al. (2006) Analysis of a family of antibodies with different half-lives in mice fails to find a correlation between affinity for FcRn and serum half-life. *Mol Immunol* **43**(9), 1462–1473.

[149] Gurbaxani, B.M. and Morrison, S.L. (2006) Development of new models for the analysis of Fc-FcRn interactions. *Mol Immunol* **43**(9), 1379–1389.

[150] Petkova, S.B. et al. (2006) Enhanced half-life of genetically engineered human IgG1 antibodies in a humanized FcRn mouse model: potential application in humorally mediated autoimmune disease. *Int Immunol* **18**(12), 1759–1769.

[151] Getman, K.E. and Balthasar, J.P. (2005) Pharmacokinetic effects of 4C9, an anti-FcRn antibody, in rats: implications for the use of FcRn inhibitors for the treatment of humoral autoimmune and alloimmune conditions. *J Pharm Sci* **94**(4), 718–729.

[152] Liu, L. et al. (2007) Amelioration of experimental autoimmune myasthenia gravis in rats by neonatal FcR blockade. *J Immunol* **178**(8), 5390–5398.

CHAPTER ELEVEN

Glycoengineered Therapeutic Antibodies

Peter Brünker, Peter Sondermann, and Pablo Umaña

Unconjugated, target-cell killing antibodies of the human IgG1 isotype are now established as successful therapeutic agents, as demonstrated by the use of ritux-imab and trastuzumab for the treatment of B cell malignancies and Her2-overex-pressing breast cancer, respectively. While both Fc-dependent and independent mechanisms can contribute to the efficacy of these drugs, it is clear that for both rituximab and trastuzumab, significant *in vivo* target cell depletion requires the Fc portion of the antibody.[1] *In vivo*, the Fc region may either engage complement activation and/or interact with Fcγ receptors that are important for cellular immune effector functions such as antibody-dependent cell-mediated cytotoxicity (ADCC), which can be mediated by various effector cells such as natural killer (NK) cells and macrophages.

Increasing evidence indicates an important role for the interaction of antibodies with FcγRIIIa. In particular, retrospective studies have correlated superior objective response rates and progression-free survival with being homozygous for the higher affinity allele of FcγRIIIa encoding a valine residue at position 158.[2–4] Only approx-imately 15% of the population is homozygous for this form of the receptor. There-fore, it may be valuable to generate therapeutic antibody variants that bind to all forms of this receptor with at least as high affinity as current IgG1 antibodies bind to FcγRIIIa-158V.

Both the polypeptide chain and the oligosaccharide component may be engi-neered in order to increase affinity for FcγRIII. We have chosen the latter path and first demonstrated that recombinant engineering of the glycosylation pattern of antibodies generates antibody glycosylation variants with increased FcγRIII binding affinity and increased ADCC.[5] As explained in more detail below, this was achieved by overexpression of a glycosyltransferase gene in Chinese hamster ovary (CHO) cells, which are the preferred and established cell host for the commercial produc-tion of therapeutic antibodies.

ANTIBODY GLYCOSYLATION VARIANTS WITH ENHANCED EFFECTOR FUNCTIONS

It has been reported that N-linked oligosaccharide structures in the Fc region of therapeutic antibodies significantly affect their biological activity.[6,7] Since antibodies are naturally glycosylated and our glycoengineering approach produces oligosaccharides found in many human glycoproteins including antibodies,[6] they are considered to be nonimmunogenic. We have also found that pharmacokinetics is not significantly affected. In Figure 11.1, the biosynthetic pathway for N-linked oligosaccharides is depicted. After several modification and trimming reactions, the finally generated carbohydrate structure is usually of the complex, fucosylated type being either zero-, mono- or bi-galactosylated when expressed in HEK 293 EBNA cells.

As also shown in Figure 11.1, the enzyme β1,4-*N*-acetyl-glucosaminyltransferase III (GnTIII) catalyzes the addition of a bisecting N-acetylglucosamine (GlcNAc) to N-linked oligosaccharides located in the Fc region of monoclonal antibodies. It has been demonstrated that overexpression of GnTIII in antibody-producing cell lines leads to the production of antibody glycovariants of the bisected, non-fucosylated type that exhibit a significantly increased ADCC activity as compared to the unmodified wild-type antibody.[5] Furthermore, it is known that GnTIII has a significant control over the N-glycosylation pathway since upon addition of a bisecting GlcNAc other important reactions during glycosylation, such as core fucosylation, are

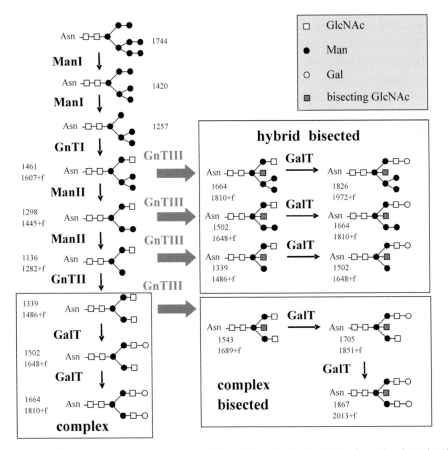

Figure 11.1. N-linked oligosaccharide biosynthetic pathway for the generation of complex, fucosylated carbohydrate structures (left part). In the right part the structures of complex and hybrid oligosaccharides containing bisecting GlcNAc are shown. The predicted mass to charge (m/z) value of the sodium associated oligosaccharide ion (in the presence or absence of core fucose) that would be obtained by MALDI/TOF-MS is indicated.

blocked.[8] Therefore, GnTIII is a favored enzyme for glycoengineering and modifying the N-glycosylation pathway. We first demonstrated that GnTIII overexpression in CHO cells within a range that did not significantly affect CHO cell growth or antibody production led to increased levels of glycoengineered antibody forms carrying bisected, non-fucosylated oligosaccharides that mediated increased ADCC activity relative to the non-glycoengineered antibody counterparts.[5,9] For stable antibody gene expression, a well-characterized commercially available, standard, though very efficient, expression vector system has been used.[10]

We have also studied additional modifications of the technology. For instance, we have engineered GnTIII in a way that the enzyme's localization in the Golgi apparatus is modified compared to the wild-type enzyme[11] and could demonstrate that the localization of GnTIII indeed has a significant impact on glycosylation. In these experiments, the catalytic domain of GnTIII (amino acids 77–546) was fused to so-called localization regions of other Golgi-resident enzymes such as GnTI, GnTII, FucT, or ManII in order to achieve an earlier localization of the chimeric GnTIII in the Golgi. These localization regions (that usually have a length of approximately 70–100 amino acid residues) consist of a cytoplasmic tail, a transmembrane region, and the actual stem region. In transient expression experiments it could be demonstrated that all the chimeric GnTIII enzymes mentioned are active in modifying carbohydrates in the Fc region of monoclonal antibodies since the majority of newly produced oligosaccharides were shown to be of the bisected type. The enzyme with the highest impact in terms of production of these oligosaccharide structures was GnTIII fused to the localization domain of human α-mannosidase II (ManII). In order to reengineer the N-glycosylation pathway in a direction to produce mainly complex, bisected non-fucosylated carbohydrate structures we found that the overexpression of wt GnTIII and ManII, as previously described,[9] yielded satisfying results. Here, the co-expression of both enzymes shifted the reaction in the desired direction toward the production of complex carbohydrate structures.[12] Antibodies carrying these glycosylation patterns also mediated significantly enhanced ADCC (compared to wild type). It has also been found that a key structural element for this enhanced ADCC is the lack of core fucosylation of bisecting GlcNAc in the carbohydrate moiety.[13,14,15] The ADCC-enhancing effect of eliminating core fucosylation in N-linked oligosaccharides also was demonstrated by generation of a recombinant CHO cell line in which the α1,6 fucosyltransferase (Fut8), which catalyzes the transfer of fucose from GDP-fucose to GlcNAc, was disrupted.[16] This modification led to the production of antibody glycosylation variants that are completely non-fucosylated and which exhibit increased ADCC activity compared to antibodies with oligosaccharides that carry the core fucose residue.

GENERATION OF STABLE, GLYCOENGINEERED ANTIBODY PRODUCTION CELL LINES

Our method of choice for the generation of cell lines with industrially robust production of glycoengineered antibodies is the constitutive co-overexpression of antibody heavy and light chain genes together with the genes encoding GnTIII and ManII in CHO cells. Following this method as previously described[9] with no further special modification, we routinely identify stable CHO clones with industrially relevant expression levels and productivity of antibody and with Fc glycosylation patterns where the majority of the N-linked sugars are of the complex, non-fucosylated type. Clones with as high as 95% of non-fucosylated oligosaccharides of the total mix of Fc-oligosaccharides, and at least 80% of these being of the complex type, can be identified following those methods.[9]

There are three different approaches for the generation of a glycoengineered antibody production cell line: In one approach, a highly productive antibody production cell line can be engineered for overexpression of GnTIII and ManII by stable transfection with suitable glycovectors. Alternatively, a pre-glycoengineered cell line with high levels of GnTIII and ManII production can be transfected with suitable, standard antibody expression vector(s). A third possibility is the simultaneous co-transfection of antibody vector and glycovector, a method that can be implemented for the generation of stable, glycoengineered antibody-producing CHO cell lines by electroporation of both vectors in a linearized form. All of the above approaches have been used to isolate production clones with the desired characteristics in terms of productivity, growth, stability, and glycosylation pattern. The generation of highly productive antibody expression cell lines with reproducible titers of 3–5 g/L in fed-batch cultivation processes lasting 2 weeks and with approximately 80% non-fucosylated complex bisected oligosaccharides is easily achievable following these methods[9] as shown in Figure 11.2.

These data indicate that by stable, constitutive overexpression of GnTIII and ManII in antibody production cell lines, it is possible to obtain high levels of complex, bisected, non-fucosylated oligosaccharides attached to the Fc region of therapeutic antibodies, even when the antibody is stably produced at very high titers. Furthermore, the antibody productivity and the glycosylation pattern is stable for at least 80 generations in the absence of any selection pressure (Figure 11.3).

GLYCOSYLATION REQUIREMENTS FOR A HIGH-AFFINITY BINDING TO FcγRIIIA

It is well accepted that the glycosylation of IgG at position Asn297 (numbering based on the Eu amino acid sequence)[17] attached to all IgG antibodies is tightly associated with the protein moiety, thereby sustaining the structural integrity of the Fc-fragment.[18] This in turn is mandatory for the affinity of IgG to all FcγRs[19,20] and their ADCC activity. However, for a long time it remained elusive that distinct carbohydrate structures on IgG molecules may also affect the mediation of effector functions. Early evidence that altered glycosylation patterns can modulate the effector functions was found using an antibody expressed in different mammalian cell lines.[7] The authors demonstrated that the antibody expressed in the rat myeloma cell line YB2/3.0[21] contained a significantly higher fraction of bisected and non-fucosylated carbohydrates, which was accompanied by a more efficient ADCC mediated by

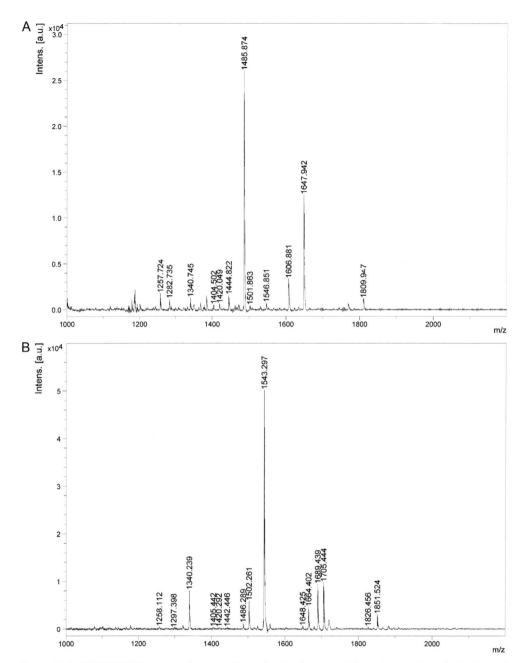

Figure 11.2. MALDI/TOF-MS spectra of neutral oligosaccharides from recombinant therapeutic antibody glycovariants. The antibodies were produced in a stable Chinese hamster ovary (CHO) production cell line that was glycoengineered to overexpress GnTIII and ManII. (A) Spectrum of neutral oligosaccharides released by PNGase F from wt, unmodified antibody. The main structures identified here are complex, fucosylated carbohydrates with different degrees of galactosylation. (B) Spectrum of oligosaccharides attached to the Fc region of glycoengineered antibodies, showing complex, bisected, non-fucosylated carbohydrates as the major products. The corresponding mass to charge values (m/z) appearing as single sodium adducts are indicated above the spectra and can be assigned according to Figure 11.1.

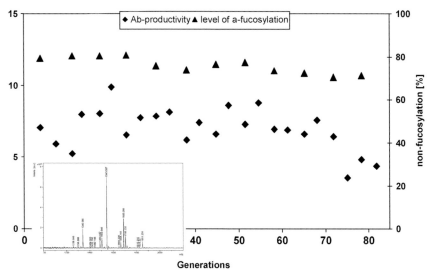

Figure 11.3. Antibody productivity as pg antibody per cell and day (pcd, ♦) and glycosylation pattern of carbohydrates released from these antibodies (▲) over a cultivation period of more than 80 generations in the absence of selective pressure. The MALDI / TOF - MS spectrum of released neutral oligosaccharides at the end of the cultivation is shown in the inset. Both the antibody productivity and the high proportion of non-fucosylated oligosaccharides is maintained over the entire cultivation process. Note that the fermentation is performed in a high-density cultivation process leading to antibody titers of 3–5 g per liter.

human NK cells that exclusively express FcγRIIIa. The first demonstration that antibody glycosylation could be recombinantly engineered to increase ADCC was obtained by overexpression of GnTIII, an enzyme catalyzing the addition of bisecting GlcNAc to the antibody's glycan moiety. This led to the increased levels of bisected, non-fucosylated antibody glycoforms mediating substantially increased ADCC.[5] Overexpression of GnTIII in mammalian cells necessarily leads to increased levels of non-fucosylated oligosaccharides, as bisected carbohydrates are not accepted as a substrate for α1,6-fucosyltransferase (Fut8; the enzyme mediates the addition of a fucose residue to the chitobiose core).[8] Further analysis suggested that non-fucosylation is the most important structural element for the observed affinity increase to FcγRIIIa,[14] although a direct contribution of the bisecting GlcNAc to the FcγRIIIa affinity was also reported.[15] In addition, it could be demonstrated that bisected and non-fucosylated carbohydrates mediate a similar enhanced ADCC regardless of whether they are of the hybrid or the complex type[11] (Figure 11.4A).

THE FcγRIIIA-V/F158 DIMORPHISM AND ITS IMPORTANCE FOR ANTIBODY-BASED THERAPIES

Retrospective pharmacogenomic studies looking at correlations between genotype for a dimorphism occurring at position 158 of FcγRIIIa[22] have indicated that an enhanced affinity of therapeutic antibodies for FcγRIIIa can be beneficial for therapeutic efficacy. This dimorphism leads to a form of FcγRIIIa bearing a valine residue at that position (FcγRIIIa-V158), while the more frequent form of FcγRIIIa

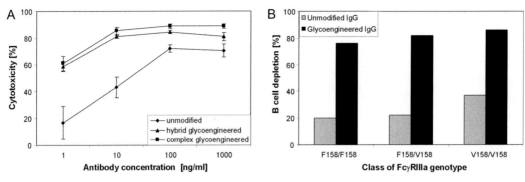

Figure 11.4. Biological activity assays of anti-CD20 antibody glycovariants. (A) ADCC using PBMCs (heterozygous FcγRIIIa-Val/Phe158 as effectors and human lymphoma Raji cells as targets. (B) B cell depletion in whole blood (different FcγRIIIa-Val/Phe158 genotype donors). 10 ng/ml anti-CD20 antibody was added for 24 h to heparinized blood. B cell depletion was calculated from the ratio of CD19-positive B cells to CD3-positive T cells.

displays a phenylalanine (FcγRIIIa-F158). Measurements by flow cytometry [22] and surface plasmon resonance[12] indicated that FcγRIIIa-F158 has a significantly lower affinity to unmodified human IgG than the high-affinity allele (Table 11.1). In several post-therapeutic pharmacogenomic studies, it turned out that patients homozygous for the high-affinity allele FcγRIIIa-V158 display a significantly better response and increased progression-free survival to an antibody therapy independent of the antibody used,[2–4,23] while a single high-affinity allele in the heterozygous patients seems to be insufficient for a better response to the therapy. It is noteworthy to mention that around 85% of the population is heterozygous or homozygous for the low-affinity allele[24,25] and therefore potentially does not respond well to an antibody-based treatment. The fact that the affinity of glycoengineered IgG1 to the low-affinity allele of FcγRIIIa is threefold higher than that of an unmodified antibody to the high-affinity allele FcγRIIIa-V158 (Table 11.1) suggests that patients carrying the low-affinity allele will significantly benefit from a treatment with a glycoengineered antibody. These results are confirmed in a whole-blood assay where the B cell depletion by a glycoengineered anti-CD20 antibody is significantly improved regardless of the genotype of the donor (Figure 11.4B).

MOLECULAR BASIS OF HIGH-AFFINITY FcγRIIIA BINDING BY GLYCOENGINEERED ANTIBODIES

The source of enhanced ADCC activity of glycoengineered antibodies could be tracked back to an increased affinity of such IgGs to FcγRIIIa[25] while the affinity to the other low-affinity FcγR (FcγRII) remains unaltered.[12] The comparison of FcγRIII and other FcγRs that all, due to their similar structure, share the same binding site on the IgG[26] reveals as the only significant difference an N-glycosylation site within the binding site to IgG at position 162.[27] Initial speculation that this glycosylation site of FcγRIII when occupied would interfere with IgG binding was investigated by the construction of a mutant receptor that is unglycosylated at position 162 by the exchange of the Asn to a Gln residue termed FcγRIIIa-V158/Q162. Surface

TABLE 11.1. Dissociation constants of IgG/FcγR complexes [12]

	WT-IgG	GE-IgG	Affinity increase by glycoengineering
FcγRIIIa-V158	0.75 μM	0.015 μM	50-fold
FcγRIIIa-F158	5 μM	0.20 μM	25-fold
FcγRIIIa-V158/Q162[a]	0.24 μM	0.20 μM	Almost unchanged (1.2-fold)
FcγRIIb	2.4 μM	2 μM	Almost unchanged (1.2-fold)

[a] N-*glycosylation* site at position 162 removed by Asn → Gln exchange.

plasmon resonance measurements revealed a threefold increase in affinity of FcγRIIIa-V158/Q162 to unmodified IgG compared with FcγRIIIa-V158 indicating a negative influence of the carbohydrate moiety probably caused by sterical hindrance upon IgG binding (Table 11.1). The surprising result, however, was that binding of the glycosylation mutant FcγRIIIa-V158/Q162 to non-fucosylated, bisected IgG showed a significantly reduced affinity [12] to the level of an unmodified IgG, suggesting that the high-affinity binding of FcγRIIIa to glycoengineered antibodies is mediated by the receptor glycosylation at position 162 in addition to the non-fucosylation of the antibody. Based on these experimental data, a model was proposed that conclusively explains the high-affinity interaction of glycoengineered IgGs with FcγRIIIa.[12] The inspection of the crystal structure of unglycosylated FcγRIII in complex with the Fc of hIgG[27] revealed that a direct interaction of the receptor's carbohydrate attached at position 162 with the fucose attachment site on the IgG seems possible. The carbohydrate moiety in IgG antibodies is strongly attached and probably well lining the protein core of the CH2 domain forming a continuous surface. Only the fucose residue present in wild-type antibodies is protruding into the open space and would prohibit a tight interaction of the receptors' carbohydrate with that region (Figure 11.5).

This model was confirmed for the Fc part by the solution of the crystal structure of a non-fucosylated Fc fragment.[28] While the overall conformations of the carbohydrates and protein moieties are similar, the main difference found is the lack of the fucose residue and the hydration mode around Tyr296 that is no longer shielded by the fucose residue. In agreement with the proposed model and the fact that a tight association of carbohydrates to the protein core is frequently mediated by aromatic amino acids, the oligosaccharide moiety of the receptor could nicely interact with Tyr296 that is usually blocked by the fucose residue in fucosylated antibodies. A comprehensive understanding of this additional, new interaction of glycoengineered antibodies with FcγRIII may allow the design of antibody variants with the potential to improve monoclonal antibody therapies in future.

OUTLOOK

Two different glycoengineered anticancer antibodies produced with the methods described here and having increased ADCC *in vitro* and *in vivo* efficacy are now

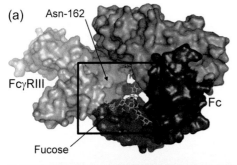

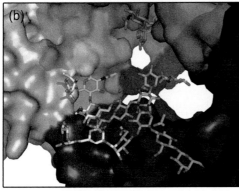

Figure 11.5. Model of the interaction of glycosylated FcγRIII with the Fc-fragment of IgG. (*Top*) Clipping of the crystal structure of non-glycosylated FcγRIII expressed in *E. coli* (green) in complex with the Fc-fragment of native (fucosylated) IgG (PDB code 1e4k27, red and blue) as indicated in the inset. The glycans attached to the Fc are shown as ball and sticks and colored accordingly. The fucose linked to the carbohydrate of the blue Fc-fragment chain is highlighted in red. (*Bottom*) Model of the interaction between a glycosylated FcγRIII and the (non-fucosylated) Fc-fragment of IgG. In this model, the carbohydrates attached at Asn 162 of FcγRIII can thoroughly interact with the non-fucosylated IgG. The figure was created using the program PYMOL (www.delanoscientific.com). [See color plate.]

being tested in clinical trials. We anticipate further application of this technology to many more therapeutic antibody candidates in the future.

REFERENCES

[1]   Clynes R.A. et al. (2000) Inhibitory Fc receptors modulate in vivo cytotoxicity against tumor targets. *Nat. Med.* **6**(4), 443–446.

[2]   Cartron G. et al. (2002) Therapeutic activity of humanized anti-CD20 monoclonal antibody and polymorphism in IgG Fc receptor FcγRIIIa gene. *Blood* **99**(3), 754–758.

[3]   Weng W.K. and Levy R. (2003) Two immunoglobulin G fragment C receptor polymorphisms independently predict response to rituximab in patients with follicular lymphoma. *J. Clin. Oncol.* **21**(21) 3940–3947.

[4]   Musolino A. et al. (2008) Immunoglobulin G fragment C receptor polymorphisms and clinical efficacy of trastuzumab-based therapy in patients with HER-2/neu-positive metastatic breast cancer. *J. Clin. Oncol.* **26**(11) 1789–1796.

[5]   Umaña P. et al. (1999) Engineered glycoforms of an antineuroblastoma IgG1 with optimized antibody-dependent cellular cytotoxic activity. *Nat. Biotech.* **17**, 176–180.

[6]   Jeffries R. et al. (1998) IgG-Fc mediated effector functions: Molecular definition of interaction sites for effector ligands and the role of glycosylation. *Immunol. Rev.* **163**, 59–76.

[7]   Lifely M.R. et al. (1995) Glycosylation and biological activity of CAMPATH-1H expressed in different cell lines and grown under different culture conditions. *J. Glycobiol.* **5**, 813–822.

[8]   Schachter H. (1986) Biosynthetic controls that determine the branching and microheterogeneity of protein-bound oligosaccharides. *Biochem. Cell. Biol.* **64**, 163–181.

[9]   Umaña P. et al. (1999) Glycosylation engineering of antibodies for improving antibody-dependent cellular cytotoxicity. US patent 6602684.

[10] Brown, M.E. et al. (1992) Process development for the production of recombinant antibodies using the glutamine synthetase (GS) system. *Cytotechnology*, **9**, 231–236.

[11]   Ferrara C. et al. (2006) Modulation of therapeutic antibody effector functions by glycosylation engineering: Influence of Golgi enzyme localization domain and co-expression of heterologous β 1,4-N-acetylglucosaminyltransferase III and Golgi α-mannosidase II. *Biotechnol. Bioeng.* **93**(5), 851–861.

[12]   Ferrara C. et al. (2006) The carbohydrate at FcγRIIIa Asn-162: An element required for high affinity binding to non-fucosylated IgG. *J. Biol. Chem.* **281**(8), 5032–5036.

[13]   Shields R.L. et al. (2002) Lack of fucose on human IgG1 N-linked oligosaccharide improves binding to human Fc gamma RIII and antibody-dependent cellular cytotoxicity. *J. Biol. Chem.* **277**(26), 26733–26740.

[14]   Shinkawa T. et al. (2003) The absence of fucose but not the presence of galactose or bisecting N-acetylglucosamine of human IgG complex-type oligosaccharides shows the critical role of enhancing antibody-dependent cellular cytotoxicity. *J. Biol. Chem.* **278**(3), 3466–3473.

[15]   Hodoniczky J. et al. (2005) Control of recombinant monoclonal antibody effector functions by Fc N-glycan remodeling in vitro. *Biotechnol. Prog.* **21**(6), 1644–1652.

[16]   Yamane-Ohnuki N. et al. (2004) Establishment of Fut8 knockout chinese hamster ovary cells: An ideal host cell line for producing completely defucosylated antibodies with enhanced antibody-dependent cellular cytotoxicity. *Biotechnol. Bioeng.* **87**(5), 614–622.

[17]   Rutishauser U. et al. (1970) The covalent structure of a human gamma G-immunoglobulin. 8. Amino acid sequence of heavy-chain cyanogen bromide fragments H5-H7. *Biochemistry.* **9**(16), 3171–3181.

[18]   Deisenhofer J. (1981) Crystallographic refinement and atomic models of a human Fc fragment and its complex with fragment B of protein A from Staphylococcus aureus at 2.9- and 2.8-A resolution. *Biochemistry.* **20**(9), 2361–2370.

[19]   Walker M.R. et al. (1989) Aglycosylation of human IgG1 and IgG3 monoclonal antibodies can eliminate recognition by human cells expressing FcγRI and/or FcγRII receptors. *Biochem. J.* **259**(2), 347–353.

[20]   Sarmay G. et al. (1992) Mapping and comparison of the interaction sites on the Fc region of IgG responsible for triggering antibody dependent cellular cytotoxicity (ADCC) through different types of human Fcγ receptor. *Mol. Immunol.* **29**(5), 633–639.

[21]   Galfrè G. and Milstein C. (1981) Preparation of monoclonal antibodies: strategies and procedures. *Methods Enzymol.* **73**(Pt B), 3–46.

[22]   Koene H.R. et al. (1997) FcγRIIIa-158V/F polymorphism influences the binding of IgG by natural killer cell FcγRIIIa, independently of the FcγRIIIa-48L/R/H phenotype. *Blood.* **90**(3), 1109–1114.

[23]   Louis E. et al. (2004) Association between polymorphism in IgG Fc receptor IIIa coding gene and biological response to infliximab in Crohn's disease. *Aliment. Pharmacol. Ther.* **19**(5), 511–519.

[24]   Wu J. et al. (1997) A novel polymorphism of FcγRIIIa (CD16) alters receptor function and predisposes to autoimmune disease. *J. Clin. Invest.* **100**(5), 1059–1070.

[25]   Okazaki A. et al. (2004) Fucose depletion from human IgG1 oligosaccharide enhances binding enthalpy and association rate between IgG1 and FcγRIIIa. *J. Mol. Biol.* **336**(5), 1239–1249.

[26]   Sondermann P. et al. (2001) Molecular basis for immune complex recognition: a comparison of Fc-receptor structures. *J. Mol. Biol.* **309**(3), 737–749.

[27]   Sondermann P. et al. (2000) The 3.2-A crystal structure of the human IgG1 Fc fragment-FcγRIII complex. *Nature.* **406**(6793), 267–273.

[28]   Matsumiya S. et al. (2007) Structural comparison of fucosylated and nonfucosylated Fc fragments of human immunoglobulin G1. *J. Mol. Biol.* **368**(3), 767–779.

PART V

ARMING ANTIBODIES

CHAPTER TWELVE

Monoclonal Antibodies for the Delivery of Cytotoxic Drugs

David J. King

Monoclonal antibodies have become an established class of anticancer therapeutics over the last few years, and yet there remains a need for increasing their efficacy, especially in solid tumor therapy. For example, trastuzumab, a humanized antibody to human epidermal growth factor receptor type 2 (HER2, ErbB-2 or HER2/neu), is an FDA-approved antibody for treatment of metastatic breast cancer. Trastuzumab therapy of metastatic breast cancer patients who express the HER2 antigen and had progressed after chemotherapy resulted in a 15% overall response rate, with 4% complete responses and a 9.1 month median duration of response.[1] In first-line treatment of metastatic breast cancer the overall response rate increased to 26%,[2] and it is only in combination with chemotherapy that higher response rates have been found. For example, a response rate of 50% was observed when trastuzumab was combined with a standard chemotherapy regimen.[3] A wide variety of different combinations of trastuzumab with chemotherapy have now been explored demonstrating the use of the antibody in combination therapy[4] and trastuzumab remains a valuable therapeutic agent. Nevertheless, results such as these have led to increased interest in improving antibody efficacy, and the use of antibodies directly attached to cytotoxic agents is being widely explored as one means of achieving this. Indeed, trastuzumab itself is now being investigated as an antibody-drug conjugate.[5]

Antibody-mediated delivery of both protein toxins and chemotherapeutic agents has been under investigation for quite some time and even predates the era of monoclonal antibodies.[6,7] Early attempts in the field failed because of a range of problems, but these are now being overcome as the technology for making drug conjugates and immunotoxins has developed. This progress has led to renewed enthusiasm for antibody-mediated delivery of cytotoxics, and now a large number of these agents are under active development, both in the clinic and at the preclinical stage.

ANTIBODY-DRUG CONJUGATES (ADCs)

Chemotherapy has been a major component of anticancer therapy for many years. The cytotoxic agents used in chemotherapy are not selective and rely largely on the premise that cancer cells will be killed more efficiently than cells in normal tissues due to their rapid rate of growth and cell division. Nonspecific toxicity is particularly prevalent in those normal tissues which are undergoing rapid proliferation, and consequently many chemotherapeutics are given at suboptimal doses for efficacy. Targeting chemotherapy by conjugation of the chemotherapeutic agent to a monoclonal antibody offers a potential solution to this issue. This is carried out with the intent of using the specificity of the monoclonal antibody to a tumor-associated antigen to deliver the chemotherapeutic agent to tumor cells and reduce exposure of normal tissues.

Early attempts in the field concentrated on the conjugation of approved chemotherapeutic agents to antibodies. A wide variety of drugs have been tested – for example, alkylating agents such as chlorambucil,[8] DNA intercalators such as daunorubicin and doxorubicin,[7] and antimitotics such as vinca alkaloids.[9] Initial problems, such as suitable chemistry for retention of activity of both the antibody and the drug, were solved, leading to some promising effects of these conjugates in animal models.[10, 11] However, it rapidly became apparent that the amount of these drugs that could be delivered to a solid tumor in humans using a monoclonal antibody conjugate was unlikely to be sufficient for effective therapy. Clinical studies have revealed that only a relatively small amount of administered antibody can be targeted to solid tumors in humans, with typical levels in the range of 0.001–0.1% injected dose per gram of tumor. A number of factors are thought to be responsible for this, including physiological barriers to extravasation and tumor penetration, heterogeneous antigen expression, and poor properties of the targeting antibody.[12] Consequently, a number of approaches have been pursued in attempts to improve ADC therapy, including attachment of more molecules of drug per antibody, or more successfully, attachment of more potent cytotoxic agents. Attachment of many molecules of drug per antibody is usually unsuccessful due to loss of antigen-binding properties of the conjugate or simply loss of solubility. Additional attempts have been made to link many molecules of drug via intermediate carriers such as dextrans, polymers, or other branched linkers,[13] although again these have suffered from poor solubility characteristics. Alternatively, antibodies have been used with some success to re-target liposomes, or nanoparticles loaded with drugs.[14]

Attention was then switched to more potent cytotoxic drugs, which are too toxic to have an acceptable therapeutic window as stand-alone agents. This approach has proven successful and led to the development of gemtuzumab ozogamicin (Mylotarg®) for the therapy of acute myeloid leukemia, which became the first, and to date the only, antibody-cytotoxic drug conjugate approved for human use.[15] Gemtuzumab ozogamicin comprises a humanized antibody to CD33 linked to calicheamicin. Calicheamicin is a member of a family of highly potent enediyne antitumor antibiotics that bind to the minor groove of DNA and lead to double strand DNA breaks and subsequent cell death.

DESIGN OF ANTIBODY-DRUG CONJUGATES

More recently, many of the parameters that are important for the production of effective and safe antibody conjugates have been identified, and a new generation

TABLE 12.1. Properties of antibody-drug conjugates to be considered in the design of conjugates for clinical evaluation

Component	Important properties for ADC development
Antibody	High specificity for tumor associated antigen
	Human or humanized (low immunogenicity)
	Stable to conjugation
	Internalizes
Drug	Potent
	Soluble
	Cellular retention
	Not subject to drug resistance
Linker	Stable in circulation
	Capable of release of active drug in tumor cells
Conjugate	Potent, highly selectively cytotoxic to antigen positive tumor cells
	Large therapeutic window *in vivo*
	Soluble and able to be formulated for administration to man

of antibody-drug conjugates is now under development. The development of effective antibody-drug conjugates is complex and requires optimization of all of the individual components of the conjugate. Table 12.1 summarizes some of the major properties that need to be considered.

THE ANTIBODY

As with any antibody therapeutic, selection of the target antigen and antibody to be used are of primary importance. In the case of drug conjugates, particular care is taken with the choice of antibody, as cross-reactivity with normal tissues could lead to delivery of the cytotoxic agent to that tissue and result in an unacceptable toxicity profile. An added barrier to effective therapy by early drug conjugates was the use of murine antibodies that led to induction of human anti-mouse antibody in treated patients and subsequent rapid clearance of the conjugate.[16] The advent of humanized and now human antibodies has largely overcome this issue, and now, provided a suitable target is identified, the identification of a high-specificity antibody of low immunogenicity should not be a major barrier.

Antibody-binding affinity can play a role in cytotoxicity of the resulting conjugates. Affinity improvement of an anti-CD22 antibody fragment was carried out, resulting in approximately a 10-fold increase in binding affinity.[17] A Pseudomonas toxin (PE38) immunotoxin was made with the resultant antibody fragment approximately 5- to 10-fold more cytotoxic to CD22 positive cells and with greatly increased activity on cells with low numbers of antigen molecules per cell.[17, 18]

Another important property of the antibody is the ability to internalize into the target cell via receptor-mediated endocytosis. If the linkage of the cytotoxic drug to the antibody is very stable, this is the primary mechanism of delivery to the target cell. Endocytosis of antibodies can take place by a number of different mechanisms,

TABLE 12.2. Selected ADCs in development for cancer therapy

Designation	Antigen	Drug	Linker	Stage	Cancer indication
Mylotarg®	CD33	Calicheamicin	Hydrazone/ hindered disulfide	FDA approved	AML
CMC-544	CD22	Calicheamicin	Hydrazone/ hindered disulfide	Phase II/III	Lymphoma and Leukemias
C242-DM1	CanAg (MUC1 glycoform)	Maytansine (DM1)	Hindered disulfide	Phase I/II	Pancreatic, colorectal, NSCLC, gastric
C242-DM4	CanAg (MUC1 glycoform)	Maytansine (DM4)	Highly hindered disulfide	Phase I/II	Pancreatic, colorectal, NSCLC, gastric
Trastuzumab-DM1	HER2	Maytansine (DM1)	Noncleavable	Phase II	Breast
SAR-3419	CD19	Maytansine (DM4)	Highly hindered disulfide	Phase I/II	Lymphoma
SGN35	CD30	MMAE	Peptide	Phase I/II	Hodgkin lymphoma
CR011	GPNMB	MMAE	Peptide	Phase II	Melanoma
CD70-MGBA	CD70	MGBA	Peptide	Preclinical	Renal and lymphoma
PSMA-MGBA	PSMA	MGBA	Peptide	Preclinical	Prostate

dependent both on the antigen and the individual antibody.[19] Two antibodies to the same antigen will not necessarily be taken into the cell at the same rate or to the same extent, and experimental studies are required to identify optimally performing antibodies for drug delivery. The internalization rate has been shown to be important for cytotoxicity of immunotoxins, more so than the absolute number of receptors present on the cell surface,[20] and inhibition of internalization of ADCs decreases activity. For example, expression of CD21 in CD19 positive cells inhibits internalization of CD19-specific ADCs and consequently reduces cytotoxicity of conjugates linked through a stable linker.[21] It is clear that valency of the ADC is important to achieve efficient cross linking of the antigen on the cell surface, and several constructs to aid internalization have been attempted. For example, conjugation of a membrane translocating peptide to an immunotoxin could increase specific cytotoxicity.[22] It has also been reported that in some cases drug conjugation itself can increase internalization. Antibodies to the B cell antigen CD20 are not well internalized into the cell, yet conjugates with the anti-mitotic agent monomethyl auristatin E (MMAE) were able to internalize and kill CD20-positive cells.[23]

As well as internalization, intracellular trafficking may also play a role. Antibodies to some antigens may be rapidly internalized and recycled to the cell surface, as appears to be the case with trastuzumab,[24] whereas others may be more rapidly routed to the lysosome for degradation, a feature that may be used advantageously in ADC linker design (discussed later in the chapter).

DRUGS

A number of highly potent drugs have been investigated for their applicability to the development of ADCs, targeting several different cellular processes. These include DNA double strand breakers such as the enediynes, which are exemplified by calicheamicin; tubulin active compounds such as maytansines and auristatins; and DNA minor groove-binding alkylating agents (MGBAs) such as duocarmycins. Primary among the desirable properties of these agents has been high potency, with the desire to exert maximal killing with only a few molecules of drug conjugated to each antibody molecule. Solubility of the drug in aqueous solution is also a major practical limitation. Cytotoxic drugs are typically hydrophobic compounds, and conjugation to antibodies can lead to aggregation of the conjugate.[25] Therefore, attempts made to identify more soluble cytotoxic drug analogs can pay off when it comes to making high-quality monomeric conjugates. Hydrophobicity and charge are also important for cellular permeability and retention. Charged drugs are generally less able to cross biological membranes and have lower potency as free drugs, but in some cases they may be advantageous for delivery by an antibody conjugate. After take-up of the ADC into the target cell, a charged drug released by ADC degradation is then trapped. For example, a comparison of ADCs with two auristatin derivatives, monomethyl auristatin E and F (MMAE and MMAF), using a number of different linkers has been carried out, MMAF being a derivative with a charged C-terminal phenylalanine.[26] Although free MMAF is relatively poorly cytotoxic, potent conjugates could be made with a large therapeutic window. Cytotoxicity of equivalent MMAE and MMAF conjugates was approximately equal despite an approximately 100-fold decrease in potency of MMAF compared to MMAE as free drug.[27] One potential consequence of this approach would be less bystander killing of cells adjacent to the target, which might be helpful for reduced toxicity but result in less potent effects against solid tumors with heterogeneous antigen expression. Activity of MMAF conjugates toward solid tumor targets may therefore be less predictable than MMAE.[26] Local drug efflux to adjacent cells has also been hypothesized to be a mechanism to explain the effectiveness of ADCs targeting the CanAg antigen against large tumors where it is heterogeneously expressed,[28] although it is now clear that linker stability plays a major role in achieving this.[29]

Drug resistance is a major issue for successful chemotherapy, and experience with the one FDA-approved ADC, gemtuzumab ozogamicin (Mylotarg®), has highlighted the same issue with antibody drug conjugates. Gemtuzumab ozogamicin has shown a response rate of 25% to 30% over a number of clinical trials, and the clinical activity clearly correlates with the drug-resistance phenotype of patients.[30] Acute myeloid leukemia (AML) blasts of responders have significantly lower levels of the MDR-1 drug-resistance protein, P-glycoprotein (pgp), than nonresponders, and it has been shown that the presence of pgp is significantly associated with poorer outcome after treatment.[31] MDR-1 associated pgp is one of a number of clinically important drug-resistance-associated proteins. It is a membrane glycoprotein that actively pumps the cytotoxic agent out of the cells and decreases intracellular accumulation.[32] These clinical findings were largely predictable from *in vitro* studies, which showed clearly that the cytotoxicity of gemtuzumab ozogamicin is greatly diminished in multidrug-resistant sublines of CD33 positive parental cell lines made either by selection or direct transfection of MDR-1. In addition, pgp inhibitors could reverse this effect, restoring the sensitivity of the sublines to the ADC suggesting that combination therapy with such inhibitors might be warranted.[33] Drugs that are not subject to pumping by drug-resistance proteins may therefore be particularly attractive for ADC development. One class of drugs that appears to be not subject to the action of a number of drug-resistance proteins, including pgp, is the duocarmycins,[34,35] and a number of ADCs using these and other MGBAs are under active development.[36–38]

LINKERS

The stability and type of linkage of the drug to the antibody can also play a role in drug resistance. For example, a calicheamicin conjugate of an Muc-1 specific antibody linked through a stable amide linkage was less subject to multidrug resistance than an equivalent hydrazone-linked conjugate and retained activity on resistant cell lines both *in vitro* and *in vivo*.[39] Intracellular routing may play a role in reducing drug efflux, as has been suggested for a doxorubicin conjugate of an antibody-targeting insulin-like growth factor receptor, which had improved activity in drug-resistant cells compared to doxorubicin alone, possibly due to lysosomal trafficking.[40] In many cases, however, alteration of the drug linkage to the antibody will result in a slightly different drug derivative being liberated inside the cell, and this may have altered substrate recognition by drug efflux pumps.

The nature of the linkage of the drug to the antibody has been a major focus of research for effective antibody-drug conjugate development. Stability of the linker to minimize systemic release of active drug is crucial for maintaining an improved therapeutic window over drug alone, and yet the linker needs to be able to efficiently release active drug at the tumor site. To overcome this dilemma, a number of different types of linkers have been widely studied, many of which attempt to take advantage of specific intracellular release mechanisms while maintaining high stability. There are four major types of linker in use today: pH-sensitive (typically hydrazones), disulfide, peptide, and noncleavable.

The pH-sensitive linkers are designed to take advantage of the reduced pH encountered by ADCs in the endosomal and lysomal compartments of the cell. A wide range of different linkers have been tested including *cis*-aconityl, semicarbazones, and acetals, but most effort has concentrated on hydrazones.[41–45] Hydrazones with a wide range of different stabilities can be made from relatively unstable to very stable. A hydrazone can be formed as a linkage between antibody carbohydrate and drug using periodate oxidation of the carbohydrate to form aldehydes and then reaction with hydrazide derivatized drugs.[45] This has the advantage of being a site-specific attachment methodology that links drug to the Fc region, well away from the antigen-binding site. However, this method allows for little flexibility in the linkage chemistry and therefore little opportunity to tune the stability of the linkage. Tuning of hydrazone stability has been shown to be important for optimal properties of the linker. A series of hydrazone linkers made during development of Mylotarg® had widely varying hydrolysis rates, with 0% to 90% of the hydrazone cleaved at neutral pH over 24 hours.[44] By also testing the stability at pH4.5 it was possible to choose one from the series that had good stability at neutral pH but rapidly released the drug at pH4.5. These properties then allowed the resulting conjugate to be extremely potent, with an IC50 of 0.04ng (calicheamicin equivalents)/ml, with several thousandfold selectivity over antigen negative cells. The conjugate was also shown to be highly effective *in vivo*, resulting in regressions of established xenograft tumors in mice, with long-term tumor-free survivors.[44]

Disulfide linkers have been used for a number of different conjugates and aim to take advantage of the increased thiol content inside the cell compared to in circulation. Disulfide linkers were originally developed for use with immunotoxins but resulted in relatively unstable linkage and therefore attention turned to the development of "hindered" disulfide linkages with a methyl or phenyl group adjacent to the disulfide.[46] Such "hindered" disulfides are more stable in circulation but still readily reduced inside the cell. Maytansine conjugates have been developed for a number of different antibodies using hindered disulfide linkers, and several of them have been taken into clinical development. DM1 is a derivative of the highly potent anti-tubulin agent maytansine, which is linked through a singly hindered disulfide containing an adjacent methyl group. Preclinical studies with DM1 conjugates have demonstrated good activity in a range of models,[28, 47] although clinical studies have suggested that stability of the linkage is less than optimal.[48, 49] In a comprehensive study aimed at improving the properties of the disulfide linker, a series of more hindered forms of the disulfide were tested and this led to the identification of DM4 with improved *in vivo* stability.[50] DM4 conjugates of the anti-CanAg antibody C242 and anti-αv integrin have been shown to be more potent than the equivalent DM1 conjugate in tumor xenograft models, possibly due to the increased circulating half-life of the more stable conjugates, leading to improved delivery.[51, 52] However, an even more hindered form of the linker resulted in conjugates with minimal activity.[52] This result may be because stability was increased too far so that the drug is not readily able to be released inside the tumor cell, or because of the differential potency of the maytansine derivative released by the more stable linkage. The potency of the derivative generated inside the cell has been shown to be crucial for activity using a noncleavable SMCC linker that creates a thioether linkage to maytansine.[51] C242 linked to maytansine in this manner was as active as the DM4 conjugate, and both forms were shown to be processed inside the cell by initial degradation of the antibody to lysine-maytansine adducts, which maintained activity; however, the DM4 conjugate could also undergo reduction to generate additional active metabolites.

Peptide linkers have also been used to generate a series of antibody conjugates with excellent preclinical activity. These are based on peptides that are cleaved by lysosomal enzymes such as cathepsin B. These have been tested with a wide range of drugs including doxorubicin, taxol, mitomycin C, and camptothecin,[53–56] but most work has focused on the auristatins MMAE and MMAF.[26, 57] A series of dipeptide linkers were tested that were able to be cleaved by cathepsin B, and phenylalanine-lysine and valine-citrulline were identified as particularly useful, being stable in circulation and able to release drug effectively inside the tumor cell.[54, 57] Lysosomal proteases can be detected in the blood, but activity is low in the circulation probably because of endogenous inhibitors and because the pH is higher than that found in the lysosomal compartment. Half-lives for peptide-linked conjugates have therefore been longer than those reported for hydrazone or disulfide linked conjugates.[58]

Other enzymatic methods of release are also being investigated. For example, linkers cleavable by beta-glucuronidase have been investigated with doxorubicin, MAAE, and MMAF.[59, 60] Beta-glucuronidase is another lysosomal enzyme that can be utilized for intracellular cleavage. Linkers cleavable by beta-glucuronidase are generally hydrophilic structures; they are under investigation as they avoid the need for hydrophobic moieties in the linker, such as the hydrophobic amino acids in the peptide linkers mentioned earlier, and therefore they may be advantageous in avoiding conjugate aggregation.[60] MMAE and MMAF conjugates made with these linkers were well tolerated and efficacious in xenograft models, although to date neither *in vivo* half-lives nor comparative studies with the equivalent peptide-linked conjugates have been reported.

Although protease sensitive and hindered disulfide linkers are designed for rapid intracellular release of the drug, there is mounting evidence that proteolytic degradation of the antibody may be a major pathway for drug release.[51,61] This has led to increased interest in linkers without a cleavable linkage, which upon degradation of the antibody result in an amino acid adduct of the drug. Such an approach is reliant upon the drug adduct retaining the cytotoxic activity of the parental drug but has the advantage of being the most stable linking approach. A conjugate of DM1 to trastuzumab has been shown to be effective in a range of animal models and has been taken into clinical studies using a noncleavable linker.[5] A noncleavable MCC linker was used to construct a conjugate of DM1 to the C242 antibody and had equivalent *in vitro* cytotoxicity to the hindered disulfides DM1 and DM4 linked to the same antibody.[29, 51] *In vivo* activity of the noncleavable conjugate was reduced compared to the DM4 ADC, likely because of reduced bystander killing of tumor cells that were poorly accessible or antigen negative. This was attributed to the cell permeability of the form of the drug released by disulfide reduction that could diffuse to tumor cells nearby, whereas the adduct formed from the noncleavable linker was unable to permeate cell membranes. Such a bystander effect might be particularly useful for targeting antigens that are heterogeneously expressed *in vivo*.[29] This approach has even been extended to antigen negative tumors *in vivo*, in which sufficient antibody accumulates through enhanced permeability and retention of the macromolecule in the tumor (EPR effect), allowing sufficient release of calicheamicin from a hydrazone-linked conjugate to result in antitumor activity.[62]

Another important parameter for antibody conjugate design is substitution ratio, or number of drug molecules attached to each antibody molecule. If sufficient potency can be achieved, keeping the substitution ratio low, and therefore minimizing the number of chemical modifications to the antibody and the number of hydrophobic moieties attached, will improve the pharmacological and physical properties of the conjugate. An interesting study with MMAE conjugates of an anti-CD30 antibody has compared conjugates with 2, 4, or 8 (E2, E4, E8) drug molecules per antibody.[63] Drugs were attached to cysteine residues following partial reduction of antibody disulfide bonds. Although potency *in vitro* was directly dependent on drug loading, the *in vivo* antitumor activity of the E4 conjugate was equivalent to the E8 conjugate at the same protein dose, and therefore half the dose of MMAE. The E2 conjugate was less active. The toxicity of the conjugates was increased in proportion to the drug loading, and consequently the E4 conjugate resulted in the best therapeutic window. This was attributed to a longer plasma half-life of the E4 conjugate, with consequent improved tumor exposure.[63] Several possible explanations for the shorter half-life of the more conjugated antibody can be postulated, including increased hydrophobicity, increased interaction with serum proteins, and greater perturbation of the antibody structure through disulfide bond reduction. A similar substitution ratio has also been shown to be optimal for maytansine conjugates.[64]

For more potent drugs it is feasible to reduce the drug loading further, with potential benefits in the physical properties of the conjugate. Conjugates with duocarmycins and other MGBAs can be made with substitution ratios of one or two that are highly efficacious with a wide therapeutic window.[36–38]

SITE-SPECIFIC ATTACHMENT

Conjugation is usually carried out to amino acid side chains – for example, to lysine residues – in a random fashion such that a distribution of chemically modified species is found in each preparation of conjugate, where different positions in the antibody may be modified each time. Although successfully used – for example, with gemtuzumab ozogamicin – this approach has several disadvantages. These include the fact that amino acids important for function of the antibody, as in antigen binding or Fc receptor binding, may be modified, particularly at higher drug loadings, and consequently, functionality of the antibody may be modified or lost. In addition, the heterogeneity of the antibody conjugate, in which a population of molecules exists with different side chains modified, complicates analysis and makes it difficult to ensure that each preparation contains the same distribution of modified species.

A potential improvement to conjugation is to attach the drug at a specific site, which is identical each time. This can be designed such that attachment to the site does not interfere with antibody functional properties and allows simplified analysis and quality control of conjugate preparations. A number of approaches have been used to accomplish this either by using naturally occurring sites in the antibody molecule or by specifically introducing additional sites through antibody engineering.

The generation of free cysteines by selective reduction of the hinge region has been used for the attachment of thiol reactive compounds to both IgG and antibody fragments – for example, to attach fluorescent compounds,[65] for attachment of chelators that can be used for site-specific radiolabeling,[66] and for drug attachment.[57] Disadvantages of this approach include the reduction of disulfide bonds that are important for maintenance of the native antibody structure. This may have detrimental effects on the functionality or stability of the resulting conjugate. Also, as several disulfide bonds are present in the antibody molecule, including two in the hinge region for human IgG1, one attaching each light chain to heavy chain, and one internal disulfide in each folded immunoglobulin domain, there remains a great deal of heterogeneity in the conjugate produced. Careful development of the reduction conditions used can control heterogeneity of the conjugates to some extent,[67] and in addition, cysteine residues can be replaced by serine to reduce the number of potential conjugation sites and subsequently reduce heterogeneity.[68]

The Fc region carbohydrate also provides a natural specific attachment site for IgG and this has been exploited in a number of antibody conjugates.[44,45] Carbohydrate is modified by periodate oxidation to generate reactive aldehydes that can then be used to attach reactive amine containing compounds by Schiff base formation. As the aldehydes can react with amine groups, reactions are carried out at low pH so that the lysine residues are protonated and unreactive. Hydrazide groups are most suitable for attachment to the aldehydes generated since they are reactive at low pH to form a hydrazone linkage. The linkage can then be further stabilized by reduction with sodium cyanoborohydride to form a hydrazine linkage. However, this approach requires relatively harsh conditions that can damage and aggregate some antibody molecules, and it also introduces the drug into a region known to be vital for efficient Fc receptor-mediated function. In addition, methionine residues present in some antibody variable regions may be particularly susceptible to oxidation by periodate, which can lead to loss of antigen-binding avidity, and in some cases histidine or tryptophan residues might also be affected. It also allows little opportunity for modulating the stability of drug linkage.

Extra cysteine residues can be introduced onto the surface of antibody constant domains to provide a specific attachment site without the need to disrupt native disulphide bonds. Introduction of specific cysteine residues in the CH1 domain of the IgG heavy chain has been shown to result in sites to which ligands can be attached without any loss of antigen binding.[69] These mutations can be used to produce site-specifically modified IgG or Fab antibody fragments and were shown not to result in antibody aggregation. Mutations in the Fc region have also been generated and used for site-specific attachment.[70] Recently, a number of additional sites in the Fab region have been identified for the introduction of cysteine residues to produce site-specific drug conjugates.[71] Trastuzumab-auristatin conjugates prepared using these mutants showed an improved therapeutic window over equivalent conjugates made by disulfide reduction, with improved *in vivo* stability.[72]

Alternative methods for site-specific attachment include the introduction of extra glycosylation sites to allow attachment via periodate oxidation. Some antibody light chains have an unusual natural glycosylation site, and thus the light chain has been used as a site to introduce a glycosylation site into antibodies that do not normally have carbohydrate attached to the light chain.[73] A third engineering strategy is to introduce extra lysine residues into the surface of the constant region domains.[74] Although this approach does not introduce a unique labeling site, lysine reactive reagents are more likely to modify the antibody at the increased concentration of lysine residues in the constant region, resulting in the retention of more antigen-binding reactivity.

EXAMPLES OF PROMISING ADCs IN DEVELOPMENT

Early work with conjugates of highly potent cytotoxic drugs led to the rapid approval of gemtuzumab ozogamicin for therapy of AML. This conjugate is linked through a pH-sensitive hydrazone bond and also contains a hindered disulfide bond that is reduced during drug activation. The high toxicity of this conjugate has been a major issue, as has drug resistance, and further trials are ongoing to find optimal treatment regimes that incorporate this agent.[75] Another agent targeted to a liquid tumor type, non-Hodgkin's lymphoma, is CMC-544, which uses calicheamicin linked to an antibody to the well-internalized antigen CD22 through the same linker. Preclinical studies with this agent have demonstrated impressive activity, and clinical studies are in progress.[76]

One exciting class of conjugates now under development use potent DNA minor-groove binding alkylating (MGBA) agents.[36–38] These compounds have a number of key advantages, including very high potency, good water solubility characteristics, and being available by entirely synthetic routes without the need for contained microbial fermentation. Molecules of this class can be extremely potent, among the most potent antitumor antibiotics known, and are natural prodrugs, which are activated only on binding to DNA.[77] After binding, MGBA agents alkylate double-stranded DNA in a sequence-selective manner, resulting in single stranded DNA breaks and subsequent cell death.[78]

Previous attempts to conjugate these molecules to antibodies have run into problems due to their insolubility in water;[79] however, new derivatives have been developed that have excellent solubility characteristics and maintain the potency of the original compounds.[36–38] Another important characteristic of MGBAs is their ability to evade the major mechanisms of drug resistance.[34] New analogs are able to retain this favorable property with excellent potency against cells expressing high levels of p-glycoprotein.[36] Prostate-specific membrane antigen (PSMA) is an antigen highly expressed on prostate cancer as well as the vasculature of other tumor types and has been the target of ADCs using maytansine[47] and auristatin;[80] it is now being developed with an ADC using a human antibody linked to an MGBA.[36] In addition, CD70, a highly selective tumor antigen on renal carcinoma, lymphoma, and a number of other tumor types, is being targeted using this approach as well as by auristatin conjugates.[38, 81]

Clinical data with disulfide-linked conjugates of DM1 have also been important for the development of ADC technology and has increased interest in reducing toxicity of conjugates through increased linker stability. CanAg is a glycoform of MUC1 that is highly expressed on a range of tumor types including colorectal, gastric, and pancreatic tumors and minimally expressed in normal tissues. The anti-CanAg antibody C242-DM1 conjugate, termed cantuzumab mertansine, was highly effective in animal models, and several clinical trials have been conducted.[48, 82] Results from these trials have shown a relatively short half-life for the conjugate, with premature release of the DM1, and have increased interest in the more hindered disulfide linkage used to make C242-DM4, which is now being studied in the clinic.[83] Similarly, a conjugate of DM1 with an antibody to PSMA, which was taken into clinical trials, suffered from the relatively unstable linker and resulted in toxicities typical of free maytansine.[49]

Stability of the linkage to maytansine was further increased to generate the trastuzumab-DM1 conjugate currently in clinical trials. This agent uses a noncleavable linker and relies on antibody degradation in the lysosome for generation of the cytotoxic moiety.[5] In a Phase I trial an encouraging response rate was seen with partial responses in 6 out of 16 patients, and Phase II studies are now under way. Peptide linkers have also been explored for trastuzumab linked to the alternative tubulin active cytotoxic, MMAF.[84] Such conjugates were efficacious in xenograft models, and conjugates made with different substitution ratios have been characterized.[84]

Clinical studies are also under way with peptide-linked conjugates of MMAE with antibodies to both CD30[85] and the melanoma-associated antigen glycoprotein nonmetastatic melanoma protein B (GPNMB).[86] Encouraging response rates have also been seen with these agents – for example, the anti-CD30 MMAE conjugate SGN-35 achieved tumor reductions in 11 of 13 Hodgkin's lymphoma patients treated at >1 mg/kg.[85] With such encouraging data there is renewed interest in the development of ADCs, particularly with more stable linkers between the antibody and cytotoxin. Such conjugates potentially harness the benefit of the long half-life and consequent tumor targeting and accumulation of the antibody without unacceptable toxicity.

REFERENCES

[1]   Cobleigh MA, Vogel CL, Tripathy D, Robert NJ, Scholl S, Fehrenbacher L, Wolter JM, Paton V, Shak S, Lieberman G, Slamon DJ (1999). Multinational study of the efficacy and safety of humanized anti-HER2 monoclonal antibody in women who have HER2-overexpressing metastatic breast cancer that has progressed after chemotherapy for metastatic disease. *J Clin Oncol* **17**, 2639–2648.

[2]   Vogel CL, Cobleigh MA, Tripathy D, Gutheil JC, Harris LN, Fehrenbacher L, Slamon DJ, Murphy M, Novotny WF, Burchmore M, Shak S, Stewart SJ, Press M (2002). Efficacy and safety of trastuzumab as a single agent in first-line treatment of HER2-overexpressing metastatic breast cancer. *J Clin Oncol* **20**, 719–726.

[3]   Slamon DJ, Leyland-Jones B, Shak S, Fuchs H, Paton V, Bajamonde A, Fleming T, Eiermann, W, Wolter J, Pegram M, Baselga J, Norton L (2001). Use of chemotherapy plus a monoclonal antibody against HER2 for metastatic breast cancer that overexpresses HER2. *N Engl J Med* **344**, 783–792.

[4] Hudis CA (2007). Trastuzumab–mechanism of action and use in clinical practice. *N Engl J Med* **357**, 39–51.

[5] Beeram M, Burris HA, Modi S, Birkner M, Girish S, Tibbitts J, Holden SN, Lutzker SG, Krop IE (2008). A phase I study of trastuzumab-DM1 (T-DM1), a first-in-class HER2 antibody-drug conjugate (ADC), in patients (pts) with advanced HER2+ breast cancer (BC). *J Clin Oncol* **26** (May 20 suppl). 1028.

[6] Moolten FL, Cooperband SR (1970). Selective destruction of target cells by diphtheria toxin conjugated to antibody directed against antigens on the cells. *Science* **169**, 68–70.

[7] Hurwitz E, Levy R, Maron R, Wilchek M, Arnon R, Sela M (1975). The covalent binding of daunomycin and adriamycin to antibodies, with retention of both drug and antibody activities. *Cancer Res* **35**, 1175–1181.

[8] Smyth MJ, Pietersz GA, McKenzie IF (1986). Potentiation of the in vitro cytotoxicity of chlorambucil by monoclonal antibodies. *J Immunol* **137**, 3361–3366.

[9] Starling JJ, Maciak RS, Law KL, Hinson NA, Briggs SL, Laguzza BC, Johnson, DA (1991). In vivo antitumor activity of a monoclonal antibody-Vinca alkaloid immunoconjugate directed against a solid tumor membrane antigen characterized by heterogeneous expression and noninternalization of antibody-antigen complexes. *Cancer Res* **51**, 2965–2972.

[10] Trail PA, Willner D, Lasch SJ, Henderson AJ, Hofstead S, Casazza AM, Firestone RA, Hellstrom I, Hellstrom KE (1993). Cure of xenografted human carcinomas by BR96-doxorubicin immunoconjugates. *Science* **261**, 212–215.

[11] Starling JJ, Maciak RS, Hinson NA, Nichols CL, Briggs SL, Laguzza BC, Smith W, Corvalan, JR (1992). In vivo antitumor activity of a panel of four monoclonal antibody-vinca alkaloid immunoconjugates which bind to three distinct epitopes of carcinoembryonic antigen. *Bioconjug Chem* **3**, 315–322.

[12] Jain M, Venkatraman G, Batra SK (2007). Optimization of radioimmunotherapy of solid tumors: biological impediments and their modulation. *Clin Cancer Res* **13**, 1374–1382.

[13] King HD, Dubowchik GM, Mastalerz H, Willner D, Hofstead SJ, Firestone RA, Lasch SJ, Trail PA (2002). Monoclonal antibody conjugates of doxorubicin prepared with branched peptide linkers: inhibition of aggregation by methoxytriethyleneglycol chains. *J Med Chem* **45**, 4336–4343.

[14] Sapra P, Tyagi P, Allen TM (2005). Ligand-targeted liposomes for cancer treatment. *Curr Drug Deliv* **2**, 369–381.

[15] Hamann PR, Hinman LM, Hollander I, Beyer CF, Lindh D, Holcomb R, Hallett W, Tsou HR, Upeslacis J, Shochat D, Mountain A, Flowers DA, Bernstein I (2002). Gemtuzumab ozogamicin, a potent and selective anti-CD33 antibody-calicheamicin conjugate for treatment of acute myeloid leukemia. *Bioconjug Chem* **13**, 47–58.

[16] Petersen BH, DeHerdt SV, Schneck DW, Bumol TF (1991). The human immune response to KS1/4-desacetylvinblastine (LY256787) and KS1/4-desacetylvinblastine hydrazide (LY203728) in single and multiple dose clinical studies. *Cancer Res* **51**, 2286–2290.

[17] Salvatore G, Beers R, Margulies I, Kreitman RJ, Pastan I (2002). Improved cytotoxic activity toward cell lines and fresh leukemia cells of a mutant anti-CD22 immunotoxin obtained by antibody phage display. *Clin Cancer Res* **8**, 995–1002.

[18] Ho M, Kreitman RJ, Onda M, Pastan I (2005). In vitro antibody evolution targeting germline hot spots to increase activity of an anti-CD22 immunotoxin. *J Biol Chem* **280**, 607–617.

[19] Conner SD, Schmid SL (2003). Regulated portals of entry into the cell. *Nature* **422**, 37–44.

[20] Recht LD, Raso V, Davis R, Salmonsen R (1996). Immunotoxin sensitivity of Chinese hamster ovary cells expressing human transferrin receptors with differing internalization rates. *Cancer Immunol Immunother* **42**, 357–361.

[21] Ingle GS, Chan P, Elliott JM, Chang WS, Koeppen H, Stephan JP, Scales SJ (2008). High CD21 expression inhibits internalization of anti-CD19 antibodies and cytotoxicity of an anti-CD19-drug conjugate. *Br J Haematol* **140**, 46–58.

[22] He D, Yang H, Lin Q, Huang H (2005). Arg9-peptide facilitates the internalization of an anti-CEA immunotoxin and potentiates its specific cytotoxicity to target cells. *Int J Biochem Cell Biol* **37**, 192–205.

[23] Law CL, Cerveny CG, Gordon KA, Klussman K, Mixan BJ, Chace DF, Meyer DL, Doronina SO, Siegall CB, Francisco JA, Senter PD, Wahl AF (2004). Efficient elimination of B-lineage lymphomas by anti-CD20-auristatin conjugates. *Clin Cancer Res* **10**, 7842–7851.

[24] Austin CD, De Maziere, AM, Pisacane PI, van Dijk, SM, Eigenbrot C, Sliwkowski MX, Klumperman J, Scheller RH (2004). Endocytosis and sorting of ErbB2 and the site of action of cancer therapeutics trastuzumab and geldanamycin. *Mol Biol Cell* **15**, 5268–5282.

[25] Hollander I, Kunz, A, Hamann PR (2008). Selection of reaction additives used in the preparation of monomeric antibody-calicheamicin conjugates. *Bioconjug Chem* **19**, 358–361.

[26] Doronina SO, Mendelsohn BA, Bovee TD, Cerveny CG, Alley SC, Meyer DL, Oflazoglu E, Toki BE, Sanderson RJ, Zabinski RF, Wahl AF, Senter PD (2006). Enhanced activity of monomethylauristatin F through monoclonal antibody delivery: effects of linker technology on efficacy and toxicity. *Bioconjug Chem* **17**, 114–124.

[27] Sutherland MS, Sanderson RJ, Gordon KA, Andreyka J, Cerveny CG, Yu C, Lewis TS, Meyer DL, Zabinski RF, Doronina SO, Senter PD, Law CL, Wahl AF (2006). Lysosomal trafficking and cysteine protease metabolism confer target-specific cytotoxicity by peptide-linked anti-CD30-auristatin conjugates. *J Biol Chem* **281**, 10540–10547.

[28] Liu C, Tadayoni BM, Bourret LA, Mattocks KM, Derr SM, Widdison WC, Kedersha NL, Ariniello PD, Goldmacher VS, Lambert JM, Blattler WA, Chari RV (1996). Eradication of large colon tumor xenografts by targeted delivery of maytansinoids. *Proc Natl Acad Sci U S A* **93**, 8618–8623.

[29] Kovtun YV, Audette CA, Ye Y, Xie H, Ruberti MF, Phinney SJ, Leece BA, Chittenden T, Blattler WA, Goldmacher VS (2006). Antibody-drug conjugates designed to eradicate tumors with homogeneous and heterogeneous expression of the target antigen. *Cancer Res* **66**, 3214–3221.

[30] Linenberger ML, Hong T, Flowers D, Sievers EL, Gooley TA, Bennett JM, Berger MS, Leopold LH, Appelbaum FR, Bernstein ID (2001). Multidrug-resistance phenotype and clinical responses to gemtuzumab ozogamicin. *Blood* **98**, 988–994.

[31] Walter RB, Gooley TA, van der Velden VH, Loken MR, van Dongen JJ, Flowers DA, Bernstein ID, Appelbaum FR (2007). CD33 expression and P-glycoprotein-mediated drug efflux inversely correlate and predict clinical outcome in patients with acute myeloid leukemia treated with gemtuzumab ozogamicin monotherapy. *Blood* **109**, 4168–4170.

[32] Kartner N, Evernden-Porelle D, Bradley G, Ling V (1985). Detection of P-glycoprotein in multidrug-resistant cell lines by monoclonal antibodies. *Nature* **316**, 820–823.

[33] Naito K, Takeshita A, Shigeno K, Nakamura S, Fujisawa S, Shinjo K, Yoshida H, Ohnishi K, Mori M, Terakawa S, Ohno R (2000). Calicheamicin-conjugated humanized anti-CD33 monoclonal antibody (gemtuzumab zogamicin, CMA-676) shows cytocidal effect on CD33-positive leukemia cell lines, but is inactive on P-glycoprotein-expressing sublines. *Leukemia* **14**, 1436–1443.

[34] Gomi K, Kobayashi E, Miyoshi K, Ashizawa T, Okamoto A, Ogawa T, Katsumata S, Mihara A, Okabe M, Hirata T (1992). Anticellular and antitumor activity of duocarmycins, novel antitumor antibiotics. *Jpn J Cancer Res* **83**, 113–120.

[35] Kobayashi E, Okamoto A, Asada M, Okabe M, Nagamura S, Asai A, Saito H, Gomi K, Hirata T (1994). Characteristics of antitumor activity of KW-2189, a novel water-soluble derivative of duocarmycin, against murine and human tumors. *Cancer Res* **54**, 2404–2410.

[36] Pan C, Gangwar S, Chen L, Rao C, Huber M, Sattari P, Do M, Dai R, Chong C, Soderberg C, Li H, Sufi B, Boyd S, Huang H, Chen H, Guerlavais V, Horgan K, Sharkov N, Cardarelli P, King DJ (2006). Human antibody conjugates of DNA minor groove-binding alkylating agents with single dose efficacy in xenograft models which retain activity in drug resistant cells. *Proc Amer Assoc Cancer Res* **47**, 1171.

[37] Rao C, Pan C, Huber M, Sattari P, Chong C, Dai R, Soderberg C, Chen L, Guerlavais V, Horgan K, Zhang A, Sufi B, Huang H, Chen H, Gangwar S, Cardarelli P, King D. (2007). Efficacy study of anti-CD19 antibody drug-conjugates in Raji tumor xenograft and systemic model. *Proc Amer Assoc Cancer Research* **48**, 4104.

[38] Terrett JA, Gangwar S, Rao-Naik C, Pan C, Guerlavais V, Huber M, Chong C, Green L, Cardarelli P, King D, Deshpande S, Rangan V, Coccia M, Lu L, Passmore D, Blansett D, Dai R, Sufi B,

Zhang Q, Chen L, Soderberg C, Kwok E, Horgan K, Cortez O, Sattari P. (2007). Single, low dose treatment of lymphoma and renal cancer xenografts with human anti-CD70 antibody-toxin conjugates, results in long term cures. *Proc Amer Assoc Cancer Res* **48**, 4112.

[39]   Hamann PR, Hinman LM, Beyer CF, Lindh D, Upeslacis J, Shochat D, Mountain A (2005). A calicheamicin conjugate with a fully humanized anti-MUC1 antibody shows potent antitumor effects in breast and ovarian tumor xenografts. *Bioconjug Chem* **16**, 354–360.

[40]   Guillemard V, Saragovi H (2004). Prodrug chemotherapeutics bypass p-glycoprotein resistance and kill tumors in vivo with high efficacy and target-dependent selectivity. *Oncogene* **23**, 3613–3621.

[41]   Schrappe M, Bumol TF, Apelgren LD, Briggs SL, Koppel GA, Markowitz DD, Mueller BM, Reisfeld RA (1992). Long-term growth suppression of human glioma xenografts by chemo-immunoconjugates of 4-desacetylvinblastine-3-carboxyhydrazide and monoclonal antibody 9.2.27. *Cancer Res* **52**, 3838–3844.

[42]   Mueller BM, Wrasidlo WA, Reisfeld RA (1990). Antibody conjugates with morpholinodoxorubicin and acid-cleavable linkers. *Bioconjug Chem* **1**, 325–330.

[43]   Gillies ER, Goodwin A, Frechet JM (2004). Acetals as pH-sensitive linkages for drug delivery. *Bioconjug Chem* **15**, 1254–1263.

[44]   Hamann PR, Hinman LM, Beyer CF, Lindh D, Upeslacis J, Flowers DA, Bernstein I (2002). An anti-CD33 antibody-calicheamicin conjugate for treatment of acute myeloid leukemia. Choice of linker. *Bioconjug Chem* **13**, 40–46.

[45]   Hinman LM, Hamann PR, Wallace R, Menendez AT, Durr FE, Upeslacis J (1993). Preparation and characterization of monoclonal antibody conjugates of the calicheamicins: a novel and potent family of antitumor antibiotics. *Cancer Res* **53**, 3336–3342.

[46]   Thorpe PE, Wallace PM, Knowles PP, Relf MG, Brown AN, Watson GJ, Blakey DC, Newell DR (1988). Improved antitumor effects of immunotoxins prepared with deglycosylated ricin A-chain and hindered disulfide linkages. *Cancer Res* **48**, 6396–6403.

[47]   Henry MD, Wen S, Silva MD, Chandra S, Milton M, Worland PJ (2004). A prostate-specific membrane antigen-targeted monoclonal antibody-chemotherapeutic conjugate designed for the treatment of prostate cancer. *Cancer Res* **64**, 7995–8001.

[48]   Tolcher AW, Ochoa L, Hammond LA, Patnaik A, Edwards T, Takimoto C, Smith L, de Bono J, Schwartz G, Mays T, Jonak ZL, Johnson R, DeWitte M, Martino H, Audette C, Maes K, Chari RV, Lambert JM, Rowinsky EK (2003). Cantuzumab mertansine, a maytansinoid immunoconjugate directed to the CanAg antigen: a phase I, pharmacokinetic, and biologic correlative study. *J Clin Oncol* **21**, 211–222.

[49]   Galsky MD, Eisenberger M, Moore-Cooper S, Kelly WK, Slovin SF, DeLaCruz A, Lee Y, Webb IJ, Scher HI (2008). Phase I trial of the prostate-specific membrane antigen-directed immunoconjugate MLN2704 in patients with progressive metastatic castration-resistant prostate cancer. *J Clin Oncol* **26**, 2147–2154.

[50]   Widdison WC, Wilhelm SD, Cavanagh EE, Whiteman KR, Leece BA, Kovtun Y, Goldmacher VS, Xie H, Steeves RM, Lutz RJ, Zhao R, Wang L, Blattler WA, Chari RV (2006). Semisynthetic maytansine analogues for the targeted treatment of cancer. *J Med Chem* **49**, 4392–4408.

[51]   Erickson HK, Park PU, Widdison WC, Kovtun YV, Garrett LM, Hoffman K, Lutz RJ, Goldmacher VS, Blattler W (2006). Antibody-maytansinoid conjugates are activated in targeted cancer cells by lysosomal degradation and linker-dependent intracellular processing. *Cancer Res* **66**, 4426–4433.

[52]   Chen Q, Millar HJ, McCabe FL, Manning CD, Steeves R, Lai K, Kellogg B, Lutz RJ, Trikha M, Nakada MT, Anderson GM (2007). Alphav integrin-targeted immunoconjugates regress established human tumors in xenograft models. *Clin Cancer Res* **13**, 3689–3695.

[53]   Dubowchik GM, Firestone RA (1998). Cathepsin B-sensitive dipeptide prodrugs. 1. A model study of structural requirements for efficient release of doxorubicin. *Bioorg Med Chem Lett* **8**, 3341–3346.

[54]   Dubowchik GM, Mosure K, Knipe JO, Firestone RA (1998). Cathepsin B-sensitive dipeptide prodrugs. 2. Models of anticancer drugs paclitaxel (Taxol), mitomycin C and doxorubicin. *Bioorg Med Chem Lett* **8**, 3347–3352.

[55]   Dubowchik GM, Firestone RA, Padilla L, Willner D, Hofstead SJ, Mosure K, Knipe JO, Lasch SJ, Trail PA (2002). Cathepsin B-labile dipeptide linkers for lysosomal release of doxorubicin from internalizing immunoconjugates: model studies of enzymatic drug release and antigen-specific in vitro anticancer activity. *Bioconjug Chem* **13**, 855–869.

[56]   Walker MA, Dubowchik GM, Hofstead SJ, Trail PA, Firestone RA (2002). Synthesis of an immunoconjugate of camptothecin. *Bioorg Med Chem Lett* **12**, 217–219.

[57]   Doronina SO, Toki BE, Torgov MY, Mendelsohn BA, Cerveny CG, Chace DF, DeBlanc RL, Gearing RP, Bovee TD, Siegall CB, Francisco JA, Wahl AF, Meyer DL, Senter PD (2003). Development of potent monoclonal antibody auristatin conjugates for cancer therapy. *Nat Biotechnol* **21**, 778–784.

[58]   Sanderson RJ, Hering MA, James SF, Sun MM, Doronina SO, Siadak AW, Senter PD, Wahl AF (2005). In vivo drug-linker stability of an anti-CD30 dipeptide-linked auristatin immunoconjugate. *Clin Cancer Res* **11**, 843–852.

[59]   de Graaf, M, Boven E, Scheeren HW, Haisma HJ, Pinedo HM (2002). Beta-glucuronidase-mediated drug release. *Curr Pharm Des* **8**, 1391–1403.

[60]   Jeffrey SC, Nguyen MT, Moser RF, Meyer DL, Miyamoto JB, Senter PD (2007). Minor groove binder antibody conjugates employing a water soluble beta-glucuronide linker. *Bioorg Med Chem Lett* **17**, 2278–2280.

[61]   Alley SC, Okeley NM, Sanderson RJ, Nanayakkara V, Campbell RL, Kline TB, Doronina SO, Jeffrey SC, Benjamin D, Senter PD (2006). Intracellular metabolism of antibody-drug conjugates: identification and quantitation of released drugs. *Proc Amer Assoc Cancer Res* **47**, 1992.

[62]   Boghaert ER, Khandke K, Sridharan L, Armellino D, Dougher M, Dijoseph JF, Kunz A, Hamann PR, Sridharan A, Jones S, Discafani C, Damle NK (2006). Tumoricidal effect of calicheamicin immuno-conjugates using a passive targeting strategy. *Int J Oncol* **28**, 675–684.

[63]   Hamblett KJ, Senter PD, Chace DF, Sun MM, Lenox J, Cerveny CG, Kissler KM, Bernhardt SX, Kopcha AK, Zabinski RF, Meyer DL, Francisco JA (2004). Effects of drug loading on the anti-tumor activity of a monoclonal antibody drug conjugate. *Clin Cancer Res* **10**, 7063–7070.

[64]   Chari RV, Martell BA, Gross JL, Cook SB, Shah SA, Blattler WA, McKenzie SJ, Goldmacher VS (1992). Immunoconjugates containing novel maytansinoids: promising anticancer drugs. *Cancer Res* **52**, 127–131.

[65]   Packard B, Edidin M, Komoriya A (1986). Site-directed labeling of a monoclonal antibody: targeting to a disulphide bond. *Biochem.* **25**, 3548–3552.

[66]   King DJ, Turner A, Farnsworth APH, Adair JR, Owens RJ, Pedley RB, Baldock D, Proudfoot KA, Lawson ADG, Beeley NRA, Millar K, Millican TA, Boyce B, Antoniw P, Mountain A, Begent RHJ, Shochat D, Yarranton GT (1994). Improved tumour targeting with chemically cross-linked recombinant antibody fragments. *Cancer Res* **54**, 6176–6185.

[67]   Sun MM, Beam KS, Cerveny CG, Hamblett KJ, Blackmore RS, Torgov MY, Handley FG, Ihle NC, Senter PD, Alley SC (2005). Reduction-alkylation strategies for the modification of specific monoclonal antibody disulfides. *Bioconjug Chem* **16**, 1282–1290.

[68]   McDonagh CF, Turcott E, Westendorf L, Webster JB, Alley SC, Kim K, Andreyka J, Stone I, Hamblett KJ, Francisco JA, Carter P (2006). Engineered antibody-drug conjugates with defined sites and stoichiometries of drug attachment. *Protein Eng Des Sel* **19**, 299–307.

[69]   Lyons A, King DJ, Owens RJ, Yarranton GT, Millican A, Whittle NR, Adair JR (1990). Site-specific attachment to recombinant antibodies via introduced surface cysteine residues. *Protein Eng* **3**, 703–708.

[70]   Stimmel JB, Merrill BM, Kuyper LF, Moxham CP, Hutchins JT, Fling ME, Kull FC (2000). Site-specific conjugation on serine-cysteine variant monoclonal antibodies. *J Biol Chem* **275**, 30445–30450.

[71]   Junutula JR, Bhakta S, Raab H, Ervin KE, Eigenbrot C, Vandlen R, Scheller RH, Lowman HB (2008). Rapid identification of reactive cysteine residues for site-specific labeling of antibody-Fabs. *J Immunol Methods* **332**, 41–52.

[72]   Junutula J, Raab H, Bhakta S, Parsons K, Clark S, Yu S, Ross S, Kim A, McDorman K, Flagella K, Spencer S, Vandlen R, Lowman HB, Mallet W, Polakis P, Sliwkowski MX, Scheller RH (2008).

Site-specific conjugation of cytotoxic drugs to antibodies substantially improves the therapeutic window. *Proc Amer Assoc Cancer Res* **49**, 2132.

[73] Leung S, Losman MJ, Govidan SV, Griffiths GL, Goldenberg DM, Hansen HJ (1995). Engineering a unique glycosylation site for site-specific conjugation of haptens to antibody fragments. *J Immunol* **154**, 5919–5926.

[74] Hemminki A, Hoffren AM, Takkinen K, Vehniainen M, Makinen ML, Pettersson K, Teleman O, Soderlund H, Teeri TT (1995). Introduction of lysine residues on the light chain constant domain improves the labelling properties of a recombinant Fab' fragment. *Protein Eng* **8**, 185–191.

[75] Stasi R, Evangelista ML, Buccisano F, Venditti A, Amadori S (2008). Gemtuzumab ozogamicin in the treatment of acute myeloid leukemia. *Cancer Treat Rev* **34**, 49–60.

[76] DiJoseph JF, Armellino DC, Boghaert ER, Khandke K, Dougher MM, Sridharan L, Kunz A, Hamann PR, Gorovits B, Udata C, Moran JK, Popplewell AG, Stephens S, Frost P, Damle NK (2004). Antibody-targeted chemotherapy with CMC-544: a CD22-targeted immunoconjugate of calicheamicin for the treatment of B-lymphoid malignancies. *Blood* **103**, 1807–1814.

[77] Searcey M (2002). Duocarmycins – natures prodrugs? *Curr Pharm Des* **8**, 1375–1389.

[78] Boger DL, Johnson DS, Yun W, Tarby CM (1994). Molecular basis for sequence selective DNA alkylation by (+)- and ent-(-)-CC-1065 and related agents: alkylation site models that accommodate the offset AT-rich adenine N3 alkylation selectivity. *Bioorg Med Chem* **2**, 115–135.

[79] Jeffrey SC, Nguyen MT, Andreyka JB, Meyer DL, Doronina SO, Senter PD (2006). Dipeptide-based highly potent doxorubicin antibody conjugates. *Bioorg Med Chem Lett* **16**, 358–362.

[80] Ma D, Hopf CE, Malewicz AD, Donovan GP, Senter PD, Goeckeler WF, Maddon PJ, Olson WC (2006). Potent antitumor activity of an auristatin-conjugated fully human monoclonal antibody to prostate-specific membrane antigen. *Clin Cancer Res* **12**, 2591–2596.

[81] Law CL, Gordon KA, Toki BE, Yamane AK, Hering MA, Cerveny CG, Petroziello JM, Ryan MC, Smith L, Simon R, Sauter G, Oflazoglu E, Doronina SO, Meyer DL, Francisco JA, Carter P, Senter PD, Copland JA, Wood CG, Wahl AF (2006). Lymphocyte activation antigen CD70 expressed by renal cell carcinoma is a potential therapeutic target for anti-CD70 antibody-drug conjugates. *Cancer Res* **66**, 2328–2337.

[82] Rodon J, Garrison M, Hammond LA, de Bono J, Smith L, Forero L, Hao D, Takimoto C, Lambert JM, Pandite L, Howard M, Xie H, Tolcher AW (2008). Cantuzumab mertansine in a three-times a week schedule: a phase I and pharmacokinetic study. *Cancer Chemother Pharmacol* **62**, 911–919.

[83] Qin A, Watermill RA, Mastico RA, Lutz RJ, O'Keefe J, Zildjian S, Mita AC, Phan AT, Tolcher AW (2008). The pharmacokinetics and pharmacodynamics of IMGN242 (huC242-DM4) in patients with CanAg-expressing solid tumors. *J Clin Oncol* **26**, May 20 suppl., 3066.

[84] Leipold DD, Jumbe N, Dugger D, Crocker L, Leach W, Sliwkowski MX, Meyer D, Senter PD, Tibbitts J (2007). Trastuzumab-MC-vc-PAB-MMAF: The effects of the Drug:Antibody Ratio (DAR) on efficacy, toxicity and pharmacokinetics. *Proc Amer Assoc Cancer Res* **48**, 1551.

[85] Younes A, Forero-Torres A, Bartlett NL, Leonard JP, Rege B, Kennedy DA, Lorenz JM, Sievers EL (2008). Objective responses in a phase I dose escalation study of SGN-35, a novel antibody-drug conjugate (ADC) targeting CD30, in patients with relapsed or refractory Hodgkin lymphoma. *J Clin Oncol* **26**, May 20 suppl., 8526.

[86] Hwu P, Sznol M, Kluger H, Rink L, Kim KB, Papadopoulos NE, Sanders D, Boasberg P, Ooi CE, Hamid O (2008). A phase I/II study of CR011-vcMMAE an antibody toxin conjugate drug in patients with unresectable stage III/IV melanoma. *J Clin Oncol* **26**, May 20 suppl. 9029.

CHAPTER THIRTEEN

Immunotherapy with Radio-immune Conjugates

Christina A. Kousparou and Agamemnon A. Epenetos

Monoclonal antibodies have been used in a variety of ways in the management of cancer including diagnosis, monitoring, and treatment of disease. The U.S. Food and Drug Administration (FDA) has approved numerous monoclonals for the treatment of cancer (Table 13.1). Among the unmodified monoclonal antibodies, Panitumumab (Vectibix), cetuximab (Erbitux) and bevacizumab (Avastin) are now marketed for metastatic colorectal cancer, trastuzumab (Herceptin) for breast cancers that overexpress HER-2 receptors, and alemtuzumab (Campath) for B cell lymphocytic leukemia (B-CLL). Several other monoclonal antibodies are in late-stage clinical trials. With the general availability of these agents, it appears that antibody-based therapeutics have an established role in clinical oncology.

Radio-immunotherapy (RIT) utilizes an antibody labeled with a radionuclide to deliver cytotoxic radiation to a target cell. In cancer therapy, a monoclonal antibody[1] (mAb) with specificity for a tumor-associated antigen is used to deliver a lethal dose of radiation to the tumor cells. The ability of the antibody to specifically bind to a tumor-associated antigen increases the dose delivered to the tumor cells while decreasing the dose to normal tissues. While antibodies armed with drug conjugates and immunotoxins kill only the targeted cell, radionuclide conjugates can exert a bystander effect, destroying adjacent cells that lack antigen expression.[2] With external beam therapy, only a limited area of the body is irradiated. However, RIT, like cytotoxic chemotherapy, is a systemic treatment that, in principle, can eliminate metastatic disease throughout the body.

A number of issues must be addressed in designing an optimal systemic radio-immunotherapeutic agent, including (1) selection of the antigenic target to which the radio-immunoconjugate will bind, (2) choice of a carrier molecule that will face the least barriers, and (3) choice of the radionuclide. We will address these issues separately.

TUMOR-ASSOCIATED ANTIGENS

The molecular abnormalities which are involved in neoplastic growth result in differences between malignant and nonmalignant cells. These differences are exemplified in the DNA, RNA, proteins and other molecules, which in turn can be found intracellularly or displayed on the surface of tumor cells. Investigators have exploited the

TABLE 13.1. Monoclonal antibodies currently used in oncology

Antibody	Antigenic target	Cancer type	FDA approval
Vectibix (Panitumumab)	EGFR	Colorectal carcinoma	2006
Erbitux (Cetuximab)	EGFR	Squamous cell carcinoma of the head and neck	2006
		Colorectal carcinoma	2004
Avastin (Bevacizumab)	VEGF	Non-small cell lung cancer	2006
		Colorectal carcinoma	2004
Campath (Alemtuzumab)	CD52	B cell chronic lymphocytic leukemia	2001
Zevalin (^{90}Y-Ibritumomab)	CD20	Non-Hodgkin's lymphoma	2001
Bexxar (I^{131}-Tositumomab)	CD20	Non-Hodgkin's lymphoma	2001
Mylotarg (Gemtuzumab Ozogamicin)	CD33	Acute myelogenous leukemia	2000
Ontak (Denileukin difitox)	CD25	Cutaneous T-cell leukemia	1999
Herceptin (Trastuzumab)	HER-2	HER-2 positive breast cancer	1998
Rituxan (Rituximab)	CD20	Non-Hodgkin's lymphoma	1997

characteristics of these molecules and have devised means to make them more visible to the immune system, or make them serve as targets for directed therapy.[3]

Antigens which could be targeted for cancer therapy would ideally have high and homogeneous expression in tumors, minimal expression in normal tissues, little or no soluble form, and accessibility from the circulation.[4] Such a combination of characteristics is, however, rarely found. Expression is often heterogeneous, and there is the potential for loss of the antigenic target due to shedding, internalization, modulation of its form, or down-regulation of its expression. In addition, the presence of the antigen on normal cells raises issues of cross-reactivity and toxicity, and compromises therapeutic effectiveness. All the factors mentioned are important issues to be considered in defining antigens on tumor cells and in designing optimum targeting strategies.

To date, a number of tumor-associated antigens have been identified.[3] Cell surface antigens or receptors on normal cells may be overexpressed in tumors. Examples include interleukin-2 (IL-2) receptors,[5] the epidermal growth factor (EGF) receptor (c-*erb*-B1)[6] and the HER-2/neu (c-*erb*-B2) antigen.[7] In certain instances, tumor cells, due to defects in their glycosylation pathways, express unusual carbohydrate moieties on their surface glycoproteins – for example polymorphic epithelial mucin (PEM).[8]

Malignant cells have the tendency to become more primitive and as a result express "oncofoetal" antigens on their surface,[9] such as carcinoembryonic antigen

(CEA)[10] and placental alkaline phosphatase (PLAP).[11] Intracellular protein targets for therapy include viral antigens and mutated proteins. In addition, targets include proteins which are not usually accessible in normal, viable cells, such as histones and cytokeratins, but are easy to target in necrotic, permeable tumor masses because of leaky vascularization.[12]

Angiogenesis, although normal during fetal growth and wound healing, is an abnormal process occurring during tumor growth and metastasis.[13] Approaches for destroying tumors by attacking their vasculature are being developed, exploiting the presence of antigens in neovascular endothelium. For example, endoglin and endosialin are two endothelial cell surface antigens that preferentially express on proliferating vascular cells, and might be exploited as targets for cytotoxic therapy.[14] Vascular endothelial growth factors (VEGFs) and their receptors have been demonstrated to produce angiogenesis reduction when targeted with blocking molecules.[15] Other angiogenic markers identified so far include three domains of fibronectin which are overexpressed in tumor-derived cells: IIICS, ED-A and ED-B.[16]

BARRIERS TO SUCCESSFUL ANTIBODY THERAPY

The most important limitation is antigen specificity. Few, if any, monoclonal antibodies react only with tumor cells and fail to react with normal tissues. Moreover, antigens that modulate and are shed into the circulation, such as CD10 in ALL, have generally proven to be poor targets for targeted therapy. An exception to this generalization has been observed with HER-2/*neu*, which has demonstrated substantial activity against breast cancer, alone and in combination with chemotherapy. The extracellular domain of HER-2/*neu* is cleaved and has been used as a marker for receptor overexpression.

Due to their size, monoclonal antibodies have slower kinetics of distribution and less tissue penetration than do conventional drugs.[17] The success of an antibody to localize to tumors depends on several factors. Biodistribution studies indicate distance from blood vessels to be a factor of importance with respect to antigen recognition and binding. In addition, central areas of bulky disease have poor blood supply and increased intratumoral fluid pressure, making them less accessible to immunoconjugates.[18] Furthermore, large masses can act as antigenic sinks, decreasing drug delivery to other tumor sites.[19] Modeling studies led Juweid and colleagues to formulate the hypothesis of the binding-site barrier, which postulated that antibody molecules could be prevented from penetrating tumors by the very fact of their successful binding to peritumoral antigen. Intracavitary therapy has been used in an attempt to improve access of antibody to tumor cells, but the antibody generally penetrates only a few millimeters beneath the serosal surface.

Heterogeneity has been observed in antigen expression within and between cancers from different individuals. Cells that lack antigen expression cannot be effectively targeted. With unconjugated antibodies that lack "bystander" activity, a combination of several reagents may be required to target all cells. This is where the use of radio-immunotargeting is advantageous.

The host's response to the foreign immunoglobulin is a major limitation. Because a large number of antibodies used clinically are derived from mice, they can induce the development of human anti-mouse antibodies (HAMAs). The presence of HAMAs can prevent effective delivery of murine monoclonal antibodies to tumor cells, particularly when multiple doses must be administered to obtain optimal antitumor activity. Genetic manipulation of murine monoclonal antibodies has been used to generate less immunogenic reagents. Chimeric (60% human) and humanized (95% human) antibodies have been engineered to retain the murine antigen-binding complementarity regions in association with human framework regions.[20] Although the immunogenicity of such antibodies can be substantially reduced and HAMA responses can be limited, their injection can still evoke an anti-idiotypic response. Unlike murine antibodies, human or humanized antibodies that contain the human Fc antibody portion trigger antibody-dependent cell-mediated cytotoxicity (ADCC) and complement-dependent cytotoxicity. The availability of antibodies derived entirely from humans, such as those isolated from combinatorial libraries using the process of phage display, has revolutionized therapeutic strategies.[21] Genetic engineering has also been used to produce single-chain antigen binding proteins that have more favorable pharmacokinetic properties than intact immunoglobulin or Fab fragments.

CHOICE OF THE RADIONUCLIDE

The third component of an optimal radio-immunotherapeutic regimen to consider is the nature of the radionuclide used. Radionuclides used in monoclonal-based therapy, their physical half-lives, emissions, and path lengths are listed in Table 13.2.

To take advantage of tumor targeting, relatively short path lengths are desirable. Consequently, radio-isotopes have been chosen that emit alpha particles or beta particles rather than gamma rays. The path of beta emissions can range from 1 to 10 millimeters and exert a bystander effect on antigen-negative neighboring cells. Alpha particles have a very short path length but a very high rate of linear energy transfer (LET). The biologic effectiveness of such high LET radiation does not require the presence of oxygen, nor does it depend on dose rate.[22] Overall, tumor response depends on multiple factors such as dose rate, cumulative radiation dose, and the actual radiosensitivity of the tumor.

Most published clinical studies used the β-emitting radionuclides ^{90}Y or ^{131}I. Such β-emitting radionuclides depend on cross-fire for their action on large tumor masses. However, as the tumor mass decreases, the benefit of the crossfire effect also decreases. With various small tumors including leukemias, the therapeutic effect of high-energy β-emitting radionuclides is limited because they yield a high dose of irradiation outside of the tumor volume as a result of the long path of the β-irradiation. For such forms of malignancy, the development of pretargeting approaches[23] focuses on α-emitting radionuclides that are the most effective agents

TABLE 13.2. Radionuclides used in monoclonal-antibody-based cancer radiotherapy regimens

Isotope	Half-life (h)	Emission	Maximum energy (keV)	Maximum particle range (mm)
[a]Iodine-131 (^{131}I)	193	Beta	610	2.0
Yttrium-90 (^{90}Y)	64	Beta	2280	12.0
Lutetium-177 (^{177}Lu)	161	Beta	496	1.5
Copper-67 (^{67}Cu)	62	Beta	577	1.8
[a]Rhenium-186 (^{186}Re)	91	Beta	1080	5.0
Rhenium-188 (^{188}Re)	17	Beta	2120	11.0
Bismuth-212 (^{212}Bi)	1	Alpha	8780	0.09
Bismuth-213 (^{213}Bi)	0.77	Alpha	>6000	<0.1
Astatine-211 (^{211}At)	7.2	Alpha	7450	0.08

[a] They also have gamma emissions.

Source: Adapted from Chester KA, Hawkins RE. Clinical issues in antibody design. *Trends Biotechnol* 1995; **13**: 294–300.

for killing tumor cells without damaging adjacent normal tissues. This separates the antibody targeting from the delivery of the radionuclide. The antibody is first targeted to the tumor followed by clearance of the residual circulating antibody that is facilitated by a clearing agent. A radioactive agent is then administered for selective capture at the tumor site. The problem of pretargeting strategies is their inherent complexity and the immunogenicity of the components, which are generally not of human origin.

Schemes for pretargeted RIT have occasionally used bispecific antibodies with specificities for both tumor and radionuclide chelator,[24] but more commonly, the very high-affinity interaction between biotin and avidin or streptavidin has been exploited. An infused antibody – streptavidin conjugate or fusion protein – is first allowed to localize to a tumor target. A clearing agent is then used to remove the remaining circulating conjugate. Delivery of a radionuclide is achieved with the use of a biotinylated chelator. The chelator, radionuclide complex, is either captured by the antibody – streptavidin bound to tumor cells – or cleared rapidly through the kidney due to its low molecular weight. Significant advantages of pretargeted therapy over conventional RIT include the much greater tumor-to-normal-tissue ratio, thereby lowering the whole-body exposure. The immunogenicity of streptavidin might, however, prevent the repeated treatment cycles that may be required for effective therapy. In addition, a rather large quantity of radionuclide must be administered to capture a small fraction of the radionuclide at the tumor target site.

β EMITTERS

In beta decay, a neutron inside the nucleus of an atom breaks down and changes to a proton, emits an electron, and then the atomic number goes up by one and the mass number remains unchanged.[25] ß rays are more suited for tumors larger than 0.5cm and are advantageous over α-particles in the sense that, because of their longer path length, not every cell needs to be targeted to be killed. The traversals of tumor cells by multiple β-particles result in enhanced killing by cross-fire, partially compensating for nonhomogeneity of antigen expression, whereas the short path length of α-particles increases the requirement for much greater homogeneity of targeting cells within a tumor. This limitation may be more significant for solid tumors, which are often poorly vascularized and have high interstitial pressure, as previously mentioned due to poor lymphatic drainage.

Although beta emissions can kill tumor cells, normal cells will also be affected by the circulating radio-isotopes to varying extents, For example, the bone marrow cells of patients who have a significant amount of lymphoma in the bone marrow are particularly sensitive to radiation damage.

^{131}I was the first isotope used in radiotherapy, but it was associated with low energy β-particles and emitted unwanted γ radiation, while the biological half-life of the conjugate in the tumor area was short due to the action of tissue dehalogenases.[26] In addition, myelosuppression followed ^{131}I-antibody treatment from the radiation dose that the bone marrow receives from the circulating conjugate. Alternatively, ^{90}Y emits only β-particles of appropriate energy for therapy, but it still presents problems associated with myelosuppression. The extent of heterogeneity of dose deposition in tumors is highly dependent on the antibody characteristics and radionuclide properties, and can enhance therapeutic efficacy through the selective dose delivery to the radiosensitive areas of the tumor. In a study by Flynn and colleagues where the aim was to assess the influence of radionuclide characteristics on the heterogeneity of dose deposition, ^{131}I generally delivered a higher dose throughout the tumor even though the dose-rate distribution for ^{90}Y was more uniform.[27]

α EMITTERS

Alpha emissions have energies in the several MeV range with a high probability to produce cytotoxic DNA double-strand breaks. The range is, however, short enough to avoid damage to nontargeted regions, but a homogeneous antibody distribution is essential if a bystander effect is to be observed on antigen-negative cells. The interest in bismuth-212 and bismuth-213 has been steadily increasing due to their availability and to the fact that with bismuth-212, the ^{212}Pb precursor (longer half-life) can be used as an *in vivo* ^{212}Bi-generator.[28] Astatine-211 has been conjugated to antibodies (rituximab) and demonstrated a very short half-life, short path length and very high tumor to normal cell toxicity ratio *in vitro*.

Other studies have shown that radio-immunotherapy of micrometastatic disease, monocellular bloodborne malignancies (such as leukemias, lymphomas), and malignancies spread on the surface of body compartments (like neoplastic meningitis) using high linear energy transfer α-particles and monoclonal antibody fragments have therapeutic advantages over β radio-immunotherapy.[29] Such micrometastases from the residual disease are life-threatening and lead to relapse and mortality from the postradical metastatic residual disease.

RADIO-IMMUNOTHERAPY IN HEMATOLOGIC MALIGNANCIES

In hematopoietic neoplasms, which are more radiosensitive, lower radiation doses can induce greater tumor responses. Lymphomas are particularly attractive targets considering their inherent radiosensitivity as well as the presence of differentiation antigens at the lymphoma cell surface. Arming anti-CD20 antibodies with radionuclides has resulted in significant antitumor responses in patients with non-Hodgkin's lymphoma (NHL). Two anti-CD20 monoclonals – Zevalin (^{90}Y-ibritumomab) and Bexxar (^{131}I-tositumomab) – were approved by the FDA in 2002 and 2003, respectively, for radio-immunotherapy of NHL patients either relapsed or refractory to chemotherapy and rituximab. Phase III clinical trials showed that in comparison to rituximab or chemotherapy, the enhanced targeted cytotoxicity provided by these radio-immuno-conjugates translated into significantly higher overall (OR) and complete remissions (CR).[30] A Phase II study with Bexxar as first-line therapy for stage III and IV follicular lymphoma resulted in CR of 75% and OR of 95%.[31]

It is important to note that prior to the introduction of rituximab and its yttrium-90 conjugate, Zevalin, there were no targeted therapies for lymphoma and the outcomes were poor for many patients. This is therefore a significant addition to the treatment options and it has been extremely effective in treating patients resistant to more conventional therapies.

Lym-1, a mAb that selectively targets malignant lymphocytes, also has induced therapeutic responses and prolonged survival in patients with NHL when labeled with iodine-131 (^{131}I).[32,33] The antibody Lym-1 is specific for a human leukocyte antigen (HLA-DR) expressed in >95% of B cell tumors. This murine mAb has not been humanized. Lym-1 has shown efficacy in patients who have failed chemotherapy, either with low-grade or aggressive forms of NHL.

The cell surface antigen CD33 is expressed on most myeloid leukemic blasts and leukemic progenitor cells. Its normal tissue expression is limited to committed normal myelomonocytic and erythroid progenitor cells and (at low levels) early hematopoietic stem cells. M195, a murine anti-CD33 mAb, has been used to deliver therapeutic doses of ^{131}I in combination with busulfan or cyclophosphamide to eliminate disease before bone marrow transplantation.[34] HuM195, a humanized version of M195, has been employed as a vehicle for the RAIT of acute and chronic myelogenous leukemia. HuM195 RAIT resulted in minor responses in 8 of 12 patients treated with ^{90}Y-conjugated mAb and 13 of 18 patients treated with ^{213}Bi-conjugated mAb.[35,36]

RADIO-IMMUNOTHERAPY IN SOLID TUMORS

Activity of radio-immunoconjugates has also been shown for solid tumors with varying success. Several molecules have been used against antigenic targets for the detection and therapy of colorectal, breast, lung, ovarian and medullary thyroid cancers.[37]

High-dose radio-immunotherapy followed by stem cell hematologic rescue has resulted in delivery of higher radiation doses to tumors. Trials involving patients with solid tumors, including breast, gastrointestinal, and prostate cancer, produced variable antitumor responses, but these were not as impressive as the responses observed in hematologic malignancies.

BREAST CANCER

Breast cancer is the second most common cause of cancer death in women in the United States. Although more than 60% of patients can now be cured by initial treatment, the rest will die of their disease. Early detection of micrometastases and improved treatment using monoclonal antibodies may provide an effective means of increasing the prospects for survival. Radiolabeled monoclonal antibodies are currently being applied for the treatment of primary or metastatic breast cancer, in experimental, preclinical, or clinical trials, in combination with traditional external beam radiotherapy and/or chemotherapy. Antigen targets have included primarily carcinoembryonic antigen (CEA), mucin (MUC1), and L6. Radioactive antibodies are applied with adjuvant autologous peripheral blood stem cells transfusion to prevent myelotoxicity. Partial or rarely complete responses to "hot" antibody treatment of breast cancer have been reported. Innovative strategies using this combined-modality treatment hold promise for better disease-free and survival rates.

BrE-3 antibody, a murine IgG1 monoclonal, reacts with an epitope on the tandem repeat of the peptide core of MUC-1.[38] A Phase I trial was performed to explore the use of [^{90}Y]BrE-3 murine Ab.[39] Although responses were observed, an immune response prevented further use of this Ab. A humanized version has been evaluated in a clinical trial, and 8 of 17 patients (47%) showed responses despite failing previous conventional therapies.[40]

The anti-MUC1 Ab m170, radiolabeled with ^{90}Y and combined with paclitaxel, has progressed to dosimetric studies with measurable tumor regression and partial responses.[41]

L6 cell surface antigen is highly expressed in breast cancer and is related to a number of cell surface proteins with similar predicted membrane topology implicated in cell growth. ^{90}Y-DOTA-peptide-ChL6 resulted in excellent tumor targeting and an effective therapeutic index in preclinical studies.[42,43]

CEA is expressed in normal tissues and in cancers, including breast carcinomas.[44] NP-4, a murine anti-CEA Ab labeled with ^{131}I, resulted in therapeutic responses in a Phase I/II study. When 57 patients were treated with [^{131}I]NP-4, modest antitumor activity was seen in 12 of 35 assessable patients, with one partial remission, four minor/mixed responses and seven instances of stabilization of progressing disease.[45]

COLORECTAL CANCER

Some of the most advanced radio-immunoconjugates relate to gastrointestinal disease. The antigens targeted in colorectal cancer include Ep-CAM, TAG-72, A33, and CEA.

The Ep-CAM receptor has been used as a target for the NR-LU-10 antibody. The results of a Phase II clinical trial of [^{90}Y]DOTA-biotin pretargeted by NR-LU-10 Ab/ streptavidin in patients with metastatic colon cancer were reported,[46] but the agent suffered from side effects such as bowel toxicity due to antigen cross-reactivity.

TAG-72 antigen has been targeted by the I^{131}-CC49 antibody but failed to produce significant clinical responses.[47] The ^{90}Y-labeled antibody was evaluated in a Phase I clinical trial to avoid dehalogenation issues, but its potential use has been hampered by high hepatic doses.[48]

The A33 antigen is a promising radioimmunotherapy target as it is highly and homogenously expressed in 95% of all colorectal carcinomas. In a Phase I trial, colorectal patients were treated with a combination of [^{131}I]huA33 and [^{125}I]huA33 one week before surgery.[49] No dose-limiting toxicity was observed and excellent tumor uptake was demonstrated. Higher doses were administered in a corresponding Phase I dose-escalation trial of [^{131}I]huA33 with excellent targeting resulting in 4 of 15 patients having stable disease.[50]

A Phase I/II clinical trial of ^{90}Y-labeled hMN14, a humanized radiolabeled Ab targeting CEA, was performed in patients with colorectal cancer between 2000 and 2004.[51] A radio-halogenated version of the same Ab, [^{131}I]labetuzumab, gave impressive results in a Phase II trial in 19 colorectal cancer patients after salvage resection of liver metastases.[52] The same antibody, yttrium-90 labeled, was used in a clinical trial in the United States but was terminated for unspecified reasons, possibly due to the unsuitability of ^{90}Y for treating limited residual disease after surgery.[53]

Another ^{90}Y-labeled anti-CEA Ab, T84.66, was tested in a Phase I trial in combination with 5-fluorouracil.[54] No objective responses were observed, but more than half of the patients shifted from progressive to stable disease.

OVARIAN CANCER

Two tumor-associated monoclonal antibodies (human milk fat globule membrane protein antibodies) HMFG1 and HMFG2 directed against MUC-1 and labeled with ^{123}I have been used to detect primary and metastatic ovarian, as well as breast, and gastrointestinal neoplasms.[55,56] ^{90}Y-labeled HMFG1 murine mAb (pemtumomab) has been used to treat patients with advanced ovarian cancer following conventional therapy.[57] Encouraging results were obtained in patients with minimal residual disease, with 50% complete remission several years after treatment. Following surgery, chemotherapy and intraperitoneal radio-immunotherapy, 78% of the 21 patients in complete remission survived for >10 years. Unfortunately, [^{90}Y]HMFG1 then failed to demonstrate a therapeutic effect in a multi-institution international randomized concurrently controlled Phase III clinical trial.

Ovarian cancer patients were also treated with intravenously administered ^{131}I-labeled chimeric monoclonal antibody MOv18.[58] Therapeutic doses could be achieved without normal organ toxicity. Immunospecific localization of antibody on antigen-expressing tumors has been demonstrated, suggesting that further studies should be carried out.[59]

Currently, there are no radiolabeled Abs in late-stage clinical development for ovarian cancer, although a number are currently in Phase I/II clinical trials, including [^{90}Y] HU3S193 at Memorial Sloan-Kettering Cancer Center and [^{90}Y] CC49 at the University of Alabama.

PROSTATE CANCER

Prostate antigenic targets have been targeted with radio-immunoconjugates with variable success. No major responses were observed in therapeutic studies targeting TAG-72 in prostate cancer patients.[60]

A particularly promising target would seem to be prostate-specific membrane antigen (PSMA) . The most well-known radiolabeled Ab to PSMA is [^{111}In] capromab pendetide (ProstaScint), which was approved 10 years ago by the FDA for imaging soft tissues, but not bone sites, of metastatic prostate cancer for presurgical staging or evaluation of PSMA relapse after local therapy.[61,62] For presurgical patients with high-risk disease but negative bone CT and MRI scans, capromab was able to identify some patients with positive nodes, thereby sparing them not-indicated surgery.

Promising results have been obtained using ^{90}Y-J591 antibody in treating hormone-refractory metastatic prostate cancer.[63] This antibody targets the extracellular domain of PSMA. Patient recruitment is ongoing for a Phase II trial to study the efficacy of [^{177}Lu]DOTA-J591 in the treatment of metastatic prostate cancer.

In the combined modality radio-immunotherapy of prostate cancer for treating disseminated disease, chemotherapeutic doses have been employed which would otherwise not be tolerated with external beam radiation. O'Donnell and colleagues [64] published the combined effects of a radio-immunoconjugate [90]yttrium-DOTA-Peptide-ChL6 with taxanes in mice. They observed a 67% cure rate, whereas no mice were cured with radio-immunotherapy alone or chemotherapy alone. The doses used are achievable in humans and are expected to provide therapeutic synergy without increased toxicity.

LUNG CANCER

Lung cancer is the most common cancer in the world. Over half a million new cases are diagnosed annually in the world's three major markets. The disease has a poor prognosis and it is the main cause of cancer death in the UK with around 37,000 deaths every year.

Verluma is a ^{99m}Tc-labeled Fab fragment for identifying advanced-stage disease in patients with small-cell lung cancer.[65,66] It was approved in 1996 but was recently abandoned because, even though Verluma could accurately determine whether the disease was limited or extensive, it sometimes failed to image tumors and additional standard diagnostic tests were required.

In 2005, a Phase I study of [^{90}Y]CC49 in advanced non-SCLC patients yielded very disappointing results, warranting the development of a humanized version of CC49.[67] There were no objective tumor responses, and both immunogenicity and hematologic toxicities were problematic.

RENAL CANCER

Metastatic renal carcinoma has been treated with a ^{131}I-labeled mouse monoclonal antibody (G250).[68] Thirty-three patients with measurable metastatic renal cell carcinoma were treated in a study by Divgi and colleagues. There were no major responses. On the basis of external imaging, ^{131}I-labeled mouse monoclonal antibody G250 showed excellent localization to all tumors that were > or = 2 cm. Seventeen of 33 patients had stable disease, with tumor shrinkage observed in two patients. Antibody immunogenicity restricted therapy to a single infusion. A follow-up Phase I dose-escalation trial showed that fractionation did not significantly improve dose-limiting hematopoietic toxicity.[69]

BRAIN CANCER

Brain cancer is one of the fastest growing and deadliest forms of cancer. According to the Central Brain Tumor Registry of the United States, each year in the United States alone, an estimated 35,500 new cases of primary brain tumors are diagnosed. Approximately 23% of all brain tumors are glioblastomas, which are only rarely cured.

In 2001, the U.S. Food and Drug Administration (FDA) has granted fast track status to Cotara$^{(TM)}$ ([^{131}I]chTNT Peregrine Pharmaceuticals, Inc.) for the treatment of recurrent glioblastoma multiforme. It is a radiolabeled monoclonal antibody that binds to the DNA exposed in necrotic zones. The clinical experience with [^{131}I]chTNT to date has been recently reviewed by Shapiro et al.[70]

Tenascin-C (TN-C) is an extracellular matrix glycoprotein that is expressed ubiquitously in high-grade gliomas but not in normal brain. A study of locoregional radio-immunotherapy of high-grade malignant gliomas was performed using anti-tenascin antibodies labeled initially with ^{131}I and then with ^{90}Y.[71] Using this technique, tumor growth could be retarded over relatively long periods of time. The glioblastoma median survival was prolonged to 25 months (^{131}I group) or 31 months (^{90}Y group). The response rate (which comprised of PR, CR, and NED) was 47.1% (glioblastoma ^{131}I group) or 40% (glioblastoma ^{90}Y group). In many cases a significant tumor shrinkage effect was observed. The use of ^{90}Y proved more favorable in bulky lesions and reduced the radioprotection problems.

Another study was performed that assessed the efficacy and toxicity of the ^{131}I-labeled murine antitenascin monoclonal antibody 81C6 and determined its true response rate among patients with newly diagnosed malignant glioma. Intratumoral administration of [^{131}I]81C6 has shown promise in a Phase I trial.[72] In a more recent Phase II study at Duke University, the efficacy and toxicity of [^{131}I]81C6 infused directly into the resection cavity (intracavitary injection) were assessed in 33 patients with previously untreated malignant glioma.[73] Median survival achieved exceeded that of historical controls treated with conventional radiotherapy and chemotherapy, confirming the efficacy of labeled 81C6 for patients with newly diagnosed malignant glioma and supporting the case for carrying out a randomized Phase III study.

A three-step avidin-biotin approach was used to target ^{90}Y-biotin to the tumor in patients with recurrent high-grade glioma.[74] Encouraging results obtained in this Phase I–II study prompted workers to apply the same approach in an adjuvant setting, to evaluate (1) time to relapse and (2) overall survival. Results indicated that radio-immunotherapy impeded tumor progression, prolonged time to relapse and increased overall survival.

PRETARGETING STRATEGIES

Radio-immunoconjugates can be specifically targeted to cancer cells through pretargeting.[75] This scheme typically requires two or three separate components. In one scheme, the antibody component is first targeted to the tumor followed by clearance of the residual circulating antibody, often facilitated by a clearing agent. A cytotoxic agent is then administered for selective capture or activation at the tumor site. Pretargeting of radionuclides to tumors is particularly attractive in that it has the potential to greatly reduce the systemic toxicity of conventional radio-immunotherapy and cytotoxic chemotherapy, respectively. The problem of pretargeting strategies is their inherent complexity and the immunogenicity of the components that are not of human origin. Pretargeting strategies have advanced markedly, but many obstacles remain to be overcome if they are to provide significant new treatment options for cancer patients.

Significant advantages of pretargeted therapy over conventional radio-immunotherapy include the much greater ratios of radioactivity in tumor versus nontumor tissues, thereby lowering the whole body exposure to radioactivity. However, the immunogenicity of molecules such as streptavidin might prevent the repeated treatment cycles that would probably be necessary for effective therapy. A further problem for pretargeted radioimmunotherapy is the large quantity of radionuclide that must be administered in comparison to the minute proportion captured at the tumor target site.

CONCLUSION

Targeted radiotherapy of cancer using monoclonal antibodies has been an attractive concept for the past 25 years. However, real interest from clinical oncologists has only been shown in the last few years following the impressive results using radio-immunotherapy to treat hematological tumors.

Key issues in radio-immunotherapy still remain to be elucidated, such as the genomic mechanism behind the cytotoxic effect observed. It has still not been clearly addressed whether cell death is due to an apoptotic or a necrotic mechanism and the reasons behind the apparent independence of extent of cell death from dose of radiation delivered. Other issues which remain controversial are the choice of radioisotope and the ideal half-life that the radio-immunoconjugate should have in order to have maximum beneficial effect at the tumor site but to cause minimum damage to normal tissues. Nevertheless, we predict, that in at least some indications, radio-immunotherapy will be increasingly employed as a useful therapeutic option either as monotherapy or as a combination with conventional chemotherapy or radiotherapy.

REFERENCES

[1]   Köhler G, Milstein C. Continuous cultures of fused cells secreting antibody of predefined specificity. *Nature* 1975; **256**: 495–7.

[2]   Chester KA, Hawkins RE. Clinical issues in antibody design. *Trends Biotechnol* 1995; **13**: 294–300.

[3]   Herlyn M, Menrad A, Koprowski H. Structure, function and clinical significance of human tumour antigens. *J Natl Cancer Inst* 1990; **82**: 1883–9.

[4]   Scott AM, Cebon J. Clinical promise of tumour immunology. *Lancet* 1997; **349**(S2): 19sII–22sII.

[5]   Hurteau JA, Woolas RP, Jacobs IJ, et al. Soluble interleukin-2 receptor alpha is elevated in sera of patients with benign ovarian neoplasms and epithelial ovarian cancer. *Cancer* 1995; **76**(9): 1615–20.

[6]   Tsutsui S, Ohno S, Murakami S, et al. EGFR, c-erbB2 and p53 protein in the primary lesions and paired metastatic regional lymph nodes in breast cancer. *Eur J Surg Oncol* 2002; **28**(4): 383–7.

[7]   Slamon DJ, Godolphin W, Jones LA, et al. Studies of the HER-2/*neu* protooncogene in human breast and ovarian cancer. *Science* 1989; **244**: 707–12.

[8]   Taylor-Papadimitriou J, Peterson JA, Arklie J, et al. Monoclonal antibodies to epithelium-specific components of the human milk fat globule membrane: production and reaction with cells in culture. *Int J Cancer* 1981; **28**: 17–21.

[9]   Blakey DC. Drug targeting with monoclonal antibodies. *Acta Oncol* 1992; **31**: 91–7.

[10] Gold P, Freedman SO. Demonstration of tumour-specific antigens in human colonic carcinomata by immunological tolerance and absorption techniques. *J Exp Med* 1965; **121**: 439.

[11] Iles RK, Ind TEJ, Chard T. Production of placental alkaline phosphatase (PLAP) and PLAP-like material by epithelial germ cell and non-germ cell tumours *in vitro. Br J Cancer* 1994; **69**: 274–8.

[12] Epstein AL, Chen FM, Taylor CR. A novel method for the detection of necrotic lesions in human cancers. *Cancer Res* 1988 15; **48**(20): 5842–8.

[13] Folkman J. Angiogenesis in cancer, vascular, rheumatoid and other disease. *Nat Med* 1995; **1**: 27–31.

[14] Rettig WJ, Garin-Chesa P, Healey JH, et al. Identification of endosialin, a cell surface glycoprotein of vascular endothelial cells in human cancer. *PNAS, USA* **89**: 10832–6.

[15] Skobe M, Rockwell P, Goldstein N, et al. Halting angiogenesis suppresses carcinoma cell invasion. *Nat Med* 1997; **3**: 1222–7.

[16] Zardi L, Carmonella B, Siri A, et al. Transformed human cells produce a new fibronectin isoform by preferential alternative splicing of a previously unobserved exon. *EMBO J* 1987; **6**: 2337–42.

[17] Weiner L. Monoclonal antibody therapy of cancer. *Semin Oncol* 1999; **26**(Suppl. 4): 43–51.

[18] Boxer GM, Begent RHJ, Kelly AMB, et al. Factors influencing variability of localisation of antibodies to carcinoembryonic antigen (CEA) in patients with colorectal carcinoma-implication for radioimmunotherapy. *Br J Cancer* 1992; **65**: 825–31.

[19] Juweid M, Swayne LC, Sharkey RM, et al. Prospects of radioimmunotherapy in epithelial ovarian cancer: results with iodine-131-labeled murine and humanized MN-14 anti-carcinoembryonic antigen monoclonal antibodies. *Gynecol Oncol* 1997; **67**: 259–71.

[20] Reichmann L, Clark M, Waldmann H, Winter G. Reshaping antibodies for therapy. *Nature* 1988; **332**: 323–7.

[21] Winter G, Griffiths AD, Hawkins RE, Hoogenboom HR. Making antibodies using bacterial phage display. *Protein Eng* 1998; **11**: 825–32.

[22] Bast RC, Zalutsky MR, Kreitman RJ, et al. Monoclonal serotherapy. In Bast RC, Kufe D, Pollock R, editors. *Cancer Medicine*. 5th ed. Hamilton, Ontario: BC Decker; 2000, pp. 860–75.

[23] Goodwin DA, Meares CF. Pretargeted peptide imaging and therapy. *Cancer Biother Radiopharm* 1999; **14**: 146–52.

[24] Chang CH, Sharkey RM, Rosel EA, et al. Molecular advances in pretargeting radioimmunotherapy with bispecific antibodies. *Mol Cancer Ther* 2002; **1**: 553–6.

[25] Kampf G. Steps towards cancer therapy with radionuclides – a review including radiation biophysical aspects. *Radiobiol Radiother (Berl)* 1990; **31**(3): 215–29.

[26] Price P, Sikora K. *Treatment of Cancer*. 3rd ed. London: Chapman and Hall, 1995.

[27] Flynn AA, Pedley RB, Green AJ, et al. Antibody and radionuclide characteristics and the enhancement of the effectiveness of radioimmunotherapy by selective dose delivery to radiosensitive areas of tumor. *Int J Radiat Biol* 2002; **78**(5): 407–15.

[28] Gansow OA, Wu C. Advanced methods for radiolabelling monoclonal antibodies with therapeutic radionuclides. In Goldenberg, DM. ed. *Cancer Therapy with Radiolabelled Antibodies*, Boca Raton, Florida: CRC Press, 1995, pp. 63–76.

[29] Behr TM, Behe M, Stabin MG., et al. High LET α versus low-LET β-emitters in RIT of solid tumours: Therapeutic efficacy and dose-limiting toxicity of Bi-213 versus Y-90-labelled CO17-1A Fab′ fragments in a human colonic cancer model. *Cancer Res* 1999, **59**: 2635–43.

[30] DeNardo GL. Treatment of non-Hodgkin's lymphoma (NHL) with radiolabeled antibodies (mAbs). *Semin Nucl Med* 2005; **35**: 202–11.

[31] Kaminski MS, Tuck M, Estes J, et al. 131I-Tositumomab therapy as initial treatment for follicular lymphoma. *N Engl J Med* 2005; **352**: 441–9.

[32] DeNardo GL, DeNardo SJ, Lamborn KR, et al. Low-dose, fractionated radioimmunotherapy for B-cell malignancies using ^{131}I – Lym-1 antibody. *Cancer Biother Radiopharm* 1998; **13**: 239–54.

[33] Schillaci O, DeNardo GL, DeNardo SJ, et al. Effect of antilymphoma antibody, 131I-Lym-1, on peripheral blood lymphocytes in patients with non-Hodgkin's lymphoma. *Cancer Biother Radiopharm* 2007, **22**(4): 521–30.

[34] Jurcic JG, Caron PC, Nikula TK, et al. Radiolabeled anti-CD33 monoclonal antibody M195 for myeloid leukemias. *Cancer Res* 1995; **55**: (23 Suppl.): 5908s–10s.

[35] Jurcic JG, Divgi CR, McDevitt MR, et al. Potential for myeloablation with yttrium-90 – HuM195 (anti-CD33): a phase I trial in advanced myeloid leukemias. *Blood* 1998; **92**: 613A(Abstr.).

[36] Jurcic JG, McDevitt MR, Sgouros G, et al. Phase I trial of targeted alpha particle therapy for myeloid leukemias with bismuth-213 – HuM195 (anti-CD33). *Proc Am Soc Clin Oncol* 1999; **18**: 7A(Abstr.).

[37] Yuliya S, Divgi J, Divgi C. Current status of therapy of solid tumors, *J Nucl Med* 2005; **46**: 141S–150S.

[38] Blank EW, Pant KD, Chan CM, et al. A novel anti-breast epithelial mucin MoAb (BrE-3). *Cancer* 1992; **5**: 38–44.

[39] Schrier DM, Stemmer SM, Johnson T, et al. High-dose ^{90}Y-Mx-diethylenetriaminepentaacetic acid (DTPA)-BrE-3 and autologous hematopoietic stem cell support (AHSCS) for the treatment of advanced breast cancer: a phase I trial. *Cancer Res* 1995; **55**: 5921s–24s.

[40] DeNardo SJ, Kramer EL, O'Donnell RT, et al. Radioimmunotherapy for breast cancer using ^{111}In/^{90}Y-BrE-3: results of a phase I clinical trial. *J Nucl Med* **38** 1997; **8**: 1180–5.

[41]   Richman CM, DeNardo SJ, O'Donnell RT, et al. Combined modality radioimmunotherapy (RIT) in metastatic prostate and breast cancer using paclitaxel and a MUC-1 monoclonal antibody, m170, linked to ^{90}Y: a phase I trial. *J Clin Oncol* 2004; **22**(14S): 2554.

[42]   DeNardo SJ, Richman CM, Goldstein DS, et al. Yttrium-90/Indium-111-DOTA-peptide-chimeric L6: pharmacokinetics, dosimetry and initial results in patients with incurable breast cancer. *Anticancer Res* 1997; **17**: 1735–44.

[43]   DeNardo SJ, Kukis DL, Miers LA, et al. Yttrium-90-DOTA-peptide ChL6 radioimmunoconjugate: efficacy and toxicity in mice bearing p53 mutant human breast cancer xenografts. *J Nucl Med* 1998; **39**: 842–9.

[44]   Ebeling FG, Stieber P, Untch M, et al. Serum CEA and CA 15-3 as prognostic factors in primary breast cancer. *Br J Cancer* 2002; **86**(8): 1217–22.

[45]   Behr TM, Sharkey RM, Juweid ME, et al. Phase I/II clinical radioimmunotherapy with an ^{131}I-labeled anti-carcinoembryonic antigen murine monoclonal antibody IgG. *J Nucl Med* 1997; **38**(6): 858–70.

[46]   Knox S, Goris ML, Tempero M, et al. Phase II trial of ^{90}Y-DOTA-biotin pre-targeted by NR-LU-10 antibody/streptavidin in patients with metastatic colon cancer. *Clin Cancer Res* 2000; **6**: 406–14.

[47]   Buchsbaum D, Khazaeli MB, Liu TP, et al. Fractionated radioimmunotherapy of human colon carcinoma xenografts with ^{131}I-labeled monoclonal antibody CC49. *Cancer Res* 1995; **55**(23 Suppl S): S5881–7.

[48]   Tempero M, Leichner P, Baranowska-Kortylewicz J, et al., High-dose therapy with ^{90}Yttrium-labeled monoclonal antibody CC49: a phase I trial. *Clin Cancer Res* 2000; **6**: 3095–102.

[49]   Scott AM, Lee FT, Jones R, et al. A phase I trial of humanized monoclonal antibody A33 in patients with colorectal carcinoma: biodistribution, pharmacokinetics, and quantitative tumor uptake. *Clin Cancer Res* 2005; **11**: 4810–7.

[50]   Chong G, Lee FT, Hopkins W, et al. Phase I trial of ^{131}I-huA33 in patients with advanced colorectal carcinoma. *Clin Cancer Res* 2005; **11**: 4818–26.

[51]   Immunomedics, Inc. Safety study of hMN14 to treat either colorectal or breast cancer. Accessed February 2007 at www.clinicaltrials.gov/ct/show/NCT00041652.

[52]   Liersch T, Meller J, Kulle B, et al. Phase II trial of carcinoembryonic antigen radioimmunotherapy with ^{131}I-labetuzumab after salvage resection of colorectal metastases in the liver: five-year safety and efficacy results. *J Clin Oncol* 2005; **23**(27): 6763–70.

[53]   Immunomedics, Inc. Safety study of ^{90}Y-hMN14 to treat colorectal cancer patients with limited residual disease after surgery. Accessed February 2007 at http://www.clinicaltrials.gov/ct/show/NCT00041691.

[54]   Wong JYC, Shibata S, Williams LE, et al. A phase I trial of ^{90}Y-anti-carcinoembryonic antigen chimeric T84.66 radioimmunotherapy with 5-fluorouracil in patients with metastatic colorectal cancer. *Clin Cancer Res* 2003; **9**: 5842–52.

[55]   Epenetos AA, Canti G, Taylor-Papadimitriou J, et al. Use of two epithelium-specific monoclonal antibodies for diagnosis of malignancy in serous effusions. *Lancet* 1982; **II**: 1004–6.

[56]   Epenetos AA, Carr D, Johnson PM, et al. Antibody-guided radiolocalisation of tumours in patients with testicular or ovarian cancer using two radioiodinated monoclonal antibodies to placental alkaline phosphatase. *Br J Cancer* 1986; **59**: 117–25.

[57]   Epenetos AA, Hird V, Lambert H, et al. Long term survival of patients with advanced ovarian cancer treated with intraperitoneal radioimmunotherapy. *Int J Gynecol Cancer* 2000; **10**(Suppl 1): 44–6.

[58]   Zanten-Przybysz I, Molthoff CF, Roos JC, et al. Radioimmunotherapy with intravenously administered ^{131}I-labeled chimeric monoclonal antibody MOv18 in patients with ovarian cancer. *J Nucl Med* 2000; **41**: 1168–76.

[59]   Coliva A, Zacchetti A, Luison E, et al. ^{90}Y labeling of monoclonal antibody MOv18 and preclinical validation for radioimmunotherapy of human ovarian carcinomas. *Cancer Immunol Immunother* 2005; **54**: 1200–13.

[60]   Meredith RF, Bueschen AJ, Khazaeli MB, et al. Treatment of metastatic prostate carcinoma with radiolabeled antibody CC49. *J Nucl Med* 1994; **35**(6): 1017–22.

[61]   Bander NH. Technology insight: monoclonal antibody imaging of prostate cancer. *Nat Clin Pract* 2006; **3**(4): 216–25.

[62]   Raj GV, Partin AW, and Polascik TJ. Clinical utility of ^{111}In-capromab pendetide immunoscintigraphy in the detection of early, recurrent prostate carcinoma after radical prostatectomy. *Cancer* 2002; **94**(4): 987–96.

[63]   Vallabhajosula S, Goldsmith SJ, Kostakoglu L, et al. Radioimmunotherapy of prostate cancer using [90]Y- and ^{177}Lu-labeled J591 monoclonal antibodies: effect of multiple treatments on myelotoxicity. *Clin Cancer Res* 2005; **11**: 7195s–7200s.

[64]   O'Donnell RT, DeNardo SJ, Miers LA, et al. Combined modality radioimmunotherapy for human prostate cancer xenografts with taxanes and 90 Yttrium-DOTA-peptide-ChL6. *The Prostate* 2002; **50**: 27–37.

[65]   Breitz HB, Tyler A, Bjorn MJ, et al. Clinical experience with ^{99m}Tc-nofetumomab merpentan (Verluma) radioimmunoscintigraphy. *Clin Nucl Ned* 1997; **22**(9): 615–20.

[66]   Machac J, Krynyckyi B, and Kim C. Peptide and antibody imaging in lung cancer. *Semin Nucl Med* 2002; **32**(4): 276–92.

[67]   Forero A, Meredith RF, Khazaeli MB, et al. Phase I study of ^{90}Y-CC49 monoclonal antibody therapy in patients with advanced non-small cell lung cancer: effect of chelating agents and paclitaxel administration. *Cancer Biother Radiopharm* 2005; **20**(5): 467–78.

[68]   Divgi CR, Bander NH, Scott AM, et al. Phase I/II radioimmunotherapy trial with iodine-131-labeled monoclonal antibody G250 in metastatic renal cell carcinoma. *Clin Cancer Res* 1998; **4**: 2729–39.

[69]   Divgi CR, O'Donoghue JA, Welt S, et al. Phase I clinical trial with fractionated radioimmunotherapy using ^{131}I-labeled chimeric G250 in metastatic renal cancer. *J Nucl Med* 2004; **45**(8): 1412–21.

[70]   Shapiro WR, Carpenter SP, Roberts K, Shan JS. ^{131}I-chTNT-1/B mAb: tumor necrosis therapy for malignant astrocytic glioma. *Expert Opin Biol Ther*, 2006; **6**(5): 539–45.

[71]   Riva P, Franceschi G, Riva N, et al. Role of nuclear medicine in the treatment of malignant gliomas: the locoregional radioimmunotherapy approach. *Eur J Nucl Med* 2000; **27**(5): 601–9.

[72]   Bigner DD, Brown M, Coleman RE, et al. Phase I studies of treatment of malignant gliomas and neoplastic meningitis with ^{131}I-radiolabeled monoclonal antibodies anti-tenascin 81C6 and anti-chondroitin proteoglycan Mel-14 F(ab')2 preliminary report. *J Neurooncol* 1995; **24**: 109–22.

[73]   Reardon D, Akabani G, Coleman RE, et al. Phase II trial of murine ^{131}I-labeled antitenascin monoclonal antibody 81C6 administered into surgically created resection cavities of patients with newly diagnosed malignant gliomas. *J Clin Oncol* 2002; **20**(5): 1389–97.

[74]   Grana C, Chinol M, Robertson C, et al. Pretargeted adjuvant radioimmunotherapy with yttrium-90-biotin in malignant glioma patients: a pilot study. *Br J Cancer* 2002; **86**(2): 207–12.

[75]   Goodwin DA, Meares CF. Pretargeted peptide imaging and therapy. *Cancer Biother Radiopharm* 1999; **14**: 146–52.

CHAPTER FOURTEEN

Immunotherapeutic Antibody Fusion Proteins

Nigel S. Courtenay-Luck and David Jones

The discovery of the monoclonal antibody technology by Milstein and Kohler paved the way for antibodies of desired specificity to be made in quantities that could enable large clinical trials, and heralded the start of the antibody targeted-therapy era. Numerous clinical trials were conducted using murine antibodies derived from the spleen cells of immunized mice and myeloma cells. A major drawback to the use of these murine, xenogeneic antibodies in man was the development of a human anti-murine antibody response (HAMA) against both the constant and variable regions of the antibody. This response rarely led to anaphylactic or other hypersensitivity reactions but did severely limit the number of administrations that could be made, and hence it often negated the therapeutic efficacy of these antibodies.

Studies in a number of laboratories paved the way to humanizing these murine antibodies (see chapter by Saldanha) and, as the advances in antibody technology increased, fully human antibodies with high affinity have been developed for clinical use. Today, antibodies are by and large combined with chemotherapeutics, and in this setting, have been shown to improve both the time to disease progression and survival in patients with a wide spectrum of tumors. Combination therapy in oncology is an established protocol, as it is necessary to target various molecular events of the tumor cell as well as antigens preferentially expressed by such tumor cells. The majority of the approved antibodies work by either blocking cell signaling, mediated by the antigen or receptor to which they bind, or by mediation of components of the recipient's immune system, such as complement resulting in complement-mediated killing (CDC) of target cells, or by eliciting antibody-mediated cell cytotoxicity (ADCC), killing through activation of cytotoxic T cells or natural killer (NK) cells.

To increase the efficacy of tumor cell lysis, large numbers of antibodies over the past 25 years have been conjugated to various agents, such as radio-isotopes, toxins, cytokines, and interleukins. The majority of these were chemically conjugated to attach the cell-killing agent to the antibody, that is, the effector to the vector. In terms of producing a product, this method of attaching a cell-killing moiety to an antibody is costly and often results in a molecule that is unstable *in vivo* and a product that is nonhomogeneous. In the literature there are hundreds of examples of chemically conjugated antibodies; the success of this approach is reflected in the fact that only one, Mylotarg, is approved. Mylotarg consists of an anti-CD33 antibody to which calicheamycin is attached; it is used for the treatment of acute myeloid leukemia.

To increase both the stability and homogeneity of these molecules, genetic approaches were developed that allowed the insertion of both the antibody and effector genes into expression vectors. After transfection into cells and the generation of stable cell lines, homogeneous preparations of immunotherapeutic antibody fusion protein could be manufactured.

Antibodies of dual specificity could also be regarded as fusion proteins, but in this section, only those that carry an active effector molecule, such as an interleukin, will be discussed.

THE DEVELOPMENT OF FUSION PROTEINS

Some 17 years ago, Hoogenboom et al.[1] published a paper showing the construction and expression of a F(ab′)2-like antibody-tumor necrosis factor (TNF) fusion protein that could both bind to antigen and elicit TNF cytotoxicity, indicating that the TNF had retained its activity in this fusion protein construct. This molecule was produced by linking the synthetic gene coding for human TNF to the heavy chain gene of an anti-transferrin receptor antibody. The resultant chimeric heavy chain-TNF genes were then introduced into a light chain secreting transfectoma cell line, which was producing the light chain of the same antibody. Cell lines were then isolated that secreted antibody-TNF fusion proteins of both the expected size and composition; these were then tested for cytotoxicity against both the murine L929 and human MCF-7 cell lines. Their results illustrated the feasibility of an antibody engineering technology to create and produce chimeric mouse-human immunotoxin-like fusion proteins. Furthermore, their results also demonstrated the ability of mammalian (myeloma) cells to express and secrete antibody-cytokine hybrid molecules with a potential use in cancer therapy.

One year later, Gillies et al.[2] demonstrated that a genetically engineered fusion protein consisting of a chimeric anti-ganglioside GD2 antibody (ch14.18) and IL-2 had the ability to enhance killing of autologous GD-2-expressing melanoma target cells by a tumor-infiltrating lymphocyte cell line (660 TIL). This work showed that fusion of IL-2 to the carboxy terminus of the immunoglobulin heavy chain did not reduce the IL-2 activity, as measured by a standard proliferation assay using either mouse or human T cell lines. This work demonstrated that pre-coating of the autologous GD-2 positive melanoma target cells with the fusion protein enhanced the killing by resting 660 TIL cells. An important observation was that the level of stimulation of killing was greater than that of uncoated cells in the presence of equivalent or higher concentrations of free IL-2.

In 1993, Savage et al.[3] demonstrated that even smaller molecules in the form of a single-chain antibody linked to Interleukin-2 (IL-2) (SCA-IL-2) could be produced. Interleukin-2 had already shown clinical utility in the treatment of both melanoma and renal cell carcinoma (RCC). The aim of this work was to illustrate the feasibility of producing a single-chain-IL-2 fusion protein that would, with the right antibody single chain, allow IL-2 to be targeted and concentrated in the tumor, maximizing the antitumor immune response while at the same time reducing the systemic toxicity seen with recombinant IL-2 alone. Reducing the toxicity was important because it so often reduced the amount of rIL-2 that could be given, negating its full potential therapeutic effect. This group also showed that these fusion proteins could be expressed and secreted in bacteria, *Escherichia Coli*, rather than mammalian cell lines, and that the purified product possessed both antigen-binding activity and the immunostimulatory properties of the rIL-2.

In the work of Savage et al., described earlier, an anti-lysozyme single-chain antibody (D1.3) was used to illustrate the feasibility of producing such Ab-IL-2 fusion proteins. This single-chain antibody of course had no clinical utility, but shortly after this, other papers described the production of clinically relevant IL-2 fusion proteins. An example of this came out of the work of Reisfeld et al.[4] at the Scripps Research Institute in La Jolla, California, who showed that IL-2 could be fused to an anti-melanoma antibody, which, *in vivo*, was effective in eradicating established hepatic and pulmonary metastasis of melanoma. Isolation of CD8+ T cells from tumor-bearing mice treated with the fusion protein exerted a major histocompatability complex (MHC) class 1 – restricted cytotoxicity against the same tumor *in vitro*. This fusion protein was also able to facilitate partial regression of large subcutaneous melanoma, which exceeded more than 5% of the animal's body weight. This group went on to publish many articles showing clearly that different antibodies targeted to antigens of therapeutic interest such as EpCAM, EGFR, DNA-histone, and GD-2 could be fused to a number of interleukins, including IL-2, IL-12, and TNF alpha; the resultant fusion proteins could be produced and used to demonstrate *in vivo* activity in various tumor models. A number of these fusion proteins would eventually find their way into clinical trials, and will be described later.

Penichet et al.[5] published data showing that murine B cell lymphoma cells (38C13) could be targeted *in vivo*, as visualized by the use of a gamma camera, and killed by an anti-idiotypic IgG3-CH3-IL-2 fusion protein. This study showed a 17-fold greater half-life of the fusion protein, compared to IL-2 alone; good localization; and enhanced antitumor activity compared with the combination of antibody and IL-2 administered together. This study demonstrated that the antitumor activity was dose dependent, with a single dose preventing tumor growth in 50% of animals and multiple doses preventing tumor growth in 87% of animals. What was surprising was that the animals receiving a single dose, and who survived, demonstrated evidence of immunologic memory, whereas the animals receiving multiple doses were ineffective in generating protective immunological memory, indicating that multiple dosing was leading to the animals' becoming tolerant of the fusion protein.

TARGETING THE ONCOFETAL ANTIGEN, ED-B

A major factor in targeting antibodies or antibody fusion proteins to the tumor is the antigen. To achieve a therapeutic effect, while reducing systemic toxicity due to the targeting of nontumor tissues, the antigen needs to be as tumor-specific as possible. Many tumor antigens are up-regulated in tumor tissue, which has led to a quantitative difference in the percentage of injected dose localizing in the tumor compared to some normal tissues, which express the antigen at much lower levels. What would really be desirable is the identification of tumor antigens that were qualitatively different and really differentiated the tumor from normal tissue, leading to a far greater specificity of targeted cancer therapy. Research groups have worked hard to identify antigens that are tumor specific against which antibodies could be raised. Some such antigens are the embryonic and oncofetal antigens; these are expressed only during the developmental phase of the embryo or fetus, respectively.

One such antigen is the oncofetal fibronectin molecule, known as extra-domain B (ED-B).[6] This antigen is found widely distributed in the tissues of the developing fetus during the first trimester of pregnancy. During the second and third trimesters, the antigen is hardly expressed by any tissues except those where growth is ongoing. A large volume of data now clearly illustrates that this oncofetal fibronectin molecule is expressed in the development of a large number of solid and hematological tumors including breast cancer.[7] This antigen has been the focus of attention for many research groups and is now known to be a marker for new blood vessels during angiogenesis.[8] The first murine monoclonal antibody to be raised against this antigen was BC-1, raised in the group of Luciano Zardi, in Genoa, Italy. A single-chain antibody known as L19[9] was developed by the group of Dario Neri in Zurich, Switzerland, and has been used widely to demonstrate the importance of this antigen as an ideal candidate for targeted therapy.

Although BC-1 was the first antibody to be raised to the ED-B antigen, it has been difficult to use in animal models for generating data that could support the clinical use of this antigen as a target for immunotherapy. Although the ED-B sequence is conserved in many animals, and expressed in mice bearing human tumors, BC-1 recognizes a cryptic epitope in fibronectin which is not conserved between mice and men; this epitope is seen in human tissues, where this 91 amino acid domain is expressed and can be used in immunohistological studies, but it is not seen in human tumor xenograft models in mice. L19 recognizes a noncryptic conserved epitope and has therefore been used in many *in vivo* studies to support the use of ED-B as a viable target for antibody therapy. The group of Dario Neri have published a large number of papers clearly illustrating the viability of targeting this antigen with L19 alone. They have also published a large volume of data showing that the L19 molecule can be used with a number of potential effector molecules, such as vascular endothelial growth factor (VEGF),[10–11] tumor necrosis factor alpha (TNF-alpha),[12] IL-12,[13] IL-10,[14] IL-15, granulocyte macrophage colony-stimulating factor (GM-CSF),[15] and IL-2.[16]

Although BC-1 has been used in fewer animal studies, for the reasons stated earlier, it was fused with IL-12 (discussed later in the chapter) and tested against a number of human tumor models in SCID mice that included the PC3mm2 prostate, A431 epidermoid carcinoma, and the HT29 colon models. In all of these models, the fusion protein consisting of humanized BC-1 fused to murine IL-12, as human IL-12 has no activity in mice, showed significant biological activity in terms of tumor growth delay.[17] A major reason for highlighting this antigen is that it has now been the subject of a number of clinical trials, which will be described later.

Many other antigens have been used as targets for fusion proteins; these include the Her-2/neu antigen, expressed in about 25% of breast cancers, and the target for the approved antibody Herceptin. This antibody was fused with IL-2 and showed a novel mechanism by which the use of tumor-specific T cells for adoptive transfer could be bypassed by use of nontumor-specific T cells in combination with the anti-Her-2/neu-IL-2 fusion protein. In addition, the authors showed that the transfer of these nontumor-specific T cells in combination with the fusion protein could eradicate established Her-2-, Her-3-, and Her-4-expressing tumors in SCID mice. These same tumors could not be eradicated by transfer of these nontumor-specific T cells plus rIL-2 or an irrelevant Ab-IL-2 fusion protein, indicating the antitumor activity was dictated by the specificity of the fusion proteins.[18]

In another study, an anti-CD-30-IL-2 and an anti-CD30-IL-12 were combined to demonstrate that fusion proteins can act in a cooperative manner to activate resting NK cells and induce gamma-interferon release. In this study, the authors proposed that the combination of these two fusion proteins could be used to treat Hodgkin's lymphoma by reversing the anergy in functional T cells and NK cells; these cells are found accumulated in the vicinity of malignant Hodgkin/Reed-Sternberg (H/RS) cells, which characterizes Hodgkin's disease.[19]

A recent study showed that the anti-Her IgG3 antibody fused to endostatin inhibits the growth of both murine and human breast tumor xenografts. The study further demonstrated that increasing the half-life of endostatin by fusing it to an antibody was far superior to using endostatin alone, which has a short half-life.[20]

CLINICAL TRIALS USING IMMUNOTHERAPEUTIC ANTIBODY FUSION PROTEINS

The literature is full of examples of fusion proteins that have been raised against a wide number of antigens and fused with a wide number of different effector molecules, such as toxins, endostatin, nucleases, and interleukins, to name just some. However, very few of these have entered large-scale clinical trials, predominantly because manufacturing productivity is not sufficient for a commercially viable product. Many of these fusion proteins required refolding, lowering even more the yield of biologically active product. This section will discuss a few of the recent or ongoing clinical trials in which the problems of productivity have clearly been overcome, generating fusion proteins that can be scaled up to proceed across all the phases of human trials required for registration as a new drug.

As mentioned earlier in this section, the work from Gillies and Reisfeld generated a number of antibody fusion proteins, of which two will be discussed here. The first known, as EMD 273066 (huKS-IL2), was developed by EMD-Lexigen Research Centre Corporation, Billerica, Massachusetts. It consisted of two molecules of IL-2 genetically fused to a humanized monoclonal antibody directed against human adenocarcinoma-associated antigen KSA, also known as EpCAM or epithelial adhesion molecule; this molecule is expressed on many epithelial cancers including prostate, colon, breast, and lung cancers. In this Phase I clinical trial, prostate cancer patients received EMD 273066, and both safety and the maximum tolerated dose (MTD) were determined.[21]

Patients were men at least 18 years of age with advanced androgen-independent prostate cancer. In this open label multicenter trial, dose EMD 273066 was administered on an inpatient basis in two treatment cycles separated by approximately 4 weeks. Each treatment cycle comprised 3 consecutive days 1 through 3 and days 29 through 31 of a once daily 4-hour intravenous infusion. The first patient received 0.4mg/m2/d, which was less than 10% of the limiting dose seen in animal toxicology studies. Dose esculation was 0.4, 0.7, 1.4, 2.8, 4.3, 6.4, and 8.5 mg/m2/d. In this study, 22 patients were enrolled, all receiving at least one infusion and 15 out of 22 receiving at least two treatment cycles. Three patients received more than two cycles with one of these receiving four treatment cycles at 1.4 mg/m2/d followed by two cycles at 2.8mg/m2/d, on the basis of a positive prostate-specific antigen (PSA) response.

From this study, it was seen that the maximum tolerated dose was 6.4 mg/m2/d, with the most common adverse events of grade 2 or above being fever, asthenia, and chills. The majority of adverse events were grade 1 or 0. Pharmacokinetic data showed high intra- and interpatient variability with a mean t1/2, which was independent of dose, ranging between 4 and 6.7 hours. Immunogenicity in the form of an anti-immunocytokine response was seen at day 8 in 14 of 20 patients. Titers did not increase during the second cycle. An anti-FcIL-2 was observed during both the first and second treatment cycles in 20 of 21 patients, although patient titers did not increase during the second cycle. What this study clearly showed was immunologic action, with NK-cell numbers and specific activity as well as ADCC activity increased after administration of EMD 273066. Lymphocyte counts reflected lymphopenia during each treatment cycle followed by rebound lymphocytosis.

In a second clinical trial carried out by the same company, a humanized, hu14.18 antibody directed toward the GD-2 antigen was fused with IL-2. In this trial, 27 pediatric patients, 26 with recurrent/refractory neuroblastoma and 1 with melanoma, were treated with this fusion protein known as EMD 273063.[22] In this study, in which the fusion protein was again administered intravenously over a 4-hour period for 3 consecutive days, a maximum tolerated dose of 12/mg/m2/d was observed. There were no deaths in the trial, but no measurable complete or partial responses were observed. For toxicities seen in this trial, 93% of patients developed grade 2 or 3 fevers and 64% had grade 2 or 3 pain (rectal pelvic, myalgia, neuropathic, abdominal, arthralgia, chest, bone, and headache); 61% of patients also experienced grade 2 hypotension. All of these toxicities were anticipated and have been seen using this antibody and IL-2. Even though no complete or partial responses were seen, three patients did show evidence of antitumor activity, and as with the previous study, immunological action was evidenced by elevated serum levels of IL-2 receptor alpha. Immune responses to the fusion protein were seen, with >60% of all patients developing anti-idiotypic antibody responses to the immunocytokine and 50% developing anti-Fc-IL-2 antibody responses, which in this study did appear to increase with subsequent courses of treatment. A Phase II clinical trial of hu14.18-IL-2 was planned using a dose of 12mg/m2/d for 3 days repeated every 28 days.

Earlier in this chapter, the significance of ED-B as an oncofetal antigen was described, and to date, two clinical trials have been or are being conducted to determine the safety and tolerability of immunocytokines directed to this antigen. The first study, conducted by Schering pharma, now known as Bayer Schering pharma, employed the use of the L19-IL-2 fusion protein developed by Dario Neri's group, and licensed from Philogen S.p.A. Siena, Italy. Although little data are available for this trial, it has been reported that the Phase I study showed immunological activity and was well tolerated, with toxicities being mild and reversible. It also revealed clinical activity in certain cancers such as renal cell carcinoma.[23]

FUSION PROTEINS CASE STUDY: AS1409

One fusion protein currently undergoing evaluation in a Phase I clinical trial is Antisoma's IgG1-interleukin 12 (IL-12) fusion protein, AS1409.[17] This is a hexameric molecule of approximately 270kDa and is currently in a Phase I clinical trial for patients with metastatic melanoma or metastatic renal cell carcinoma. The antibody is a humanized version of a murine BC1 that has previously been used in clinical trials and in an imaging study.[24] As stated earlier, the huBC1 antibody targets a splice variant of fibronectin that contains (EDB) extra domain B.[25] This is an oncofetal isoform of fibronectin, which is expressed on a number of solid tumors including breast, colorectal, renal, head and neck, melanoma, glioblastoma, and lung as well as on neovasculature.[26] There is minimal expression of EDB fibronectin on normal adult tissues (though it may be found for example on the endometrium in the proliferative phase). EDB fibronectin is an attractive target because it is found on tumor cells, blood vessels of tumors, and extracellular matrix of tumors. Fibronectin has a modular structure and exists as multiple isoforms as a result of alternative mRNA splicing. It plays a role in many cellular functions including cell migration and adhesion, blood clotting, and tissue repair. The actual epitope recognized by huBC1 is not within the EDB domain itself but is found in domain seven; only when the EDB domain is present is the epitope exposed. The use of EDB-FN as a tumor marker has been demonstrated in several preclinical and clinical studies.[24,27,28]

Human IL-12 is a heterodimeric glycoprotein comprising a p35 and a p40 subunit. IL-12 bridges innate and adaptive immunity and has been used in a number of clinical trials for the treatment of cancer.[29–30] It is of particular importance in the oncology setting as it elicits a three-pronged attack on tumor cells, causing direct killing of cancer cells as well as being antimetastatic and anti-angiogenic. It is a key activator of cell-mediated responses, priming Th1 cell responses and stimulating activity and proliferation of NK cells and cytotoxic T cells. These effects are closely associated with its ability to induce expression of interferon gamma (IFNγ). This leads to induction of secondary cytokines including interferon gamma-inducible protein 10 (IP10) and monokine induced by IFNγ (Mig). Together these have the effect of up-regulating MHC class I and II molecules (enhancing antigen processing and presentation) as well as inhibiting angiogenesis and extracellular matrix remodeling (reducing tumor invasion and blood vessel formation). IL-12 is thus expected to kill remaining tumor cells and destroy tumor vasculature.

IL-12 has been used in the clinic in cancer trials both as a single agent and in combination with other agents. Many trials have been in the cytokine-responsive indications of melanoma and renal cell carcinoma,[31–32] where some responses have been observed, though other indications have also been tested. Trials in lymphoma and Kaposi's sarcoma patients have given some notable responses, but the results to date have been largely disappointing.[30] It is anticipated that by directly targeting the IL-12 to tumor cells and tumor vasculature, a much enhanced response and therapeutic index will be observed. Furthermore, trials to date have demonstrated that IL-12 is toxic at elevated concentrations and it is again hoped that AS1409 will exhibit reduced systemic activity, but with enhanced activity localized at the tumor.

Production

AS1409 was engineered so that the DNA encoding the p35 subunit of IL-12 was appended to the 3′ end of the DNA encoding the IgG heavy chain and these two molecules are expressed as a single polypeptide.[17] The antibody light chain and p40 subunit are co-expressed in the same cell and thus are able to associate with this fusion protein by disulfide bond formation, and the complete protein can fold into the active conformation. At the heavy chain–p35 fusion junction, the DNA was further engineered to remove a potential site of proteolysis and also to remove a potential T cell epitope (identified in silico).

AS1409 is expressed in murine NS0 cells. The NS0 cell line was first transfected with a plasmid that expresses the p40 subunit using a neomycin resistance (G418) marker. This cell line was then transfected with a plasmid that expresses both the light chain of huBC1 and the heavy chain of huBC1 fused to the p35 subunit. This plasmid contained a dihydrofolate reductase (methotrexate) marker. The molecular weight of the hexameric polypeptide is approximately 260kDa, but in addition, the antibody heavy chain and both subunits of IL-12 are glycosylated, further increasing the total molecular mass of AS1409. Cell lines were generated in serum-containing medium; these were subjected to two rounds of subcloning and then adapted to serum-free suspension culture. From these, a lead production cell line was selected based on productivity, stability, and growth, and cell banks were generated. When grown in a chemically defined medium in a fed-batch bioreactor, productivities in excess of 0.5g/L were achieved, though this was considerably higher with the addition of complex feeds, suggesting further process development could further improve productivity. It is of note, however, that IL-12 is dosed at very low concentrations (<1μg/kg), hence high productivity was not a key driver for AS1409.

The downstream purification process was successfully developed as for an antibody, comprising Protein A affinity chromatography followed by anion exchange (in flow-through mode on a membrane) and a final polishing cation exchange step. The formulated, vialed AS1409 is stable at 4°C (and ongoing stability studies indicate no loss of structural integrity or activity after at least 2 years).

    Activity of the interleukin moiety of AS1409 may be measured by stimulation of human PBMCs (or an NK cell line) to produce IFNγ. Assays demonstrate a 10-fold reduction in the activity of AS1409 compared to IL-12 alone, which is most likely due to steric effects. This, however, may be seen as beneficial, as IL-12 alone has been demonstrated to have a maximal tolerated dose (MTD) of around 0.5μg/kg.[32] A reduction in activity allows higher dosing and simplifies the dosing regime. Antigen binding by the antibody is largely unaffected by the presence of the cytokine.

In vivo efficacy

IL-12 fusion proteins have previously exhibited efficacy in murine models.[33–35] *In vivo* efficacy has also been demonstrated using a surrogate molecule comprising huBC1 fused to murine IL-12 (as human IL-12 is not active in mice; see ref.[17] This fusion protein huBC1-muIL-12 has been used in several different xenograft models and one set of data is shown in Figure 14.1. This shows response seen in a human prostate cell line (PC3mm2) in nude mice. Different doses are given to account for differences in IL-12 activity of the different constructs and also to compensate for molarity. From the data it can be seen that the fusion protein has superior activity over IL-12 alone or the co-administered individual components of the fusion protein in the reduction of tumor growth. Furthermore, these models may underestimate the potential effects of AS1409 because the only source of BC-1 antigen in the models is transplanted human tumor cells; patients will have tumor cells plus tumoral vasculature and stroma. In addition, the SCID and nude mouse models lack a full

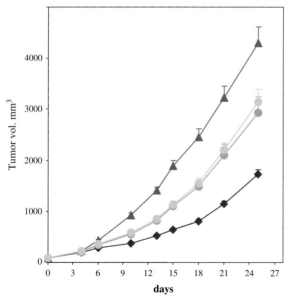

Figure 14.1. Efficacy of AS1409 in a PC3mm2 subcutaneous model [See color plate.].
▲ Phosphate-buffered saline
◆ huBC1-muIL-12 20μg x 7 daily doses
● huBC1 10μg & muIL-12 1.5μg x 7 daily doses
◐ muIL-12 1.5μg x 7 daily doses

repertoire of immune cells; thus it could be expected that the efficacy of huBC1-huIL-12 would be far greater in humans. Similarly, in a lung colony xenograft model, control mice showed extensive lung microtumors, whereas lungs from mice treated with surrogate AS1409 were essentially free of microtumors. These data are described in Lo et al.[17]

DISCUSSION

Although a number of examples of the emerging generation of antibody immunocytokines have been discussed here, the literature is full of other examples of effector molecules being added recombinantly to antibodies such as enzymes, as in ADEPT, discussed in this book. A major drawback to their use in the clinic has been the inability to scale up production, with many only being produced at between 1 and 10 mg/liter, which is clearly not commercially viable; it is almost impossible to obtain sufficient quantities to carry out large-scale clinical trials.

The case study provided in this section is intended to provide the reader with an example of how many of the manufacturing problems, which severely limit the application of such molecules, have been overcome. In all the examples of fusion proteins in clinical trials, manufacturing is carried out at a commercially viable scale. There is no doubt that further manufacturing progress will be made in this field, which should result in an even greater number of antibody fusion proteins coming through to clinical trials.

Much still needs to be elucidated regarding immunotherapy of cancer with cytokines and cytokine fusion proteins. Most clinical studies with IL-12 to date have not given startling responses, and this might be due to down-regulation of the IL-12 receptor and possibly also to the immune system negative regulatory feedback pathways. The role of regulatory T cells in cancer as well as complex cross-talk and interacting immune regulatory pathways may also be key to the efficacy of cytokines.[36,37] The correct balance in the perturbation, down-regulation, and activation of different immune regulatory proteins may require considerable optimization, but cytokine treatment seems to be an increasingly attractive option for the treatment of cancer. It is anticipated that fusion proteins having at least two cytokines – for example IL-12 and IL-2 – will enter clinical trials in order to improve the clinical results seen to date with the use of a single interleukin. It may also be possible to increase clinical efficacy by using improved single interleukin-antibody fusion proteins such as AS1409, which is at the vanguard of targeted immunotherapeutics. The results of the ongoing trial with this fusion protein are keenly awaited.

REFERENCES

[1] Hoogenboom HR et al: *Mol Immunol.* 1991 Sept; **28**(9):1027–37.
[2] Gillies SD et al: *Proc Natl Acad Sci USA.* 1992 Feb. 15; **89**(4):1428–32.

[3]   Savage P et al: *Br J Cancer.* 1993 Feb; **67**(2):304–10.

[4]   Reisfeld RA et al: *Melanoma Res.* 1997 Aug 7; suppl 2:S99–106.

[5]   Penichet ML et al: *J Interferon Cytokine Res.* 1998 Aug; **18**(8):597–607.

[6]   Carnemolla B et al: *J Cell Biol.* 1989 Mar; **108**(3):1139–48.

[7]   Kaczmarek J et al: *Int J Cancer.* 1994 Oct 1; **59**(1):11–16.

[8]   Castellani P et al: *Int J Cancer.* 1994 Dec 1; **59**(5):612–8.

[9]   Pini A et al: *J Biol Chem.* 1998 Aug 21; **273**(34):21769–76.

[10]   Halin C et al: *Int J Cancer.* 2002 Nov 10; **102**(2):109–16.

[11]   Afanasieva TA et al: *Gene Ther.* 2003 Oct; **10**(21):1850–9.

[12]   Borsi L et al: *Blood.* 2003 Dec 15; **102**(13):4384–92.

[13]   Gafner V et al: *Int J Cancer.* 2006 Nov; **119**(9):2205–12.

[14]   Trachsel E et al: *Arthritis Res Ther.* 2007; **9**(1):R9.

[15]   Kaspar M et al: *Cancer Res.* 2007 May 15; **67**(10):4940–8.

[16]   Carnemolla B et al: *Blood.* 2002 Mar 1; **99**(5):1659–65.

[17]   Lo K-M et al: *Cancer Immunol Immunother.* 2007; **56**:447–57.

[18]   Lustgarten J. *Cancer Immunol Immunother.* 2003 Dec; **52**(12):751–60.

[19]   Hombach A et al: *Int J Cancer.* 2005 Jun 10; **115**(2):241–7.

[20]   Cho HM et al: *Mol Cancer Ther.* 2005 Jun; **4**(6):956–67.

[21]   Ko YJ et al: *J Immunother.* 2004 May–Jun; **27**(3):232–9.

[22]   Osenga KL et al: *Clin Cancer Res.* 2006 Mar 15; **12**(6):1750–9.

[23]   Curigliano G et al: *J Clin Oncol.* 2007 June 20 suppl; **25**(185):3057.

[24]   Mariani G et al: *Cancer.* 1997; **80**:2484.

[25]   Carnemolla B et al: *J Biol Chem.* 1992; **267**:24689.

[26]   Midulla M et al: *Cancer Res.* 2000; **60**:164.

[27]   Mariani G et al: *Cancer.* 1997; **80**:2378.

[28]   Castellani P et al: *Am J Pathol.* 2002; **161**:1695.

[29]   Weiss JM et al: *Expert Opin Biol Ther.* 2007; **7**:1705.

[30]   Del Vecchio, M et al: *Clin Cancer Res.* 2007; **13**:4677.

[31]   Gollob JA et al: *Clin Cancer Res.* 2000; **6**:1678.

[32]   Gollob JA et al: *J Clin Oncol.* 2003; **21**:2564.

[33]   Gillies S et al: *J Immunol.* 1998; **160**:6195.

[34]   Peng LS et al: *J Immunol.* 1999; **163**:250.

[35]   Halin C et al: *Nat Biotechnol.* 2002; **20**:264.

[36]   Smyth MJ et al: *J Immunol.* 2006; **176**:1582.

[37]   King IL and Degal BM. *J Immunol.* 2005; **175**:641.

PART VI

NOVEL ANTIBODY FORMATS

CHAPTER FIFTEEN

Alternative Antibody Formats

Fabrice Le Gall and Melvyn Little

During evolution, antibodies have acquired several invaluable properties that are now being exploited for clinical applications. First, they can bind a wide variety of target molecules with exquisite specificity. This property can be used to block the action of ligands such as TNFα in patients with rheumatoid arthritis or the Her-2 receptor in patients with breast cancer. In contrast to this mode of action, antibodies can also imitate ligand binding and stimulate various signaling pathways. Antibodies binding to CD20, for example, can induce apoptotic signals in the malignant cells of patients with non-Hodgkin's lymphoma. Additional effector functions are provided by the Fc domains, which can induce cell lysis by binding to complement (CDC) or by binding to Fc receptors on natural killer cells and macrophages (ADCC). An additional binding domain for the neonatal receptor on endothelial cells facilitates their uptake and recycling, enabling antibody therapeutics to remain in the circulation for many weeks.

To optimize the properties of an antibody for a particular indication or for use as a diagnostic, it would be preferable to improve or even delete particular characteristics. For example, to achieve better tumor penetration or a better tumor-to-blood ratio for visualizing metastases, it would be preferable to have a relatively small antibody fragment with a fairly short half-life. On the other hand, the antibody should not be too small in order to avoid a rapid clearance immediately after its application. It would also be very advantageous for certain clinical applications to improve the effector functions. For example, the affinity of the Fc domains for their receptors has been increased by various means (see Part IV, Antibody Effector Functions). In another approach, multivalent and bispecific antibody formats have been developed that facilitate a more effective recruitment of immune effector cells for lysing tumor cells. The design and use of novel alternative antibody formats are described in this chapter.

RECOMBINANT ANTIBODIES COMPRISING ONLY VARIABLE DOMAINS

Single-Domain Antibodies

In 1989, a library comprising only the Vh domains of human immunoglobulins was successfully screened for specific binders (Ward et al., 1989). A few years later, a novel type of mammalian antibody was discovered in the serum of camels that contained only heavy chain variable domains (Hamers-Casterman et al., 1993). Therapeutic products based on such single antibody domains are now being developed as so-called dAbs by Domantis (acquired by GlaxoSmithKline) and nanobodies by Ablynx, respectively. In the case of human single antibody domains, mutations were introduced at the Vh/Vl contact site to decrease its hydrophobic character by substitutions with hydrophilic amino acids. Libraries generated from these mutated domains have been successfully screened by phage display for dAbs binding to therapeutically interesting targets (Holt et al., 2003). High affinity single-domain antibodies have also been obtained from the B lymphocytes of camels or llamas after immunization.

Serum Half-life

High yields of single-domain antibodies are obtained from bacteria, which could result in a significant reduction in the cost of goods. Furthermore, they should be able to penetrate tumors or bind to antigens in poorly accessible parts of the body much better than full-length antibodies. However, this advantage will be lost if they are cleared very rapidly from the circulation. One approach to increasing the half-life would be to fuse several domains using peptide linkers to create multivalent and even multispecific antibodies. Small dual-specific antibodies, for example, have been constructed that bind a combination of targets specific for a particular cancer. However, even molecules with four linked units are still too small to prevent a high rate of clearance through the kidneys. It may therefore be necessary to fuse them to other antibody fragments or to other moieties that can prolong their serum half-life. Single-domain antibodies fused to serum albumin, for example, have half-lives similar to that of serum albumin itself (Holt et al., 2008). Alternatively, polyethylene glycol can be covalently attached by either random or site-specific PEGylation chemistry (Chapman, 2002).

For a detailed description of single-domain antibodies (sdAbs), see the chapter in this book by Muyldermans et al.

Single-chain Fv antibodies

Single-chain Fv (scFv) molecules, first described in 1988 (Huston et al., 1988), are 25–30 kDa proteins composed of heavy chain variable (Vh) and light chain variable (Vl) domains usually connected by a flexible peptide linker of 15 to 20 amino acids (Figure 15.1). As in the case of single-domain antibodies, the relatively small scFv are rapidly cleared from the bloodstream through the kidneys. Several methods have been used to modify the pharmacokinetics and/or the pharmacodynamic properties of the scFv. In one approach, for example, the half-life of an anti-GM-CSF scFv was extended by a factor of 30 in a mouse model after site-specific PEGylation using a branched 40 kDa PEG-polymer (Krinner et al., 2006).

In another approach, two (scFv')$_2$ fragments have been joined to make a bivalent product of approximately 50–55 kDa (Figure 15.1). For example, scFvs containing an

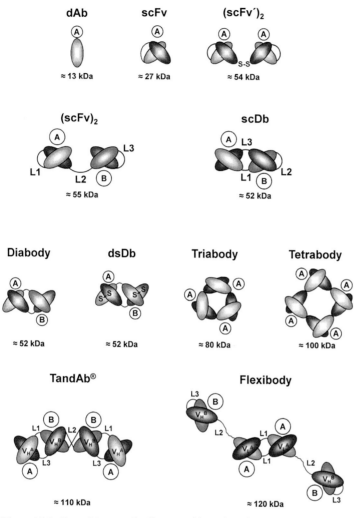

Figure 15.1. Recombinant antibodies comprising only variable domains.

additional C-terminal cysteine were linked either by chemical coupling (Adams et al., 1993) or by spontaneous oxidation of the free sulfhydryl groups in the periplasm of *Escherichia coli* (Kipriyanov et al., 1994) (Figure 15.1). Affinity measurements demonstrated that covalently linked (scFv')$_2$ have binding constants quite close to those of the parental monoclonal antibodies and fourfold higher than scFv monomers (Kipriyanov et al., 1994). *In vivo*, bivalent (scFv')$_2$ fragments demonstrated longer blood retention and higher tumor accumulation in comparison to scFv monomers (Adams et al., 1993).

Bivalent scFvs can also be genetically engineered by introducing a peptide linker between the two scFv units (Figure 15.1). This middle linker does not have much influence on the structure as a whole and can vary in length as long as the antigen-binding sites remain intact (Mack et al., 1995). Both scFvs can be identical or different, yielding monospecific bivalent or bispecific bivalent molecules, respectively. For example, so-called bispecific T cell engagers (BiTE®) directed against both a tumor associated antigen and CD3 appear to be particularly effective for the recruitment of T cells to lyse tumor cells (Baeuerle et al., 2003; Löffler et al., 2000; Mack et al., 1995). One such construct directed against CD19 on B lymphocytes has been developed by Micromet (Munich, Germany) for the treatment of non-Hodgkin's lymphoma. It is able to redirect and activate unstimulated primary T cells against CD19$^+$ lymphoma cells with high efficacy *in vitro* and *in vivo*, and is being evaluated in an ongoing Phase I clinical trial in non-Hodgkin's lymphoma. An upcoming Phase II clinical trial for the treatment of acute lymphoblastic leukemia will shortly be initiated.

Diabody Constructs

If the linker between the Vh and Vl domains of an scFv construct is shortened below about 10 amino acids, the two variable domains are sterically hindered from forming an Fv binding unit. The two domains can then only pair with their corresponding partner domains on a second molecule leading to the formation of a 50 kDa non-covalent scFv dimer "diabody" (Figure 15.1), which can either be monospecific or bispecific (Holliger et al., 1993; Kipriyanov et al., 1998). It has been shown by crystallographic analysis that the two antigen-binding sites of a diabody are located on opposite sides, assembled in either a Vh-to-Vl (Perisic et al., 1994) or Vl-to-Vh (Carmichael et al., 2003) orientation, such that they are able to cross link two cells. The stability of diabodies has been enhanced by introduction of a disulfide bridge or "knob-into-hole" mutations into the Vh/Vl interface (FitzGerald et al., 1997; Zhu et al., 1997) (Figure 15.1) or by introducing a linker between the two diabody-forming units to form a single-chain diabody (Kipriyanov et al., 1999; Kipriyanov et al., 2003; Kontermann et al., 1999) (Figure 15.1).

For binding to two different targets, the diabody is a heterodimer, since Vh of one specificity has to be linked by a short peptide to Vl of the second specificity in order to facilitate inter-chain pairing of the corresponding Vh and Vl domains. One disadvantage, however, is that nonfunctional homodimers can also form in addition to the desired heterodimers. One solution to avoid the formation of nonfunctional homodimers is to link the the two dimerizing chains with a peptide comprising at least 12 amino acids that is long enough to permit the corresponding variable domains to form an antigen-binding unit (Figure 15.1). It has been demonstrated that head-to-tail folding and formation of functional single-chain diabodies readily occurs, at least in *Escherichia coli* (Kipriyanov et al., 2003). Moreover, the single-chain diabody (scDb) format facilitates the production of relatively stable bispecific constructs from weakly associated Fv fragments (Kipriyanov et al., 2003).

Diabodies, scDb, and (scFv)$_2$ have significantly improved half-lives compared to scFv. In a tumor-bearing mouse model, a prolonged tumor retention *in vivo* and higher tumor-to-blood ratios were reported for diabodies over scFv monomers (Adams et al., 1998). An anti-CEA x anti-CD3 bispecific antibody in both an (scFv)$_2$ and an scDb format prolonged the half-life by a factor 4 and 6.5, respectively, when compared to a monovalent scFv (Müller et al., 2007). In order to increase the pharmacokinetic properties of the CEA × CD3 scDb still further, the effect of N-glycosylation and PEGylation were tested (Stork et al., 2008). One, four, or seven N-glycosylation sites were introduced at the C-terminus of the scDb. The glycosylated scDb showed a moderate increase in its half-life compared to the unmodified scDb (terminal half-life increased by a factor 1.1 to 1.6). In the same study, conjugation of a branched 40 kDa PEG-polymer showed an increase in the terminal half-life by a factor 2.3.

If the peptide linker between the Vh and Vl domains of a monospecific dimeric diabody is shortened to only a few amino acids or is completely eliminated, one often observes the formation of trimers ("triabody," ~90 kDa (Kortt et al., 1997)) or tetramers ("tetrabody," ~120 kDa (Le Gall et al., 1999; Todorovska et al., 2001)) (Figure 15.1). A comparison of the *in vitro* cell-binding characteristics of the diabody, triabody, and tetrabody specific for CD19 on B lymphocytes demonstrated 1.5- and 2.5-fold higher affinities of the diabody and tetrabody in comparison to the scFv monomer (Le Gall et al., 1999). This increased avidity of the tetrabody combined with its larger size could prove to be particularly advantageous for tumor imaging and radio-immunotherapy.

Tetravalent TandAb® and Flexibody

As discussed earlier, a polypeptide comprising four neighboring variable domains can form both two linked single-chain Fvs (scFv) or a single-chain diabody depending on the respective lengths of the three peptide linkers. If all three of the linkers are too short to facilitate intra-chain pairing of any of the variable domains, they can only pair with the variable domains of another polypeptide chain. Depending on the order of the domains along the chain, head-to-tail dimerization of the two identical chains can lead to the formation of a tetravalent homodimer (Kipriyanov et al., 1999) (Figure 15.2). The structure of these so-called TandAb®s is stabilized by the tight intermolecular association of four cognate VH/VL pairs. Depending on the origin of the variable domain, the TandAb® can be a mono- or bispecific molecule and can bind tetravalently to the same antigen or bivalently to two different antigens, respectively. In comparison to the diabody and (scFv)$_2$ molecules, the TandAb® is twice as large with a molecular weight of about 105 kDa.

The TandAb® appears to be ideally suited for recruiting immune effector cells to lyse tumor cells since it has two binding sites for each specificity and its size is well above the limit for first pass renal clearance. An anti-CD19 x anti-CD3 bispecific TandAb® recruiting T cells to kill CD19 positive cells showed a lower clearance rate compared to the bispecific diabody, a higher apparent affinity for both antigens and enhanced biological activity both *in vitro* and *in vivo* (Cochlovius et al., 2000; Kipriyanov et al., 1999).

If the linker separating the first two variable domains of a four-domain polypeptide is long enough, they will fold to form a cognate scFv pair. The two last domains, however, can only bind to corresponding domains on another polypeptide if the linker between them is too short for intra-chain pairing. The resulting tetravalent homodimer has been called a flexibody because of its relatively flexible and

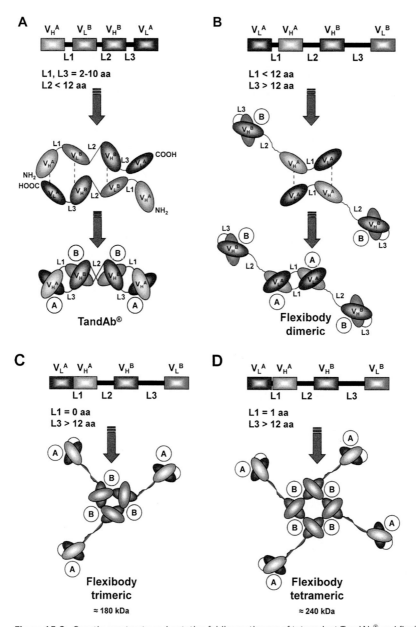

Figure 15.2. Genetic constructs and putative folding pathways of tetravalent TandAb® and flexibody. Starting as a four-domain gene product, tetravalent eight-domain constructs arise through the intermolecular pairing of the complementary Vh and Vl domains of the same specificity to form a TandAb® (A) or a flexibody (B). In the case of the flexibody, intermolecular pairing is preceded by intramolecular pairing of one of the adjacent amino- or carboxy-terminal Vh and Vl domains. The diabody mulitmer motif of the flexibody can give rise to hexavalent and octavalent antibodies if very short or zero linkers are used (C and D).

extended structure when compared to a TandAb® (Le Gall et al., patent WO-030250189) (Figure 15.2). Flexibodies can potentially form trimers and tetramers if a diabody multimerization motif with very short linkers is used as in the examples described earlier for the anti-CD19 diabody molecules (Figure 15.2). An anti-CD19 x anti-CD3 bispecific flexibody appeared to possess higher avidity and enhanced activity in mediating T cell cytotoxicity against CD19$^+$ leukemia cells than both the bivalent and single-chain diabody (Le Gall et al., patent WO-030250189).

RECOMBINANT ANTIBODIES BASED ON VARIABLE AND CONSTANT DOMAINS

One or all of the constant domains of a full-length IgG can be used as a basis for generating antibody fragments and antibody fusions to develop novel approaches for diagnosis and therapy. Several antibody Fv binding units can be fused to either the N- or C-terminal ends of both the heavy and light chain constant domains to create multivalent and multispecific antibodies (Figure 15.3).

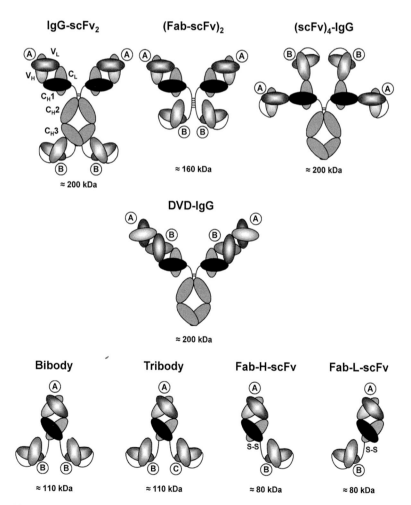

Figure 15.3. Recombinant antibodies comprising both variable and constant domains based on IgG and Fab formats.

IgG, Fab Fusions

An scFv has been genetically fused either to the C_H3 domain of an IgG molecule or to the hinge region of a Fab to form IgG-scFv$_2$ and (Fab-scFv)$_2$, respectively (Figure 15.3). *In vivo*, the IgG-scFv$_2$ antibody showed a terminal half-life of 3.8 days, two times longer than (Fab-scFv)$_2$, but shorter than an IgG3 (5 days) (Coloma et al., 1997). However, the scFv has a lower affinity for its antigen, which may be due to steric hindrance from the rest of the IgG. Moreover, the IgG-scFv$_2$ showed reduced ability to bind C1q and was unable to effect complement cell-mediated lysis.

In an alternative approach, two scFvs of different specificities were fused to the N-termini of the first constant heavy chain (C_H1) and the constant light chain (C_L) of an IgG to form two polypeptides, scFv^A-C_H1-Hinge-C_H2-C_H3 and scFv^B-C_L, respectively (Zuo et al., 2000). Co-expression of these polypeptides in mammalian cells resulted in the formation of a covalently linked bispecific heterotetramer, (scFv)$_4$-IgG (Figure 15.3), as a result of the natural pairing between the constant domain of the light and heavy chains. A fully human (scFv)$_4$-IgG antibody directed against both epidermal growth factor receptor (EGFR) and the insulin-like growth factor receptor (IGFR) was able to significantly inhibit tumor cell proliferation *in vitro* (Lu et al., 2004). More recently, a dual-variable-domain IgG (DVD-Ig) was described in which two variable domains have been linked in tandem in each heavy and light chain (Figure 15.3) (Wu et al., 2007). This antibody, which is specific for both IL-12 and IL-18, could be produced in reasonable quantities in mammalian cells on a laboratory scale and was able to block cytokine action as efficiently as a combination of the two parental antibodies.

Somewhat smaller bispecific (Bibody) and even trispecific (Tribody) trivalent molecules were generated by the fusion of scFvs to Fd and L-chains of a Fab fragment (Schoonjans et al., 2000) (Figure 15.3). Very similar bispecific Fab-scFv fragments have been generated by genetically fusing an scFv to the C-terminus of either the light chain or the heavy chain of a Fab fragment of different antigen-binding specificities to generate Fab-L-scFv and Fab-H-scFv antibodies, respectively (Lu et al., 2002; Schoonjans et al., 2000) (Figure 15.3).

All the Fab molecules described earlier are derived from two gene products. The production of a Fab as a single gene product has been achieved by genetic fusion of the Fd and L-chain with a flexible linker (scFab') (Inoue et al., 1997).

C_H3, C_H4, Fc fusions

As an alternative approach to fusing Fv binding domains with full-length immunoglobulin or Fabs, scFvs have been fused to either the complete Fc domain or to single constant domains. For example, an scFv has been genetically fused with the first constant domain of the heavy chain and the constant domain of the light chain to facilitate the formation of heterodimers (Müller et al., 1998; Zuo et al., 2000) [(scFv)$_2$-Fab] (Figure 15.4).

An scFv molecule was also fused to the human IgG1 C_H3 domain to form a so-called minibody (Hu et al., 1996) (Figure 15.4). Due to the strong interactions between the C_H3 domains, the scFv-C_H3 molecule dimerizes to form a stable

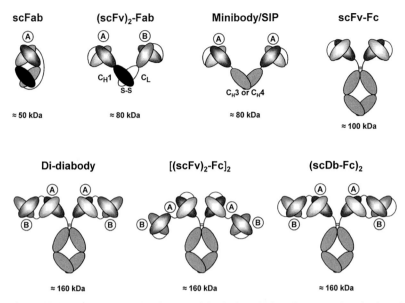

Figure 15.4. Recombinant antibodies comprising both variable and constant domains based on C_H3, C_H4 and Fc fragments.

molecule of about 80 kDa. An iodinated anti-CEA minibody demonstrated excellent tumor uptake (Hu et al., 1996; Wu et al., 2000) and a prolonged blood clearance compared to its scFv and diabody counterparts in nude mice bearing a CEA-positive tumor xenograft (Wu et al., 1996, 1999). Another minibody was similarly constructed using the variable genes of an anti-p185^{HER-2} antibody (Olafsen et al., 2004). Both minibodies showed similar blood clearance but lower tumor uptake. Minibodies with different specificities displayed similar pharmacokinetics but the tumor uptake varied depending on the particular specificity.

An alternative dimerization domain is the human IgE C_H4 domain, which was used to create a variant of the minibody called SIP (small immunoprotein) (Borsi et al., 2002) (Figure 15.4). Compared to (scFv)$_2$ and IgG1 formats (Berndorff et al., 2005; Tijink et al., 2006) in tumor-bearing mice, a SIP targeting the extra domain B of fibronectin, a marker for tumor angiogenesis, was identified as the best antibody format for radiotherapy (Borsi et al., 2002).

Based on the (scFv)$_2$ and single-chain diabody formats described, tetravalent bispecific IgG-like molecules have been created by the fusion of bispecific (scFv)$_2$ or scDb to the human Fc region to generate [(scFv)$_2$-Fc]$_2$ and (scDb-Fc)$_2$ antibodies, respectively (Alt et al., 1999; Park et al., 2000) (Figure 15.4). An additional diabody variant was also engineered to increase its molecular weight by fusing a Vl$_A$-Vh$_B$ peptide to the Fc chain (Vl$_A$-Vh$_B$-Hinge-C_H2-C_H3) of a human IgG1 and by co-secretion of a corresponding Vl$_B$-Vh$_A$ peptide to generate a so-called di-diabody (Lu et al., 2005) (Figure 15.4). However, this latter construct, in contrast to the [(scFv)$_2$-Fc]$_2$ and (scDb-Fc)$_2$ antibodies, is the product of two genes. Thus, in the case of the EGFR x IGFR bispecific di-diabody, in addition to the formation of active tetravalent bispecific antibodies, nonactive scFv-Fc dimers were detected that were devoid of the Vl$_A$-Vh$_B$ peptide (Lu et al., 2005).

Fusions to the Fc domain should result in products with relatively long serum half-lives through interaction with the neonatal Fc receptor (FcRn). However, for some applications, such as imaging, a shorter half-life may be more desirable. In the case of an scFv-Fc molecule (Figure 15.4), modulation of the half-life was accomplished by mutating the Fc-FcRn binding site (Kenanova et al., 2005). ScFv-Fc mutants were obtained that showed half-lives ranging from 7.96 to 83.4 hours compared to a half-life of 12 days for the wild type (Kenanova et al., 2005).

CONCLUSIONS

A variety of antibody fragments and novel antibody formats are now available for fine-tuning the desired pharmacokinetic and pharmacodynamic properties. These antibodies are able to provide multivalent binding for higher avidity and multispecific binding for a more effective tumor targeting. For diagnostic purposes, the optimal tumor: blood ratio will depend not only on Ab size but also on affinity of the antibody, accessibility of the antigen, and type of radioactive isotope. For therapeutic purposes, antibody formats can be chosen for binding simultaneously to a combination of targets that are specific for particular tumors. Bispecific formats can also be employed for the efficient recruitment of various immune effector cells to lyse tumor cells. Furthermore, by using bispecific formats devoid of constant domains, an extensive cross linking of Fc receptors leading to unwanted side effects through the excessive release of cytokines can be avoided. In certain cases, antibodies able to gain access to cryptic targets or that are cleared fairly rapidly are advantageous. Several of the individual formats described in this chapter may therefore be a source of future clinical products with optimal properties for a particular therapeutic need.

REFERENCES

Adams GP, McCartney JE, Tai MS, Oppermann H, Huston, JS, Stafford WF, Bookman M.A., Fand, I., Houston LL, Weiner LM: Highly specific *in vivo* tumor targeting by monovalent and divalent forms of 741F8 anti-c-erbB-2 single-chain Fv. *Cancer Res.* (1993) **53**:4026–4034.

Adams GP, Schier R, McCall AM, Crawford RS, Wolf EJ, Weiner LM, Marks JD: Prolonged *in vivo* tumour retention of a human diabody targeting the extracellular domain of human HER2/neu. *Br. J. Cancer.* (1998) **77**:1405–1412.

Alt M, Müller R, Kontermann RE: Novel tetravalent and bispecific IgG-like antibody molecules combining single-chain diabodies with the immunoglobulin gamma1 Fc or CH3 region. *FEBS Lett.* (1999) **454**:90–94.

Baeuerle PA, Kufer P, Lutterbüse R: Bispecific antibodies for polyclonal T-cell engagement. *Curr. Opin. Mol. Ther.* (2003) **5**:413–419.

Berndorff D, Borkowski S, Sieger S, Rother A, Friebe M, Viti F, Hilger CS, Cyr JE, Dinkelborg LM: Radioimmunotherapy of solid tumors by targeting extra domain B fibronectin: identification of the best-suited radioimmunoconjugate. *Clin. Cancer Res.* (2005) **11**:7053s–7063s.

Borsi L, Balza E, Bestagno M, Castellani P, Carnemolla B, Biro A, Leprini A, Sepulveda J, Burrone O, Neri D, Zardi L: Selective targeting of tumoral vasculature: comparison of different formats of an antibody (L19) to the ED-B domain of fibronectin. *Int. J. Cancer.* (2002) **102**:75–85.

Carmichael JA, Power BE, Garrett TP, Yazaki PJ, Shively JE, Raubitschek AA, Wu AM, Hudson PJ: The crystal structure of an anti-CEA scFv diabody assembled from T84.66 scFvs in VL-to-VH orientation: implications for diabody flexibility. *J. Mol. Biol.* (2003) **326**:341–351.

Chapman AP: PEGylated antibodies and antibody fragments for improved therapy: a review. *Adv. Drug Deliv. Rev.* (2002) **54**:531–545.

Clynes RA, Towers TL, Presta LG, Ravetch JV: Inhibitory Fc receptors modulate *in vivo* cytoxicity against tumor targets. *Nat. Med.* (2000) **6**:443–446.

Cochlovius B, Kipriyanov SM, Stassar MJ, Schuhmacher J, Benner A, Moldenhauer G, Little M: Cure of Burkitt's lymphoma in severe combined immunodeficiency mice by T cells, tetravalent CD3 x CD19 tandem diabody, and CD28 costimulation. *Cancer Res.* (2000) **60**:4336–4341.

Coloma MJ, Morrison SL: Design and production of novel tetravalent bispecific antibodies. *Nat. Biotechnol.* (1997) **15**:159–163.

FitzGerald K, Holliger P, Winter G: Improved tumour targeting by disulphide stabilized diabodies expressed in Pichia pastoris. *Protein Eng.* (1997) **10**:1221–1225.

Hamers-Casterman C, Atarhouch T, Muyldermans S, Robinson G, Hamers C, Songa EB, Bendahman N, Hamers R: Naturally occurring antibodies devoid of light chains. *Nature* (1993) **363**:446–448.

Holliger P, Prospero T, Winter G: "Diabodies": small bivalent and bispecific antibody fragments. *Proc. Natl. Acad. Sci. USA* (1993) **90**:6444–6448.

Holt LJ, Herring C, Jespers LS, Woolven BP, Tomlinson IM: Domain antibodies: proteins for therapy. *Trends Biotechnol.* (2003) **21**:484–490.

Holt LJ, Basran A, Jones K, Chorlton J, Jespers LS, Brewis ND, Tomlinson IM: Anti-serum albumin domain antibodies for extending the half-lives of short lived drugs. *Protein Eng. Des. Sel.* (2008) **21**:283–288.

Hu S, Shively L, Raubitschek A, Sherman M, Williams LE, Wong JY, Shively JE, Wu AM: Minibody: a novel engineered anti-carcinoembryonic antigen antibody fragment (single-chain Fv-CH3) which exhibits rapid, high-level targeting of xenografts. *Cancer Res.* (1996) **56**:3055–3061.

Huston JS, Levinson D, Mudgett-Hunter M, Tai MS, Novotný J, Margolies MN, Ridge RJ, Bruccoleri RE, Haber E, Crea R, et al.: Protein engineering of antibody binding sites: recovery of specific activity in an anti-digoxin single-chain Fv analogue produced in Escherichia coli. *Proc. Natl. Acad. Sci. USA* (1988) **85**:5879–5883.

Inoue Y, Ohta T, Tada H, Iwasa S, Udaka S, Yamagata H: Efficient production of a functional mouse/human chimeric Fab′ against human urokinase-type plasminogen activator by Bacillus brevis. *Appl. Microbiol. Biotechnol.* (1997) **48**:487–492.

Kenanova V, Olafsen T, Crow DM, Sundaresan G, Subbarayan M, Carter NH, Ikle DN, Yazaki PJ, Chatziioannou AF, Gambhir SS, Williams LE, Shively JE, Colcher D, Raubitschek AA, Wu AM: Tailoring the pharmacokinetics and positron emission tomography imaging properties of anti-carcinoembryonic antigen single-chain Fv-Fc antibody fragments. *Cancer Res.* (2005) **65**:622–631.

Kipriyanov SM, Dübel S, Breitling F, Kontermann RE, Little M: Recombinant single-chain Fv fragments carrying C-terminal cysteine residues: production of bivalent and biotinylated miniantibodies. *Mol. Immunol.* (1994) **31**:1047–1058.

Kipriyanov SM, Moldenhauer G, Strauss G, Little M: Bispecific CD3 x CD19 diabody for T cell-mediated lysis of malignant human B cells. *Int. J. Cancer* (1998) **77**:763–772.

Kipriyanov SM, Moldenhauer G, Schuhmacher J, Cochlovius B, Von der Lieth CW, Matys ER, Little M: Bispecific tandem diabody for tumor therapy with improved antigen binding and pharmacokinetics. *J. Mol. Biol.* (1999) **293**:41–56.

Kipriyanov SM, Moldenhauer G, Braunagel M, Reusch U, Cochlovius B, Le Gall F, Kouprianova OA, Von der Lieth CW, Little M: Effect of domain order on the activity of bacterially produced bispecific single-chain Fv antibodies. *J. Mol. Biol.* (2003) **330**:99–111.

Kontermann RE, Müller R: Intracellular and cell surface displayed single-chain diabodies. *J. Immunol. Methods* (1999) **226**:179–188.

Kortt AA, Lah M, Oddie GW, Gruen CL, Burns JE, Pearce LA, Atwell JL, McCoy AJ, Howlett GJ, Metzger DW, Webster RG, Hudson PJ: Single-chain Fv fragments of anti-neuraminidase antibody NC10 containing five- and ten-residue linkers form dimers and with zero-residue linker a trimer. *Protein Eng.* (1997) **10**:423–433.

Krinner EM, Hepp J, Hoffmann P, Bruckmaier S, Petersen L, Petsch S, Parr L, Schuster I, Mangold S, Lorenczewski G, Lutterbüse P, Buziol S, Hochheim I, Volkland J, Mølhøj M, Sriskandarajah M, Strasser M, Itin C, Wolf A, Basu A, Yang K, Filpula D, Sørensen P, Kufer P, Baeuerle P, Raum T. A human monoclonal IgG1 potently neutralizing the pro-inflammatory cytokine GM-CSF. *Protein Eng. Des Sel.* (2006) **19**:461–470.

Le Gall F, Kipriyanov SM, Moldenhauer G, Little M: Di-, tri- and tetrameric single chain Fv antibody fragments against human CD19: effect of valency on cell binding. *FEBS Lett.* (1999) **453**:164–168.

Le Gall F, Kipriyanov S, Reusch U, Moldenhauer G, Little M: Dimeric and multimeric antigen-binding structure. *Patent WO-03025018* (2003) Affimed Therapeutics AG.

Löffler A, Kufer P, Lutterbuse R, Zettl F, Daniel PT, Schwenkenbecher JM, Riethmüller G, Dörken B, Bargou RC: A recombinant bispecific single-chain antibody, CD19 x CD3, induces rapid and high lymphoma-directed cytotoxicity by unstimulated T lymphocytes. *Blood* (2000) **95**:2098–2103.

Lu D, Jimenez X, Zhang H, Bohlen P, Witte L, Zhu Z: Fab-scFv fusion protein: an efficient approach to production of bispecific antibody fragments. *J. Immunol. Methods* (2002) **267**:213–226.

Lu D, Zhang H, Ludwig D, Persaud A, Jimenez X, Burtrum D, Balderes P, Liu M, Bohlen P, Witte L, Zhu Z: Simultaneous blockade of both the Epidermal Growth Factor Receptor and the Insulin-like Growth Factor Receptor signaling pathways in cancer cells with a fully human recombinant bispecific antibody. *J. Biol. Chem.* (2004) **279**:2856–2865.

Lu D, Zhang H, Koo H, Tonra J, Balderes P, Prewett M, Corcoran E, Mangalampalli V, Bassi R, Anselma D, Patel D, Kang X, Ludwig DL, Hicklin DJ, Bohlen P, Witte L, Zhu Z: A fully human recombinant IgG-like bispecific antibody to both the epidermal growth factor receptor and the insulin-like growth factor receptor for enhanced antitumor activity. *J. Biol Chem.* (2005) **280**:19665–19672.

Mack M, Riethmüller G, Kufer P: A small bispecific antibody construct expressed as a functional single-chain molecule with high tumor cell cytotoxicity. *Proc. Natl. Acad. Sci. USA* (1995) **92**: 7021–7025.

Müller KM, Arndt KM, Strittmatter W, Plückthun A: The first constant domain (CH1 and CL) of an antibody used as heterodimerization domain for bispecific miniantibodies. *FEBS Lett.* (1998) **422**:259–264.

Müller D, Karle A, Meissburger B, Höfig I, Stork R, Kontermann RE: Improved pharmacokinetics of recombinant bispecific antibody molecules by fusion to human serum albumin. *J. Biol. Chem.* (2007) **282**:12650–12660.

Olafsen T, Tan GJ, Cheung CW, Yazaki PJ, Park JM, Shively JE, Williams LE, Raubitschek AA, Press MF, Wu AM: Characterization of engineered anti-p185HER-2 (scFv-CH3)2 antibody fragments (minibodies) for tumor targeting. *Protein Eng. Des. Sel.* (2004) **17**: 315–323.

Park SS, Ryu CJ, Kang YJ, Kashmiri SV, Hong HJ: Generation and characterization of a novel tetravalent bispecific antibody that binds to hepatitis B virus surface antigens. *Mol. Immunol.* (2000) **37**:1123–1130.

Perisic O, Webb PA, Holliger P, Winter G, Williams RL: Crystal structure of a diabody, a bivalent antibody fragment. *Structure* (1994) **2**:1217–1226.

Schoonjans R, Willems A, Schoonooghe S, Fiers W, Grooten J, Mertens N: Fab chains as an efficient heterodimerization scaffold for the production of recombinant bispecific and trispecific antibody derivatives. *J. Immunol.* (2000) **165**:7050–7057.

Stork R, Zettlitz KA, Müller D, Rether M, Hanisch FG, Kontermann RE: N-glycosylation as novel strategy to improve pharmacokinetic properties of bispecific single-chain diabodies. *J. Biol. Chem.* (2008) Epub ahead of print.

Tijink BM, Neri D, Leemans CR, Budde M, Dinkelborg LM, Stigter-van Walsum M, Zardi L, van Dongen GA: Radioimmunotherapy of head and neck cancer xenografts using 131I-labeled antibody L19-SIP for selective targeting of tumor vasculature. *J. Nucl. Med.* (2006) **47**:1070–1074.

Todorovska A, Roovers RC, Dolezal O, Kortt AA, Hoogenboom HR, Hudson PJ: Design and application of diabodies, triabodies and tetrabodies for cancer targeting. *J. Immunol. Methods* (2001) **248**:47–66.

Ward ES, Güssow D, Griffiths AD, Jones PT, Winter G: Binding activities of a repertoire of single immunoglobulin variable domains secreted from Escherichia coli. *Nature* (1989) **341**:544–546.

Wu AM, Chen W, Raubitschek A, Williams LE, Neumaier M, Fischer R, Hu SZ, Odom-Maryon T, Wong JY, Shively JE: Tumor localization of anti-CEA single-chain Fvs: improved targeting by non-covalent dimers. *Immunotechnology* (1996) **1**:21–36.

Wu AM, Williams LE, Zieran L, Padma A, Sherman M, Bebb GG, Odom-Maryon T, Wong JYC, Shively JE, Raubitschek AA: Anti-carcinoembryonic antigen (CEA) diabody for rapid tumor targeting and imaging. *Tumor Targeting* (1999) **4**:47–58.

Wu AM, Yazaki PJ: Designer genes: recombinant antibody fragments for biological imaging. *Q.J. Nucl. Med.* (2000) **44**:268–283.

Wu C, Ying H, Grinnell C, Bryant S, Miller R, Clabbers A, Bose S, McCarthy D, Zhu RR, Santora L, Davis-Taber R, Kunes Y, Fung E, Schwartz A, Sakorafas P, Gu J, Tarcsa E, Murtaza A, Ghayur T: Simultaneous targeting of multiple disease mediators by a dual-variable-domain immunoglobulin. *Nat. Biotechnol.* (2007) **25**:1290–1297.

Zhu Z, Presta LG, Zapata G, Carter P: Remodeling domain interfaces to enhance heterodimer formation. *Protein Sci.* (1997) **6**:781–788.

Zuo Z, Jimenez X, Witte L, Zhu Z: An efficient route to the production of an IgG-like bispecific antibody. *Protein Eng.* (2000) **13**:361–367.

CHAPTER SIXTEEN

Single-Domain Antibodies

Serge Muyldermans, Gholamreza Hassanzadeh Ghassabeh,
and Dirk Saerens

The antigen-binding entity of an antibody, reduced in size to one single domain, is referred to as a "single-domain antibody." Various strategies have been explored with variable success to arrive at functional single-domain antibodies. The potential of single-domain antibodies, as research tools or in medicine, is reflected by the three companies – founded in Europe – with a mission to bring these molecules to the market. Domantis using human VH-derived single-domain antibodies started in 2000 and was bought by GSK for £300M in December 2007. Haptogen employing shark single-domain antibodies was acquired by Wyeth, and Ablynx focusing on llama-derived single-domain antibodies received over €70M in three rounds of venture capitalist investments and another €80M on the Euronext stock market in November 2007. Regarding therapeutic applications, Arana Therapeutics in Australia entered a Phase 2 clinical trial with its single-domain antibody derivative. In this chapter, we will review (1) the various antibodies used for generating single-domain antibodies, (2) the properties of single-domain antibodies that create an added value for use in immunotherapy, and (3) a number of therapeutic applications.

THE DEVELOPMENT OF SINGLE-DOMAIN ANTIBODIES

Antibodies comprise two identical heavy chain polypeptides (H) carrying chains of carbohydrates and two identical light chain proteins (L). Their ability to bind specifically to an antigen is dictated by the paired variable regions of the heavy (VH) and the light (VL) chain (Figure 16.1). Efforts to obtain stable, minimal-sized antigen-binding fragments resulted in the construction of improved single chain antibodies (scFv) containing a synthetic linker between the VH and VL polypeptides (Worn et al., 2001). In an independent research program, a single-domain antibody (sdAb) format was proposed as a favored alternative. From early experiments it was known that isolated heavy chains of anti-hapten antibodies retain some antigen-binding capacity in the absence of the light chains (Haber et al., 1966; Utsumi et al., 1964). This finding was in line with the observation that the complementarity determining region (CDR3) of the VH domain is the most diverse antigen-binding loop and largely determines the antigen specificity. Unfortunately, attempts to obtain the

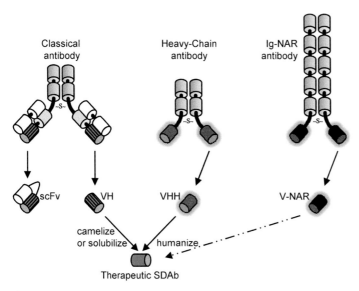

Figure 16.1. Schematic representation of the domain composition of classical antibodies, camelid heavy chain antibodies, and shark Ig-NAR antibodies. Single-domain antibody fragments (VH, VHH and V-NAR, respectively) can be derived from these antibodies and can be further engineered (camelized, solubilized, humanized) to generate therapeutic single-domain antibodies.

smallest antigen-binding unit in a VH format from classical antibodies ran into difficulties, partially due to the poor solubility of isolated VH molecules – although some successful attempts have been reported (Ward et al., 1989). In a radical attempt to produce a more soluble and even smaller binding unit, the VH domain was shortened to a synthetic sequence of 61 amino acids that lacked both the FR4 and the CDR3 of the VH domain (Pessi et al., 1993).

Sources of sdAbs

sdAbs from Sharks

As regularly happens when researchers try to solve a problem, nature has already gone twice through a similar exercise a long time ago and has provided the solution in cartilaginous fish and in *Camelidae*. Indeed, cartilaginous fish (i.e., wobbegong or nurse shark) possess an ancestral type of antibody that lacks the light chain (Diaz et al., 2002). This antibody is composed of a homodimer of a heavy chain (Figure 16.1), and each N-terminal domain, called V-NAR, is active in antigen binding. Therefore, it is possible to immunize these shark species and to clone the V-NAR repertoire from which to select the antigen-binding V-NARs. Proof of principle was shown using chicken lysozyme or human translocase receptor Tom70 as antigen – a single-domain antibody was isolated that binds the antigen with low nM affinity (Dooley et al., 2003; Nuttall et al., 2003). Even the crystal structures of the V-NAR and the V-NAR-lysozyme complex were solved, which demonstrated that V-NAR has only two CDRs (Stanfield et al., 2004; Streltsov et al., 2005).

sdAbs from Camelids

Much later in evolution, the homodimeric H-chain antibody format was "reinvented" by nature and evolved in *Camelidae* (*Camelus dromedarius, Camelus bactrianus, Lama glama, Lama vicugna, Lama guanaco, Lama alpaca*). Evolutionary studies (Nguyen et al., 2002) on the IgG sequences confirm that these special antibodies emerged after these species of the suborder *Tylopoda* split from the species of *Ruminantia* and *Suiformes*, the other suborders within the order of *Artiodactyl*. Of special note, camelids produce both classical antibodies and the so-called heavy chain antibodies (hcAbs). The hcAbs are devoid of light chains, their H-chain lacks the first constant domain (CH1), and the V domain (known as VHH) is distinct from the VH-domain of a classical H2L2 antibody (De Genst et al., 2006a) (Figure 16.1). Although both V domains share the same folding pattern of two β-pleated sheets, one of 4 β-strands and one of 5 β-strands, the conserved hydrophobic amino acids that are normally involved in VL interactions are solvent exposed in VHH and substituted by hydrophilic amino acids, which is believed to improve the solubility. In addition, the variability in the antigen-binding loops is extended at the N-terminal end of the CDR1 and comprises more amino acids in CDR3 of the dromedary (although a significant number of llama-VHHs do not show this enlarged CDR3 region). The *Camelidae* species can be immunized like any other mammal to raise an antigen-specific immune response, and subsequently, their VHH repertoire can be cloned from this, antigen-specific VHHs can be isolated, usually by phage display. Multiple high-affinity VHHs against a wide variety of antigens have been obtained from such "immune" libraries, and many VHH-antigen interactions have been characterized in detail, including X-ray crystallography (De Genst et al., 2006b).

sdAbs from Human VH Domains

For human immunotherapy, there is an enormous pressure to employ molecules that are as close as possible in sequence to human proteins. In contrast to VHH where "humanization" seems possible (Conrath et al., 2005), this might be more difficult to achieve for V-NARs. An alternative approach to avoid humanization of a VHH consists of selecting antigen-specific sdAbs from a synthetic library employing a human VH scaffold with favorable solubility properties. Davies and Riechmann (1995) were the first to employ human-derived VH libraries to search for antigen-specific sdAbs. In fact, to overcome the solubility problems of the isolated human VH, they first "camelized" this human VH before generating a synthetic library on this scaffold (Figure 16.1). For the camelization of the human VH they substituted the hydrophobic amino acids within the FR2 region to mimic the hydrophilic amino acids of VHH in that region.

Reiter et al. (1999) introduced another approach. They first selected an autonomous VH from a large pool of mouse VHs carrying natural mutations that render the domain more soluble than its homologues (Figure 16.1). A synthetic library was then generated on this autonomous scaffold. This strategy was adapted by Domantis to produce large synthetic libraries of human VH single domains from which to retrieve potent antigen-specific binders.

Finally, using combinatorial phage-displayed libraries with randomized amino acids at key positions in the framework-2 region and CDR3 of the human VH-4D5, Barthelemy et al. (2008) identified optimal mutations to generate a soluble, stable, well-expressed human VH. Remarkably, the mutations were different from those found in natural camelid VHHs and could not be predicted. The *in vitro*-evolved autonomous VHs have their solvent-exposed hydrophobic residues in the former light chain interface substituted by structurally compatible hydrophilic residues, whereas the CDR3 region remained unchanged. It is to be expected that this and similarly derived scaffolds will now be employed in the near future to generate synthetic libraries. Indeed, these examples indicate that nearly all protein scaffolds can be considered as a basis for generating synthetic libraries. For example, soluble VL has also been employed to generate synthetic libraries as well as related domains with an immunoglobulin fold such as human VL, CTLA4, or human fibronectin domains (Fn3) (Koide et al., 1998).

Immune, Naïve, and Synthetic sdAb Libraries

Cartilaginous fish and camelids can be immunized before the "immune" V-NAR or VHH repertoire is cloned to isolate affinity-matured antigen-specific sdAbs. If the antigen is difficult to prepare, DNA vaccination can be a possibility or total cell extracts can be used to immunize or vaccinate (Saerens et al., 2008a). However, the obvious downside of an immunization step remains the requirement of a relative large batch of (recombinant) antigen to immunize the animals. Sometimes this antigen is not available (e.g., transmembrane proteins) or toxic. In these instances, it is difficult to immunize an animal and to generate an immune library, and one would definitely benefit from the availability of naïve or synthetic VHH or V-NAR libraries. Naïve libraries are obtained by cloning the VHH or V-NAR repertoire from nonimmunized llamas or sharks, respectively. For synthetic libraries, the codons for amino acids occurring in the CDR loops are randomized. Large "single pot" libraries have been constructed on V-NAR and VHH scaffolds and used successfully to isolate antigen-specific binders after phage display panning (Goldman et al., 2006; van Koningsbruggen et al., 2003; Liu et al., 2007a,b; Muruganandam et al., 2002; Nuttall et al., 2003; Shao et al., 2007; Verheesen et al., 2006b; Yau et al., 2003).

The antigen-binding human VHs can only be retrieved from synthetic libraries. Normally, the cloned VH repertoire of an immunized, vaccinated, or infected human (i.e., an "immune" VH library) will not contain high affinity, antigen-specific sdAbs as the absence of the VL partner, which in combination with the VH was affinity-matured against the immunogen, will curtail the affinity and specificity. However, this might change in the future, as transgenic mice have been engineered that produce functional hcAbs. In one transgenic mouse, two llama

VHH germline genes and the human D, J, and Cμ and/or Cγ constant regions with their CH1 domain deleted were joined in the same locus (Janssens et al., 2006). The other transgenic mice were L-chain knockouts, further engineered to carry a CH1-CH2 truncated Cμ gene (Zou et al., 2007). Experiments with such mice might provide deeper insights in hcAb generation and show the way to assemble new transgenic mice with a modified human H-chain locus that will produce specific human hcAbs.

Selection of Antigen-specific sdAbs

Several strategies have been employed to identify antigen-specific sdAbs. The most popular technique is to express the VHH, V-NAR, or human VH on phage and select the binders directly on antigen, either immobilized on immunotubes or microtiter plates, or coupled to streptavidin-coated beads after biotinylation. This is a robust technique and versatile to select for particular properties (e.g., binders stable under harsh conditions) and works particularly well for immune, naïve, and synthetic libraries. In an alternative strategy, the selections were optimized in a yeast display system. This has the advantage that during the selections, besides enrichment for the antigen-specific binders, enrichment also occurs for those clones that express well in this host, which is an important aspect if extremely large amounts of sdAb are required later (Frenken et al., 2000).

In principle, ribosome display could also be used to screen for antigen-specific sdAbs in a library. In fact, this selection technique was employed to identify binders with an increased affinity or with an enhanced stability compared to the original sdAb. Variations were introduced by either spiked oligonucleotide mutagenesis in the CDR region or by random mutagenesis following the molecular evolution technique with DNase I cutting of the polymerase chain reaction (PCR) fragment followed by reassembly by PCR (van der Linden et al., 2000; Yau et al., 2003).

Immune libraries contain an increased number of antigen-specific clones within the bank as a result of the *in vivo* proliferation of B cells during immunization. Since titers of close to 1% antigen-specific clones might be obtained after hyperimmunization, it should become feasible to screen for the antigen-specific clones by colony hybridization with radioactive-labeled antigen. Likewise, simple colony picking by a robot and testing each individual clone separately in an ELISA might be envisaged. Such approaches discriminate between antigen binders and nonbinders; however, they fail to indicate which clones provide binders of highest affinity or best expression levels. It could be argued, however, that affinity maturation during immunization ensures that only B cells carrying high-affinity antigen receptors will survive and proliferate, so that all the isolated sdAbs will be good binders. A protocol was therefore developed that avoids the cumbersome construction of a library (Nanoclone®, Ablynx). In this approach, llamas were first hyperimmunized to increase the titer of B cells expressing antigen-specific hcAbs. These antigen-specific B cells were selected on fluorescence-assisted cell sorter (FACS) with a combination of fluorescent markers for the B cells carrying hcAbs and fluorescent antigen. Individual cells were sorted in individual wells of micro-titer plates and the encoded VHH was amplified by a single cell RT-PCR and cloned. It is claimed that this approach yields a better range of sdAbs – and even of higher affinity – than those isolated from an immune library using phage display.

ADVANTAGEOUS PROPERTIES OF sdAbs FOR IMMUNOTHERAPY

Expression

If the selected antibody fragment can be expressed at high levels, this is an advantage, although less important for an immunotherapeutic. All reports indicate that the sdAbs perform very well in this respect, independent of whether they are expressed in bacterial cultures grown in shaker flasks or in fermentation setups. Expression in yeast (*Saccharomyces* or *Pichia*) also seems to be extremely economic, and it is estimated that a cost of €100 per g of sdAb is possible, which is 10–100 times cheaper than scFv production (Frenken et al., 2000; Rahbarizadeh et al., 2006; Thomassen et al., 2002). Recently, high-yield expression of VHH in plants was reported (Ismaili et al., 2007), although production in plants is not yet the first choice for the manufacture of an immunotherapeutic.

Stability and Solubility

High stability and solubility are critical parameters since stable antibody fragments perform better in tumor targeting and are expected to have a longer shelf life. They can also be transported or stored under nonrefrigerated or non-thermo stabilized conditions. The V-NARs seem to be resistant to high concentrations of urea, whereas the camelid VHHs and optimized human VH sdAbs are usually resistant to elevated temperatures and high concentrations of chaotropic denaturants such as guanidinium. HCl (Barthelemy et al., 2008; Dumoulin et al., 2002). It was even reported that some llama-derived sdAbs retain their antigen-binding activity after a prolonged incubation at 90°C (van der Linden et al., 1999). This high thermostability or good refolding property following heat denaturation has been exploited to design a VHH purification protocol (Olichon et al., 2007). Incubating the periplasmic extract for 20 minutes at 90°C apparently aggregated all contaminating proteins so that pure VHHs were recovered in solution after a simple centrifugation step, without the involvement of ion exchange or affinity chromatographic steps. Interestingly, the thermostability of the VHHs could be increased even further by ~10°C after introducing an extra disulfide bond in their scaffold between amino acid positions 54 and 78 (Saerens et al., 2008b).

Apart from these qualities, the camelid sdAbs also seem to be resistant to acidic conditions and proteases, suggesting that they might pass the gut in an active form. This is an important asset as it would allow a straightforward oral administration of an sdAb-based immunotherapeutic (Harmsen et al., 2006).

Affinity, Specificity, and Recognition of Unique Epitopes

In general, the affinity (expressed as equilibrium dissociation constant KD in nM) of binders that are retrieved from synthetic libraries is correlated with the size of the bank. As a rule of thumb, to have a reasonable success of isolating binders with nM affinity one should start with an effective bank size of approximately 10^9–10^{10} individual clones. In contrast, the immune camelid sdAb libraries of 10^6–10^7 individual clones routinely yield antigen binders that recognize their cognate target with nM (or even sub-nM) affinities, due to the *in vivo* affinity maturation during immunization and the cloning of the intact antigen-binding site as one single PCR product. (Note that the cloning of an immune library from classical antibodies disrupts the affinity-matured antigen-binding site as the VL and VH gene fragments are amplified separately and subsequently reassembled randomly into all possible pairs. Large banks are therefore required in order to isolate the original affinity-matured VH-VL pair). For large naïve and synthetic sdAb libraries, the binders that are normally isolated have affinities around 200 nM. These affinities can be subsequently improved after randomizing some of the synthetic codons (or codons in their vicinity) in combination with phage display or, preferably, ribosome display selections (van der Linden et al., 2000; Yau et al., 2003). However, this *in vitro* affinity maturation step takes time and the outcome remains unpredictable. It is therefore probably safer to invest a short time in immunizing a camelid (or shark) and to generate an immune sdAb library from which nM affinity binders are routinely isolated.

The "specificity" of antibodies is an ill-defined characteristic. However, it is our feeling that the specificity of the sdAbs is as good as that attained by classical antibodies or scFv. Some of our sdAbs against chicken lysozyme cross-react with turkey lysozyme, but evidently these antigens share a high degree of sequence identity. On other occasions, one single amino acid difference in the epitope can be sufficient to prevent antigen recognition. For example, it has been shown that an *in vivo* affinity-matured sdAb against GFP (KD of 230 pM) fails to bind to CFP that differs by only two amino acid substitutions (N147I and M154T). The single point mutation revertant of CFP where "I" at position 147 was backmutated to "N" was recognized by the sdAb, whereas the other revertant at codon 154 was not (Rothbauer et al., 2008).

A unique property of sdAbs is that they seem to preferentially recognize the catalytic site of enzymes. This was demonstrated for sdAbs derived from dromedaries and particularly for enzyme targets having a large catalytic cleft (e.g., 6 out of 8 sdAbs against chicken lysozyme bind into the active site) (De Genst et al., 2006b) and less so for enzymes with a more planar active site (e.g., only 1 out of 6 sdAbs inhibited lactamase). Remarkably, this could not be repeated with llama sdAbs (Ferrari et al., 2007), whereas other groups confirmed that sdAbs from llamas act as enzyme inhibitors (Jobling et al., 2003).

Fast Lead Identification

The time from target selection until the Investigative New Drug (IND) filing should be kept to a minimum. It is expected that the discovery time of the lead candidate which takes 3 to 6 years in cases of conventional antibodies can be reduced by 1 to 4 years with sdAbs from immune libraries. The possibility of a prior immunization and the cloning of the intact affinity-matured antigen-binding fragment in one single exon is an advantage of sdAbs from immune libraries over synthetic libraries and over other antibody formats, as lengthy *in vitro* affinity maturation steps are avoided.

Minimal-Sized Antibody

Smaller molecules tend to be less immunogenic. This has been confirmed with a sdAb of camelid origin in mice (Cortez-Retamozo et al., 2002). The camelid sdAb already possesses a high degree of sequence identity with human VH and can even be "humanized" using the sequence of a human VH as a lead (Conrath et al., 2005). It is therefore expected that such humanized sdAb and also human VHs will not be immunogenic when administered in man.

The small size of the sdAbs ensures a rapid distribution throughout the body, a good tissue penetration, and a fast renal clearance, which together are beneficial properties for noninvasive *in vivo* targeting. However, for maximal therapeutic effect, a longer half-life of the drug in the patient is necessary. For this purpose, the rapidly cleared monomeric sdAbs should be engineered to increase their size above the renal clearance cutoff or by targeting to long-lived serum proteins. This is achieved either by pegylation (Harmsen et al., 2007) or by reconstitution of the therapeutic sdAb with an Fc into an hcAb, or by conjugation with another sdAb recognizing serum albumin (Coppieters et al., 2006; Holt et al., 2008; Roovers et al., 2007) or an IgG (Harmsen et al., 2005).

Generation of Multidomain Constructs

The small and strict monomeric behavior of an sdAb makes it an ideal entity to construct complex entities that combine multiple specificities for "multi-tasking" purposes. With this objective, the sdAb has been reconstituted in hcAbs to acquire bivalent entities with longer blood half-life and exerting natural effector functions such as antibody-dependent cell-mediated cytotoxicity (ADCC) and complement-dependent cytotoxicity (CDC) (Figure 16.2). Other innovative constructs such as biparatopic, bivalent, trivalent, pentavalent, and even decavalent constructs (Zhang et al., 2004) have been created aiming at an increase in potency or a gain in function by higher avidity or the possibility to cross link antigens (Figure 16.2). The inclusion of an sdAb against a prominent serum protein in the multispecific sdAb construct is an elegant strategy to increase the serum half-life of a rapidly cleared therapeutic (Coppieters et al., 2006; Holt et al., 2008; Roovers et al., 2007).

Other interesting sdAbs with a strong potential to be part of larger multitasking entities are the sdAb against human cerebromicrovascular endothelial cells and FcγRIII (Behar et al., 2008; Muruganandam et al., 2002). Entities with the former sdAb can transmigrate across a model *in vitro* human blood-brain barrier, whereas constructs with the latter sdAb can recruit FcγRIII expressing killer cells to target and destroy tumor cells.

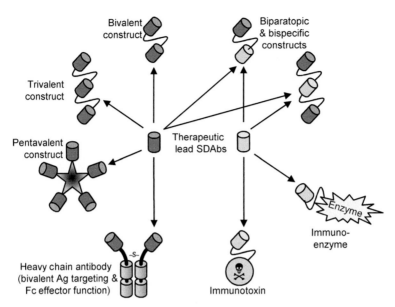

Figure 16.2. Various multidomain constructs that have been generated from therapeutic sdAbs.

Finally, the linkage of sdAbs with an enzyme or a toxic protein (Figure 16.2) generated a versatile tool to combat cancer cells or parasite infections (Baral et al. 2006; Cortez-Retamozo et al., 2004).

IMMUNOTHERAPEUTIC APPLICATIONS

Direct Neutralization of Toxic Molecules

Antibodies or Fab'2-derivatives have been used for many years in serotherapy. However, in instances where antibodies are too large and Fc effector functions are pointless, smaller derivatives might perform better. Especially in scorpion or snake envenoming, the sdAb might be a preferred serotherapeutic because its size and biodistribution match closely that of the toxins; hence, a higher neutralization capacity could be achieved in mouse models (Hmila et al., 2008). It has been postulated that for complex snake venoms a mixture of monomeric sdAbs and pentamerized sdAbs might be preferable to obtain improved toxin neutralization (Stewart et al., 2007).

Panning of a nonimmune llama VHH library against the lipopolysaccharide (LPS) of *Neisseria meningitis* allowed El Khattabi et al. (2006) to identify an sdAb with specificity for the inner core of LPS. This sdAb exhibits a broad specificity for LPS from various bacteria and blocks the binding of LPS to target cells of the immune system so that it could become a therapeutic against LPS-mediated sepsis.

Since stable sdAbs could prevent, *in vitro*, the unfolding of unstable amyloidogenic protein variants, it is anticipated that they could also reduce their aggregation that ultimately leads to the formation and deposition in tissues of toxic amyloid fibrils (Dumoulin et al., 2003). More important still, a camel sdAb against the A-β 1–42 peptide causing Alzheimer could distinguish Aβ amyloid fibrils from disaggregated Aβ peptide and Aβ oligomers. The sdAb stabilizes the Aβ protofibrils and inhibits the formation of amyloid fibrils (Habicht et al., 2007). Evidently, these sdAbs have an attractive therapeutic potential for treating amyloidosis disorders such as Alzheimer's and Parkinson's disease. Likewise, the intracellularly expressed sdAb recognizing the nuclear polyA binding protein 1 (PABPN1) could inhibit the aggregation of its target and even reduce the presence of already existing aggregates (Verheesen et al., 2006a). As the PABPN1 aggregation causes oculopharyngeal muscular dystrophy, it is hoped that such sdAb might be developed into a next generation therapeutic against this group of protein aggregation disorders.

Combating Pathogenic Infections

Although the sdAb often has a small footprint on its antigen, hitting the correct epitope can by itself be sufficient to neutralize or to prevent proliferation of the target cells, even in the absence of any antibody Fc effector function. sdAbs with such activities have been isolated against P2 bacteriophages and shown to protect *Lactococcus lactis* from phage-induced lysis (de Haard et al., 2005). In the same vein, the daily administration of an untagged sdAb against *Streptococcus mutants* led to a significantly reduced development of smooth surface caries supporting their prophylactic activity (Kruger et al., 2006).

The presence of an sdAb against the matrix domain protein p15 from porcine endogenous retrovirus Gag polyprotein blocks the retrovirus production (Dekker et al., 2003). Employment of such sdAbs might eliminate the risk of transmission of infectious diseases if tissues and organs from pigs are to be used in xenotransplantation.

Van der Vaart et al. (2006) isolated rotavirus-specific llama sdAbs with the capacity to reduce the morbidity of rotavirus-induced diarrhea in mice. Such sdAbs produced by lactobacilli either in a secreted or surface-attached form markedly shortened disease duration, severity, and the viral load in mice infected with rotavirus (Pant et al., 2006). Similar treatments might have a significant impact on the course of an often fatal childhood rotavirus infection.

Apart from these direct pathogen-neutralizing sdAbs, some sdAbs need to be tagged with a moiety that is toxic for the pathogen. The linkage of a truncated human-ApoLI, which lyses the human serum-resistant East African trypanosomes, to an sdAb that recognizes a conserved carbohydrate present on various trypanosome serotypes formed a strong trypanolytic compound that clears the parasites in mouse models (Baral et al., 2006). Likewise, a synthetic antimicrobial peptide was conjugated to an *S.mutans*-targeting sdAb to maximize the lethal effect on the targeted bacteria (Szynol et al., 2006).

Eliminating Cancer Cells

Therapeutic sdAbs are also in the pipeline to combat cancer. Obvious targets are the epidermal growth factor receptor (EGFR) and carcino-embryonic antigen (CEA).

From an "immune" library, an sdAb was isolated that specifically competes with the epidermal growth factor (EGF) for binding to EGFR without acting as an agonist (Coppieters et al., 2006). It was further demonstrated that this untagged sdAb blocked EGF-mediated signaling and EGF-induced cell proliferation and inhibited the growth of A431-derived solid tumors.

A human sdAb isolated against Etk – a nonreceptor protein tyrosine kinase expressed in a variety of hematopoietic, epithelial, and endothelial cells where it participates in several cellular processes such as proliferation, differentiation, and motility – could block its kinase activity (Paz et al., 2005). The intracellular expression of this sdAb inhibited the Etk kinase activity and retarded the clonogenic cell growth. Although such sdAbs might not be immediately applicable in cancer treatment, they might reveal novel targets for future cancer intervention.

However, it is clear that in most cases, one would benefit from the attachment of a toxin or an effector moiety to the sdAb to eliminate malignant cells. Lidamycin is one such promising candidate. This macromolecule consists of a labile enediyne chromophore and a noncovalently bound apoprotein. When fused to an sdAb with specificity toward type IV collagenase, the fusion became a potent cancer-targeting drug with marked anti-angiogenic activity *in vitro* and an extreme cytotoxicity to hepatoma cancer cells in mouse models (Miao et al., 2007). The fusion is also more effective than the lidamycin alone.

It is not necessary to couple the toxic molecule directly to the tumor-targeting sdAb to generate cancer therapeutics. In a different two-step approach, an sdAb against the tumor associated CEA was conjugated to *Enterobacter cloacae* β-lactamase (Figure 16.2), an enzyme that converts a harmless prodrug into a potent phenylenediamine mustard toxin. The conjugate showed an excellent tumor-targeting capacity to tumor xenografts, and the subsequent prodrug therapy was able to eradicate the solid tumor entirely without a relapse (Cortez-Retamozo et al., 2004).

Anti-thrombotic Agents

Several sdAbs against Von Willebrand factor (VWF) have been identified. Some of these, which recognize specifically the activated form of VWF that interacts spontaneously with platelets, could be used as a tool to distinguish between acquired and congenital thrombotic thrombocytopenic purpura (TTP) (Hulstein et al., 2005). However, more important yet are those that inhibit platelet activation and adhesion to collagen at high shear rate as these sdAbs could prevent thrombus formation and vessel occlusion. A bivalent sdAb, ALX-0081, with two identical anti-VWF domain A1 sdAbs have been developed at Ablynx (www.ablynx.com) into a promising new anti-thrombotic agent. Preclinical tests demonstrated an improved efficacy and safety profile over approved drugs. The intravenous administration of ALX-0081 envisaged for the acute treatment of TTP patients has been successfully tested in a Phase 1a clinical trial with healthy persons and in a Phase 1b clinical trial in patients with stable angina undergoing elective percutaneous coronary intervention.

Rheumatoid Arthritis

The interleukin-1 receptor antagonist (IL-1ra), an approved protein for treatment of rheumatoid arthritis (RA), is a potent inhibitor of IL-1 signaling. It has a short half-life *in vivo* due to its small size. Therefore, a human sdAb against serum albumin was identified and conjugated to IL-1ra to prolong the half-life of the fusion protein by retention on albumin. In this case, the sdAb is not the therapeutic compound but it is a partner that assists in obtaining a superior efficacy (Holt et al., 2008).

The introduction of tumor necrosis factor (TNF)-blocking compounds provides an effective but highly expensive drug to treat rheumatoid arthritis (RA). At Arana Therapeutics (www.arana.com) an hcAb was reconstituted with an sdAb against TNF and a human Fc (Figure 16.2). This compound, named ART 621, performs as well as a blockbuster anti-TNF antibody product on the market. Furthermore, it is a stable compound with a prolonged action and favorable tissue location. The product has entered into a Phase II clinical trial for testing against plaque psoriasis.

Antagonistic anti-TNF llama sdAbs were also isolated (Coppieters et al., 2006). In a murine collagen-induced arthritis model, the bivalent construct of the sdAb was over 500 times more potent than the monovalent form. In other settings, the antagonistic effect of antihuman TNF exceeds that of Infliximab or Adalimumab. And the inclusion of an sdAb against serum albumin prolonged the *in vivo* half-life and promoted its targeting to inflamed joints in the murine CIA model of RA.

REFERENCES

Baral, T.N., S. Magez, et al. (2006). Experimental therapy of African trypanosomiasis with a nanobody-conjugated human trypanolytic factor. *Nat Med* **12**, 580–584.

Barthelemy, P.A., H. Raab, et al. (2008). Comprehensive analysis of the factors contributing to the stability and solubility of autonomous human VH domains. *J Biol Chem* **283**, 3639–3654.

Behar, G., S. Siberil, et al. (2008). Isolation and characterization of anti-FcgammaRIII (CD16) llama single-domain antibodies that activate natural killer cells. *Protein Eng Des Sel* **21**, 1–10.

Conrath, K., C. Vincke, et al. (2005). Antigen binding and solubility effects upon the veneering of a camel VHH in framework-2 to mimic a VH. *J Mol Biol* **350**, 112–125.

Coppieters, K., T. Dreier, et al. (2006). Formatted anti-tumor necrosis factor alpha VHH proteins derived from camelids show superior potency and targeting to inflamed joints in a murine model of collagen-induced arthritis. *Arthritis Rheum* **54**, 1856–1866.

Cortez-Retamozo, V., N. Backmann, et al. (2004). Efficient cancer therapy with a nanobody-based conjugate. *Cancer Res* **64**, 2853–2857.

Cortez-Retamozo, V., M. Lauwereys, et al. (2002). Efficient tumor targeting by single-domain antibody fragments of camels. *Int J Cancer* **98**, 456–462.

Davies, J., L. Riechmann (1995). Antibody VH domains as small recognition units. *Biotechnol* **13**, 475–479.

De Genst, E., D. Saerens, et al. (2006a). Antibody repertoire development in camelids. *Dev Comp Immunol* **30**, 187–198.

De Genst, E., K. Silence, et al. (2006b). Molecular basis for the preferential cleft recognition by dromedary heavy-chain antibodies. *Proc Natl Acad Sci USA* **103**, 4586–4591.

de Haard, H.J., S. Bezemer, et al. (2005). Llama antibodies against a lactococcal protein located at the tip of the phage tail prevent phage infection. *J Bacteriol* **187**, 4531–4541.

Dekker, S., W. Toussaint, et al. (2003). Intracellularly expressed single-domain antibody against p15 matrix protein prevents the production of porcine retroviruses. *J Virol* **77**, 12132–12139.

Diaz, M., R.L. Stanfield, et al. (2002). Structural analysis, selection, and ontogeny of the shark new antigen receptor (IgNAR): identification of a new locus preferentially expressed in early development. *Immunogenetics* **54**, 501–512.

Dooley, H., M.F. Flajnik, et al. (2003). Selection and characterization of naturally occurring single-domain (IgNAR) antibody fragments from immunized sharks by phage display. *Mol Immunol* **40**, 25–33.

Dumoulin, M., A.M. Last, et al. (2003). A camelid antibody fragment inhibits the formation of amyloid fibrils by human lysozyme. *Nature* **424**, 783–788.

Dumoulin, M., K. Conrath, et al. (2002). Single-domain antibody fragments with high conformational stability. *Protein Sci* **11**, 500–515.

El Khattabi, M., H. Adams, et al., (2006). Llama single-chain antibody that blocks lipopolysaccharide binding and signaling: prospects for therapeutic applications. *Clin Vaccine Immunol* **13**, 1079–1086.

Ferrari, A., M.M. Rodriguez, et al. (2007). Immunobiological role of llama heavy-chain antibodies against a bacterial beta-lactamase. *Vet Immunol Immunopathol* **117**, 173–182.

Frenken, L.G., R.H. van der Linden, et al. (2000). Isolation of antigen specific llama VHH antibody fragments and their high level secretion by Saccharomyces cerevisiae. *J Biotechnol* **78**, 11–21.

Goldman, E.R., G.P. Anderson, et al. (2006). Facile generation of heat-stable antiviral and antitoxin single domain antibodies from a semisynthetic llama library. *Anal Chem* **78**, 8245–8255.

Haber, E., F.F. Richards (1966). The specificity of antigenic recognition of antibody heavy chain. *Proc R Soc Lond B Biol Sci* **166**, 176–187.

Habicht, G., C. Haupt, et al. (2007) Directed selection of a conformational antibody domain that prevents mature amyloid fibril formation by stabilizing Aβ protofibrils. *Proc Natl Acad Sci USA* **104**, 19232–19237.

Harmsen, M.M., C.B. van Solt, et al. (2005). Prolonged in vivo residence times of llama single-domain antibody fragments in pigs by binding to porcine immunoglobulins. *Vaccine* **23**, 4926–4934.

Harmsen, M.M., C.B. van Solt, et al., (2006). Selection and optimization of proteolytically stable llama single-domain antibody fragments for oral immunotherapy. *Appl Microbiol Biotechnol* **72**, 544–551.

Harmsen, M.M., C.B. van Solt, et al. (2007). Passive immunization of guinea pigs with llama single-domain antibody fragments against foot-and-mouth disease. *Vet Microbiol* **120**, 193–206.

Hmila, I., R.B. Abdallah, et al. (2008) VHH, bivalent domains and chimeric heavy chain-only antibodies with high neutralizing efficacy for scorpion toxin AahI. *Mol Immunol* **45**, in press.

Holt, L.J., A. Basran, et al. (2008). Anti-serum albumin domain antibodies for extending the half-lives of short lived drugs. *Protein Eng Des Sel* **21**, 283–288.

Hulstein, J.J., P.G. de Groot, et al. (2005). A novel nanobody that detects the gain-of-function phenotype of von Willebrand factor in ADAMTS13 deficiency and von Willebrand disease type 2B. *Blood* **106**, 3035–3042.

Ismaili, A., M. Jalali-Javaran, et al. (2007). Production and characterization of anti-(mucin MUC1) single-domain antibody in tobacco (Nicotiana tabacum cultivar Xanthi). *Biotechnol Appl Biochem* **47**, 11–19.

Janssens, R., S. Dekker, et al. (2006). Generation of heavy-chain-only antibodies in mice. *Proc Natl Acad Sci USA* **103**, 15130–15135.

Jobling, S.A., C. Jarman, et al. (2003). Immunomodulation of enzyme function in plants by single-domain antibody fragments. *Nat Biotechnol* **21**, 77–80.

Koide, A., C.W. Bailey, et al. (1998). The fibronectin type III domain as a scaffold for novel binding proteins. *J Mol Biol* **284**, 1141–1151.

Kruger, C., A. Hultberg, et al. (2006). Therapeutic effect of llama derived VHH fragments against Streptococcus mutans on the development of dental caries. *Appl Microbiol Biotechnol* **72**, 732–737.

Liu, J.L., G.P. Anderson, et al. (2007a). Selection of cholera toxin specific IgNAR single-domain antibodies from a naive shark library. *Mol Immunol* **44**, 1775–1783.

Liu, J.L., G.P. Anderson, et al. (2007b). Isolation of anti-toxin single domain antibodies from a semi-synthetic spiny dogfish shark display library. *BMC Biotechnol* **7**, 78.

Miao, Q.F., X.Y. Liu, et al. (2007). An enediyne-energized single-domain antibody-containing fusion protein shows potent antitumor activity. *Anticancer Drugs* **18**, 127–137.

Muruganandam, A., J. Tanha, et al. (2002). Selection of phage-displayed llama single-domain antibodies that transmigrate across human blood-brain barrier endothelium. *Faseb J* **16**, 240–242.

Nuttall, S.D., U.V. Krishnan, et al. (2003). Isolation and characterization of an IgNAR variable domain specific for the human mitochondrial translocase receptor Tom70. *Eur J Biochem* **270**, 3543–3554.

Nguyen, V.K., C. Su, et al. (2002). Heavy-chain antibodies in Camelidae; a case of evolutionary innovation. *Immunogenetics* **54**, 39–47.

Olichon, A., D. Schweizer, et al. (2007). Heating as a rapid purification method for recovering correctly-folded thermotolerant VH and VHH domains. *BMC Biotechnol* **7**, 7.

Pant, N., A. Hultberg, et al. (2006). Lactobacilli expressing variable domain of llama heavy-chain antibody fragments (lactobodies) confer protection against rotavirus-induced diarrhea. *J Infect Dis* **194**, 1580–1588.

Paz, K., L.A. Brennan, et al. (2005). Human single-domain neutralizing intrabodies directed against Etk kinase: a novel approach to impair cellular transformation. *Mol Cancer Ther* **4**, 1801–1809.

Pessi, A., E. Bianchi, et al. (1993). A designed metal-binding protein with a novel fold. *Nature* **362**, 367–369.

Rahbarizadeh, F., M.J. Rasaee, et al. (2006). Over expression of anti-MUC1 single-domain antibody fragments in the yeast Pichia pastoris. *Mol Immunol* **43**, 426–435.

Reiter, Y., P. Schuck, et al. (1999). An antibody single-domain phage display library of a native heavy chain variable region: isolation of functional single-domain VH molecules with a unique interface. *J Mol Biol* **290**, 685–698.

Roovers, R.C., T. Laeremans, et al. (2007). Efficient inhibition of EGFR signaling and of tumour growth by antagonistic anti-EFGR nanobodies. *Cancer Immunol Immunother* **56**, 303–317.

Rothbauer, U., K. Zolghadr, et al. (2008). A versatile nanotrap for biochemical and functional studies with fluorescent fusion proteins. *Mol Cell Proteomics* **7**, 282–289.

Saerens, D., B. Stijlemans, et al. (2008a). Parallel selection of multiple anti-infectome nanobodies without access to purified antigens. *J Immunol Methods* **329**, 138–150.

Saerens, D., K. Conrath, et al. (2008b). Disulfide bond introduction for general stabilization of immunoglobulin heavy-chain variable domains. *J Mol Biol* **377**, 478–488.

Shao, C.Y., C.J. Secombes, et al. (2007). Rapid isolation of IgNAR variable single-domain antibody fragments from a shark synthetic library. *Mol Immunol* **44**, 656–665.

Stanfield, R.L., H. Dooley, et al. (2004). Crystal structure of a shark single-domain antibody V region in complex with lysozyme. *Science* **305**, 1770–1773.

Stewart, C.S., C.R. MacKenzie, et al. (2007). Isolation, characterization and pentamerization of alpha-cobrotoxin specific single-domain antibodies from a naive phage display library: preliminary findings for antivenom development. *Toxicon* **49**, 699–709.

Streltsov, V.A., J.A. Carmichael, et al. (2005). Structure of a shark IgNAR antibody variable domain and modeling of an early-developmental isotype. *Protein Sci* **14**, 2901–2909.

Szynol A., J.J. de Haard, et al. (2006). Design of a peptibody consisting of the antimicrobial peptide dhvar5 and a llama variable heavy-chain antibody fragment. *Chem Biol Drug Des* **67**, 425–431.

Thomassen, Y.E., W. Meijer, et al. (2002). Large-scale production of VHH antibody fragments by Saccharomyces cerevisiae. *Enzyme Microb. Technol.* **30**, 273–278.

Utsumi, S., F. Karush (1964). The Subunits of Purified Rabbit Antibody. *Biochemistry* **3**, 1329–1338.

van der Linden, R.H., B. de Geus, et al. (2000). Improved production and function of llama heavy chain antibody fragments by molecular evolution. *J Biotechnol* **80**, 261–270.

van der Linden, R.H., L.G. Frenken, et al. (1999). Comparison of physical chemical properties of llama VHH antibody fragments and mouse monoclonal antibodies. *Biochim Biophys Acta* **1431**, 37–46.

van der Vaart, JM., N. Pant, et al. (2006). Reduction in morbidity of rotavirus induced diarrhoea in mice by yeast produced monovalent llama-derived antibody fragments. *Vaccine* **24**, 4130–4137.

van Koningsbruggen, S., H. de Haard, et al. (2003). Llama-derived phage display antibodies in the dissection of the human disease oculopharyngeal muscular dystrophy. *J Immunol Methods* **279**, 149–161.

Verheesen, P., A. de Kluijver, et al. (2006a). Prevention of oculopharyngeal muscular dystrophy-associated aggregation of nuclear polyA-binding protein with a single-domain intracellular antibody. *Hum Mol Genet* **15**, 105–111.

Verheesen, P., A. Roussis, et al. (2006b). Reliable and controllable antibody fragment selections from Camelid non-immune libraries for target validation. *Biochim Biophys Acta* **1764**, 1307–1319.

Ward, E.S., D. Gussow, et al. (1989). Binding activities of a repertoire of single immunoglobulin variable domains secreted from Escherichia coli. *Nature* **341**, 544–546.

Worn, A., A. Pluckthun (2001). Stability engineering of antibody single-chain Fv fragments. *J Mol Biol* **305**, 989–1010.

Yau, K.Y., M.A. Groves, et al. (2003). Selection of hapten-specific single-domain antibodies from a non-immunized llama ribosome display library. *J Immunol Methods* **281**, 161–175.

Zhang, J., J. Tanha, et al. (2004). Pentamerization of single-domain antibodies from phage libraries: a novel strategy for the rapid generation of high-avidity antibody reagents. *J Mol Biol* **335**, 49–56.

Zou X., M.J. Osborn, et al. (2007) Heavy chain-only antibodies are spontaneously produced in light chain-deficient mice. *J Exp Med* **204**, 3271–3283.

CHAPTER SEVENTEEN

Engineering of Non-CDR Loops in Immunoglobulin Domains

Florian Rüker and Gordana Wozniak-Knopp

The immune system creates binding sites of high specificity and affinity in the variable domains of antibodies by generating sequence and consequently structural diversity in the complementarity-determining region (CDR) loops, which are located at the N-terminal ends of these domains. Sequence variations in the CDR loops of an antibody generally do not have a significant influence on the overall structure of the variable domain that carries them. This feature of variable domains is actually observed in a more general sense in immunoglobulin-like domains, which are known to have a similar general shape in the core beta-barrel and high structural variability in the loops. Furthermore, overall sequence similarity of domains with an immunoglobulin fold is mainly below 25%, while their structural similarity is high, with a root mean square (rms) deviation of Cα atoms always below 3.9 Å (Halaby et al., 1999).

We therefore set out to explore whether this inherent stability and conservation of the immunoglobulin fold allows loops of immunoglobulin domains other than the CDR loops to accommodate sequence variation without negatively impacting the overall structure and stability of the protein. As shown in Figure 17.1, the candidate loops of an IgG1 for this kind of engineering are manifold, including the N- and C-terminal loops of the constant domains as well as C-terminal loops of the variable domains.

In the examples described in this chapter, we engineered the AB and the EF loops of the third constant domain (CH3) of human IgG1 by randomizing a number of residues and also by inserting random sequences in the loops, thereby generating new binding sites. Results on the design, manufacture, and characterization of such domains are presented here.

DESIGN OF LIBRARIES BASED ON THE HUMAN IgG1 CH3 DOMAIN

For designing the CH3 domain libraries, several criteria were applied in order to choose those residues in the sequence that should be randomized to create the new binding surface. Solvent accessibility and relative structural independence of the residues located in the AB and in the EF loop were judged based on the crystal structure of an Fc fragment of human IgG1 (PDB code 1OQO). The degree of

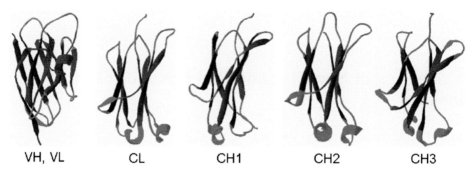

VH, VL   CL   CH1   CH2   CH3

Figure 17.1. Ribbon presentation of the domains of an IgG1. Non-CDR loops are indicated in red, CDR loops in green, and the beta sandwich core in blue. The structures are aligned such that the N-terminal ends are on the top and the C-terminal ends are on the bottom. [See color plate.]

evolutionary conservation of the residues was evaluated using the ConSurf Server (Landau et al., 2005) and was taken as a further guide for selecting the residues to be mutated. Finally, it was ensured that together, the mutated residues form a coherent patch on the surface of the CH3 domain. The following eight residues were randomized for the generation of a CH3 library: 359, 360, 361, 413, 414, 415, 418, and 419 (EU numbering). Due to structural considerations, Arg 416 and Trp 417 were left unmutated. In addition to randomizing the denoted residues in the sequence, we constructed two additional libraries in which insertions of three and five residues, respectively, were made in the EF loop (CH3 + 3 and CH3 + 5 libraries). Together, the randomized positions in these three libraries yield a coherent surface of approximately 700, 1,000, and 1,200 Å^2, respectively, which compares well with the surface areas buried in Fab-antigen interactions, which typically range from 600 to 900 Å^2 (Coley et al., 2007). A schematic presentation of the secondary structure of the CH3 domains, highlighting the randomized positions, is given in Figure 17.2.

ISOLATION OF CH3 DOMAIN MUTANTS BINDING TO LYSOZYME

As a first example for the isolation of specifically binding CH3 domains, hen egg white lysozyme (HEL) was chosen as a target. The libraries (CH3, CH3 + 3, and CH3 + 5) were cloned in the phagemid vector pHEN1 (Hoogenboom et al., 1991) and displayed on the surface of filamentous phage M13 as N-terminal fusion proteins with protein III using standard protocols (Clackson, 2004). After three panning rounds on HEL, enriched inserts were pool-amplified by a polymerase chain reaction (PCR), cloned in the *E. coli* expression vector pBAD/myc-His (Invitrogen), and expressed in soluble form in *E. coli*. Periplasmic lysates were tested in ELISA for specific binding to HEL. Approximately 5% of the tested clones gave a positive signal in this ELISA (see Figure 17.3), indicating that it was possible to isolate CH3 domains with mutations in structural loops that give rise to novel binding properties.

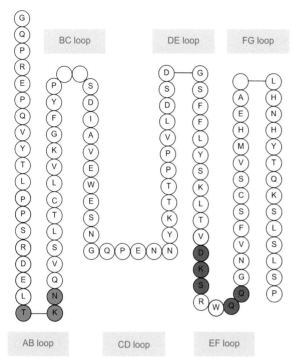

Figure 17.2. The fold of the CH3 domain of human IgG1 presented in perlchain form (Ruiz and Lefranc, 2002). Residues that were randomized in the CH3 libraries are indicated in blue and red, respectively. [See color plate.]

ISOLATION OF A CD20-BINDING CH3 DOMAIN

CH3 domains binding specifically to CD20 were selected by panning the CH3 libraries described above against a peptide mimotope to human CD20 that was previously described (Perosa et al., 2005). After three panning rounds, sequences of selected CH3 domain mutants were rescued by PCR, cloned into the expression vector pET27b (Novagen), and expressed in *E. coli* BL21 (DE3). Four hundred clones were individually screened for binding to the CD20 mimotope in an ELISA using periplasmic lysates. In order to further characterize positive clones, soluble CH3 domains were expressed and purified via their His-Tag by immobilized metal affinity chromatography (IMAC) and tested for their ability to stain the CD20 positive cell line Daudi. One clone, D83, which yielded strong signals in this FACS analysis, was used in a cell-binding experiment in competition with the anti-CD20 antibody Rituximab (Figure 17.4). D83 binding to Daudi cells was observed at 1 µg/ml and could be inhibited with increasing Rituximab concentrations. An isotype control for Rituximab did not inhibit D83 binding, demonstrating the specific interaction of clone D83 with CD20 on Daudi cells.

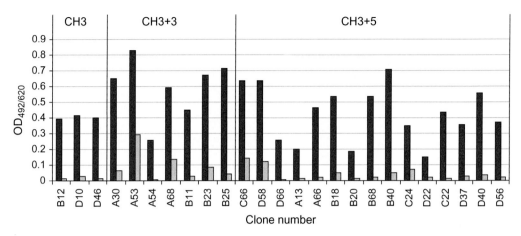

Figure 17.3. ELISA screening of soluble CH3-domain mutants isolated from periplasmic lysates of *E. coli*. Source libraries from which the clones were derived are given in the top line. Lysozyme signals: black bars; blank signals: gray bars.

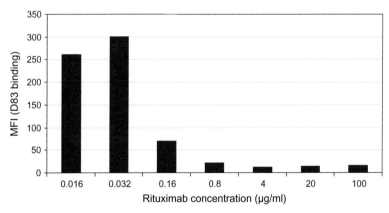

Figure 17.4. Competition of CH3 domain D83 versus Rituximab for binding to human CD20-positive Daudi cells. The reduction of the mean fluorescent intensity (MFI; y-axis) of D83 stained cells in response to increasing Rituximab concentration (x-axis) is shown.

Fcab AS A SCAFFOLD: A CONCEPT

Evidence that target binding sites can be engineered into the structural loops of IgG1 CH3 domains led to the anticipation that this is also possible when the CH3 domains are placed in the context of an Fc fragment. This would yield target binding molecules that, at a size of only approximately 50 kD, also possess all attractive properties of complete antibodies such as their ability to bind to molecules triggering effector functions (e.g., Fcγ receptors, C1q), and, due to the presence of the FcRn binding site, also display the long *in vivo* half-life of antibodies. Such **Fc** molecules with **a**ntigen-**b**inding properties were named Fcab.

INTEGRIN-BINDING F_{CAB}: PRODUCTION AND
PURIFICATION OF F_{CAB}-RGD

As a model for any Fcab with target binding sites engineered by random mutagenesis of the structural loops of IgG1 CH3 domains, we designed Fcab-RGD. This protein encompasses hinge, CH2, and CH3 domains, and harbors the grafted peptide sequence CRGDCL (Koivunen et al., 1993) in the EF loop of the human IgG1 CH3 domain. The RGD motif has been shown to confer binding to human $\alpha_V\beta_3$ integrin. Fcab-RGD was cloned into the mammalian expression vector pCEP4 (Invitrogen) and expressed in human embryonic kidney (HEK293) cells. The protein was purified by protein A affinity chromatography in a one-step process.

Eluted Fcab-RGD was dialyzed against PBS and analyzed by SDS-PAGE under nonreducing conditions. Coomassie staining revealed a single band with an approximate molecular weight of 55 kD. Under reducing conditions, a single band at about half the molecular weight was detected. This indicates that both Fcab-wt as well as Fcab-RGD were purified in a single-affinity chromatography step to a purity greater than 98% and that both proteins were expressed as homodimers, linked by the disulfide bridges in the hinge region.

To assess the various binding properties of Fcabs, binding studies to antigen and effector molecules were performed. Additionally, binding to the neonatal Fc receptor (FcRn) mediating the long half-life of immunoglobulins and to protein A were evaluated by surface plasmon resonance (SPR) measurement.

BINDING TO $\alpha_V\beta_3$ INTEGRIN

The inserted RGD sequence is expected to confer binding to $\alpha_V\beta_3$ integrin, which was tested in a plate-trapped antigen ELISA. Fcab-RGD bound to human $\alpha_V\beta_3$ integrin was detected with Protein A-HRP conjugate. Results of this ELISA are shown in Figure 17.5 and indicate that the interaction between Fcab-RGD and $\alpha_V\beta_3$ integrin was specific.

BINDING TO EFFECTOR MOLECULES

Binding of human FcγRI, the high-affinity Fcγ receptor CD64, and of human complement 1q (C1q) was assessed by coating Fcab-RGD and by adding either C1q or soluble CD64 cross linked with the respective detection antibody (Figure 17.6). The human IgG1 antibody Herceptin as well as human plasma-derived IgG Fc served as positive controls. Fcab-RGD was able to bind the effector molecules in a similar manner as observed for Fc and Herceptin.

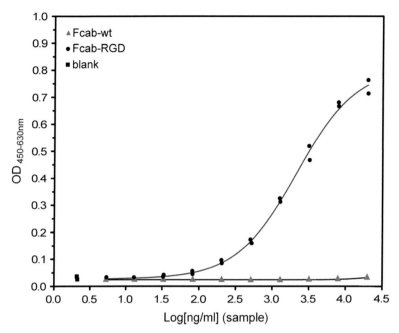

Figure 17.5. Integrin binding ELISA. Fcab-RGD (circles) shows a sigmoidal binding curve to human $\alpha_V\beta_3$ integrin in response to increasing protein concentrations. Fcab-wt (triangles) does not bind to human $\alpha_V\beta_3$ integrin.

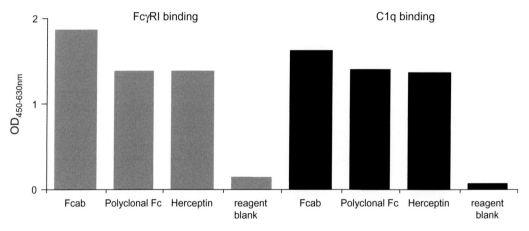

Figure 17.6. Binding of FcγRI (gray bars) and C1q (black bars) to plate-immobilized Fcab-RGD, polyclonal Fc isolated from human plasma IgG and the human IgG1 antibody Herceptin.

BINDING TO PROTEIN A AND TO FcRn

SPR analysis was used to assess the binding of Fcabs to protein A and FcRn. Fcabs and control Fc were injected at different concentrations on a protein A-coated CM5 chip and the on and off signals were overlayed. Both the dose-dependent signals as well as similar on and off rates were observed for the Fcabs and plasma-derived Fc (data not shown). Binding of antibodies and lone Fc fragments to FcRn occurs in a strictly pH-dependent manner at acidic pH 6, while at a pH of 7.4 the ligand is released

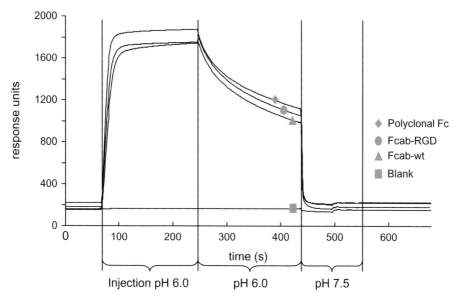

Figure 17.7. Fcab binding to FcRn analyzed by SPR. The pH dependent FcRn binding is observed for Fcab-RGD and control proteins. Symbols are placed on top of the curves as follows – diamond: polyclonal Fc; circle: Fcab-RGD; triangle: Fcab-wt; square: blank.

(Raghavan et al., 1995). As can be seen in Figure 17.7, the pH-dependent binding of FcRn to Fcab-RGD is similar to that observed for Fcab-wt and plasma-derived Fc.

STABILITY OF Fcab *IN VIVO*

The exceptionally long half-life of antibodies *in vivo* is due primarily to their binding to FcRn and to their resistance to serum proteases (Brown et al., 1970). Fcab-RGD, Fcab-wt, and plasma-derived Fc exhibited similar *in vitro* binding characteristics to human FcRn in our SPR experiments (Figure 17.7). Furthermore, high resistance to serum proteases was observed by *in vitro* incubation in human serum at 37°C (data not shown). We therefore evaluated the half-life of Fcab-RGD *in vivo* in mice. Although the half-life of human antibodies or Fc is known to be significantly lower in mice than in humans, this is a commonly accepted model that allows extrapolation to the behavior observed in humans (Datta-Mannan et al., 2007).

The two recombinant proteins Fcab-RGD and Fcab-wt were purified via a single-step protein A affinity chromatography, dialyzed against PBS and applied to mice by tail vein injection. Plasma-derived Fc was used as a control. Over a period of 14 days, blood samples were repeatedly taken from the mice and the residual concentration of the injected proteins was determined via a sensitive ELISA specific for human Fc. As shown in Figure 17.8, Fcab-wt showed a half-life of 41 hours and Fcab-RGD a half-life of 61 hours, which compared well to the mean value of 46 hours for plasma-derived Fc. Thus, the modification in loops of constant domains in Fc fragments is possible without impairing the *in vitro* and *in vivo* stability of the proteins.

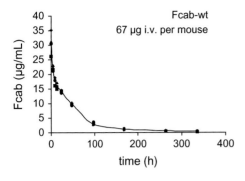

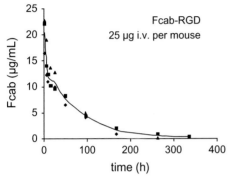

Figure 17.8. Half-life of human Fc and Fcabs *in vivo* in mice. Human Fc and HEK-produced Fcab-wt and Fcab-RGD were applied intravenously to C6D2F1 mice at the indicated amounts. Blood samples were taken after 1, 5, 9, and 14 hours, and after 1, 2, 4, 7, 11, and 14 days and protein concentrations determined by ELISA. The data for the individual mice in the experimental series were plotted in the graph. A bi-exponential curve was fitted to these data, allowing the calculation of half-life values.

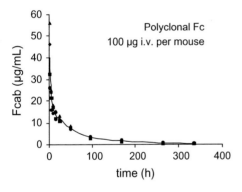

APPLICATIONS AND OUTLOOK

From the results described, we conclude that modification of loops of constant immunoglobulin domains such as the CH3 domain is possible through random mutagenesis of the structural loops and can efficiently lead to the generation of Fcabs – that is, Fc fragments with novel, engineered-binding properties – while maintaining the pharmacokinetic and effector molecule-binding properties of such domains. We anticipate that Fcabs will not only be used as stand-alone molecules. For example, fusion of an Fcab with an Fab via the hinge region allows the introduction of additional valencies for target binding or a second binding specificity into a complete monoclonal antibody.

Preliminary data in our lab have shown that C-terminal loops of CL and of CH1 domains can be engineered in a similar manner, opening the route toward Fab fragments with added binding specificities and valencies. The technology described here is therefore not limited to the engineering of C-terminal loops of the CH3 domain of human IgG1 but can probably be applied to immunoglobulin domains of any type and species.

We thank Austria Wirtschaftsservice for funds provided under its "Preseed" program, the Austrian Research Promotion Agency (FFG) for funds provided under its "BRIDGE" program (project 813002 "Modular Antibody Design Based on Immunoglobulin Libraries"), and f-star for funds provided as the industry partner in connection with the "BRIDGE" program. We thank all colleagues from f-star GmbH for their valuable contributions to this work.

REFERENCES

Brown WR, Newcomb RW, Ishizaka K. Proteolytic degradation of exocrine and serum immunoglobulins. *J Clin Invest*. 1970 Jul;**49**(7):1374–80.

Clackson T (ed). *Phage display, a practical approach*. Oxford Univ. Press, 2004 (Practical approach series; 266).

Coley AM, Gupta A, Murphy VJ, Bai T, Kim H, Anders RF, Foley M, Batchelor AH. Structure of the malaria antigen AMA1 in complex with a growth-inhibitory antibody. *PLoS Pathog*. 2007 Sep 7;**3**(9):1308–19.

Datta-Mannan A, Witcher DR, Tang Y, Watkins J, Jiang W, Wroblewski VJ. Humanized IgG1 variants with differential binding properties to the neonatal Fc receptor: relationship to pharmacokinetics in mice and primates. *Drug Metab Dispos*. 2007 Jan;**35**(1):86–94.

Halaby DM, Poupon A, Mornon J. The immunoglobulin fold family: sequence analysis and 3D structure comparisons. *Protein Eng*. 1999 Jul;**12**(7):563–71.

Hoogenboom HR, Griffiths AD, Johnson KS, Chiswell DJ, Hudson P, Winter G. Multi-subunit proteins on the surface of filamentous phage: methodologies for displaying antibody (Fab) heavy and light chains. *Nucleic Acids Res*. 1991 Aug 11;**19**(15):4133–7.

Koivunen E, Gay DA, Ruoslahti E. Selection of peptides binding to the alpha 5 beta 1 integrin from phage display library. *J Biol Chem*. 1993 Sep 25;**268**(27):20205–10.

Landau M, Mayrose I, Rosenberg Y, Glaser F, Martz E, Pupko T, Ben-Tal N. ConSurf 2005: the projection of evolutionary conservation scores of residues on protein structures. *Nucleic Acids Res*. 2005 Jul 1;**33**(Web Server issue):W299–302.

Perosa F, Favoino E, Caragnano MA, Dammacco F. CD20 mimicry by a mAb rituximab-specific linear peptide: a potential tool for active immunotherapy of autoimmune diseases. *Ann N Y Acad Sci*. 2005 Jun;**1051**:672–83.

Raghavan M, Bonagura VR, Morrison SL, Bjorkman PJ. Analysis of the pH dependence of the neonatal Fc receptor/immunoglobulin G interaction using antibody and receptor variants. *Biochemistry*. 1995 Nov 14;**34**(45):14649–57.

Ruiz M, Lefranc MP. IMGT gene identification and Colliers de Perles of human immunoglobulins with known 3D structures. *Immunogenetics*. 2002 Feb;**53**(10–11):857–83.

PART VII

ANTIGEN-BINDING REPERTOIRES OF NON-IMMUNOGLOBULIN PROTEINS

CHAPTER EIGHTEEN

Alternative Scaffolds: Expanding the Options of Antibodies

Andreas Plückthun

In the language of modern biotechnology, monoclonal antibodies (Köhler & Milstein, 1975) were the first "library" of proteins that was available, and the immune system was the first "selection" technology by which a specific binder could be obtained. However, only the subsequent introduction of molecular biology into this field allowed a true control over the molecules (reviewed, e.g., in Plückthun & Moroney, 2005; Weiner & Carter, 2003). This development of technologies was largely driven by the desire to use antibodies therapeutically, since the extraordinarily strong immune response to a nonhuman antibody in humans had put an end to essentially all of these endeavors. As will be illustrated in the following paragraphs, technological developments intended to solve this problem made not only the use of an animal immune system, but, ironically, also the antibody molecule itself dispensable.

Three fundamental approaches have been developed to arrive at antibody molecules that are able to evade the human immune surveillance and which, at least from this perspective, may become potential therapeutics. The first approach, termed "humanization" (Jones et al., 1986), converts an existing murine antibody obtained by immunization into an analogous one with as much human sequence as possible. Another approach, a technical tour de force, was to introduce human antibody genes into a mouse and inactivate or delete the murine loci, such that an immunized mouse would then produce antibodies after immunization that essentially consisted of human sequences (Fishwild et al., 1996; Mendez et al., 1997). Finally, a third approach made the antibody completely independent of an animal's immune system: it consisted of establishing methods for rapidly producing recombinant antibodies in various formats, creating first a repertoire of the antibody genes outside the animal, and second a selection technology with which the antibodies (and their genes) could be enriched from the library (Burton et al., 1991; Hoogenboom & Winter, 1992; Knappik et al., 2000; Marks et al., 1991; Mondon et al., 2008; Skerra & Plückthun, 1988; Vaughan et al., 1996). For these antibody repertoires, either the natural immune repertoire is polymerase chain reaction (PCR) amplified, or fully synthetic repertoires are created. For the selection technology, display technologies such as phage display, ribosome display, and surface display on bacteria and yeast (Bass et al., 1990; Boder & Wittrup, 1997; Hanes & Plückthun, 1997; McCafferty et al., 1990; Smith, 1985) are most widely used and have proven most successful. Over the years, many more selection technologies (Levin & Weiss, 2006) have been developed, all of which cannot be reviewed here.

It is with this last approach, using a synthetic antibody repertoire and a selection technology, that an endeavor that originally set out to mimic the immune system "in the test tube" finally became independent of using antibodies at all. In other words, the same technology enabling the selection of antibodies from libraries can in principle be used to select any protein from any synthetic library for specific binding. It might be worth pointing out that the concept of selection from libraries with phage display had actually first been demonstrated with synthetic peptide libraries, before it was applied to antibodies (Cwirla et al., 1990; Devlin et al., 1990; Scott & Smith, 1990; Smith, 1985).

STATUS QUO: SIX HALLMARKS OF ANTIBODIES THAT OTHER BINDING PROTEINS NEED TO ADDRESS

While, technically, almost any protein can be subjected to library creation and selection, there are clear criteria that should be met by a useful binding molecule. It is probably useful to critically analyze the antibody molecule in this respect, especially from a standpoint of its use as a therapeutic entity. Other proteins will have to equalize or surpass these properties, but researchers are free to choose molecular means by which this can be achieved. Six properties of antibodies can be denoted that other molecules will have to address:

1. *Wide range of targets and epitopes:* Regarding the range of molecules and epitopes that can be bound, the antibody-combining site is extremely versatile. This has to do with the fact that the six loops that constitute the CDRs can vary greatly in length, and some in relative disposition, allowing the creation of a pocket (e.g., to engulf an amino acid side chain or any other molecular entity protruding from the target), a groove (e.g., to harbor a linear oligomer, such as a peptide or an unstructured part from a protein, or an oligosaccharide), a rather flat surface (to bind to another flat surface on a target protein), or even a protrusion (which sticks into a cavity in the target) (Almagro, 2004; Ramsland & Farrugia, 2002). Each of these binding modes has been achieved with different non-antibody scaffolds just as well (see below), but probably at this time, all these options are not possible with the use of only one molecular scaffold. It may well be that these particular binding modes lead to epitope preferences on the target. However, this is not really an impediment, since different libraries with different randomized parts can be created, as can different loop lengths, or even different specialized scaffolds.

2. *High affinity and specificity:* Antibodies can bind their targets with very high affinity. This is achieved by an iterative affinity maturation (Di Noia & Neuberger, 2007; Peled et al., 2008) in the B cells, but high affinity is certainly not a guaranteed outcome from immunization. The iterative evolution strategy of the immune system was the inspiration to create similar approaches in a cell-free system, as realized in the cell-free evolution technology of ribosome display (Hanes & Plückthun, 1997) or mRNA display (Lipovsek et al., 2007; Roberts & Szostak, 1997). These cell-free techniques can be applied to well-folding non-antibody scaffolds (Xu et al., 2002; Zahnd

et al., 2007a) and single-chain antibody Fv fragments alike (Luginbühl et al., 2006; Zahnd et al., 2004). Of course, directed evolution can also be combined with other selection technologies, such as phage display (Pearce et al., 1999; Schier et al., 1996) or yeast display (Boder et al., 2000), but perhaps somewhat more laboriously, since *in vitro* randomization (e.g., error-prone PCR) and library transformation have to be alternated. In summary, with modern technology it is possible to re-create the generation of high affinity and high specificity *in vitro*, thus imitating affinity maturation of antibodies, and it can be applied to non-antibody proteins just as well.

3. *Long half-life:* Intact IgGs have a proverbially long serum half-life. There are two molecular features that play a decisive role for this property. First, antibodies (like all high-abundance serum proteins) are too large to be filtered through the glomerular filters of the kidneys. The pores are thought to be 60 nm fenestrations in the epithelial cell layer, which are, however, filled with negatively charged proteoglycans, and this cell layer is covered by a glycocalyx toward the blood side, further restricting the effective size and introducing charge selectivity (Haraldsson et al., 2008). The next layer, the glomerular basement membrane, followed by a layer of podocytes, may also contribute to the size restriction. There is no sharp cutoff molecular size, but molecules up to 25 kDa will largely be filtered, while molecules above 65 kDa will be almost completely retained. While IgG molecules are safely above this size, Fab fragments are just at the critical size and scFv molecules are clearly below this limit. Second, when the antibody is taken up by vascular endothelium, which engulfs all serum proteins by endocytosis, it is largely recycled, and not degraded. This is due to the interaction with the neonatal FcRn receptor (also termed Brambell receptor after its discoverer), which is expressed in hepatocytes, endothelial cells, and phagocytic cells of the reticuloendothelial system, the main locations of protein catabolism. By this mechanism, the half-life of IgG is increased by a factor of 10 compared to IgG half-life in transgenic animals lacking this receptor (Junghans, 1997; Telleman & Junghans, 2000). The other molecule that shows an unusually long half-life and uses an analogous mechanism is serum albumin (Chaudhury et al., 2003).

Most non-Ig binding proteins will be below the critical size limit and, almost certainly, will not have a built-in mechanism for half-life extension. To increase half-life, one will thus have to resort to one of the following measures: (1) dramatically increase the hydrodynamic radius by attachment of a tail, most commonly polyethylene glycol (Caliceti & Veronese, 2003; Chapman et al., 1999; Greenwald et al., 2003; Yang et al., 2003), (2) attach a binding region specific for a molecule which by itself has a long half-life, usually serum albumin or IgG (Dennis et al., 2002, 2007; Holt et al., 2008; Kawe et al., unpublished; Silverman et al., 2005; Tolmachev et al., 2007), or (3) fuse an Fc region or serum albumin. For the interaction with the FcRn, glycosylation of the Fc region is not needed (Ghetie & Ward, 2002). Nonetheless, the production of such a fusion protein will usually have to be carried out in mammalian cells for higher folding yields of the disulfide-containing Fc region, abrogating many of the advantages of alternative scaffolds.

It must be pointed out that a long half-life is by no means always desired. A typical case in point is *in vivo* diagnostics; another one may be the use of radio-isotopes or toxin conjugates, which need to be cleared rapidly to limit off-target toxicity. In these applications, most non-Ig-scaffolds already have the right size.

4. *Bivalency:* Immunoglobulin molecules are bivalent, or of even higher valency. The physiological reason is, of course, that this leads to a gain of functional affinity (avidity) if the target epitope is arranged in multivalent form, as on the surface of viral or bacterial pathogens, which after all are the natural targets of the antibody molecule. Importantly, this has no consequence when the target is monomeric and can even create problems when, in a therapeutic setting, a surface receptor molecule is targeted, as an undesired agonist activity can be induced. A fascinating discovery, whose molecular basis became clear only very recently (van der Neut Kolfschoten et al., 2007), showed that the Fc part of the human IgG4 molecules are unstable in the presence of trace amounts of thiols, such as glutathione that occurs in traces in blood: they dissociate and re-equilibrate with each other such that all human IgG4 molecules appear to be bispecific and that a therapeutic IgG4 would equilibrate with unexpected partners – a scenario that must be carefully considered for this class of molecules.

Bivalency, when needed, can of course be engineered into other protein classes. There are several ways of achieving this. Conceptually the simplest is to covalently link the molecules by a flexible linker. This requires that they fold well in such an assembly and that the target epitopes are arranged in such a way that they can actually be reached by the bivalent molecules. The next strategy is to fuse the binding molecule of interest to a module that dimerizes by itself. Numerous modules have been described (see, e.g., Plückthun & Pack, 1997, for a review of some examples), and the use of the Fc part is just one particular example. Importantly, because of the many options, in principle, a far wider range of molecular arrangements is possible than in the IgG configuration of binding sites, from higher valency to multi-specificity, from head-to-head over head-to-tail to tail-to-tail linkage.

5. *Effector functions:* The antibody is an adapter molecule. It "connects" a variable binding site specific for the pathogen with a constant part that binds to immune effector cells, carrying different types of Fc receptors (Nimmerjahn & Ravetch, 2007a,b) to induce antibody-dependent cellular cytotoxicity (ADCC). In addition, it can bind to the complement component C1q to induce complement-dependent cytotoxicity (CDC) (Wang & Weiner, 2008).

The key assumption that drives the field of alternative binding molecules is that the Fc-mediated triggering of ADCC and CDC, while extremely powerful in some cases, will not be sufficient to combat all diseases. It follows that other – adapted or artificial – effector mechanisms can, and need to be, engineered for numerous applications in human health care. And if this is so, then the need to use antibodies for the sole purpose of targeting is not apparent. As will be discussed at length in the remainder of this chapter, other molecules can be used as the "variable" part, with engineering, expression, and manufacture being in many cases much more straightforward than with antibodies or their fragments.

6. *A – generally – low immunogenicity of human antibodies:* Very few aspects of therapeutic molecules have been as hotly debated as the issue of immunogenicity. This is mostly because there are comparatively few certain facts, inviting

speculations and alleging immunogenicity or the lack of it, depending on which side of the fence one is on with regard to a particular molecule.

What is clear is that *any* type of protein, including fully human antibodies in human patients, can be in principle immunogenic, as found, for example, in adalimumab (Humira™) (Bender et al., 2007), but each individual case is still almost impossible to predict. In an extremely simplified summary, the lack of an immune response can be thought to be due to one of two scenarios:

First, the protein is recognized as "self," in that no MHC-presented peptide triggers a T cell, the thymus having eliminated those T cells that would recognize any peptide-MHC complex carrying a "self"-peptide. Second, not a single peptide of the foreign protein can be presented, by not fitting in any MHC molecule and/or a lack of appropriate processing. More likely is a composite scenario, where some peptides are presented but are recognized as "self" (being similar enough to those of the human proteome), while others are not presented. A great part of the antibody sequence is shared between all antibodies and thus "self," but every individual molecule, depending on its sequence, can potentially bear T cell epitopes and thus potentially raise an immune response, as in the case of adalimumab (Humira) (Bender et al., 2007).

How serious the problem of an immune response against a therapeutic protein is in patients depends on the outcome of such an immune response. In some cases, nothing happens as a result of an immune response, at least in the absence of chronic application. In others, the therapeutic molecule is neutralized, preventing multiple applications but not acute treatments. For example, in the case of adalimumab (Humira), different studies reached different conclusions over whether there is a connection between an immune response and reduced clinical efficacy of this fully human antibody (summarized in Bender et al., 2007). Only the third case must be avoided at all costs: if the immune response, induced by the recombinant protein and/or stimulated by impurities acting as adjuvants, leads to cross-reactivity with the body's own proteins, a very serious condition may result. A well-known example is the red cell aplasia resulting from an induced immune response against some preparations of recombinant human erythropoietin (Casadevall et al., 2005; Ryan et al., 2006), and this immune response then turns against the body's own erythropoietin.

THE OPPORTUNITIES: THE SHORTCOMINGS OF ANTIBODIES IN THERAPY

Nature's design of the immunoglobulin molecule appears to be close to perfect when it is used as originally intended, namely, as an adapter molecule in fighting infectious agents: bivalent binding to a surface (typically, a microbial cell or a virus) and recruiting effector cells for ADCC and/or activating the complement system for CDC, and at the same time exploiting a long half-life. (The intricate levels of spatio-temporal immune regulation, requiring different constant regions and different receptors, will not even be mentioned here). However, most *recombinant* antibodies currently considered for human therapy are not intended for infectious diseases. Therefore, the properties of the protein molecule must be individually considered, and almost always a tailor-made collection of properties can be engineered to adapt it to the needs of a particular medical application.

Conversely, even in the realm of infectious diseases, there is nothing that could not be achieved with other molecules as well, if they have been properly engineered for specificity, affinity, valency, and desired effector function. It may not be so compelling, however, to compete with antibodies on their home turf. Furthermore, in most infectious diseases, vaccination is the holy grail – that is, to bring the body to produce precisely the required antibodies itself – and passive immunization will always have to be measured against this promise.

WHEN BINDING IS ENOUGH

In some cases of therapeutic applications, no other feature of the antibody is needed other than specific binding. This would be the case in blocking a monovalent target in solution, when often ADCC and CDC are even undesirable. In these cases, the only redeeming feature of the Fc region is its mediation of a long half-life, which may translate to less frequent dosing. However, this property of the Fc region can also be achieved by other half-life extension strategies (summarized above). In other words, there is no problem with using an antibody, but also no definite requirement. Some popular examples, such as titrating cytokines with recombinant alternative binders, will be discussed below.

EFFECTIVENESS VERSUS COST

However, in other disease settings the whole antibody function is required, such as in several anticancer applications, where the effector functions of the Fc part are utilized. Nonetheless, a shortcoming of several antibodies used in oncology, in the form of IgGs, appears to be their unfavorable balance between effectivity and cost. A case in point is Herceptin™, which unquestionably provides an improvement for patient health, but showed only 8 complete responses among 222 patients with metastatic breast cancer observed in the pivotal trial (Cobleigh et al., 1999), with objective response rates in monotherapy only between 12% and 34% (Nahta & Esteva, 2006), and even in combination with chemotherapy the median time to disease progression was only 7 months.

In addition to the rather moderate clinical benefit of some antitumor antibodies generated so far, the costs of production are rather high due to their intricate molecular composition. This could, in the long run, jeopardize the support of these treatments by the public health service. As an example, both Avastin™ and Erbitux™ are no longer made available by the National Health Service of the UK at this time, with other countries and antibodies likely to follow. Importantly, when the natural effector functions are required, the IgG molecule cannot be "simplified": disulfide bonds and glycosylation are both essential for immune effector functions mediated by the binding of the Fc region to the Fc receptor (Jefferis et al., 1998; Krapp et al., 2003), as is of course the 4-chain nature of the molecule for creating the binding site and bivalent structure.

It implicitly follows that the next-generation therapeutics will have to address both effectivity and cost. Almost certainly, therefore, the IgG format by itself will be insufficient for many applications, and alterations may be needed. At this point, however, it is no longer necessary to use an antibody as a starting point.

In the following, molecular features will be summarized that are not intrinsic to the IgG molecule but could provide additional biological activity to binding molecules and expand the range of possible applications that become possible. It will become apparent that for those applications, alternative binding molecules may provide a more convenient engineering platform than either IgGs or other antibody fragment derivatives. Several such constructs have, of course, already been realized with alternative scaffolds, and some will be mentioned in the section below. Before going into the details of the scaffolds, it may be more useful, however, to first conceptualize the approaches.

FORMATS BEYOND THE IgG: AN OPPORTUNITY FOR NEW SCAFFOLDS

1. Bispecific Binding Molecules

Bispecific binding proteins can become attractive in several scenarios. First, they would bridge two cells, and thereby enforce an interaction. Probably one of the most widely studied applications is the recruitment of a cytotoxic cell (a cytotoxic T cell, or a natural killer cell) (Müller & Kontermann, 2007). Recently, encouraging results have been obtained for application of such bispecific molecules in non-Hodgkin's lymphoma (Bargou et al., 2008), while clinical efficacy data for solid tumors have not been reported yet.

In a related approach, bispecific molecules could be used to increase specificity for a particular cell type. If it were possible for the binding epitopes of two adjacent receptors to be oriented in such a way that bridging by a specific molecule is geometrically possible, and if the binding to each were of low affinity, then the binding of such a bispecific molecule would be expected to be of high affinity (I. Tomlinson et al., various seminar discussions). It is clear that only a small subset of epitopes will be appropriate for this approach. Nonetheless, this approach might be able to increase the selectivity for particular cell types, when the antigen is expressed at low levels in other cells. The same approach can also be used if both epitopes are on the same protein, even though this will enhance only the functional affinity, not the selectivity for certain cell types.

Another application of bispecific molecules would be their use as alternatives to a cocktail (reviewed in Presta, 2008), where several functionally redundant proteins must be targeted. However, as defined antibody cocktails are gradually gaining acceptance (Wiberg et al., 2006), it will be interesting to see how cocktails will measure up to linked molecules on the regulatory front.

Many technical approaches have been taken to engineer bispecific antibodies in the IgG format (Fischer & Leger, 2007; Müller & Kontermann, 2007; Marvin & Zhu,

2005; Presta, 2008; Ridgway et al., 1996), yet none of them appears particularly convenient to carry out. The challenge is that the antibody-combining site is again made up from two chains, which, when recombined with the wrong light chain, lead to nonfunctional molecules. Nonetheless, asymmetric IgG molecules (Marvin & Zhu, 2005) have been engineered, and it remains to be seen how facile these approaches will be when implemented in large-scale production systems.

Recombinant antibody fragments have been used to solve this problem of creating bispecific antibodies with new molecular formats (Fischer & Leger, 2007; Müller & Kontermann, 2007; Plückthun & Pack, 1997). Notably in the single-chain Fv format, the connection of both parts of the antibody-combining site is covalent, and thus the assembly problem is simplified. To generate bispecific molecules, a dimerization module can be fused to the C-terminus (Plückthun & Pack, 1997) to generate mini-antibodies. Alternatively, two scFv can be fused in series, but since the *in vivo* folding of many antibody domains is often accompanied by some aggregation, these molecules tend to also lead to illicit pairing of VH and VL domains that usually makes their expression in mammalian cells mandatory (Bargou et al., 2008). Finally, linkers between VL and VH can be chosen that are too short to allow monomeric assembly, creating so-called diabodies (Holliger et al., 1993) and their bispecific and higher valency derivatives (Hudson & Kortt, 1999; Kipriyanov, 2002).

Despite the conceptual elegance of these methods, because of the great variation between the biophysical properties of antibody variable domains (Ewert et al., 2003), it is not guaranteed that the approaches are generic for every combination of binding sites to be tested. It follows that robust scaffolds, which may result in high-yielding assemblies of essentially all combinations of binders to be tested for biological activity, would be particularly attractive and potentially allow further exploitation of these biological approaches.

2. Protein-radio-isotope Conjugates

Radio-immunotherapy, the delivery of radioactivity to the site of a tumor, has a long history (Dearling & Pedley, 2007; Jain et al., 2007) and has shown promise largely in the area of lymphomas and leukemias, while challenges remain in solid tumors. Two antibody-radio-isotope conjugates are on the market, both for the treatment of non-Hodgkin's lymphoma, namely, ibritumomab tiuxetan (Zevalin) and tositumomab (Bexxar). Zevalin and Bexxar carry yttrium-90 and iodine-131, respectively, but both are mouse antibodies. In the radio-immunotherapy setting, one of the main challenges is maximizing the dosage of radioactivity reaching the targeted tumor cells without delivering dangerous levels of nonspecific radiation to vital organs and tissues, notably the bone marrow, the site where hematopoietic stem cells, the precursors of all blood cells, are produced. This balancing act requires that the antibody must have a relatively short half-life, which is the reason that, historically, murine antibodies have been favored in this setting. They do not interact with the human FcRn. Interestingly, large quantities of the unlabeled antibody must be administered prior to or concomitantly with the radioconjugate to improve targeting. The relatively low dose that is sufficient for treating hematopoietic malignancies reduces adverse side effects and may be the reason that for this disease a useful therapeutic window can be found.

While it is unclear at the present time whether a sufficient therapeutic window can also be found for solid tumors – that is, a dose with enough radioactivity delivered to the tumor while keeping bone marrow toxicity (and potentially other off-target toxicities) at bay – it is clear that no intrinsic feature of an antibody is needed to deliver the radio-isotope. This field is thus wide open for other protein molecules. Those scaffolds that can conveniently be engineered to be site-specifically equipped with a radioligand (typically a metal chelate that would be attached to a unique cysteine remote from the binding site) and that can still be produced efficiently would seem especially well suited for this approach, assuming that uptake and half-life can be engineered over wide ranges.

3. Small Molecule Toxin Conjugates

Similar to radio-immunotherapy, the idea of coupling a small molecule toxin to a targeting protein was first tested with whole antibodies (reviewed by Carter & Senter, 2008). A case in point is gemtuzumab ozogamicin (Mylotarg), the only antibody-based drug derived from this approach to reach the market. Mylotarg is a chimeric anti-CD33 antibody conjugated to the highly potent enediyne drug calicheamicin, and is approved in the United States but not the EU, for the treatment of acute myeloid leukemia (Voutsadakis, 2002). The target for such toxin conjugates should be an internalizing surface protein, as most small molecule drugs act as inhibitors of cell replication and therefore need to reach the cytoplasm or nucleus to exert their effect (Trail et al., 2003).

There are two reasons that IgGs may not be the preferred molecules for this approach. First, chemical consistency is nontrivial to achieve, neither with coupling of the drug to sugars, to lysines, or to the cysteines from the partially reduced hinge region (Carter & Senter, 2008). Second, the long half-life of whole IgGs may again increase toxicity to nontarget tissues and thereby create side effects that decrease the therapeutic window. It thus appears that other scaffolds can well take the place of the targeting moiety, as no particular features of the antibody (other than the binding site) are needed. As outlined above in the case of radiolabeled antibodies, the optimal targeting molecule will have to be tailored together with the toxin. Most importantly, the elimination pathway of the toxin conjugate, be it through the kidney or liver, may have a bearing on the dose-limiting toxicity. Whether a long half-life is desirable at all will depend on the exact targeting modalities. With the wide range of possibilities available, this seems to be an area of great promise for scaffold proteins.

4. Protein Toxin Fusions

A conceptually similar approach as the chemical coupling of a small molecule toxin is the conjugation of protein toxins to antibodies (Kreitman, 2006). Such toxins, typically from plants or bacteria, are enzymes that catalytically inactivate essential cellular processes such as translation. By covalently modifying a translation factor or the ribosome itself in an enzymatic process, a single enzyme molecule can be sufficient to kill a cell (Falnes & Sandvig, 2000; Perentesis et al., 1992; Stirpe, 2004). The best clinically studied members of this group are *Pseudomonas* exotoxin A, a tripartite protein that enzymatically ADP-ribosylates translation elongation factor 2, and ricin, derived from the plant *Ricinus communis*, which modifies a critical nucleotide in eukaryotic ribosomal RNA. The natural toxins are produced with their own, unspecific uptake mechanism that allows them to infect any cell, exploiting receptor molecules ubiquitously expressed on mammalian cells. By deleting these cell-binding domains and replacing them by an internalizing binding protein, tumor-selective killing can be achieved. The antibody thus mediates uptake of the enzyme by tumor cells. As the targeting moiety is only required for specific binding, alternative binding proteins are again very well suited for this approach, and especially those scaffolds with superior production properties can give rise to alternative targeted toxins.

5. Other Fusion Proteins, Such as Immunocytokines

Over the last few years, the use of immunostimulatory cytokines has been investigated to enhance the immune response to a tumor. In order to localize the cytokine to the tumor, fusion proteins with antibodies have been made. Constructs investigated include interleukin-2, interleukin-12, granulocyte macrophage-colony stimulating factor (GM-CSF), and members of the TNF superfamily (Gillies et al., 2002a,b; Helguera et al., 2002; Osenga et al., 2006; Sondel et al., 2003). As is the case with bispecific antibodies, where so far encouraging data have only been reported for lymphoma (see earlier discussion), the main challenge in the use of immunocytokines in the treatment of solid tumors will be to prevent systemic engagement of the cytokine receptor by the cytokine part of the conjugate in the absence of the antibody binding to the tumor, as this is the most likely source of adverse side effects mainfest as the uncontrolled release of cytokines by inflammatory cells. The severity of the problem will depend on the complex interplay of pharmacokinetics of the fusion protein, and on whether it preferentially localizes to the tumor or prematurely to the cytokine receptor on the "unwanted" target cells. Nonetheless, this is again an area where alternative targeting proteins can play an important role, as no function other than antigen binding would be used. In fact, many fusion proteins will be substantially easier to produce with well-behaving alternative scaffolds. The desired half-life will very much depend on the application and can be engineered accordingly.

6. Immunoliposomes

Nanoscale drug delivery systems, including liposomes, polymers, and other nanoparticles have been investigated for improved delivery of cancer therapeutics (Park et al., 2004). Of these drug delivery systems, liposome encapsulated agents, particularly liposomal anthracyclines, have been most widely used, but of course a host of other agents lend themselves to this kind of delivery. Most frequently, PEGylated (or STEALTH) liposomes have been developed, using whole antibodies or scFv fragments as targeting agents (Hussain et al., 2007; Noble et al., 2004). Whole antibodies are not preferred in this approach due to their ability to bind to Fc receptors on effector cells.

Well-folding, stable, and easily derivatized scaffolds (especially with single cysteines) would allow a much wider range of coupling conditions, including high temperature or solvent mixtures, thereby increasing the number of different types of nanocontainers and nanoparticles that can be used. Here, it appears that scaffolds with these properties might have an advantage over at least some antibody fragments, which do not withstand these conditions.

THE NEED FOR FACILE ENGINEERING

Importantly, many of the above applications, several of which have not progressed beyond preclinical work, are very demanding in terms of the epitope that needs to be targeted, the affinity window that needs to be reached, and specificity. This usually requires many different binders to be tested, often in constructs with multiple arrangements. This in turn necessitates a system in which the protein can be produced conveniently and variants are rapidly accessible in good yields. It seems that at the present time, *E. coli* is unbeatable for this purpose. For this reason alone, scaffolds that express well, where only small *E. coli* cultures are sufficient to obtain mg amounts of a large number of candidates in parallel for testing, are at a huge advantage. While there has been enormous progress with antibody fragments made in *E. coli* in this respect over the years (reviewed, e.g., in Monsellier & Bedouelle, 2006; Wörn & Plückthun, 2001), the very high levels obtained with some non-Ig scaffolds (see, e.g., Binz et al., 2004) do not appear to be generally reachable with antibodies or antibody fragments at present. Importantly, this difference is even magnified when it comes to more demanding fusion proteins and conjugates, because of aggregation. The examples summarized above should serve to illustrate only some of the potential applications of such more demanding constructs.

SOME GENERAL CONSIDERATIONS FOR SCAFFOLD SELECTION

As has been outlined in the introductory section, the technology development in the field of recombinant and, later, synthetic antibody libraries has made it possible, almost ironically, that the immunoglobulin molecule is no longer needed, since synthetic library design and selection can now be applied to any protein. This, of course, immediately leads to the question of which protein scaffold should be used. So far, all protein scaffolds have been derived from natural proteins. Nonetheless, it can be foreseen that once *de novo* design (Butterfoss & Kuhlman, 2006) has become more robust, *ab initio* designed scaffolds might also be used as the basis for libraries. In an even more distant future, the full rational design of a binding protein to a target is also conceivable (meaning the fold *and* the specific binding site), but it should be remembered that the structure of the great majority of interesting targets is simply not known. Even with known folds and known targets, protein flexibility and plasticity is an enormous challenge, such that work on designing complementary interfaces that will actually fold in reality is only just beginning. At the time of writing, combinatorial and evolutionary methods based on protein libraries with an underlying known structure of the scaffold appear still to be the only practical way to generate a specific, high-affinity binder against a given target within a reasonable time. The choice of scaffold to be used for designing protein libraries has been inspired by the following considerations, which are not mutually exclusive:

Similarity to antibodies – The first group of scaffolds can be characterized as those where similarity to antibody variable domains was desired. The immunoglobulin domain is a β-sandwich structure with a conserved disulfide bond between the two β-sheets, which supports three hypervariable loops. In antibodies from most species, two of these domains come together, such that six loops make up the binding site. The loops differ not only in sequence but also in length, giving rise to a wider range of shapes in the antigen-contacting surface. It should be pointed out that a fully synthetic library with significant length diversity in several loops is somewhat more laborious to construct (Knappik et al., 2000; Koide et al., 2007; Lee et al., 2004), and therefore, this has usually not been implemented in scaffold libraries. Representatives of the first group of antibody structure–inspired scaffolds are the 10th domain of type 3 fibronectin (^{10}FN3, FNfn10), (whose library members have been dubbed trinectin, adnectin, or monobody) or lipocalins (whose library members have been dubbed anticalins), which will both be discussed in more detail later in the chapter.

A completely unexpected development was that, after libraries of leucine-rich repeat proteins and ankyrin repeat proteins (see later in the chapter) had already been published (Binz et al., 2003; Stumpp et al., 2003), leucine-rich repeat proteins were discovered to be the basis of the adaptive immune system in jawless fish (Pancer et al., 2004; Pancer & Cooper, 2006). Repeat proteins have an extended, rather rigid structure and are built from closely packed repeating units of secondary structure (Kobe & Kajava, 2000). Thus, these repeat proteins have in essence been "validated" as a perfectly suitable basis of a diversified immune response. Perhaps one therefore needs to broaden the term "similarity to antibodies" beyond the IgG domain fold.

Favorable biophysical properties – Another consideration has been the search for superior biophysical properties. This mandates a search for a stable starting position for constructing the library. In the case of designed ankyrin repeat proteins (DARPins), there is actually no evidence that *natural* proteins with ankyrin repeats are particularly stable. However, by using a method termed consensus design (Forrer et al., 2004), the information contained in all the thousands of ankyrin repeat sequences can be exploited, and an "idealized" fold can be constructed (discussed later). Such designed proteins indeed turn out to have extremely favorable biophysical properties and express to very high levels in the cytoplasm of any host cell. Other scaffolds, such as the engineered domain of *Staphylococcus aureus* Protein A (Nord et al., 1997), β-crystallin (Ebersbach et al., 2007), fibronectin (Koide et al., 1998; Xu et al., 2002), and many others can also be expressed in soluble form in the cytoplasm.

The success of minimalist randomization strategies, where only binary codes are being used (discussed later) and loops are often not even varied in length, shows the enormous importance of library quality and biophysical properties. At the expense of diversity, notably the absence of long destabilizing loops, the structure of proteins derived from such methods is maintained. Thus, different lines of investigation underline the key importance of stable starting structures.

Avoidance of potential antigenicity – There are at least two critical components to protein immunogenicity. The first is a lack of protein aggregation (being equivalent to superior biophysical properties, described earlier), in order to prevent a T cell independent activation of B cells, and the second is an absence of T cell epitopes. It is useful to stress that in *any* library of proteins, irrelevant of whether a scaffold is called "human" or not, each member of the library may potentially present new such linear T cell epitopes, due to the randomized regions. A related factor is the frequency of antigen presentation in the MHC molecule, which may also be related to protein stability due to the required proteolytic processing, but this is not yet well understood.

Very small domains with three disulfide bonds (so-called LDL-A modules or A-domains) that occur, for example, in the low-density lipoprotein receptor (Koduri & Blacklow, 2001), have been investigated in this respect (Silverman et al., 2005), as it has been proposed that their processing might be ineffective leading to low immunogenicity in the case tested. Alternatively, a scaffold with a rather limited number of different linear peptides, such as realized in designed repeat proteins (Binz et al., 2004), holds the same promise, as among the pool of diverse binders that represent the outcome of a typical selection usually a number of high-affinity binders free of T cell epitopes can be obtained.

Scaffolds that already have a similar function as desired – Some scaffolds are not meant as a generic engine to generate binders to any target but to a particular subset of proteins. It is reasonable, for example, when trying to inhibit a particular protease, to start from a protease inhibitor template (see, e.g., Dimasi et al., 1997; Markland et al., 1996; Röttgen & Collins, 1995; Tanaka et al., 1999) and to adapt this to the protease target under consideration, especially to inhibit plasma proteases in applications such as angiodema and in potential anti-inflammatory applications (Attucci et al., 2006; Williams & Baird, 2003). After all, evolution has provided a set of solutions to the problem of how a catalytic site of a protease can be blocked by a protein, which can avoid being catalytically cleaved like a substrate. Conversely, the specificity of particular peptide-binding modules can be exploited to detect other proteins carrying variants of the recognition sequence. SH2 domains have been used to find binders for phosphorylated peptides (Malabarba et al., 2001), SH3 domains have been used to detect proline-rich peptides containing a polyproline II helix conformation (Hiipakka & Saksela, 2002; Panni et al., 2002), and PDZ domains were used to select binders for peptides with a free C terminus (Junqueira et al., 2003; Reina et al., 2002; Schneider et al., 1999; Sidhu et al., unpublished).

Scaffolds for displaying a constrained peptide – Finally, those scaffolds should be mentioned whose only function is to display a loop, but in a conformation that this constrained peptide can bind to a pocket in the target protein. A case in point is thioredoxin (Borghouts et al., 2005; Klevenz et al., 2002), which has been used for this purpose as a well-expressed protein, where a peptide can be inserted into the fold without destabilizing the structure too much, even though this destabilitation differs greatly between constructs. Clearly, there are many more proteins suitable for such an approach.

ENGINEERING DIVERSITY INTO DIFFERENT SCAFFOLDS

When choosing the scaffold, the randomization strategy must be considered at the same time. In many cases, structures of natural members of the protein family will be known, providing information on where the protein scaffold tends to interact with its target. In other cases, one can work by analogy: Fibronectin, for example, has an architecture related to immunoglobulins, and hence a randomization of residues in the CDR-like loops appears attractive (Koide et al., 1998; Xu et al., 2002). However, the transposition of the CDR-loop concept to scaffolds with unrelated architectures may be delicate, as the example of GFP shows, which appears not to tolerate highly diverse β-strand connecting loops (Abedi et al., 1998).

Depending on the scaffold, diversity can be introduced within one single protruding loop (Borghouts et al., 2005; Klevenz et al., 2002; Norman et al., 1999), which binds into cavities of the target. Alternatively, adjacent loops can be randomized. We may conceptually distinguish the cases that the loops are rather short, and in fact form a contiguous surface, or that they are long and open up a cavity in the binding protein, giving it a concave shape, as, for example, in fibronectin domains or lipocalins (Beste et al., 1999; Karatan et al., 2004; Vogt & Skerra, 2004; Xu et al., 2002). However, there is no sharp distinction between them and the transition is rather fluid.

Finally, a surface of a secondary structure element (e.g., a β-sheet or the surface of an α-helix bundle) may be randomized as, for example, in protein A (Nord et al., 1997) or β-crystallin (Ebersbach et al., 2007).

All of these sequence alterations almost invariably destabilize the scaffold, with the consequence that a certain fraction of the library, depending on the quality of the design, may become aggregation-prone. In the case of loops, the insertion of a longer loop than in the original framework will involve a higher entropic cost in folding the molecule. A shorter loop, on the other hand, may not reach the target or provide insufficient variety. In the case of secondary structure elements, introduction of a few amino acids with a low propensity for this secondary structure may be tolerated, but a higher fraction will destabilize the structure, or if an extended hydrophobic patch is generated, may lead to aggregation. The same is true, of course, if a hydrophobic patch is generated from adjacent loops.

To counteract these problems, it is essential that the stability of the "master" framework is as high as possible and that despite the stability losses incurred by (random) sequence alterations, very stable proteins can still be obtained. This can be illustrated in the case of the designed ankyrin repeat proteins (DARPins): to arrive at an optimal starting position, an engineering strategy that had already proven useful in antibody engineering approaches was used: consensus design (Forrer et al., 2003; Knappik et al., 2000). The underlying idea of consensus design is that structurally important residues are more conserved than other residues in families of homologous proteins (Steipe et al., 1994). In contrast, residues involved in the binding of a particular partner will be "averaged out" over the family, as every member of the family will bind to a different target. The design of a protein based on a protein family consensus sequence should hence lead to an "idealized" protein. As it is a statistical approach, consensus design is particularly well suited to protein scaffolds derived from protein families with many homologous members. In the case of repeat proteins, this can be multiplied by the number of repeats in each protein. To illustrate the power of this approach, using an idealized "full-consensus" ankyrin repeat, proteins resistant to boiling and saturated guanidine hydrochloride were obtained when more than three repeats were present between capping repeats (Wetzel et al., 2008). To randomize the binding surface, which consists of adjacent helices and loops (discussed later), a library can be used using trinucleotide building blocks (Virnekäs et al., 1994), which in the case of designed ankyrin repeat proteins was devoid of prolines, glycines, and cysteines. The randomization strategy in this example is thus a composite of those mentioned earlier: the surface of adjacent helices and short loops is randomized, resulting in a very extended (depending on repeat number), moderately concave surface.

While it has been found that binders to many, if not most, targets can be obtained using proteins such as those discussed in more detail later, it is not clear how diverse the epitopes recognized on these targets are, as this is something that cannot easily be determined in high throughput. If, for example, a flat surface is randomized, the binding to a flat epitope on a folded protein may clearly be favored over binding to extended peptide epitopes or small molecules, which require a pocket or groove to bind to (Beste et al., 1999) and vice versa.

EXAMPLES OF SCAFFOLDS INVESTIGATED IN SOME DETAIL

This chapter cannot make an effort to be comprehensive, and the author apologizes to those whose elegant work may be inadequately adumbrated. By necessity, this chapter relies on studies that have been published and may thus underrepresent important work for which this is not the case. In 2005, we made an attempt to provide a comprehensive listing of alternative scaffolds, concentrating on those not derived from immunoglobulins (of any species) (Binz et al., 2005). Because of the rapid development of the field, a comprehensive update would be out of date the minute this book is in print.

Staphylococcus Protein A Domains ("Affibodies")

One of the first scaffolds to be investigated was an engineered domain B of *Staphylococcus* protein A (SpA) (Nord et al., 1997). This three α-helical bundle protein of 58 amino acids can be expressed well in the cytoplasm of *E. coli*. The randomization of the 13 residues of this domain that are naturally involved in human Fc binding allowed the construction of combinatorial phage display libraries that have been used to generate binders to a variety of targets.

The crystal and NMR structures of the complex between an affibody and its target, another affibody, have been obtained (Högbom et al., 2003; Wahlberg et al., 2003) (Figure 18.1a). The studies show that most of the randomized surface of this "anti-idiotypic" affibody was involved in the 6 μM affinity interaction. NMR studies revealed that this particular affibody seems to be a molten globule that folds only

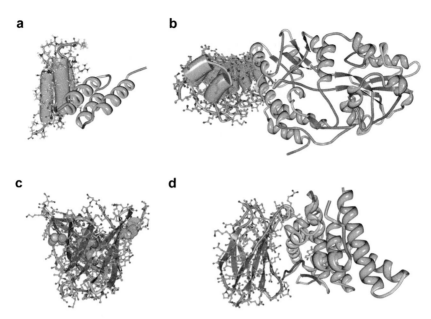

Figure 18.1. Representative structures of non-antibody binders in complex with their target. The figure attempts to emphasize the different secondary structures of the different scaffolds. Structures were obtained from the PDB. The selected binder is shown with its side chains, and helices as cylinders, the target without side chains and helices as ribbons. (a) Affibody in complex with its target, here another affibody (PDB ID 2B87), (b) DARPin in complex with Maltose Binding Protein (PDB ID 1SVX), (c) Anticalin in complex with fluorescein (shown as space filling model in the center); the two disulfide bonds of the lipocalin are also shown in space filling representation on the top left and top right (PDB ID 1N0S), (d) Monobody in complex with the human estrogen receptor alpha ligand-binding domain (PDB ID 2OCF). [See color plate.]

upon binding to its target, protein Z (Dincbas-Renqvist et al., 2004; Lendel et al., 2004; Wahlberg et al., 2003), which may explain the comparatively low affinity, despite the extended interaction surface in this example. Another affibody selected against human CD28 was shown to block the co-stimulatory interaction between CD28 and CD80 expressing cells, hence being a candidate for immune suppressive intervention (Sandström et al., 2003). The micromolar affinity of the anti-CD28 affibody was improved for cell binding by fusion to an Fc region which provides bivalency.

Initially, affinities around micromolar were obtained that had to be improved by secondary affinity maturation projects. More recently, nanomolar affinities were reached directly, and an affibody with specificity to HER2 could be further affinity-matured to a K_D of 22 pM (Orlova et al., 2006). These affibodies to HER2, because of their small size, hold promise as imaging reagents (Engfeldt et al., 2007; Orlova et al., 2007). Different radionuclides (e.g. [76]Br, ^{125}I, ^{111}In, [114m]I, ^{99m}Tc, and [211]At) have been attached via different principles (Nygren, 2008). In a first clinical study, microdoses (<100 μg) of both ^{68}Ga-labeled and ^{111}In-labeled DOTA-labeled anti-HER2 affibody material were injected into patients with recurrent breast cancer. Using SPECT, small HER2-positive metastases were reported to be detectable (Baum et al., 2006). Using different isotopes and half-life extension strategies, such molecules are also being evaluated for radiotherapy (Tolmachev et al., 2007). The affibody technology is commercialized by Affibody AB (www.affibody.com).

The three-helix bundle domain is a "benign" protein and can thus be fused to many other proteins. For example, a head-to-tail dimeric version of an anti-HER2 affibody protein has been inserted into the H1 loop of the knob structure in adenovirus type 5 (Ad5) fibers (Magnusson et al., 2007) or even as a replacement for the knob domain (Belousova et al., 2008). Virus particles containing such fibers were demonstrated to infect cells via HER2 receptors rather than via the normal Coxsackie B virus and Ad receptor (CAR) route. Perhaps such and similar vectors can be further developed into vehicles for gene therapy.

DESIGNED ANKYRIN REPEAT PROTEINS ("DARPins")

Repeat proteins are, besides antibodies, other natural scaffolds that are abundant and used for sets of diverse natural specific binding proteins, notably inside the cell. Ankyrin repeat (AR), armadillo repeat (ARM), leucine-rich repeat (LRR), and tetratricopeptide repeat (TPR) proteins are the most prominent members of this protein class. Repeat proteins are composed of homologous structural units (repeats) that stack to form elongated domains (Kobe & Kajava, 2000) leading to large target interaction surfaces. They lose very little entropy upon binding, as they are rigid and do not possess flexible loops that would only rigidify upon complex formation. This rigidity probably partially explains the high frequency with which binders with subnanomolar affinities have been selected.

Ankyrin repeat proteins (Li et al., 2006) are built from tightly joined repeats of (usually) 33 amino acid residues. Each repeat forms a structural unit consisting of a β-turn followed by two antiparallel α-helices. Libraries of designed ankyrin repeat proteins (DARPins) have been developed for the generation of binding molecules (Binz et al., 2003). In this case, the chosen approach was different from most other scaffold approaches in that no existing AR protein was used as scaffold, but DARPin libraries of varying repeat numbers, between capping repeats that provide a hydrophilic surface, were generated using a consensus-designed AR module as a building block (Forrer et al., 2003; Forrer et al., 2004). This consensus strategy led to remarkably stable proteins (Interlandi et al., 2008; Kohl et al., 2003; Wetzel et al., 2008). Because of the absence of cysteines and low aggregation tendencies, they seem very well suited not only for the generation of novel fusion proteins and conjugates for extracellular targeting but also for intracellular applications.

DARPins can be expressed in soluble form in the cytoplasm of *Escherichia coli* constituting up to 30% of total cellular protein (200 mg per liter of shake-flask culture, and over 10 grams per liter in a fermenter [U. Horn et al., unpublished results]), while to isolate 1 mg of pure protein in high throughput purification only a few ml of *E. coli* are needed (Steiner et al., 2008).

Binders have been mostly selected by ribosome display, a cell-free technology that allows a true evolution of the library (Zahnd et al., 2007a), and this can also be combined with protein fragment complementation (Amstutz et al., 2006). Alternatively, DARPins have been selected by phage display, which is of interest when selecting under more stringent conditions or on whole cells. In this case, a special signal sequence is required to direct the protein to the signal recognition particle (SRP) translocation pathway of *E. coli* (Steiner et al., 2006) to efficiently present it on the phage particle, since DARPins fold too fast for the Sec-dependent signal sequences normally used on standard phagemid vectors. Without any affinity maturation, binders with sub-nanomolar affinities could be isolated directly from the library (Steiner et al., 2008).

Specific DARPin binders were isolated against a number of rather diverse targets – for example, maltose-binding protein (MBP) (Binz et al., 2004) – several MAP kinases (Amstutz et al., 2005) (P. Parizek, L. Kummer et al., unpublished), several G-protein coupled receptors (GPCRs) (Milovnik et al., 2009; Batyuk, Mohr et al., unpublished), Caspase-2 (Schweizer et al., 2007), telomeric repeats of DNA (O. Scholz et al., unpublished), and many therapeutic targets including EpCAM (P. Martin-Killias et al., unpublished), EGF-R (Steiner et al., 2008), HER2 (Steiner et al., 2008; Zahnd et al., 2006; Zahnd et al., 2007b), HER3 (Y. Boersma et al., unpublished), and HER4 (Steiner et al., 2008), or antibody Fc regions (Steiner et al., 2008), among others. All binders showed affinities in the sub-nanomolar or low nanomolar range, and possessed very favorable biophysical properties.

Several crystal structures of selected DARPin-target complexes (see, e.g., Binz et al., 2004; Kohl et al., 2005; Schweizer et al., 2007; Sennhauser et al., 2007) (Figure 18.1b) show that the selected binding interface forms highly specific interactions, very similar in size and number to those in high-affinity antibody-antigen interactions. Because of their rigidity, they also lend themselves to co-crystallization with membrane proteins (Huber et al., 2007; Sennhauser et al., 2007). Moreover, in some cases, enzyme inhibitors have been selected (Amstutz et al., 2005; Kawe et al., 2006; Kohl et al., 2005; Schweizer et al., 2007), and the mechanism could be deduced as one of induced allostery on the target.

Using HER2 as a target, tumor localization experiments of proteins labeled with $^{99m}Tc(CO)_3$ of the His tag (Waibel et al., 1999) showed excellent targeting, with very high tumor-to-blood ratios, which was apparently a function of the picomolar affinity and the small size of the protein (Zahnd, Stumpp, Kawe, Dreier, Nagy, Waibel et al., unpublished). Similarly, fusion proteins with, for example, *Pseudomonas* exotoxin A gave highly specific killing of only antigen-positive tumor cells, relative to normal or tumor cells not expressing the antigen, in models with EpCAM and with HER2-specific DARPins (Martin-Killias, Wyss, Stefan, Binz, Zangemeister-Wittke, Jost, Morrison, Tamaskovic et al., unpublished). The very low aggregation tendency of DARPins and the restricted diversity of the framework part of the sequence has another important consequence: the first property secures against T cell independent activation of the immune system; the second guarantees that in every selection, where normally a wide range of different sequences is obtained, there are always some molecules obtained devoid of T cell epitopes. This gives a good prognosis for applications of DARPins in human therapy. The DARPin technology is commercialized by Molecular Partners AG (www.molecularpartners.com).

FIBRONECTIN TYPE III DOMAINS ("TRINECTINS," "MONOBODIES")

In contrast to most other β-sandwich proteins, fibronectin type III domains do not have disulfide bonds and can, therefore, be used under oxidizing and reducing conditions alike. The 10th type III domain of fibronectin (also named ^{10}FN3, FNfn10) (Karatan et al., 2004; Xu et al., 2002) has been used as a scaffold by several groups ("Trinectins," "Monobodies"). This 94 amino acid protein is well expressed in soluble form in the cytoplasm of bacteria and thermodynamically stable.

In early work, fibronectins with a novel binding specificity to ubiquitin with an affinity in the micromolar range could be generated from a library with two randomized loops by phage display (Koide et al., 1998). With a similar library, binders to Src SH3 domain with micromolar affinities were also selected (Karatan et al., 2004). Clones with the typical SH3 domain 1 binding motif PXXP were found, but also a sequence containing no PXXP motif. In another approach with a different library having the three loops fully randomized, and by using mRNA display as a selection technology, binders in the nanomolar range were reported after nine selection rounds against TNFα (Xu et al., 2002). From these nanomolar binders, picomolar binders could be evolved with further affinity maturation steps (Xu et al., 2002). With a similar approach, binders to VEGF-R2 were selected, but the increase in affinity during affinity maturation was associated with a significant loss of stability and solubility, which could be improved again by structure-based engineering (Parker et al., 2005).

The fibronectin scaffold was also successfully used in a yeast two-hybrid approach, indicating that the framework could be of interest for intracellular applications (Koide et al., 2002).

More recently, phage display libraries were constructed, with a minimal alphabet, following similar experiments with synthetic Fab fragment libraries (Fellouse et al., 2004; Fellouse et al., 2005). The potential binding site (i.e., 3 loops with length variation, with a total diversity of ca. 10^{10}) was randomized to allow either only Tyr and Ser, or Tyr, Ser, and one other amino acid (Gilbreth et al., 2008; Koide et al., 2007). Binders to MBP could be crystallized when fused to MBP and helped to define the binding interactions. High-affinity binders could thus be obtained from large libraries with all loops randomized, either completely or with a reduced set of amino acids (Figure 18.1d). High affinity binders could also be obtained from a much smaller library, but with a rather complete sampling akin to CDR walking by using yeast surface display (Lipovsek et al., 2007). Interestingly, the highest affinity variant selected a disulfide bond between adjacent loops, illustrating the importance of rigidity for very tight binding.

Using mRNA display, a VEGF binder was isolated that was reported as the first member of this family to enter Phase I clinical trial (www.adnexus.com) with a view to eventual applications in anti-angiogenesis tumor therapy.

LIPOCALINS ("ANTICALINS")

Lipocalins are conical β-barrel proteins with about 160–180 amino acids with a ligand binding pocket surrounded by four loops. These loops show structure divergence in natural lipocalins. Small hydrophobic compounds, such as vitamins, hormones, and secondary metabolites, such as retinol, retinoic acid, or bilin, are the natural ligands of lipocalins. Because of the disulfide bonds present in most lipocalins, members of this family and their library derivatives are typically produced in the bacterial periplasm, similar to antibody scFv fragments.

Different lipocalin variants (also termed "anticalins") with new compound specificities such as fluorescein (Beste et al., 1999), benzyl butyl phthalate (Mercader & Skerra, 2002), and the toxic digoxigenin (Schlehuber et al., 2000) for which the selected binder might represent a therapeutic antidote could be isolated from a phage display library. This was achieved by randomizing amino acids in contact with the ligands, pointing toward the inside of the cup-shaped protein (Figure 18.1c). In contrast, by randomizing amino acids in the loops exposed at the protein surface, binding to protein targets could be achieved (Vogt & Skerra, 2004). For example, binders to cytotoxic T-lymphocyte antigen-4 (CTLA-4) (CD152), which inhibits T cell-mediated immune response, have been isolated (Schlehuber & Skerra, 2005). Such binders might be tested as immunostimulatory molecules in cancer therapy. A binder to vascular endothelial growth factor, an angiogenesis factor, has also been reported (Hohlbaum & Skerra, 2007), which might be tested for treatment of age-related macular degeneration (AMD) or in cancer therapy. In summary, lipocalins have been shown to be useful for binding either small molecules or proteins, depending on where the sequence is randomized. The anticalin technology is commercialized by Pieris (www.pieris-ag.com).

LDL-A-MODULES ("AVIMERS")

A family of very small domains of about 40 amino acids, held together by three disulfide bonds and a fourfold coordinated Ca^{2+} ion, formed the basis for the library of scaffolds termed Avimers. The domains are the so-called LDL-A-modules (or A-domains), being derived from various receptors, such as, for example, the low-density lipoprotein receptor, where they occur in tandem arrangement of a number of these modules. In contrast to the repeat proteins, where repeats are rigidly connected, the modules are flexibly linked, like beads on a string. Libraries were constructed encoding a domain of about 40 amino acids, with 12 conserved and 28 variable positions, and were selected by phage display. In order to derive a higher functional affinity, several of these domains need to be strung together to achieve multivalent binding at several epitopes on the target.

The selected proteins described (Silverman et al., 2005) were expressed in soluble form in *E. coli*, and appear to spontaneously oxidize with air to form the required disulfides. In contrast, the natural LDL-A modules form inclusion bodies (North & Blacklow, 1999) and were reported to require refolding in the presence of Ca^{2+}, and they appear to be sensitive to certain mutations. It will be interesting to see what range of sequences is commensurate with the LDL-A module fold.

A Phase I clinical trial was initiated with IL6 as a target (Avidia, acquired by Amgen [www.amgen.com]), where three linked modules chelated the cytokine molecule, and multivalent binders to other targets were described. IL6 is part of the acute phase response leading to inflammation, and the anti-IL6 avimer might have possible uses in preventing symptoms of autoimmune diseases such as Crohn's disease.

THE FUTURE

When therapeutic antibodies first arrived, they were compared to the well-established small molecule drugs, and questions about the persistence of this phenomenon and the size of this market were raised by the skeptics. Today, therapeutic antibodies have become a mainstay of the pharmaceutic industry. However, the overwhelming majority of the molecules that are on the market, and even those that are in clinical trials, are still of the IgG format. Nevertheless, non-antibody-binding proteins have made the transition to the clinic already. It is therefore a reasonable prediction that in the future, there will be three main classes of therapeutic entities: small molecules, classic antibodies, and other engineered binding proteins. The latter may carry small-molecule payloads or other tailor-made effector functions, thus creating a continuum between these molecular classes.

Protein engineering, creating complex proteins to specifications, may turn out to be one of the most powerful ways to tackle some complex diseases. It may not be easy to create molecules better than IgGs to fight infectious diseases. It seems almost certain, however, that for many other disease settings, proteins will eventually be created which combine predesigned specificity with novel tailor-made effector mechanisms.

Acknowledgments

The author is indebted to Drs. Peter Lindner, Patricia Martin-Killias, Daniel Scott, Rastislav Tamaskovic, and Prof. Uwe Zangemeister-Wittke for critical reading of the manuscript.

REFERENCES

Abedi, M.R., Caponigro, G. & Kamb, A. (1998). Green fluorescent protein as a scaffold for intracellular presentation of peptides. *Nucleic Acids Res.* **26**, 623–630.

Almagro, J.C. (2004). Identification of differences in the specificity-determining residues of antibodies that recognize antigens of different size: implications for the rational design of antibody repertoires. *J. Mol. Recognit.* **17**, 132–143.

Amstutz, P., Binz, H.K., Parizek, P., Stumpp, M.T., Kohl, A., Grütter, M.G., Forrer, P. & Plückthun, A. (2005). Intracellular kinase inhibitors selected from combinatorial libraries of designed ankyrin repeat proteins. *J. Biol. Chem.* **280**, 24715–24722.

Amstutz, P., Koch, H., Binz, H.K., Deuber, S.A. & Plückthun, A. (2006). Rapid selection of specific MAP kinase-binders from designed ankyrin repeat protein libraries. *Protein Eng. Des. Sel.* **19**, 219–229.

Attucci, S., Gauthier, A., Korkmaz, B., Delepine, P., Martino, M.F., Saudubray, F., Diot, P. & Gauthier, F. (2006). EPI-hNE4, a proteolysis-resistant inhibitor of human neutrophil elastase and potential anti-inflammatory drug for treating cystic fibrosis. *J. Pharmacol. Exp. Ther.* **318**, 803–809.

Bargou, R., Leo, E., Zugmaier, G., Klinger, M., Goebeler, M., Knop, S., Noppeney, R., Viardot, A., Hess, G., Schuler, M., Einsele, H., Brandl, C., Wolf, A., Kirchinger, P., Klappers, P., Schmidt, M., Riethmüller, G., Reinhardt, C., Baeuerle, P.A. & Kufer, P. (2008). Tumor regression in cancer patients by very low doses of a T cell-engaging antibody. *Science* **321**, 974–977.

Bass, S., Greene, R. & Wells, J.A. (1990). Hormone phage: an enrichment method for variant proteins with altered binding properties. *Proteins* **8**, 309–314.

Baum, R., Orlova, A., Tolmachev, V. & Feldwisch, J. (2006). Receptor PET/CT and SPECT using an affibody molecule for targeting and molecular imaging of HER2 positive cancer in animal xenografts and human breast cancer patients. *J. Nucl. Med.* **47**(suppl. 1), 108P.

Belousova, N., Mikheeva, G., Gelovani, J. & Krasnykh, V. (2008). Modification of adenovirus capsid with a designed protein ligand yields a gene vector targeted to a major molecular marker of cancer. *J. Virol.* **82**, 630–637.

Bender, N.K., Heilig, C.E., Droll, B., Wohlgemuth, J., Armbruster, F.-P. & Heilig, B. (2007). Immunogenicity, efficacy and adverse events of adalimumab in RA patients. *Rheumatol. Int.* **27**, 269–274.

Beste, G., Schmidt, F.S., Stibora, T. & Skerra, A. (1999). Small antibody-like proteins with prescribed ligand specificities derived from the lipocalin fold. *Proc. Natl. Acad. Sci. USA* **96**, 1898–1903.

Binz, H.K., Amstutz, P., Kohl, A., Stumpp, M.T., Briand, C., Forrer, P., Grütter, M.G. & Plückthun, A. (2004). High-affinity binders selected from designed ankyrin repeat protein libraries. *Nat. Biotechnol.* **22**, 575–582.

Binz, H.K., Amstutz, P. & Plückthun, A. (2005). Engineering novel binding proteins from nonimmunoglobulin domains. *Nat. Biotechnol.* **23**, 1257–1268.

Binz, H.K., Stumpp, M.T., Forrer, P., Amstutz, P. & Plückthun, A. (2003). Designing repeat proteins: well-expressed, soluble and stable proteins from combinatorial libraries of consensus ankyrin repeat proteins. *J. Mol. Biol.* **332**, 489–503.

Boder, E.T., Midelfort, K.S. & Wittrup, K.D. (2000). Directed evolution of antibody fragments with monovalent femtomolar antigen-binding affinity. *Proc. Natl. Acad. Sci. USA* **97**, 10701–10705.

Boder, E.T. & Wittrup, K.D. (1997). Yeast surface display for screening combinatorial polypeptide libraries. *Nat. Biotechnol.* **15**, 553–557.

Borghouts, C., Kunz, C. & Groner, B. (2005). Peptide aptamers: recent developments for cancer therapy. *Expert Opin. Biol. Ther.* **5**, 783–797.

Burton, D.R., Barbas, C.F., 3rd, Persson, M.A., Koenig, S., Chanock, R.M. & Lerner, R.A. (1991). A large array of human monoclonal antibodies to type 1 human immunodeficiency virus from combinatorial libraries of asymptomatic seropositive individuals. *Proc. Natl. Acad. Sci. USA* **88**, 10134–10137.

Butterfoss, G.L. & Kuhlman, B. (2006). Computer-based design of novel protein structures. *Annu. Rev. Biophys. Biomol. Struct.* **35**, 49–65.

Caliceti, P. & Veronese, F.M. (2003). Pharmacokinetic and biodistribution properties of poly(ethylene glycol)-protein conjugates. *Adv. Drug Deliv. Rev.* **55**, 1261–1277.

Carter, P.J. & Senter, P.D. (2008). Antibody-drug conjugates for cancer therapy. *Cancer J.* **14**, 154–169.

Casadevall, N., Eckardt, K.U. & Rossert, J. (2005). Epoetin-induced autoimmune pure red cell aplasia. *J. Am. Soc. Nephrol.* **16** Suppl. 1, S67–69.

Chapman, A.P., Antoniw, P., Spitali, M., West, S., Stephens, S. & King, D.J. (1999). Therapeutic antibody fragments with prolonged in vivo half-lives. *Nat. Biotechnol.* **17**, 780–783.

Chaudhury, C., Mehnaz, S., Robinson, J.M., Hayton, W.L., Pearl, D.K., Roopenian, D.C. & Anderson, C.L. (2003). The major histocompatibility complex-related Fc receptor for IgG (FcRn) binds albumin and prolongs its lifespan. *J. Exp. Med.* **197**, 315–322.

Cobleigh, M.A., Vogel, C.L., Tripathy, D., Robert, N.J., Scholl, S., Fehrenbacher, L., Wolter, J.M., Paton, V., Shak, S., Lieberman, G. & Slamon, D.J. (1999). Multinational study of the efficacy and safety of humanized anti-HER2 monoclonal antibody in women who have HER2-overexpressing metastatic breast cancer that has progressed after chemotherapy for metastatic disease. *J. Clin. Oncol.* **17**, 2639–2648.

Cwirla, S.E., Peters, E.A., Barrett, R.W. & Dower, W.J. (1990). Peptides on phage: a vast library of peptides for identifying ligands. *Proc. Natl. Acad. Sci. USA* **87**, 6378–6382.

Dearling, J.L.J. & Pedley, R.B. (2007). Technological advances in radioimmunotherapy. *Clin. Oncol. (R. Coll. Radiol).* **19**, 457–469.

Dennis, M.S., Jin, H., Dugger, D., Yang, R., McFarland, L., Ogasawara, A., Williams, S., Cole, M.J., Ross, S. & Schwall, R. (2007). Imaging tumors with an albumin-binding Fab, a novel tumor-targeting agent. *Cancer Res.* **67**, 254–261.

Dennis, M.S., Zhang, M., Meng, Y.G., Kadkhodayan, M., Kirchhofer, D., Combs, D. & Damico, L.A. (2002). Albumin binding as a general strategy for improving the pharmacokinetics of proteins. *J. Biol. Chem.* **277**, 35035–35043.

Devlin, J.J., Panganiban, L.C. & Devlin, P.E. (1990). Random peptide libraries: a source of specific protein binding molecules. *Science* **249**, 404–406.

Di Noia, J.M. & Neuberger, M.S. (2007). Molecular mechanisms of antibody somatic hypermutation. *Annu. Rev. Biochem.* **76**, 1–22.

Dimasi, N., Martin, F., Volpari, C., Brunetti, M., Biasiol, G., Altamura, S., Cortese, R., De Francesco, R., Steinkühler, C. & Sollazzo, M. (1997). Characterization of engineered hepatitis C virus NS3 protease inhibitors affinity selected from human pancreatic secretory trypsin inhibitor and mini-body repertoires. *J. Virol.* **71**, 7461–7469.

Dincbas-Renqvist, V., Lendel, C., Dogan, J., Wahlberg, E. & Härd, T. (2004). Thermodynamics of folding, stabilization, and binding in an engineered protein-protein complex. *J. Am. Chem. Soc.* **126**, 11220–11230.

Ebersbach, H., Fiedler, E., Scheuermann, T., Fiedler, M., Stubbs, M.T., Reimann, C., Proetzel, G., Rudolph, R. & Fiedler, U. (2007). Affilin-novel binding molecules based on human gamma-β-crystallin, an all beta-sheet protein. *J. Mol. Biol.* **372**, 172–185.

Engfeldt, T., Tran, T., Orlova, A., Widström, C., Feldwisch, J., Abrahmsen, L., Wennborg, A., Karlström, A.E. & Tolmachev, V. (2007). 99mTc-chelator engineering to improve tumour targeting properties of a HER2-specific Affibody molecule. *Eur. J. Nucl. Med. Mol. Imaging* **34**, 1843–1853.

Ewert, S., Huber, T., Honegger, A. & Plückthun, A. (2003). Biophysical properties of human antibody variable domains. *J. Mol. Biol.* **325**, 531–553.

Falnes, P.O. & Sandvig, K. (2000). Penetration of protein toxins into cells. *Curr. Opin. Cell Biol.* **12**, 407–413.

Fellouse, F.A., Li, B., Compaan, D.M., Peden, A.A., Hymowitz, S.G. & Sidhu, S.S. (2005). Molecular recognition by a binary code. *J. Mol. Biol.* **348**, 1153–1162.

Fellouse, F.A., Wiesmann, C. & Sidhu, S.S. (2004). Synthetic antibodies from a four-amino-acid code: a dominant role for tyrosine in antigen recognition. *Proc. Natl. Acad. Sci. USA* **101**, 12467–12472.

Fischer, N. & Leger, O. (2007). Bispecific antibodies: molecules that enable novel therapeutic strategies. *Pathobiology* **74**, 3–14.

Fishwild, D.M., O'Donnell, S.L., Bengoechea, T., Hudson, D.V., Harding, F., Bernhard, S.L., Jones, D., Kay, R.M., Higgins, K.M., Schramm, S.R. & Lonberg, N. (1996 Jul.). High-avidity human IgG kappa monoclonal antibodies from a novel strain of minilocus transgenic mice. *Nat. Biotechnol.* **14**, 845–851.

Forrer, P., Binz, H.K., Stumpp, M.T. & Plückthun, A. (2004). Consensus design of repeat proteins. *ChemBioChem* **5**, 183–189.

Forrer, P., Stumpp, M.T., Binz, H.K. & Plückthun, A. (2003). A novel strategy to design binding molecules harnessing the modular nature of repeat proteins. *FEBS Lett.* **539**, 2–6.

Ghetie, V. & Ward, E.S. (2002). Transcytosis and catabolism of antibody. *Immunol. Res.* **25**, 97–113.

Gilbreth, R.N., Esaki, K., Koide, A., Sidhu, S.S. & Koide, S. (2008). A dominant conformational role for amino acid diversity in minimalist protein-protein interfaces. *J. Mol. Biol.* **381**, 407–418.

Gillies, S.D., Lan, Y., Brunkhorst, B., Wong, W.K., Li, Y. & Lo, K.M. (2002a). Bi-functional cytokine fusion proteins for gene therapy and antibody-targeted treatment of cancer. *Cancer Immunol. Immunother.* **51**, 449–460.

Gillies, S.D., Lo, K.M., Burger, C., Lan, Y., Dahl, T. & Wong, W.K. (2002b). Improved circulating half-life and efficacy of an antibody-interleukin 2 immunocytokine based on reduced intracellular proteolysis. *Clin. Cancer Res.* **8**, 210–216.

Greenwald, R.B., Choe, Y.H., McGuire, J. & Conover, C.D. (2003). Effective drug delivery by PEGylated drug conjugates. *Adv. Drug Deliv. Rev.* **55**, 217–250.

Hanes, J. & Plückthun, A. (1997). *In vitro* selection and evolution of functional proteins by using ribosome display. *Proc. Natl. Acad. Sci. USA* **94**, 4937–4942.

Haraldsson, B., Nyström, J. & Deen, W.M. (2008). Properties of the glomerular barrier and mechanisms of proteinuria. *Physiol. Rev.* **88**, 451–487.

Helguera, G., Morrison, S.L. & Penichet, M.L. (2002). Antibody-cytokine fusion proteins: harnessing the combined power of cytokines and antibodies for cancer therapy. *Clin. Immunol.* **105**, 233–246.

Hiipakka, M. & Saksela, K. (2002). Capacity of simian immunodeficiency virus strain mac Nef for high-affinity Src homology 3 (SH3) binding revealed by ligand-tailored SH3 domains. *J. Gen. Virol.* **83**, 3147–3152.

Högbom, M., Eklund, M., Nygren, P.-Å. & Nordlund, P. (2003). Structural basis for recognition by an *in vitro* evolved affibody. *Proc. Natl. Acad. Sci. USA* **100**, 3191–3196.

Hohlbaum, A.M. & Skerra, A. (2007). Anticalins: the lipocalin family as a novel protein scaffold for the development of next-generation immunotherapies. *Expert Rev. Clin. Immunol.* **3**, 491–501.

Holliger, P., Prospero, T. & Winter, G. (1993). "Diabodies": small bivalent and bispecific antibody fragments. *Proc. Natl. Acad. Sci. USA* **90**, 6444–6448.

Holt, L.J., Basran, A., Jones, K., Chorlton, J., Jespers, L.S., Brewis, N.D. & Tomlinson, I.M. (2008). Antiserum albumin domain antibodies for extending the half-lives of short lived drugs. *Protein Eng. Des. Sel.* **21**, 283–288.

Hoogenboom, H.R. & Winter, G. (1992). By-passing immunisation. Human antibodies from synthetic repertoires of germline VH gene segments rearranged in vitro. *J. Mol. Biol.* **227**, 381–388.

Huber, T., Steiner, D., Röthlisberger, D. & Plückthun, A. (2007). In vitro selection and characterization of DARPins and Fab fragments for the co-crystallization of membrane proteins: The Na(+)-citrate symporter CitS as an example. *J. Struct. Biol.* **159**, 206–221.

Hudson, P.J. & Kortt, A.A. (1999). High avidity scFv multimers; diabodies and triabodies. *J. Immunol. Methods* **231**, 177–189.

Hussain, S., Plückthun, A., Allen, T.M. & Zangemeister-Wittke, U. (2007). Antitumor activity of an epithelial cell adhesion molecule targeted nanovesicular drug delivery system. *Mol. Cancer Ther.* **6**, 3019–3027.

Interlandi, G., Wetzel, S.K., Settanni, G., Plückthun, A. & Caflisch, A. (2008). Characterization and further stabilization of designed ankyrin repeat proteins by combining molecular dynamics simulations and experiments. *J. Mol. Biol.* **375**, 837–854.

Jain, M., Venkatraman, G. & Batra, S.K. (2007). Optimization of radioimmunotherapy of solid tumors: biological impediments and their modulation. *Clin. Cancer. Res.* **13**, 1374–1382.

Jefferis, R., Lund, J. & Pound, J.D. (1998). IgG-Fc-mediated effector functions: molecular definition of interaction sites for effector ligands and the role of glycosylation. *Immunol. Rev.* **163**, 59–76.

Jones, P.T., Dear, P.H., Foote, J., Neuberger, M.S. & Winter, G. (1986). Replacing the complementarity-determining regions in a human antibody with those from a mouse. *Nature* **321**, 522–525.

Junghans, R.P. (1997). Finally! The Brambell receptor (FcRB). Mediator of transmission of immunity and protection from catabolism for IgG. *Immunol. Res.* **16**, 29–57.

Junqueira, D., Cilenti, L., Musumeci, L., Sedivy, J.M. & Zervos, A.S. (2003). Random mutagenesis of PDZ(Omi) domain and selection of mutants that specifically bind the Myc proto-oncogene and induce apoptosis. *Oncogene* **22**, 2772–2781.

Karatan, E., Merguerian, M., Han, Z., Scholle, M.D., Koide, S. & Kay, B.K. (2004). Molecular recognition properties of FN3 monobodies that bind the Src SH3 domain. *Chem. Biol.* **11**, 835–844.

Kawe, M., Forrer, P., Amstutz, P. & Plückthun, A. (2006). Isolation of intracellular proteinase inhibitors derived from designed ankyrin repeat proteins by genetic screening. *J. Biol. Chem.* **281**, 40252–40263.

Kipriyanov, S.M. (2002). Generation of bispecific and tandem diabodies. *Methods Mol. Biol.* **178**, 317–331.

Klevenz, B., Butz, K. & Hoppe-Seyler, F. (2002). Peptide aptamers: exchange of the thioredoxin-A scaffold by alternative platform proteins and its influence on target protein binding. *Cell. Mol. Life Sci.* **59**, 1993–1998.

Knappik, A., Ge, L., Honegger, A., Pack, P., Fischer, M., Wellnhofer, G., Hoess, A., Wölle, J., Plückthun, A. & Virnekäs, B. (2000). Fully synthetic human combinatorial antibody libraries (HuCAL) based on modular consensus frameworks and CDRs randomized with trinucleotides. *J. Mol. Biol.* **296**, 57–86.

Kobe, B. & Kajava, A.V. (2000). When protein folding is simplified to protein coiling: the continuum of solenoid protein structures. *Trends Biochem. Sci.* **25**, 509–515.

Koduri, V. & Blacklow, S.C. (2001). Folding determinants of LDL receptor type A modules. *Biochemistry* **40**, 12801–12807.

Kohl, A., Amstutz, P., Parizek, P., Binz, H.K., Briand, C., Capitani, G., Forrer, P., Plückthun, A. & Grütter, M.G. (2005). Allosteric inhibition of aminoglycoside phosphotransferase by a designed ankyrin repeat protein. *Structure (Camb)* **13**, 1131–1141.

Kohl, A., Binz, H.K., Forrer, P., Stumpp, M.T., Plückthun, A. & Grütter, M.G. (2003). Designed to be stable: Crystal structure of a consensus ankyrin repeat protein. *Proc. Natl. Acad. Sci. USA* **100**, 1700–1705.

Köhler, G. & Milstein, C. (1975). Continuous cultures of fused cells secreting antibody of predefined specificity. *Nature* **256**, 495–497.

Koide, A., Abbatiello, S., Rothgery, L. & Koide, S. (2002). Probing protein conformational changes in living cells by using designer binding proteins: application to the estrogen receptor. *Proc. Natl. Acad. Sci. USA* **99**, 1253–1258.

Koide, A., Bailey, C.W., Huang, X. & Koide, S. (1998). The fibronectin type III domain as a scaffold for novel binding proteins. *J. Mol. Biol.* **284**, 1141–1151.

Koide, A., Gilbreth, R.N., Esaki, K., Tereshko, V. & Koide, S. (2007). High-affinity single-domain binding proteins with a binary-code interface. *Proc. Natl. Acad. Sci. USA* **104**, 6632–6637.

Krapp, S., Mimura, Y., Jefferis, R., Huber, R. & Sondermann, P. (2003). Structural analysis of human IgG-Fc glycoforms reveals a correlation between glycosylation and structural integrity. *J. Mol. Biol.* **325**, 979–989.

Kreitman, R.J. (2006). Immunotoxins for targeted cancer therapy. *AAPS J.* **8**, E532–551.

Lee, C.V., Liang, W.C., Dennis, M.S., Eigenbrot, C., Sidhu, S.S. & Fuh, G. (2004). High-affinity human antibodies from phage-displayed synthetic Fab libraries with a single framework scaffold. *J. Mol. Biol.* **340**, 1073–1093.

Lendel, C., Dincbas-Renqvist, V., Flores, A., Wahlberg, E., Dogan, J., Nygren, P.-Å. & Härd, T. (2004). Biophysical characterization of Z(SPA-1) – a phage-display selected binder to protein A. *Protein Sci.* **13**, 2078–2088.

Levin, A.M. & Weiss, G.A. (2006). Optimizing the affinity and specificity of proteins with molecular display. *Molecular Biosystems* **2**, 49–57.

Li, J., Mahajan, A. & Tsai, M.-D. (2006). Ankyrin repeat: a unique motif mediating protein-protein interactions. *Biochemistry* **45**, 15168–15178.

Lipovsek, D., Lippow, S.M., Hackel, B.J., Gregson, M.W., Cheng, P., Kapila, A. & Wittrup, K.D. (2007). Evolution of an interloop disulfide bond in high-affinity antibody mimics based on fibronectin type III domain and selected by yeast surface display: molecular convergence with single-domain camelid and shark antibodies. *J. Mol. Biol.* **368**, 1024–1041.

Luginbühl, B., Kanyo, Z., Jones, R.M., Fletterick, R.J., Prusiner, S.B., Cohen, F.E., Williamson, R.A., Burton, D.R. & Plückthun, A. (2006). Directed evolution of an anti-prion protein scFv fragment to an affinity of 1 pM and its structural interpretation. *J. Mol. Biol.* **363**, 75–97.

Magnusson, M.K., Henning, P., Myhre, S., Wikman, M., Uil, T.G., Friedman, M., Andersson, K.M., Hong, S.S., Hoeben, R.C., Habib, N.A., Stahl, S., Boulanger, P. & Lindholm, L. (2007). Adenovirus 5 vector genetically re-targeted by an Affibody molecule with specificity for tumor antigen HER2/neu. *Cancer Gene Ther.* **14**, 468–479.

Malabarba, M.G., Milia, E., Faretta, M., Zamponi, R., Pelicci, P.G. & Di Fiore, P.P. (2001). A repertoire library that allows the selection of synthetic SH2s with altered binding specificities. *Oncogene* **20**, 5186–5194.

Markland, W., Ley, A.C., Lee, S.W. & Ladner, R.C. (1996). Iterative optimization of high-affinity proteases inhibitors using phage display. 1. Plasmin. *Biochemistry* **35**, 8045–8057.

Marks, J.D., Hoogenboom, H.R., Bonnert, T.P., McCafferty, J., Griffiths, A.D. & Winter, G. (1991). By-passing immunization. Human antibodies from V-gene libraries displayed on phage. *J. Mol. Biol.* **222**, 581–597.

Marvin, J.S. & Zhu, Z. (2005). Recombinant approaches to IgG-like bispecific antibodies. *Acta Pharmacol. Sin.* **26**, 649–658.

McCafferty, J., Griffiths, A.D., Winter, G. & Chiswell, D.J. (1990). Phage antibodies: filamentous phage displaying antibody variable domains. *Nature* **348**, 552–554.

Mendez, M.J., Green, L.L., Corvalan, J.R., Jia, X.C., Maynard-Currie, C.E., Yang, X.D., Gallo, M.L., Louie, D.M., Lee, D.V., Erickson, K.L., Luna, J., Roy, C.M., Abderrahim, H., Kirschenbaum, F., Noguchi, M., Smith, D.H., Fukushima, A., Hales, J.F., Klapholz, S., Finer, M.H., Davis, C.G., Zsebo, K.M. & Jakobovits, A. (1997). Functional transplant of megabase human immunoglobulin loci recapitulates human antibody response in mice. *Nat. Genet.* **15**, 146–156.

Mercader, J.V. & Skerra, A. (2002). Generation of anticalins with specificity for a nonsymmetric phthalic acid ester. *Anal. Biochem.* **308**, 269–277.

Milovnik, P., Ferrari, P., Sarkar, C.A. & Plückthun, A. (2009). Selection and characterization of DARPins specific for the neurotensin receptor 1. *Protein Eng. Des. Sel.*, in press.

Mondon, P., Dubreuil, O., Bouayadi, K. & Kharrat, H. (2008). Human antibody libraries: a race to engineer and explore a larger diversity. *Front. Biosci.* **13**, 1117–1129.

Monsellier, E. & Bedouelle, H. (2006). Improving the stability of an antibody variable fragment by a combination of knowledge-based approaches: validation and mechanisms. *J. Mol. Biol.* **362**, 580–593.

Müller, D. & Kontermann, R.E. (2007). Recombinant bispecific antibodies for cellular cancer immunotherapy. *Curr. Opin. Mol. Ther.* **9**, 319–326.

Nahta, R. & Esteva, F.J. (2006). HER2 therapy: molecular mechanisms of trastuzumab resistance. *Breast Cancer Res.* **8**, 215.

Nimmerjahn, F. & Ravetch, J.V. (2007a). Fc-receptors as regulators of immunity. *Adv. Immunol.* **96**, 179–204.

Nimmerjahn, F. & Ravetch, J.V. (2007b). Antibodies, Fc receptors and cancer. *Curr. Opin. Immunol.* **19**, 239–245.

Noble, C.O., Kirpotin, D.B., Hayes, M.E., Mamot, C., Hong, K., Park, J.W., Benz, C.C., Marks, J.D. & Drummond, D.C. (2004). Development of ligand-targeted liposomes for cancer therapy. *Expert Opin. Ther. Targets* **8**, 335–353.

Nord, K., Gunneriusson, E., Ringdahl, J., Ståhl, S., Uhlén, M. & Nygren, P.-Å. (1997). Binding proteins selected from combinatorial libraries of an α-helical bacterial receptor domain. *Nat. Biotechnol.* **15**, 772–777.

Norman, T.C., Smith, D.L., Sorger, P.K., Drees, B.L., O'Rourke, S.M., Hughes, T.R., Roberts, C.J., Friend, S.H., Fields, S. & Murray, A.W. (1999). Genetic selection of peptide inhibitors of biological pathways. *Science* **285**, 591–595.

North, C.L. & Blacklow, S.C. (1999). Structural independence of ligand-binding modules five and six of the LDL receptor. *Biochemistry* **38**, 3926–3935.

Nygren, P.-Å. (2008). Alternative binding proteins: affibody binding proteins developed from a small three-helix bundle scaffold. *FEBS J.* **275**, 2668–2676.

Orlova, A., Magnusson, M., Eriksson, T.L., Nilsson, M., Larsson, B., Hoiden-Guthenberg, I., Widström, C., Carlsson, J., Tolmachev, V., Stahl, S. & Nilsson, F.Y. (2006). Tumor imaging using a picomolar affinity HER2 binding affibody molecule. *Cancer Res.* **66**, 4339–4348.

Orlova, A., Tran, T., Widström, C., Engfeldt, T., Eriksson Karlström, A. & Tolmachev, V. (2007). Preclinical evaluation of [111In]-benzyl-DOTA-Z(HER2:342), a potential agent for imaging of HER2 expression in malignant tumors. *Int. J. Mol. Med.* **20**, 397–404.

Osenga, K.L., Hank, J.A., Albertini, M.R., Gan, J., Sternberg, A.G., Eickhoff, J., Seeger, R.C., Matthay, K.K., Reynolds, C.P., Twist, C., Krailo, M., Adamson, P.C., Reisfeld, R.A., Gillies, S.D. & Sondel, P.M. (2006). A phase I clinical trial of the hu14.18-IL2 (EMD 273063) as a treatment for children with refractory or recurrent neuroblastoma and melanoma: a study of the Children's Oncology Group. *Clin. Cancer Res.* **12**, 1750–1759.

Pancer, Z., Amemiya, C.T., Ehrhardt, G.R., Ceitlin, J., Gartland, G.L. & Cooper, M.D. (2004). Somatic diversification of variable lymphocyte receptors in the agnathan sea lamprey. *Nature* **430**, 174–180.

Pancer, Z. & Cooper, M.D. (2006). The evolution of adaptive immunity. *Annu. Rev. Immunol.* **24**, 497–518.

Panni, S., Dente, L. & Cesareni, G. (2002). In vitro evolution of recognition specificity mediated by SH3 domains reveals target recognition rules. *J. Biol. Chem.* **277**, 21666–21674.

Park, J.W., Benz, C.C. & Martin, F.J. (2004). Future directions of liposome- and immunoliposome-based cancer therapeutics. *Semin. Oncol.* **31**, 196–205.

Parker, M.H., Chen, Y., Danehy, F., Dufu, K., Ekstrom, J., Getmanova, E., Gokemeijer, J., Xu, L. & Lipovsek, D. (2005). Antibody mimics based on human fibronectin type three domain engineered for thermostability and high-affinity binding to vascular endothelial growth factor receptor two. *Protein Eng. Des. Sel.* **18**, 435–444.

Pearce, K.H., Jr., Cunningham, B.C., Fuh, G., Teeri, T. & Wells, J.A. (1999). Growth hormone binding affinity for its receptor surpasses the requirements for cellular activity. *Biochemistry* **38**, 81–89.

Peled, J.U., Kuang, F.L., Iglesias-Ussel, M.D., Roa, S., Kalis, S.L., Goodman, M.F. & Scharff, M.D. (2008). The biochemistry of somatic hypermutation. *Annu. Rev. Immunol.* **26**, 481–511.

Perentesis, J.P., Miller, S.P. & Bodley, J.W. (1992). Protein toxin inhibitors of protein synthesis. *BioFactors* **3**, 173–184.

Plückthun, A. & Moroney, S.E. (2005). Modern antibody technology: The impact on drug development. In *Modern Biopharmaceuticals* (Knäblein, J., ed.), Vol. 3, pp. 1147–1186. Wiley-VCH, Weinheim.

Plückthun, A. & Pack, P. (1997). New protein engineering approaches to multivalent and bispecific antibody fragments. *Immunotechnology* **3**, 83–105.

Presta, L.G. (2008). Molecular engineering and design of therapeutic antibodies. *Curr. Opin. Immunol.* **20**, 460–470.

Ramsland, P.A. & Farrugia, W. (2002). Crystal structures of human antibodies: a detailed and unfinished tapestry of immunoglobulin gene products. *J. Mol. Recognit.* **15**, 248–259.

Reina, J., Lacroix, E., Hobson, S.D., Fernandez-Ballester, G., Rybin, V., Schwab, M.S., Serrano, L. & Gonzalez, C. (2002). Computer-aided design of a PDZ domain to recognize new target sequences. *Nat. Struct. Biol.* **9**, 621–627.

Ridgway, J.B., Presta, L.G. & Carter, P. (1996). "Knobs-into-holes" engineering of antibody CH3 domains for heavy chain heterodimerization. *Protein Eng.* **9**, 617–621.

Roberts, R.W. & Szostak, J.W. (1997). RNA-peptide fusions for the in vitro selection of peptides and proteins. *Proc. Natl. Acad. Sci. USA* **94**, 12297–12302.

Röttgen, P. & Collins, J. (1995). A human pancreatic secretory trypsin inhibitor presenting a hypervariable highly constrained epitope via monovalent phagemid display. *Gene* **164**, 243–250.

Ryan, M.H., Heavner, G.A., Brigham-Burke, M., McMahon, F., Shanahan, M.F., Gunturi, S.R., Sharma, B. & Farrell, F.X. (2006). An in vivo model to assess factors that may stimulate the generation of an immune reaction to erythropoietin. *Int. Immunopharmacol.* **6**, 647–655.

Sandström, K., Xu, Z., Forsberg, G. & Nygren, P.-Å. (2003). Inhibition of the CD28-CD80 co-stimulation signal by a CD28-binding affibody ligand developed by combinatorial protein engineering. *Protein Eng.* **16**, 691–697.

Schier, R., Bye, J., Apell, G., McCall, A., Adams, G.P., Malmqvist, M., Weiner, L.M. & Marks, J.D. (1996). Isolation of high-affinity monomeric human anti-c-erbB-2 single chain Fv using affinity-driven selection. *J. Mol. Biol.* **255**, 28–43.

Schlehuber, S., Beste, G. & Skerra, A. (2000). A novel type of receptor protein, based on the lipocalin scaffold, with specificity for digoxigenin. *J. Mol. Biol.* **297**, 1105–1120.

Schlehuber, S. & Skerra, A. (2005). Lipocalins in drug discovery: from natural ligand-binding proteins to "anticalins." *Drug Discov. Today* **10**, 23–33.

Schneider, S., Buchert, M., Georgiev, O., Catimel, B., Halford, M., Stacker, S.A., Baechi, T., Moelling, K. & Hovens, C.M. (1999). Mutagenesis and selection of PDZ domains that bind new protein targets. *Nat. Biotechnol.* **17**, 170–175.

Schweizer, A., Roschitzki-Voser, H., Amstutz, P., Briand, C., Gulotti-Georgieva, M., Prenosil, E., Binz, H.K., Capitani, G., Baici, A., Plückthun, A. & Grütter, M.G. (2007). Inhibition of caspase-2 by a designed ankyrin repeat protein: specificity, structure, and inhibition mechanism. *Structure* **15**, 625–636.

Scott, J.K. & Smith, G.P. (1990). Searching for peptide ligands with an epitope library. *Science* **249**, 386–390.

Sennhauser, G., Amstutz, P., Briand, C., Storchenegger, O. & Grütter, M.G. (2007). Drug export pathway of multidrug exporter AcrB revealed by DARPin inhibitors. *PLoS Biol.* **5**, e7.

Silverman, J., Liu, Q., Bakker, A., To, W., Duguay, A., Alba, B.M., Smith, R., Rivas, A., Li, P., Le, H., Whitehorn, E., Moore, K.W., Swimmer, C., Perlroth, V., Vogt, M., Kolkman, J. & Stemmer, W.P. (2005). Multivalent avimer proteins evolved by exon shuffling of a family of human receptor domains. *Nat. Biotechnol.* **23**, 1556–1561.

Skerra A. & Plückthun, A. (1988). Assembly of a functional immunoglobulin Fv fragment in *Escherichia coli. Science* **240**, 1038–1041.

Smith, G.P. (1985). Filamentous fusion phage: novel expression vectors that display cloned antigens on the virion surface. *Science* **228**, 1315–1317.

Sondel, P.M., Hank, J.A., Gan, J., Neal, Z. & Albertini, M.R. (2003). Preclinical and clinical development of immunocytokines. *Curr. Opin. Investig. Drugs* **4**, 696–700.

Steiner, D., Forrer, P. & Plückthun, A. (2008). Efficient Selection of DARPins with Sub-nanomolar Affinities using SRP Phage Display. *J. Mol. Biol* **382**, 1211–1227.

Steiner, D., Forrer, P., Stumpp, M.T. & Plückthun, A. (2006). Signal sequences directing cotranslational translocation expand the range of proteins amenable to phage display. *Nat. Biotechnol.* **24**, 823–831.

Steipe, B., Schiller, B., Plückthun, A. & Steinbacher, S. (1994). Sequence statistics reliably predict stabilizing mutations in a protein domain. *J. Mol. Biol.* **240**, 188–192.

Stirpe, F. (2004). Ribosome-inactivating proteins. *Toxicon* **44**, 371–383.

Stumpp, M.T., Forrer, P., Binz, H.K. & Plückthun, A. (2003). Designing repeat proteins: modular leucine-rich repeat protein libraries based on the mammalian ribonuclease inhibitor family. *J. Mol. Biol.* **332**, 471–487.

Tanaka, A.S., Silva, M.M., Torquato, R.J., Noguti, M.A., Sampaio, C.A., Fritz, H. & Auerswald, E.A. (1999). Functional phage display of leech-derived tryptase inhibitor (LDTI): construction of a library and selection of thrombin inhibitors. *FEBS Lett.* **458**, 11–16.

Telleman, P. & Junghans, R.P. (2000). The role of the Brambell receptor (FcRB) in liver: protection of endocytosed immunoglobulin G (IgG) from catabolism in hepatocytes rather than transport of IgG to bile. *Immunology* **100**, 245–251.

Tolmachev, V., Orlova, A., Pehrson, R., Galli, J., Baastrup, B., Andersson, K., Sandstrom, M., Rosik, D., Carlsson, J., Lundqvist, H., Wennborg, A. & Nilsson, F.Y. (2007). Radionuclide therapy of HER2-positive microxenografts using a 177Lu-labeled HER2-specific Affibody molecule. *Cancer Res.* **67**, 2773–2782.

Trail, P.A., King, H.D. & Dubowchik, G.M. (2003). Monoclonal antibody drug immunoconjugates for targeted treatment of cancer. *Cancer Immunol. Immunother.* **52**, 328–337.

van der Neut Kolfschoten, M., Schuurman, J., Losen, M., Bleeker, W.K., Martinez-Martinez, P., Vermeulen, E., den Bleker, T.H., Wiegman, L., Vink, T., Aarden, L.A., De Baets, M.H., van de Winkel, J.G.J., Aalberse, R.C. & Parren, P.W.H.I. (2007). Anti-inflammatory activity of human IgG4 antibodies by dynamic Fab arm exchange. *Science* **317**, 1554–1557.

Vaughan, T.J., Williams, A.J., Pritchard, K., Osbourn, J.K., Pope, A.R., Earnshaw, J.C., McCafferty, J., Hodits, R.A., Wilton, J. & Johnson, K.S. (1996). Human antibodies with sub-nanomolar affinities isolated from a large non-immunized phage display library. *Nat. Biotechnol.* **14**, 309–314.

Virnekäs, B., Ge, L., Plückthun, A., Schneider, K.C., Wellnhofer, G. & Moroney, S.E. (1994). Trinucleotide phosphoramidites: Ideal reagents for the synthesis of mixed oligonucleotides for random mutagenesis. *Nucleic Acids Res.* **22**, 5600–5607.

Vogt, M. & Skerra, A. (2004). Construction of an artificial receptor protein ("anticalin") based on the human apolipoprotein D. *ChemBioChem* **5**, 191–199.

Voutsadakis, I.A. (2002). Gemtuzumab Ozogamicin (CMA-676, Mylotarg) for the treatment of CD33+ acute myeloid leukemia. *Anti-Cancer Drugs* **13**, 685–692.

Wahlberg, E., Lendel, C., Helgstrand, M., Allard, P., Dincbas-Renqvist, V., Hedqvist, A., Berglund, H., Nygren, P.-Å. & Härd, T. (2003). An affibody in complex with a target protein: structure and coupled folding. *Proc. Natl. Acad. Sci. USA* **100**, 3185–3190.

Waibel, R., Alberto, R., Willuda, J., Finnern, R., Schibli, R., Stichelberger, A., Egli, A., Abram, U., Mach, J.P., Plückthun, A. & Schubiger, P.A. (1999). Stable one-step technetium-99m labeling of His-tagged recombinant proteins with a novel Tc(I)-carbonyl complex. *Nat. Biotechnol.* **17**, 897–901.

Wang, S.Y. & Weiner, G. (2008). Complement and cellular cytotoxicity in antibody therapy of cancer. *Expert Opin. Biol. Ther.* **8**, 759–768.

Weiner, L.M. & Carter, P. (2003). The rollercoaster ride to anti-cancer antibodies. *Nat. Biotechnol.* **21**, 510–511.

Wetzel, S.K., Settanni, G., Kenig, M., Binz, H.K. & Plückthun, A. (2008). Folding and unfolding mechanism of highly stable full-consensus ankyrin repeat proteins. *J. Mol. Biol.* **376**, 241–257.

Wiberg, F.C., Rasmussen, S.K., Frandsen, T.P., Rasmussen, L.K., Tengbjerg, K., Coljee, V.W., Sharon, J., Yang, C.Y., Bregenholt, S., Nielsen, L.S., Haurum, J.S. & Tolstrup, A.B. (2006). Production of target-specific recombinant human polyclonal antibodies in mammalian cells. *Biotechnol. Bioeng.* **94**, 396–405.

Williams, A. & Baird, L.G. (2003). DX-88 and HAE: a developmental perspective. *Transfus. Apher. Sci.* **29**, 255–258.

Wörn, A. & Plückthun, A. (2001). Stability engineering of antibody single-chain Fv fragments. *J. Mol. Biol.* **305**, 989–1010.

Xu, L., Aha, P., Gu, K., Kuimelis, R.G., Kurz, M., Lam, T., Lim, A.C., Liu, H., Lohse, P.A., Sun, L., Weng, S., Wagner, R.W. & Lipovsek, D. (2002). Directed evolution of high-affinity antibody mimics using mRNA display. *Chem. Biol.* **9**, 933–942.

Yang, K., Basu, A., Wang, M., Chintala, R., Hsieh, M.C., Liu, S., Hua, J., Zhang, Z., Zhou, J., Li, M., Phyu, H., Petti, G., Mendez, M., Janjua, H., Peng, P., Longley, C., Borowski, V., Mehlig, M. & Filpula, D. (2003). Tailoring structure-function and pharmacokinetic properties of single-chain Fv proteins by site-specific PEGylation. *Protein Eng.* **16**, 761–770.

Zahnd, C., Amstutz, P. & Plückthun, A. (2007a). Ribosome display: selecting and evolving proteins in vitro that specifically bind to a target. *Nat. Methods* **4**, 269–279.

Zahnd, C., Pécorari, F., Straumann, N., Wyler, E. & Plückthun, A. (2006). Selection and characterization of Her2 binding-designed ankyrin repeat proteins. *J. Biol. Chem.* **281**, 35167–35175.

Zahnd, C., Spinelli, S., Luginbühl, B., Amstutz, P., Cambillau, C. & Plückthun, A. (2004). Directed in vitro evolution and crystallographic analysis of a peptide binding scFv antibody with low picomolar affinity. *J. Biol. Chem.* **279**, 18870–18877.

Zahnd, C., Wyler, E., Schwenk, J.M., Steiner, D., Lawrence, M.C., McKern, N.M., Pecorari, F., Ward, C.W., Joos, T.O. & Plückthun, A. (2007b). A designed ankyrin repeat protein evolved to picomolar affinity to Her2. *J. Mol. Biol.* **369**, 1015–1028.

PART VIII

PROLONGATION OF SERUM HALF-LIFE

Polymer Fusions to Increase Antibody Half-Lives: PEGylation and Other Modifications

Sam P. Heywood and David P. Humphreys

PEGylation of proteins has been performed for over 30 years (Abuchowski et al., 1977a,b). Although the details such as polyethylene glycol (PEG) size, structure, synthesis, purification, and reactive chemistries have changed, the basic aims of the method remain the same. These aims are to improve the biophysical and pharmaceutical characteristics of proteins by modifying pharmacokinetics (circulating serum half-life); increasing resistance to proteolysis; reducing antigenicity and immunogenicity; and in some instances, increasing solubility and reducing propensity to aggregate. These improvements have been demonstrated successfully in the clinic with a variety of proteins including enzymes, cytokines, and antibodies. In this chapter we will introduce the aspects of PEGylation common to all proteins before dealing with their specific application to antibodies and antibody fragments.

POLYMERS FOR PROTEIN CONJUGATION

Many potential therapeutic proteins have characteristics that can be improved by conjugation to large water-soluble polymers. Tailoring of these characteristics is required in order to generate the most effective therapeutic. Alteration of a protein's characteristics may also expand its use, for example, from single use in acute indications to repeat dosing in chronic indications. Conjugation of both small molecule and protein-based drugs to a diverse range of polymers has been investigated in order to improve their therapeutic profile. Polymers investigated include those based on amino acids such as poly-GGGGS, polyglutamate, and polyaspartate (Jultani et al., 1997; Schlapschy et al., 2007; Zunino et al., 1982); those based on carbohydrates such as oxidized dextran, carboxymethyl dextran, starch, and polysialic acid (Baudys et al., 1998; Fagnani et al., 1990; Gregoriadis et al., 2000); and completely synthetic polymers such as poly(N-vinylpyrrolidone), poly(N-acryloil-morpholine), polyoxyethylated glycerol, hydroxypropyl methacrylamide, polymethacrylate, bow tie dendrimers, and PEG (Caliceti et al., 1999; Kaneda et al., 2004; Soucek et al., 2002). Although many of these polymers have found use in the area of protein modification, particularly antibody fragment modification, PEG has become the polymer of choice. This is because PEG improves the characteristics of drugs without any major drawbacks. The successful use of PEGylation led to the development of an increasingly sophisticated range of commercially available PEG polymers of higher quality, greater functionality, and varied size. This period of co-development cemented the use of PEG as the polymer of choice for protein modification.

PEG STRUCTURE AND SYNTHESIS

PEG is a simple repeating polymer of the formula $-(CH_2-CH_2-O)_n-$. Historically the term PEG was used for lower molecular weight polymers, whereas larger molecular weight polymers were termed polyethylene oxide. However, in the field of protein modification the polymer is generally termed PEG regardless of its size. PEGs of >1kDa molecular weight are generally used for protein modification because they are large enough to impart the required change to *in vivo* characteristics upon the protein and also lack toxicity. PEG of >1kDa molecular weight are generally regarded as safe for use in therapeutics by regulatory authorities, whereas lower molecular weight PEGs (<400Da) are degraded by alcohol dehydrogenase in the liver to toxic metabolites (Working et al., 1997). The PEG polymer is very flexible and has a high propensity for water, binding two to three water molecules per repeat. It is the combination of these factors that greatly increases the apparent size of the polymer and leads to the advantageous characteristics exploited in therapeutics.

Several variations of PEG polymerization chemistry are possible, but for PEG destined for use in therapeutic conjugates, one chemistry has prevailed. Starting with methanol, methoxy ethanol, or methoxyethoxy ethanol, ethylene oxide is polymerized onto the terminal -OH group by an anionic ring-opening mechanism. The reaction results in a methoxy terminated PEG (mPEG). However, due to trace amounts of water present in the reaction, the product is contaminated by a significant amount of diol. Diols are PEGs with an -OH at each end, and because polymerization can proceed at both ends, they tend to be large and heterogeneous. Diol is commonly removed by first converting its two -OH groups to carboxylic acids and then separating these di-carboxylic acid species from the mono-carboxylic-mPEG by ion exchange chromatography. The polymerization reaction onto the intended starting material is highly controllable and results in mPEG with a low polydispersity.

Polydispersity is an important feature of PEG and is essentially a measure of the spread of its molecular weight. A polydispersity of 1 shows that all the polymers are of exactly the same size. This would be preferred for clinical use but is not achievable with current polymerization technologies for PEGs >1kDa (Loiseau et al., 2004). Therefore, regulatory agencies demand the use of PEG with the lowest polydispersity. The most homogenous high molecular weight PEGs commercially available have a polydispersity of ~1.02. Expressed another way, the spread at half peak height for a 20kDa PEG of this polydispersity is 19.8–20.2kDa. PEG of 20kDa with a polydispersity of <1.05 has been commercially available for many years, but it is only more recently that low polydispersity PEGs up to 40kDa have become available.

Although methoxy terminated PEGs are commonly available and have become the industry standard, low polydispersity hydroxy terminated PEG is also available at commercial scale.

Historically, in order to generate larger PEGs (i.e., >20kDa) with low polydispersity, linear PEG chains were combined, as this approach made best use of the lowest polydispersity PEG building blocks available. One strategy was to link two to four PEG chains to make "branched" structures, where the PEGs were linked via lysine, glycerol, triazine, pentaerythritol, or other moieties (Matsushima et al., 1980; Monfardini et al., 1995; Nektar Therapeutics; NOF Corporation). The main feature of these molecules is that the linear PEG chains are attached to a core linker. Another combination strategy is to link three or more PEGs in a "comb" structure. These structures have a second linear polymer to which the linear PEG chains are attached. Examples of comb structures include eight PEG chains linked to a hexa-glycerol backbone or 2kDa PEG chains linked to a polymethacrylate backbone (NOF Corporation, Han et al., 2007). A third combination strategy is to link three or more PEGs via an "umbrella" structure. These structures have a multiple bifurcating network, the termini of which have PEG attached. Examples of umbrella structures include polyester bow tie dendrimer-PEG and poly-bifurcating lysine-PEG (Gillies et al., 2005).

PEG is universally regarded as having very low inherent immunogenicity. This is evidenced by the low abundance and low titer of preexisting antibodies in human sera (Richter & Åkerblom, 1984). Only by use of strong adjuvants or by coupling of PEG to highly immunogenic proteins and peptides can stronger immune responses against PEG be generated (Richter & Åkerblom, 1983). Indeed, the lack of IgG antibodies against PEG has until recently hindered their use in anti-PEG immune-detection (Wunderlich et al., 2007).

THE EFFECT OF PEGYLATION ON ANTIBODIES AND ANTIBODY FRAGMENTS

Protection from Proteolytic Degradation

Full-length antibodies were the first of this class of protein to be PEGylated, with the aim of reducing their susceptibility to proteolytic degradation in order to dose orally. 2kDa and 8kDa PEGs were randomly coupled via primary amines to immunoglobulin sera in such a way that antigen binding, complement fixation, and Fc receptor binding were minimally affected. The resulting PEGylated proteins were shown to have reduced susceptibility to pepsin, trypsin, and chymotrypsin *in vitro* (Cunningham-Rundles et al., 1992). It is commonly held that the disproportionately large hydrated volume of distribution or "hydration shell" of PEG molecules may simply act to sterically block access of proteases to the antibody. Protection from proteolysis is not specific to antibodies, since earlier work had shown that bovine catalase was significantly protected from trypsin, chymotrypsin, and *Streptomyces griseus* protease by PEGylation (Abuchowski et al., 1977a).

Reduced Antigenicity and Immunogenicity

This feature of PEGylation is one that is perhaps less important with respect to antibodies because current selection and engineering techniques deliver humanized and human antibodies that are of inherently low immunogenic potential. However, as antibody technology is now developing beyond these "natural" therapeutics to camelid/shark V_{HH} regions and various non-Ig fold antibody mimetics, PEGylation in order to minimize immunogenicity may once again become a more important aspect. Any reduction in the immunogenic potential of a therapeutic protein is always welcome and PEGylation offers a quick and simple means to reduce the potential immunogenicity of antibody:enzyme and antibody:toxin fusion proteins.

Examples of PEGylation affecting immunogenicity include a human monoclonal IgG that was immunogenic in mice being rendered nonimmunogenic when randomly PEGylated with an average of 13 or 30 molecules of 6.4kDa PEG per IgG (Wilkinson et al., 1987). Similarly, a monoclonal murine IgG modified with an average of 10 or 17 molecules of 6kDa dextran showed reduced immunogenicity and retained normal pharmacokinetics in rabbits (Fagnani et al., 1990). This suggests that the protective effect is not specific to PEG per se, but rather that it relates to the conjugation of highly solvated polymers. Fab fragments derived from two different rat IgGs were found to be immunogenic in mice until PEGylated with two molecules of 20kDa PEG at the hinge cysteines (Trakas & Tzartos, 2001). Clinical development of an immunotoxin of a mouse scFv genetically fused to the 38kDa form of *Pseudomonas* exotoxin A was hampered by the formation of neutralizing human antimouse antibody (HAMA) and anti-exotoxin antibody responses until PEGylated with either a single 5kDa or 20kDa PEG (Tsutsumi et al., 2000).

The general ability of PEGylation to reduce the immunogenic potential of proteins has been further demonstrated with non-antibody therapeutics. For example, when *Escherichia coli* L-asparaginase was heavily modified with 5kDa PEG this resulted in a large reduction in its immunogenicity in mice (Kamisaki et al., 1981). The immune response in mice, elicited when repeatedly dosed with bovine adenosine deaminase, was significantly reduced when the protein was modified with 5kDa PEG (Davis et al., 1981). An FDA approved version of a PEGylated adenosine deaminase (pegadamase bovine, Adagen®) is marketed for the treatment of severe combined immune deficiency (reviewed by Vellard, 2003). More recently, recombinant human IFN-β-1b has been extensively engineered to achieve optimal PEGylation, stability, solubility, aggregation, immunogenicity, and *in vivo* exposure (a composite of pharmacokinetics and activity). The immunogenicity of human IFN-β-1b in rats was drastically reduced by conjugation of 20kDa or 40kDa PEG (Basu et al., 2006).

Pharmacokinetics of Antibody Fragments

Perhaps the major reason for PEGylation of antibody-derived proteins, such as antibody fragments, has been to increase their serum half-life. Antibody fragments are made for a number of reasons and by a number of different methods, but they generally lack the Fc portion of the antibody that confers extended serum half-life (see Humphreys, 2003, for a review of antibody fragment structure, use, and production). Full-length glycosylated IgG typically have a half-life in humans of 12–14 days. This is mainly due to the FcRn-mediated protection and recycling of antibodies conferred by the Fc. In contrast, antibody fragments generally have half-lives in the order of 0.5–1 days. Absolute residence times are antibody fragment-dependent due to a mixture of factors including, size, shape, degree of immunogenicity, isoelectric point, affinity, location, and tissue distribution of antigen. A study in mice found residence times in the body of 8.5, 0.5, and 0.2 days for IgG, F(ab′)2 and Fab versions of the MOPC21 antibody, respectively (Covell et al., 1986). Similar patterns and magnitudes have also been observed in rat, dog, and cynomolgous monkey models (Brown et al. 1987; Chapman et al., 1999; Keyler et al., 1991; King et al., 1994; Milenic et al., 1991). Quantitative PK data for human Fab in human subjects are scarce but there is a wealth of comparative data in animal models for Fab and Fab-PEG. These can be extrapolated using the principle of allometric interspecies scaling, which predicts a $t\frac{1}{2}\beta$ of 16 hours for a Fab in a 70kg human (Grene-Lerouge et al., 1996). A murine:human chimeric Fab (abciximab, ReoPro®) was shown to have a $t\frac{1}{2}\alpha$ of 0.5 hours in humans; however, Fab was still detectable in the circulation for up to 15 days due to binding to its platelet-borne antigen. A murine:human chimeric F(ab′)$_2$ Mov18 was shown to have a half-life of 20 hours in human volunteers (Buist et al., 1993). A humanized radiolabeled Fab was shown to have a $t\frac{1}{2}\alpha$ of 1 hour and a terminal elimination of 12 hours in humans (Macfarlane et al., 2006). Sheep-derived Fab fragments have been shown to have half-lives of 16–20 hours (Ujhelyi & Robert, 1995), while horse-derived F(ab′)$_2$ fragment have been shown to have a $t\frac{1}{2}\alpha$ of 0.2 hours and a $t\frac{1}{2}\beta$ of 161 hours in healthy human volunteers (Vázquez et al., 2005; reviewed by Gutierrez et al., 2003). Collectively, these data suggest that Fab and F(ab′)$_2$ are likely to have serum half-lives in the order of 12–24 hours in humans.

Rapid distribution and clearance can be of benefit in some clinical applications. Fab are found to have nearly three times the volume of distribution of IgG, and achieve equilibration with this volume nearly 10 times faster (Bazin-Redureau et al., 1997). This means that Fab and other small fragments find particular utility in radio-imaging, as ADEPT clearance agents, and anti-toxin and anti-poisoning treatments. Fab have been taken successfully to the clinic but only in indications where long PK may be irrelevant or unwanted. Examples include ReoPro®, Lucentis®, CroFab®, DigiFab®, Digibind®, Alacramyn®, Verluma®, CEA-Scan® and Myoscint®.

Therapeutic monoclonal antibodies often target chronic indications, and in this setting a reasonably long circulating half-life is a substantial contributor to efficacy. PEGylation of antibody fragments with high molecular weight PEG has been successfully used in order to achieve such a half-life. Addition of a 40kDa branched PEG to Fab caused a ~13-fold increase in AUC (area under the curve) in rats (Chapman et al., 1999) and a 15–35-fold increase in terminal $t\frac{1}{2}$ in rabbits (Koumenis et al., 2000; Leong et al., 2001). The effect of the same PEGylation strategy assessed in cynomolgous monkeys conferred a half-life to a Fab that was ~78% of that of an IgG (Chapman et al., 1999). A graphical comparison between Fab and Fab-PEG half-life in cynomolgous monkeys is also available (Knight et al., 2004). A Fab modified with a 40kDa branched PEG has been shown to have an elimination half-life of 12–14 days in humans (Rolan et al., 2008). This is in stark contrast to the 0.5–1 day elimination half-life both observed and predicted for Fab in humans and serves to highlight the large impact that PEGylation can have in the clinical performance of therapeutic molecules. Most of the pharmacokinetic data that illustrate the magnitude of the increase in half-life due to PEGylation have been generated in animal models and hence should only be taken as a guide to the potential increase in half-life in humans.

In other clinical situations, antibody fragments with intermediate half-lives are beneficial. For example, tumor targeting for therapy or imaging has been shown to benefit from precise fine-tuning of the PEG size. Both of these aspects are described in more detail later in the chapter.

PEGylation of Antibody Fragments to Achieve Long Serum Half-lives

Early methods for antibody fragment PEGylation resulted in random attachment of low molecular weight PEG molecules. This was a natural consequence of the types of PEG molecules and reactive groups that were available at the time. It soon became apparent that random PEGylation with multiple PEG molecules suffered from a number of practical weaknesses. First, the uncontrolled and random nature of the PEGylation means that the product of the PEGylation reaction is heterogeneous, in terms of both the number and point of attachment of the PEG molecules. For example, reaction conditions can be set up such that on average 5 PEG molecules are attached on a protein that has 10 possible sites of attachment (e.g., lysines). Although most of the reaction product will have 5 PEGs attached, there will be a significant proportion of protein that has more than or less than 5 PEGs. Furthermore, these 5 PEG molecules can and will be attached at different positions on the protein. In practice, steric and other biochemical factors mean that a strong bias can be exhibited toward a subset of the target reactive side chains. A high degree of modification is generally found to affect the activity of the antibody fragments, resulting in reduced antigen affinity. This negative effect can be due to steric hindrance and is proportional to the size of PEG and the extent of modification. Alternatively, it can be due to a complete inactivation of a proportion of molecules within the product mixture. For example, PEGylation of a key lysine within a CDR can render the antibody inactive. Unless these molecules can be removed during purification they will effectively dilute out the active molecules in the final product mixture. By careful control of the degree of modification, it has been possible to control the extent of affinity loss for antibody fragments (Chapman et al., 1999; Koumenis et al., 2000). Even if monoPEGylation is the aim, a random coupling strategy can still result in positional isoforms of differing functionality that may be difficult to analyze or separate chromatographically (Bailon et al., 2001).

There have been numerous attempts to overcome these issues using protein engineering. Mutagenesis has been used to reduce the number of surface-exposed lysines in the protein of interest, hence limiting the number of possible final variants (Onda et al., 2003; Yoshioka et al., 2004). Solvent-exposed and structurally unimportant disulphide bonds can be reduced and both cysteines PEGylated by bisalkylation (Balan et al., 2007; Brocchini et al., 2006; Shaunak et al., 2006). However, the approach that has proven to be universally most useful for site-specific PEGylation of antibody fragments is the reaction of maleimide with free thiols of solvent-exposed cysteines. This has been employed most successfully with Fab and scFv fragments. Fab fragments are PEGylated at natural or engineered hinge cysteines (Chapman et al., 1999; Knight et al., 2004; Leong et al., 2001) while scFvs are PEGylated at an engineered C-terminal or linker-encoded single cysteine (Albrecht et al., 2004; Albrecht et al., 2006; Krinner et al., 2006; Kubetzko et al., 2006; Natarajan et al., 2005; Yang et al., 2003; Xiong et al., 2006). scFv-cKappa fusions (scAb) have also been site-specifically PEGylated in this way (Mabry et al., 2005).

The attraction of targeting engineered hinge cysteines is an absolute control over the number of PEG molecules and their point of attachment. This means that the PEG can be kept away from the CDRs and also that analytical challenges are minimized. MonoPEGylation at a single hinge cysteine with (branched) 40kDa PEG is the strategy that has been used successfully during the development of Cimzia® (certolizumab pegol), a humanized anti-TNFα for treatment of Crohn's disease and rheumatoid arthritis (Rose-John & Schooltink, 2003). This molecule has been administered to thousands of patients and clinical efficacy has been demonstrated (Schreiber et al., 2007). Fab contain a solvent exposed inter-chain disulphide bond; consequently, hinge-specific monoPEGylation is a trade-off between reductive strength of the reaction and the efficiency and fidelity of the conjugation (Mozier, 2003). The efficiency and fidelity of Fab PEGylation can be further improved by engineered removal of the inter-chain disulphide bond cysteines leaving just the single hinge thiol as a target. Alternatively, Fab fragments lacking hinge cysteines can be engineered leaving the structurally dispensable inter-chain disulphide bond cysteines as the sole targets for reduction and diPEGylation (Humphreys et al., 2007). With both of these approaches, highly specific PEGylation has been demonstrated, with conjugation efficiencies of up to 90%. The efficiency of the reaction can be of considerable financial importance when manufacturing at the kilogram scale.

The primary effect of PEGylation on antibody fragment pharmacokinetics is thought to be due to an increase in hydrodynamic size. Addition of PEG has a much larger effect on apparent molecular weight than would be expected from the theoretical addition of the PEG alone. For example, one linear 40kDa PEG-F(ab′)$_2$ conjugate had a theoretical molecular weight of 135kDa but its apparent molecular weight, as determined by size exclusion chromatography, was about 1600kDa (Koumenis et al., 2000). Similarly, a scFv conjugated to 20kDa PEG had a theoretical mass of ~50kDa but an apparent molecular weight of >200kDa (Kubetzko et al., 2005). The renal filtration threshold is generally described as being 50–70kDa (or 25Å–42Å) for proteins, although the threshold is also affected by molecular dimensions, shape, rigidity, and charge (Chang et al., 1975; Maack et al., 1979; Rabkin & Dahl, 1993). This means that many antibody fragment formats are efficiently filtered out into the urine by the kidney. Addition of a hydrodynamically large and flexible molecule such as PEG simply reduces the probability that the protein to which it is attached will be filtered each time that it passes through the kidney. Positively charged proteins and peptides can also interact electrostatically with the kidney basement membrane where they can be degraded by proteases. This charge-based interaction is thought to become increasingly important as the protein size nears that of the "pore size" of the kidney (Bray et al., 1984; Kobayashi et al., 1999). Hence the sizes of Fab and F(ab′)$_2$ mean that they may be subjected to this clearance mechanism in addition to filtration. Since PEGylation has been shown to make proteins less susceptible to proteolysis and immune surveillance, it is possible that the PEG shields the Fab from degradation in the kidney.

PEGylation to Increase Tumor Localization

The short biodistribution times ($t_{1/2}\alpha$ distribution half-life) of antibody fragments facilitates rapid access to extra-vascular antigens and tumor penetration, while rapid clearance from circulation via kidney filtration means that it is possible to achieve high tumor:blood ratios in a short time period. Both of these properties are important for tumor imaging, especially when imaging is performed with radio-isotopes with short half-lives and when it needs to be performed rapidly or within an in-patient clinical setting.

The first imaging molecules were monoclonal IgGs but they quickly evolved toward smaller molecules with shorter serum half-lives (Pedley et al., 1994). The very short half-life of fragments was then enhanced with moderate levels of PEGylation (Delgado et al., 1996; Kitamura et al., 1990). ScFv and its dimeric (diabody, di-scFv) and tetrameric (scFv-helix) derivatives offer a spectrum of sizes and avidities and some of these have been compared in detail against other antibody fragments and IgG (Williams et al., 2001). Fine-tuning through PEGylation was demonstrated by an anti-CEA diabody conjugated to a single 3.4kDa PEG, which improved performance in imaging beyond that of the previously preferred "mini-body" molecule (Li et al., 2006). Another study suggested that addition of a single 20kDa PEG to an scFv resulted in increased tumor accumulations that were in excess of those achievable through protein multimerization alone (Kubetzko et al., 2006). Improved pharmacokinetic and antitumor characteristics were achieved when an unPEGylated scFv-toxin fusion was conjugated with 5kDa or 20kDa PEG (Tsutsumi et al., 2000).

Together these and other studies suggest that PEG has a positive effect on tumor localization beyond that caused by the effect on molecular size and serum persistence. Support for this is found in the concept of the tumor "enhanced permeability and retention" (EPR) effect (Matsumura & Maeda, 1986). The disorganized and leaky neo-vasculature of tumors leads to a hyper-permeability to circulating macromolecules. With a lack of effective tumor lymphatic drainage, this can result in an accumulation of macromolecules including large proteins, PEG, and other polymers (reviewed by Duncan, 2003).

Effect of PEGylation on Antibody Fragment-binding Kinetics

Several groups have noted that PEGylation of small fragments, such as scFvs and diabodies, with too large or too many PEG molecules can lead to a loss of *in vitro* affinity due to a small reduction in the rate of association or "on-rate" (Krinner et al., 2006; Kubetzko et al., 2005; Kubetzko et al., 2006; Li et al., 2006). Recent improvements in the understanding of the properties of PEG molecules go a considerable way to clarifying this issue. Addition of a single 40kDa PEG or addition of one, two, or three molecules of 20kDa PEG at the hinge region of Fab fragments has been shown to have no measurable effect on antigen binding *in vitro* using surface plasmon resonance (Chapman et al., 1999; Humphreys et al., 2007; Koumenis et al., 2000; Leong et al., 2001). In contrast, a number of reports show that site-specific addition of 20kDa PEG to scFv reduces the affinity for antigen by ~5-fold and that this reduction is solely due to changes in the "on-rate" as measured with surface plasmon resonance (Krinner et al., 2006; Kubetzko et al., 2005; Kubetzko et al., 2006; Li et al., 2006). Kubetzko (2005) elegantly showed by both experimentation and modeling that the decrease in on-rate for scFv was solely due to intra- and inter-molecular blocking of scFv access to antigen by PEG and was not due to increased diffusion rate or decreased protein quality. The variation in affinity measurements can be explained if one takes into account the different sizes and shapes of Fab, scFv, PEG, and assay format. For example, Fab are longer and have a more inflexible rodlike shape than scFv. This means that for a Fab PEGylated at the hinge, there is a greater chance that the PEG molecule will be kept away from the CDRs. Also, in most published works, the 40kDa PEG attached to Fab is actually composed of two 20kDa PEGs; hence, the steric impact of such a PEG molecule may be more like that of a 20kDa PEG. scFv has been calculated as having a size of ~7.8nm while 20kDa PEG has a size of ~14nm; therefore, there is a clear opportunity for steric hindrance to occur (Kubetzko et al., 2005). Fab are twice as large as scFv and so are less likely to be affected by 20kDa PEG.

   Some affinity measurements with scFv-PEG have been performed with antigen coupled directly onto the surface of a measurement chip. This kind of "antigen down" assay format presents the opportunity for increasingly reduced access to antigen during the dynamic association phase of binding. This is sometimes referred to as the "random car-parking problem." In contrast, affinity measurements with Fab-PEG tend to have been performed by first capturing Fab-PEG onto the surface of a measurement chip using an anti-Fab immune reagent before passing antigen across the complex in solution phase. This "antigen up" format is less likely to suffer from "random car-parking" of the antigen. Neither assay format is more correct, but assay format clearly warrants careful consideration when performing affinity measurements.

PEG as a Linker Molecule

Many researchers have tried to covalently couple drugs to antibody fragments in order to augment their efficacy in tumor killing and cell depletion strategies. However, many of the drugs conjugated to antibodies and their fragments have low solubility and so can trigger protein aggregation. Low molecular weight PEG molecules (e.g., 0.5–1.0kDa) are often used as a "linker" between the antibody and the drug in an attempt to increase the overall solubility of the conjugate (Hurwitz 1983; McDonagh et al., 2006; Suzawa et al., 2002).

PROTEIN: PEG CONJUGATION CHEMISTRY

To achieve conjugation of PEG to protein, a number of different coupling chemistries and reactive groups are available. These have varying degrees of selectivity for the different target groups that act as points of attachment. Possible points of attachment include the N- or C-termini; the amino acid side chain groups of lysine, cysteine, tyrosine, histidine, arginine, aspartate, glutamate, serine, and threonine; and carbohydrate moieties. The attachment of PEG can be achieved enzymatically as well as chemically. Enzyme catalyzed conjugations using transglutaminase attach PEG to glutamate side chains (Sato, 2002), whereas the intein system attaches PEG to the C-terminus. The reactive functionalities can be combined to generate hetero/ homo, di-, and tri-functional PEGs and can be located both proximally and distally with respect to the polymer chain.

Some of the common chemistries used in the attachment of PEG to protein are:

1. Propinaldehyde for conjugation under acidic conditions to the N-terminus for site-specific attachment.

2. N-hydroxysuccinimide ester variants for random attachment to the side chain amine of a lysine residue.

3. Hydrazine for conjugation to periodate oxidized carbohydrate or periodate oxidized N-terminal serines or threonines.

4. Succinimidyl carbonate or bezotriazole carbonate for a slow release conjugation to histidine residues.

5. Maleimide, vinyl sulfone, iodoacetamide, or orthopyridyl disulphide for the conjugation to the thiol of a cysteine residue.

6. Bis-sulphones for conjugative bridging of both cysteines of a reduced disulphide bond.

The most popular PEGylation site for antibody fragments is a single engineered surface-accessible cysteine residue. As noted previously, the native intra domain disulphide cysteines are buried within the inherently stable immunoglobulin folds and so are not accessible for reduction and hence PEGylation. Single-chain Fv fragments with a cysteine residue introduced at the C-terminus have been reduced and conjugated to a range of PEG sizes, using maleimide and o-pyridyl disulphide chemistry. Both mono- and di-homofunctional PEGs have been used to create scFv-PEG and di-scFv-PEG (Kubetzko et al., 2006; Natarajan et al., 2005). Fab fragments with a single cysteine in an engineered hinge have been PEGylated by reduction of the cysteine to a thiol and use of mono- and di-maleimide functional PEGs (Chapman et al., 1999; Chapman, 2002). Reaction conditions for PEGylation of antibody

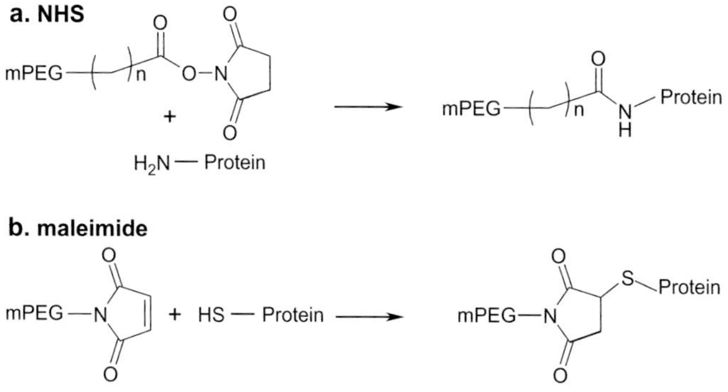

a. NHS

b. maleimide

Figure 19.1. Structures of the two most commonly used reactive groups in PEGylation.

fragments should be efficient and simple. For random PEGylation of lysine with NHS-PEG (Figure 19.1a), the antibody fragment (1–10mg/ml pH8) is mixed in a non-amine-containing buffer (e.g., phosphate, HEPES, TRICINE) with a slight molar excess of NHS-PEG reagent. The extent of PEGylation will depend on the relative molar excess of NHS-PEG used.

Random PEGylation results in a diverse range of products, and the purification and characterization of these can be challenging. In addition, the PEG may block the binding site of the antibody during conjugation, leading to a progressive loss of affinity. For site-specific PEGylation of cysteine with maleimide-PEG (Figure 19.1b), the cysteine must be in the free thiol form. Cysteines may be "capped" with small thiol-reactive compounds such as glutathione and cysteine during the production and purification process (Begg & Speicher, 1999). Therefore, solvent-accessible cysteines introduced by protein engineering should be reduced with a mono-thiol (e.g., 2-mercaptoethylamine, 2-mercaptoethanol), di-thiol (e.g., 1,4-dithiothreitol, 1,4-dithioerythritol), or phosphine (e.g., tris[2-carboxyethyl] phosphine, tris[hydroxy-propyl] phosphine) reducing agent. If the introduced solvent-accessible cysteine is the only solvent-accessible cysteine, then the phosphine and di-thiol reducing agents will be the most efficient in the reduction to a free thiol. In contrast, if there are also native solvent-accessible disulphide bonds (such as in Fab), then the mono-thiol reducing agents are most effective at selectively reducing the introduced cysteine and leaving the native disulphide intact. Finally, if the intended point of attachment is a solvent-accessible disulphide, then phosphine-reducing agents are most efficient. These are only general guidelines, and the specific conditions, in particular pH and reductant concentration, are best determined empirically. In the simplest form, where there is only one surface-accessible cysteine, a 2-fold molar excess of Tris(2-carboxyethyl) phosphine (TCEP) is added to the antibody fragment at 1–10mg/ml pH6 in an EDTA containing buffer. The TCEP can then be removed by diafiltration or gel filtration, or a large excess of maleimide-PEG added. To achieve monoPEGylation in the order of >80% efficiency from a 1:1 molar ratio of reactants, the TCEP should be removed.

Purification of specific PEGylation products from reactants and side products can also be challenging, but high resolution ion exchange chromatography can be successfully employed to achieve this. In general the "cleaner" the PEGylation reaction, the easier the separation. There are three ways in which the PEGylation reaction can be improved to ease the purification process. First, increase the amount of product in relation to all other species. This can be achieved by efficient preparation of the site of attachment and identification of the most favorable reaction conditions. Use of large molar excesses of PEG in the PEGylation reaction can aid purification by increasing the amount of product formed. However, any large excesses must be balanced against the cost of the PEG lost into the "waste" stream. Second, the higher the molecular weight of the PEG used in the conjugation, the greater the chromatographic separation between PEGylated and unPEGylated species will be. Third, use of a site-specific strategy limits the number of isoforms of PEGylated product formed in the reaction. This prevents the generation of a series of closely eluting peaks that inevitably lead to a reduction in product recovery. It follows that high-efficiency monoPEGylation with high molecular weight PEG is easier to purify than low-efficiency random PEGylation with low molecular weight PEG.

The characterization of PEGylated antibody fragments is also challenging. Sodium dodecyl sulphate polyacrylamide gel electrophoresis (SDS-PAGE) is a commonly used analytical technique, but proteins and PEG migrate differently on gels; and so when combined, the migration patterns of PEGylated proteins are difficult to predict. The bands for PEGylated proteins are also broader than for the corresponding unPEGylated protein. It is possible to visualize PEG in an SDS-PAGE gel using a barium chloride and iodine/iodide stain. However this stain is neither sensitive nor stable. Finally, random PEGylation reactions will result in a laddering pattern of the products on SDS-PAGE. The heterogeneity (polydispersity) of the PEG also presents a problem for mass spectrometric analysis. The spread of PEG sizes makes accurate molecular weight determination difficult and can also mask the mass change of other post-translational modifications to the protein. Due to its lack of a useful spectral absorption, the best technique for PEG detection during chromatography is refractive index change. However, this tends to limit the elution to isocratic gradients since changes in the refractive index signal caused by the buffer gradient can mask any change in signal produced by the PEG. The techniques described here primarily give information about the protein, PEG, or ratio of PEG to protein and so can be used to quantify the extent of PEGylation. However, they give little information on the site(s) of PEG attachment. Extensive protease mapping combined with amino acid sequencing of the peptides attached to the PEG after digestion is often required. Simplifying the complexity of this analysis is an additional benefit of site-specific PEGylation.

PEG CLEARANCE AND VISCOSITY

PEG up to ~20KDa is cleared *in vivo* to the urine whereas PEG >20KDa is cleared to both feces and urine. Chronic high dose administration of PEG has been shown to lead to the transient appearance of PEG containing vacuoles in the liver, kidney, and other tissues (Bendele et al., 1998; Webster et al., 2007). These vacuoles resolve spontaneously when PEG dosing is stopped and do not appear to compromise the function of the tissue.

PEG viscosity increases significantly with increasing size and concentration. Therefore, high concentration formulations of protein-PEG conjugates are likely to be more viscous than the unPEGylated antibody fragment. Although this may have an impact on the concentration of the final drug formulation, concentration is also affected by considerations around the proposed route and method of administration.

SUMMARY

PEGylation is a well-established and safe method for improving a number of biophysical and pharmaceutical properties of therapeutic proteins. There are at least six approved non-antibody PEGylated therapeutic proteins and one approved PEGylated antibody fragment in the clinic. Some have been in use for over 15 years, in a variety of disease indications, dose sizes, and routes of administration. It is clear that PEGylation has the ability to both alter and improve the properties of antibody fragments. Since antibody fragments have some unique and beneficial characteristics that are distinct from those of full-length glycosylated antibodies, these two technologies have become highly complementary. Therapeutic antibodies tend to be administered in higher doses than other therapeutic proteins and hence are manufactured at very large scale, something that demands the highest process efficiencies possible. This has been the main driver for the improvements and refinements in PEGylation technology described in this chapter. Site-specific addition of high molecular weight PEG in order to increase serum half-life or low molecular weight PEG to improve tumor accumulation are techniques that we expect will become more commonplace in the clinic in the future.

REFERENCES

Abuchowski, A., T. Van Es, N.C. Palczuk, and F.F. Davis. 1977a. Alteration of immunological properties of bovine serum albumin by covalent attachment of polyethylene glycol. *J. Biol. Chem.* **252**:3578–3581.

Abuchowski, A., J.R. McCoy, N.C. Palczuk, T. Van Es, and F.F. Davis. 1977b. Effect of covalent attachment of polyethylene glycol on immunogenicity and circulating life of bovine liver catalase. *J. Biol. Chem.* **252**:3582–3586.

Albrecht, H., P.A. Burke, A. Natarajan, C.Y. Xiong, M. Kalicinsky, G.L. Denardo, and S.J. Denardo. 2004. Production of soluble scFvs with C-terminal-free thiol for site-specific conjugation or stable dimeric scFvs on demand. *Bioconj. Chem.* **15**:16–26.

Albrecht, H., G.L. Denardo, and S.J. Denardo. 2006. Monospecific bivalent scFv-SH: effects of linker length and location of an engineered cysteine on production, antigen binding activity and free SH accessibility. *J. Immunol. Meth.* **310**:100–116.

Bailon, P., A. Palleroni, C.A. Schaffer, C.L. Spence, W.J. Fung, J.E. Porter, G.K. Ehrlich, W. Pan, Z.X. Xu, M.W. Modi, A. Farid, and W. Berthold. 2001. Rational design of a potent, long-lasting form of interferon: A 40kDa branched polyethylene glycol-conjugated interferon α-2a for the treatment of hepatitis C. *Bioconj. Chem.* **12**:195–202.

Balan, S., J.W. Choi, A. Godwin, I. Teo, C.M. Laborde, S. Heidelberger, M. Zloh, S. Shaunak, and S. Brocchini. 2007. Site-specific PEGylation of protein disulfide bonds using a three carbon bridge. *Bioconj. Chem.* **18**:61–76.

Basu, A., A.L. Et, and D. Filpula. 2006. Structure-function engineering of interferon-β-1b for improving stability, solubility, potency, immunogenicity, and pharmacokinetic properties by site-selective mono-PEGylation. *Bioconj. Chem.* **17**:618–630.

Baudys, M., D. Letourneur, F. Liu, D. Mix, J. Jozefonvicz, and S.W. Kim. 1998. Extending insulin action *in vivo* by conjugation to carboxymethyl dextran. *Bioconj. Chem.* **9**:176–183.

Bazin-Redureau, M.I., C.B. Renard, and J.M.G. Scherrmann. 1997. Pharmacokinetics of heterologous and homologous immunoglobulin G, F(ab′)$_2$ and Fab after intravenous administration in the rat. *J. Pharmaceut. Pharmacol.* **49**:277–281.

Begg, G.E., and D.W. Speicher. 1999. Mass spectrometry detection and reduction of disulfide adducts between reducing agents and recombinant proteins with highly reactive cysteines. *J. Biomol. Techniques.* **10**:17–20.

Bendele, A., J. Seely, C. Richey, G. Sennello, and G. Shopp. 1998. Short communication: renal tubular vacuolation in animals treated with polyethylene-glycol-conjugated proteins. *Toxicological Sci.* **42**:152–157.

Bray, J., B.G. Robinson, and J. Byrne. 1984. Influence of charge on filtration across renal basement membranes on films *in vitro*. *Kidney Interntl.* **25**:527–533.

Brocchini, S., S. Balan, A. Godwin, J.W. Choi, M. Zloh, and S. Shaunak. 2006. PEGylation of native disulphide bonds in proteins. *Nature Protocols.* **1**:2241–2252.

Brown, B.A., R.D. Corneau, P.L. Jones, F.A. Libertore, W.P. Neacy, H. Sands, and B.M. Gallagher. 1987. Pharmacokinetics of the monoclonal antibody B72.3 and its fragments labelled with either ^{125}I or [111]In. *Cancer Res.* **47**:1149–1154.

Buist, M.R., P. Kenemans, W. Den Hollander, J.B. Vermorken, C.J.M. Molthoff, C.W. Burger, T.J.M. Helmerhorst, J.P.A. Baak, and J.C. Roos. 1993. Kinetics and tissue distribution of the radiolabeled chimeric monoclonal antibody Mov18 IgG and F(ab′)$_2$ fragments in ovarian carcinoma patients. *Cancer Res.* **53**:5413–5418.

Caliceti, P., O. Schiavon, and F.M. Veronese. 1999. Biopharmaceutical properties of uricase conjugated to neutral and amphiphilic polymers. *Bioconj. Chem.* **10**:638–646.

Chang, R.L.S., I.F. Ueki, J.L. Troy, W.M. Deen, C.R. Robertson, and B.M. Brenner. 1975. Permselectivity of the glomerular capillary wall to macromolecules. *Biophysical J.* **15**:887–906.

Chapman, A.P., P. Antoniw, M. Spitali, S. West, S. Stephens, and D.J. King. 1999. Therapeutic antibody fragments with prolonged *in vivo* half-lives. *Nature Biotechnol.* **17**:780–783.

Chapman, A.P. 2002. PEGylated antibodies and antibody fragments for improved therapy: a review. *Adv. Drug Del. Reviews.* **54**:531–545.

Covell, D.G., J. Barbet, O.D. Holton, C.D.V. Black, R.J. Parker, and J.N. Weinstein. 1986. Pharmacokinetics of monoclonal Immunoglobulins γ1, F(ab′)$_2$, and Fab′ in Mice. *Cancer Res.* **46**:3969–3978.

Cunningham-Rundles, C., Z.H.O.U. Zhuo, B. Griffith, and J. Keenan. 1992. Biological activities of polyethylene-glycol immunoglobulin conjugates. *J. Immunol. Meth.* **152**:177–190.

Davis, S., A. Abuchowski, Y.K. Park, and F.F. Davis. 1981. Alteration of the circulating life and antigenic properties of bovine adenosine deaminase in mice by attachment of polyethylene glycol. *Clin. Exp. Immunol.* **46**:649–652.

Delgado, C., R.B. Pedley, A. Herraez, R. Boden, J.A. Boden, P.A. Keep, K.A. Chester, D. Fisher, R.H.J. Begent, and G.E. Francis. 1996. Enhanced tumour specificity of an anti-carcinoembrionic antigen Fab fragments by poly(ethylene glycol) (PEG) modification. *Brit. J. Cancer.* **73**:175–182.

Duncan, R. 2003. The dawning era of polymer therapeutics. *Nature Rev.* **2**:347–360.

Fagnani, R., M.S. Hagan, and R. Bartholomew. 1990. Reduction of immunogenicity by covalent modification of murine and rabbit immunoglobulins with oxidized dextrans of low molecular weight. *Cancer Res.* **50**:3638–3645.

Gillies, E.R., E. Dy, J.M.J. Frechet, and F.C. Szoka. 2005. Biological evaluation of polyester dendrimer: poly(ethylene oxide) "bow-tie" hybrids with tunable molecular weight and architecture. *Mol. Pharmaceutics.* **2**:129–138.

Gregoriadis, G., A. Fernandes, M. Mital, and B. McCormack. 2000. Polysialic acids: potential in improving the stability and pharmacokinetics of proteins and other therapeutics. *Cellular Mol. Life Sci.* **57**:1964–1969.

Grene-Lerouge, N.A.M., M.I. Bazin-Redureau, M. Debray, and J.M.G. Scherrmann. 1996. Interspecies scaling of clearance and volume of distribution for digoxin-specific Fab. *Toxicol. Appl. Pharmacol.* **138**:84–89.

Gutiérrez, J.M., G. Leon, and B. Lomonte. 2003. Pharmacokinetic-pharmacodynamic relationships of immunoglobulin therapy for envenomation. *Clin. Pharmacokinetics.* **42**:721–741.

Han, H.D., A. Lee, T. Hwang, C.K. Song, H. Seong, J. Hyun, and B.C. Shin. 2007. Enhanced circulation time and antitumour activity of doxorubicin by comb-like polymer-incorporated liposome. *J. Controlled Rel.* **120**:161–168.

Humphreys, D.P., S.P. Heywood, A. Henry, L. Ait-Lhadj, P. Antoniw, R. Palframan, K.J. Greenslade, B. Carrington, D.G. Reeks, L.C. Bowering, S. West, and H.A. Brand. 2007. Alternative antibody Fab fragment PEGylation strategies: combination of strong reducing agents, disruption of the interchain disulphide bond and disulphide engineering. *Prot. Eng. Des. Sel.* **20**: 227–234.

Humphreys, D.P. 2003. Production of antibodies and antibody fragments in *Escherichia coli* and a comparison of their functions, uses and modification. *Cur. Opin. Drug Dis. Devel.* **6**:188–196.

Hurwitz, E. 1983. Specific and nonspecific macromolecule-drug conjugates for the improvement of cancer chemotherapy. *Biopolymers.* **22**:557–567.

Jultani, A., C. Li, M. Ozen, M. Yadav, S. Yu, S. Wallace, and S. Pathak. 1997. Paclitaxel and water-soluble poly(L-glutamic acid)-paclitaxel, induce direct chromosomal abnormalities and cell death in a murine metastatic melanoma cell line. *Anticancer Res.* **17**:4269–4274.

Kamisaki, Y., H. Wada, T. Yagura, A. Matsushima, and Y. Inada. 1981. Reduction in immunogenicity and clearance rate of *Escherichia coli* L-asparaginase by modification with monomethoxypolyethylene glycol. *J. Pharmacol. Exp. Therapeutics.* **216**:410–414.

Kaneda, Y., Y. Tsutsumi, Y. Yoshioka, H. Kamada, Y. Yamamoto, H. Kodaira, S. Tsunoda, T. Okamoto, Y. Mukai, H. Shibata, S. Nakagawa, and T. Mayumi. 2004. The use of PVP as a polymeric carrier to improve plasma half-life of drugs. *Biomaterials.* **25**:3259–3266.

Keyler, D.E., D.M. Salerno, M.M. Mukakami, G. Ruth, and P.R. Pentel. 1991. Rapid administration of high-dose human antibody Fab fragments to dogs: pharmacokinetics and toxicity. *Fund. Appl. Toxicol.* **17**:83–91.

King, D.J., A. Turner, A.P.H. Farnsworth, J.R. Adair, R.J. Owens, B. Pedley, D. Baldock, K.A. Proudfoot, A.D.G. Lawson, N.R.A. Beeley, K. Millar, T.A. Millican, B.A. Boyce, P. Antoniw, A. Mountain, R.H.J. Begent, D. Shochat, and G.T. Yarranton. 1994. Improved tumour targeting with chemically cross-linked recombinant antibody fragments. *Cancer Res.* **54**:6176–6185.

Kitamura, K., T. Takahashi, K.I. Takashina, T. Yamaguchi, A. Noguchi, H. Tsurumi, T. Tokokuni, and S.I. Hakomori. 1990. Polyethylene glycol modification of the monoclonal antibody A7 enhances its tumour localization. *Biochem. Biophys. Res. Comms.* **171**:1387–1394.

Knight, D.M., R.E. Jordan, M. Kruszynski, S.H. Tam, J. Gile-Komar, G. Treacy, and G.A. Heavner. 2004. Pharmacodynamic enhancement of the anti-platelet antibody Fab abciximab by site-specific PEGylation. *Platelets.* **15**:409–418.

Kobayashi, H., N. Le, I.S. Kim, M.K. Kim, J.E. Pie, D. Drumm, D.S. Paik, T.A. Waldmann, C.H. Paik, and J.A. Carrasquillo. 1999. The pharmacokinetic characteristics of glycolated humanized anti-Tac Fabs are determined by their isoelectric points. *Cancer Res.* **59**:422–430.

Koumenis, I., Z. Shahrokh, S. Leong, V. Hsei, L. Deforge, and G. Zapata. 2000. Modulating pharmacokinetics of an anti-interleukin-8 F(ab')$_2$ by amine-specific PEGylation with preserved bioactivity. *Interntl. J. Pharmaceutics.* **198**:83–95.

Krinner, E.M., J. Hepp, P. Hoffmann, S. Bruckmaier, L. Petersen, S. Petsch, L. Parr, I. Schuster, S. Mangold, G. Lorenczewski, M. Strasser, C. Itin, A. Wolf, A. Basu, K. Yang, D. Filpula, P. Sorensen, P. Kufer, P. Baeuerle, and T. Raum. 2006. A highly stable polyethylene glycol-conjugated human single-chain antibody neutralizing granulocyte-macrophage colony stimulating factor at low nanomolar concentration. *Prot. Eng. Des. Sel.* **19**:461–470.

Kubetzko, S., C.A. Sarkar, and A. Plückthun. 2005. Protein PEGylation decreases observed target association rates via a dual blocking mechanism. *Mol. Pharmacol.* **68**:1439–1454.

Kubetzko, S., E. Balic, R. Waibel, U. Zangemeister-Wittke, and A. Plückthun. 2006. PEGylation and multimerization of the anti-p185HER-2 single chain Fv fragment 4D5. *J. Biol. Chem.* **46**:35186–35201.

Leong, S.R., L. Deforge, L. Presta, T. Gonzalez, A. Fan, M. Reichert, A. Chuntharapai, K.J. Kim, D.B. Tumas, W.P. Lee, P. Gribling, B. Snedecor, H. Chen, V. Hsei, M. Schoenhoff, V. Hale, J. Deveney, I. Koumenis, E. and G. Zapata. 2001. Adapting pharmacokinetic properties of a humanised anti-interleukin-8 antibody for therapeutic applications using site-specific PEGylation. *Cytokine.* **16**:106–119.

Li, L., P.J. Yazaki, A.L. Anderson, D. Crow, D. Colcher, A.M. Wu, L.E. Williams, J.Y.C. Wong, A. Raubitschek, and J.E. Shively. 2006. Improved biodistribution and radioimmunoimaging with poly(ethylene glycol)-DOTA-conjugated anti-CEA diabody. *Bioconj. Chem.* **17**:68–76.

Loiseau, F.A., K.K. Hii, and A.M. Hill. 2004. Multigram synthesis of well defined extended bifunctional polyethylene glycol (PEG) chains. *J. Organic Chem.* **69**:639–647.

Maack, T., V. Johnson, S.T. Kau, J. Figueredo, and D. Sigulem. 1979. Renal filtration, transport, and metabolism of low-molecular-weight proteins: A review. *Kidney Interntl.* **16**:251–270.

Mabry, R., M. Rani, R. Geiger, G.B. Hubbard, R. Carrion, K. Brasky, J.L. Patterson, G. Georgiou, and B.L. Iverson. 2005. Passive protection against anthrax by using a high affinity antitoxin antibody fragment lacking an Fc region. *Infect. Immunity.* **73**:8362–8368.

Macfarlane, D.J., R.C. Smart, W.W. Tsui, M. Gerometta, P.R. Eisenberg, and A.M. Scott. 2006. Safety, pharmacokinetic and dositmetry evaluation of the proposed thrombus imaging agent ^{99m}Tc-DI-DD-3B6/22-80B3 Fab. *Eur. J. Nucl. Med. Molec. Imaging.* **33**:648–656.

Matsumura, Y., and H. Maeda. 1986. A new concept for macromolecular therapeutics in cancer chemotherapy: mechanism of tumoritropic accumulation of proteins and the antitumour agents SMANCS. *Cancer Res.* **46**:6387–6392.

Matsushima, A., H. Nishimura, Y. Ashihara, Y. Yakata, and Y. Inada. 1980. Modification of *E. coli* asparaginase with 2,4-bis (o-methoxypolyethylene glycol)-6-chloro-s-triazine (activated PEG2); disappearance of binding towards anti-serum and retention of enzymatic activity. *Chem. Letts.*: 773–776.

McDonagh, C.F., E. Turcot, L. Westendorf, J.B. Webster, S.C. Alley, K. Kim, J. Andreyka, I. Stone, K.J. Hamblett, J.A. Francisco, and P. Carter. 2006. Engineered antibody-drug conjugates with defined sites and stoichiometries of drug attachment. *Prot. Eng. Des. Sel.* **19**:299–307.

Milenic, D.E., T. Yokota, D.R. Filpula, M.A.J. Finkelman, S.W. Dodd, J.F. Wood, M. Whitlow, P. Snoy, and J. Schlom. 1991. Construction, binding properties, metabolism, and tumour targeting of a single chain Fv derived from the pancarcinoma monoclonal antibody CC49. *Cancer Res.* **51**:6363–6371.

Monfardini, C., O. Schiavon, P. Caliceti, M. Morpurgo, J.M. Harris, and F.M. Veronese. 1995. A branched monomethoxypoly (ethylene glycol) for protein modification. *Bioconj. Chem.* **6**:62–69.

Mozier, N.M. 2003. Antibody PEG positional isomers, compositions comprising same and use thereof. WO 03/099226 A2.

Natarajan, A., C.Y. Xiong, H. Albrecht, G.L. Denardo, and S.J. Denardo. 2005. Characterization of site-specific scFv PEGylation for tumor-targeting pharmaceuticals. *Bioconj. Chem.* **16**:113–121.

Onda, M., J.J. Vincent, B. Lee, and I. Pastan. 2003. Mutants of immunotoxin anti-Tac (dsFv)-PE38 with variable number of lysine residus as candidates for site-specific chemical modification. 1. Properties of mutant molecules. *Bioconj. Chem.* **14**:480–487.

Pedley, R.B., J.A. Boden, R. Boden, R.H.J. Begent, A. Turner, A.M.R. Haines, and D.J. King. 1994. The potential for enhanced tumour localisation by poly (ethylene glycol) modification of anti-CEA antibody. *Brit. J. Cancer.* **70**:1126–1130.

Rabkin, R., and Dahl, D.C. 1993. Hormones and the kidney. In *Diseases of the Kidney* (5th ed), edited by Schrier, R.B. and Gottschalk, C.W. Boston: Little, Brown and Company, pp. 283–334.

Richter, A.W., and E. Åkerblom. 1983. Antibodies against polyethylene glycol produced in animals by immunisation with monomethoxy polyethylene glycol modified proteins. *Interntl. Arch. Allergy Appl. Immunol.* **70**:124–131.

Richter, A.W., and E. Åkerblom. 1984. Polyethylene glycol reactive antibodies in man: titer distribution in allergic patients treated with monomethoxy polythylene glycol modified allergens of placebo, and in healthy blood donors. *Interntl. Arch. Allergy Appl. Immunol.* **74**:36–39.

Rolan, P., M. Baker, F. Stringer, and S. Stephens. 2008. Pharmacokinetics of certolizumab pegol (CDP870), a PEGylated Fab anti-TNFα monoclonal antibody. *Brit. J. Clin. Pharmacol.* in press.

Rose-John, S., and H. Schooltink. 2003. CDP-870 Celltech/Pfizer. *Curr. Opin. Investl. Drugs.* **4**:588–592.

Sato, H. 2002. Enzymatic procedure for site-specific pegylation of proteins. *Adv. Drug Del. Rev.* **54**:487–504.

Schlapschy, M., I. Theobald, H. Mack, M. Schottelius, H.J. Wester, and A. Skerra. 2007. Fusion of a recombinant antibody fragment with a homo-amino-acid polymer: effects on biophysical properties and prolongues plasma half-life. *Prot. Eng., Des. Sel.* **20**:273–284.

Schreiber, S., M. Khaliq-Kareemi, I.C. Lawrance, O.Ø. Thomsen, S.B. Hanauer, J. McColm, R. Bloomfield, and W.J. Sandborn. 2007. Maintenance therapy with certolizumab pegol for crohn's disease. *New Eng. J. Med.* **357**:239–250.

Shaunak, S., A. Godwin, J.W. Choi, S. Balan, E. Pedone, D. Vijayarangam, S. Heidelberger, I. Teo, M. Zloh, and S. Brocchini. 2006. Site-specific PEGylation of native disulfide bonds in therapeutic proteins. *Nat. Chemical Biol.* **2**:312–313.

Soucek, J., P. Pouckova, J. Strohalm, D. Plocova, D. Hlouskova, M. Zadinova, and K. Ulbrich. 2002. Poly(N-2(2-hydroxypropyl)methylacrylamide) conjugates of bovine pancreatic ribonuclease (RNase A) inhibit growth of human melanoma in nude mice. *J. Drug Targeting.* **10**:175–183.

Suzawa, T., S. Nagamura, H. Saito, S. Ohta, N. Hanai, J. Kanazawa, M. Okabe, and M. Yamasaki. 2002. Enhanced tumor cell selectivity of adriamycin-monoclonal antibody conjugate via a poly(ethylene glycol)-based cleavable linker. *J. Controlled Rel.* **79**:229–242.

Trakas, N., and S.J. Tzartos. 2001. Conjugation of acetylcholine receptor-protecting Fab fragments with polyethylene glycol results in a prolonged half-life in the circulation and reduced immunogenicity. *J. Neuroimmunol.* **120**:42–49.

Tsutsumi, Y., M. Onda, S. Nagata, B. Lee, R.J. Kreitman, and I. Pastan. 2000. Site-specific chemical modification with polyethylene glycol of recombinant immunotoxin anti-Tac(Fv)-PE38 (LMB-2) improves antitumour activity and reduces animal toxicity and immunogenicity. *Pro. Natl. Acad. Sci., U.S.A.* **97**:8548–8553.

Ujhelyi, M.R., and S. Robert. 1995. Pharmacokinetic aspects of digoxin-specific Fab therapy in the management of digitalis toxicity. *Clin. Pharmacokinetics.* **28**:483–493.

Vázquez, H., A. Chávez-Haro, W. García-Ubbelohde, R. Mancilla-Nava, J. Paniagua-Solís, A. Alagón, and C. Sevcik. 2005. Pharmacokinetics of a F(ab′)$_2$ scorpion antivenom in healthy human volunteers. *Toxicon.* **46**:797–805.

Vellard, M. 2003. The enzyme as drug: application of enzymes as pharmaceuticals. *Curr. Opin. Biotechnol.* **14**:444–450.

Webster, R., E. Didier, P. Harris, N. Siegel, J. Stadler, L. Tilbury, and D. Smith. 2007. PEGylated proteins: evaluation of their safety in the absence of definitive metabolism studies. *Drug Metab. Disposition.* **35**:9–16.

Wilkinson, I., C.J.C. Jackson, G.M. Lang, V. Holford-Stevens, and A.H. Sehon. 1987. Tolerogenic polyethylene glycol derivatives of xenogeneic monoclonal immunoglobulins. *Immunol. Letters.* **15**:17–22.

Williams, L.E., A.M. Wu, P.J. Yazaki, A. Liu, A.A. Raubitschek, J.E. Shively, and T.Y.C. Wong. 2001. Numerical selection of optimal tumour imaging agents with application to engineered antibodies. *Canc. Biotherapy Radiopharmaceut.* **16**:25–35.

Working, P.K., M.S. Newman, and J. Johnson. 1997. Safety of poly(ethylene glycol) and poly(ethylene glycol) derivatives. In *Poly(ethylene glycol) Chemistry and Biological Applications,* edited by Harris, J.M., and Zalipsky, S. Washington: ACS Books, pp. 45–57.

Wunderlich, D.A., M. Macdougall, D.V. Mierz, J.G. Toth, T.M. Buckholz, K.J. Lumb, and H.V. Vasa-
vada. 2007. Generation and characterisation of a monoclonal IgG antibody to polyethylene glycol.
Hybridoma. **26**:168–172.

Xiong, C.Y., A. Natarjan, X.B. Shi, G.L. Denardo, and S.J. Denardo. 2006. Development of tumour
targeting anti-MUC-1 multimer: effects of di-scFv unpaired cysteine location on PEGylation and
tumour binding. *Prot. Eng. Des. Sel.* **19**:359–367.

Yang, K., A. Basu, M. Wang, R. Chintala, M.C. Hsieh, J. Hua, J. Zhou, M. Li, H. Phyu, G. Petti, H. Phyi,
G. Petti, M. Mendez, H. Janjua, P. Peng, C. Longley, V. Borowski, M. Mehlig, and D. Filpula. 2003.
Tailoring structure-function and pharmacokinetic properties of single-chain Fv proteins by site-
specific PEGylation. *Prot. Eng.* **16**:761–770.

Yoshioka, Y., Y. Tsutsumi, S. Ikemizu, Y. Yamamoto, H. Shibata, T. Nishibata, Y. Mukai, T. Okamoto,
M. Taniai, M. Kawamura, Y. Abe, S. Nakagawa, S. Nagata, Y. Yamagata, and T. Mayumi. 2004.
Optimal site-specific PEGylation of mutant TNF-α improves its antitumour potency. *Biochem.
Biophys. Res. Comms.* **315**:808–814.

Zunino, F., F. Giuliani, G. Davi, T. Dasdis, and R. Gambetta. 1982. Anti-tumour activity of daunorubicin linked to poly-L-aspartic acid. *Interntl. J. Cancer.* **30**:465–470.

CHAPTER TWENTY

Extending Antibody Fragment Half-Lives with Albumin

Jan Terje Andersen and Inger Sandlie

Albumin is the most abundant protein in serum and acts as a multifunctional carrier for many endogenous small molecules, as diverse as fatty acids, metals, bilirubin, amino acids, and vitamins that ensure wide biodistribution of these compounds throughout the body. In addition, its remarkably long half-life of 19 days in humans makes albumin a versatile and preferred carrier for small molecule and protein therapeutics. A receptor-mediated pathway controlled by the neonatal Fc receptor (FcRn) has recently been shown to be essential for regulation of the long half-life of albumin as well as IgG. This new discovery will strongly influence the further development of albumin-fused and albumin-targeting diagnostics and therapeutics.

The IgG class has a remarkably long serum half-life of 21 days in humans.[1,2] The utility of the mAbs spans across clinical settings such as treatment of cancer, chronic inflammatory and autoimmune diseases as well as transplantation and cardiovascular disease.[3–6] Such treatments require large quantities of mAbs; a restriction that limits their use is the manufacturing cost in mammalian production systems.[7] The most promising alternatives are production in yeast and bacteria of Ab derived fragments such as the Fab, F(ab')$_2$ and single-chain Fv (ScFv) (Figure 20.1A–C). These lack the Fc part and Fc-associated functions, which may be favorable when complement activation and FcγR-mediated effector functions are inconvenient. However, elimination of the Fc also removes the half-life extending mechanism mediated by interaction of Fc with FcRn.[8] For instance, the half-life of Fab and F(ab')$_2$ fragments is only about 1% to 5% of that of intact IgG.[6,9] Thus, the "naked" fragments have limited value because of rapid elimination from the body, a consequence of extremely fast renal filtration.

Pharmacokinetics are influenced by molecular size and the ability to recycle via FcRn. Molecular size is crucial since smaller size improves diffusion rate, extravasation, and tissue penetration; larger size abrogates clearance through the kidney and thus increases half-life. In this review, we briefly describe the biology of FcRn and how FcRn regulates IgG and albumin homeostasis. We then summarize and discuss how different strategies are used to link therapeutics to albumin, either directly, by fusion or covalent linking, or indirectly, by targeting to albumin using "albumin affinity tags."

FcRn INTERACTS WITH IgG AND ALBUMIN

FcRn is structurally related to classical major histocompatibility complex class (MHC) I molecules and consists of a unique heavy chain non-covalently associated

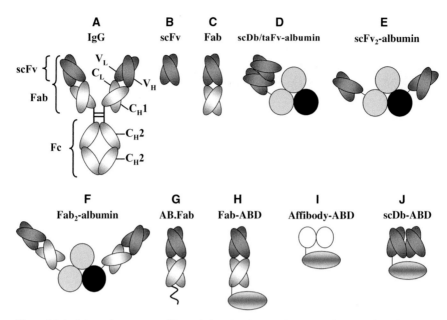

Figure 20.1. Schematic structure of intact IgG and various engineered antibody-derived fragments targeting albumin or fused to albumin. (A) Intact IgG, (B) scFv, (C) Fab, (D) scDb/tcFv-albumin, (E) scFv$_2$-albumin, (F) Fab$_2$-albumin, (G) AB.Fab, (H) Fab-ABD, (I) affibody-ABD, and (J) scDb-ABD.

with the common β2-microglobulin (β2m) subunit.[10–12] MHC class I molecules bind and present peptides to CD8+ T cells via the peptide binding groove created by the folded heavy chain.[13] The corresponding binding groove in the FcRn structure is occluded and this prevents binding of peptides.[10–12] Instead, FcRn has evolved to bind IgG and albumin at distal binding sites on the α2-domain of the heavy chain.[14–16] An illustration of human FcRn with its ligand binding sites for IgG and serum albumin is shown in Figure 20.2A. Both interactions are highly pH dependent, with binding at acidic pH (6.0–6.5) and no binding at physiological pH.[14,15,17,18] The pH stringency is mediated by protonation of conserved histidine residues at the transition from pH 7.4 to an acidic pH.

The FcRn-IgG interaction has been extensively characterized by site-directed mutagenesis and crystallographic mapping and shown to be dependent on histidine residues at the C$_H$2-C$_H$3 interface (H310 and H435; Figure 20.2B) that interact with exposed negatively charged residues on the FcRn α2-domain (Figure 20.2A).[11,12,19,20] Simultaneously, domain III (DIII) of albumin may bind to a putative cluster of conserved residues on the opposite side of the α2-domain.[15,17] Mutation of a central histidine residue (H166) within this cluster totally disrupts binding to albumin at acidic pH (Figure 20.2A) but retains its ability to interact with IgG.[15] Furthermore, H166 is conserved across species in all known FcRn heavy chain sequences, an observation that supports a role for H166 in the interaction with albumin. The exact mapping of the binding site for FcRn on DIII of albumin is still lacking, however.

Although IgG and albumin interact with FcRn by the same pH dependent histidine-mediated mechanism, they have totally different binding affinities.[15,17] While FcRn interacts with albumin monovalently with low micromolar affinity, the

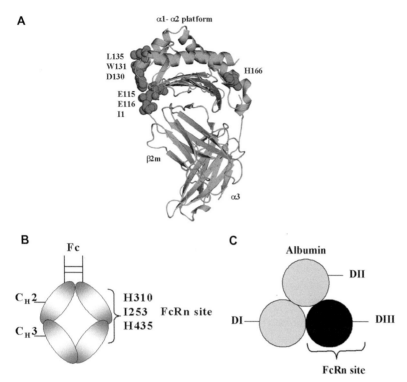

A

α1- α2 platform

L135
W131
D130

H166

E115
E116
I1

β2m

α3

B

Fc

C_H2

C_H3

H310
I253   FcRn site
H435

C

Albumin

DII

DI

DIII

FcRn site

Figure 20.2. FcRn, IgG Fc, and albumin. (A) The crystal structure of shFcRn with the localization of the amino acids essential for IgG (E115, E116, D130, W131, and L135) and albumin (H166) binding highlighted. The heavy chain is shown in green and the β2m in orange. (B) IgG Fc. Amino acids (H310, H435 and I253) at the Fc elbow region involved in binding to FcRn are highlighted. (C) Albumin consists of three domains denoted DI, DII, and DIII. The putative FcRn binding site on DIII is in black. The figure in (A) was designed using pyMOL with the crystallographic data of the shFcRn crystal.[12] [See color plate.]

interaction with IgG has been demonstrated to follow more complex binding kinetics with a high nanomolar affinity. The biological consequence, if any, of this distinct difference is unknown.

FcRn REGULATES IgG AND ALBUMIN HOMEOSTASIS

F. W. Rogers Brambell (1901–1970) was the first to postulate the existence of a cell-bound receptor responsible for both specific maternofetal transmission and serum protection of IgG.[21,22] Furthermore, Brambell and others demonstrated that both processes were dependent on the Fc part of IgG and not the Fabs.[22–24] Several observations during the following decades supported Brambell's hypothesis, and indeed, a membrane-spanning receptor, FcRn, was identified.[14,25] Initially, cloning of the rodent FcRn from the intestine of neonatal rats and subsequent crystallographic studies uncovered the pH dependent FcRn-IgG interaction site.[10,11,19,20,26] Furthermore, the human form of FcRn was cloned and crystallographic studies showed its great homology to rodent FcRn.[12,27] Functional studies of mutant murine IgGs showed that impaired FcRn binding correlates with lowered serum half-life.[28]

The generation of mice deficient in either the FcRn heavy chain or β2m conclusively demonstrated the significance of FcRn in IgG homeostasis.[29–34] Importantly, this new knowledge has been used to improve the serum persistence of small therapeutic proteins. Genetic fusions between such molecules and Fc have been made, and extending the half-life greatly increased their drug efficiency.[34–39] The close correlation between IgG serum persistence and stringent pH dependent affinity for FcRn has led to engineering of a new family of therapeutic Abs with half-lives longer than that of endogenous IgG.[40–43] Furthermore, a spectrum of mAbs with low or intermediate affinity for FcRn has been generated that rapidly clear from the circulation,[44,45] a feature demonstrated to be optimal for Ab-based tumor imaging.[45,46]

The interaction between FcRn and albumin was discovered by chance during purification of recombinant soluble human FcRn on an IgG coupled column when bovine albumin co-eluted with the receptor.[18] Subsequently, studies showed that human FcRn was able to bind human albumin in a pH-dependent manner as described.[15,17,18] This observation revived an old hypothesis postulated by Brambell's contemporaries, Schultze and Heremans.[47] They proposed that the presence of a receptor similar to the one studied by Brambell could account for the long half-life and concentration-dependent rate of degradation observed for albumin, as albumin has an unexpectedly long serum half-life of ~19 days in humans.[48] Notably, they suggested that a distinct albumin specific receptor, different from the one specific for IgG, could rescue albumin from degradation. However, we and others[15,17] have conclusively shown that FcRn is a bifunctional receptor that binds both IgG and albumin, at different sites and in a noncooperative manner. FcRn deficient mice lacking either the FcRn heavy chain or the β2m catabolized albumin twice as fast as wild-type mice.[18] In this context, it is interesting that the rare disease, human familial hypercatabolic hypoproteinemia, is characterized by very low serum levels of both IgG and albumin.[49] Investigation of two affected individuals showed that while the FcRn heavy chain encoding gene sequence was normal, the β2m encoding gene contained a single nucleotide mutation that altered the coding from alanine to proline (A11P) in the signal sequence.[50] Transfection of the β2m A11P mutant gene into a β2m deficient cell line decreased FcRn expression by 80% compared to wild-type β2m, which strongly suggests that the albumin receptor defined by Schultze and Heremans is identical to the receptor described by Brambell.

THE FcRn RECYCLING PATHWAY

IgG and albumin are present in the plasma at high concentrations, 12 mg/ml and 40 mg/ml, respectively.[5,6,48] Therefore, both molecules are continually taken up by plasma-exposed cells via fluid phase endocytosis. Unlike other endocytosed proteins, both are salvaged from lysosomal degradation by FcRn-mediated recycling.[14,16,25] Originally, the process was thought to take place in the vascular endothelium that covers several organs in addition to the bloodstream.[16,51,52] However, as FcRn has been documented to be widely expressed in organs such as liver[14,53,54] and kidneys[14,55,56] in addition to placenta,[27,57–63] and lately, in different immune cells,[14, 64–66] it is at present not clear whether FcRn at all tissue sites contributes to the homeostatic regulation of its ligands. Recently, Akilesh et al.[14] found FcRn to be highly expressed in bone marrow-derived cells and antigen-presenting cells in various tissues; using bone marrow chimeras, they showed that these significantly contribute to IgG protection. In this study, the homeostatic regulation of albumin was not addressed. It is conceivable that other sites highly exposed to circulating IgG and albumin, like the liver and kidney, also contribute to protection of the ligands.

Studies in endothelial cell lines show that FcRn binds IgG in acidified sorting endosomes and diverts it away from unbound proteins.[67–70] The FcRn-IgG complexes reside in tubular extensions from the sorting endosome that create rapidly mobile compartments.[67,68,70] Next, the complexes are exocytosed via the secretory pathway back to the cell surface where the physiological pH of the blood (pH 7.2–7.4) facilitates release into the circulation. A simplified overview of the FcRn-mediated recycling pathway is shown (Figure 20.3). Interestingly, Ober et al.[67,68] have shown that FcRn may transport IgG to the membrane using either of two distinct pathways. The classical pathway is characterized by complete fusion of the secretory compartment with the cell membrane. In the second route, only partial and repetitive cell membrane fusion, the so-called "kiss-and-run" pathway, is apparent.

PHARMACEUTICAL UTILIZATION OF SERUM ALBUMIN

Albumin is responsible for the colloidal osmotic pressure and buffers the pH of the blood.[48] In addition, albumin acts as a multifunctional carrier for many endogenous small molecules such as bilirubin, fatty acids, metals, amino acids, vitamins, and

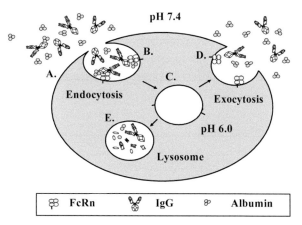

Figure 20.3. The FcRn-mediated recycling pathway. Circulating IgG and albumin (A) are continually taken up by fluid phase endocytosis (B) and enter weakly acidified compartments where FcRn resides. FcRn captures IgG and albumin in a pH-dependent manner facilitated by the acidic milieu in endosomes (C), and both ligands are thereby diverted away from the lysosomal degradation pathway and exocytosed to the cell membrane (D). When exocytotic vesicles fuse with the cell membrane, the increase in pH induces release of IgG and albumin back into the circulation. If the FcRn recycling pathway is saturated, unbound ligands are diverted to lysosomes for proteolytic degradation (E).

selected exogenous compounds, and thereby contributes to the wide distribution of all these throughout the body.[48] Albumin is normally a non-glycosylated single polypeptide (585 amino acids) with a molecular weight of 67 kDa, and crystallographic studies have shown that it mainly consists of α helices linked by flexible loops and stabilized via 17 conserved disulfide bridges.[71] It forms a heart-shaped structure with three homologous domains denoted DI, DII, and DIII. A schematic illustration of albumin is shown in Figure 20.2C. Noteworthy is the existence of rare polymorphic albumin variants with amino acid substitutions, splice-site or frame-shift mutations that may cause truncation or elongation of DIII.[72] The variants often have altered biodistribution and half-life compared to normal circulating albumin.[73]

Purified albumin is widely used as a stabilizing component in pharmaceutical products such as vaccines.[48,74,75] Clinically, albumin has been used to treat acute circulatory conditions like hypoalbuminemia, shock due to blood loss, burns and surgery.[48] The albumin preparations used are obtained from blood donors, but alternative industrial methods to obtain recombinant albumin are now being explored using yeast as the host organism.[75,76]

The remarkably long half-life of albumin was well recognized before its relationship with FcRn was discovered, and was utilized to enhance the *in vivo* effect of therapeutic substances. Specifically, substances of interest were covalently coupled to albumin. Tumors are known to have increased fluid phase endocytosis compared to healthy tissue and use circulating serum albumin as a major nitrogen and energy source.[48,77] This has been utilized for tumor targeting of therapeutics to achieve high tumor accumulation, low liver uptake, and extended half-life. One illustrating example is albumin covalently coupled to methotrexate (albumin-MTX).[78–82]

In addition to covalent coupling to albumin itself, approaches focusing on non-covalent association with albumin by way of covalent coupling to an "albumin affinity tag" have shown promising results. Albumin binds and transports endogenous fatty acids,[48,83] a property that has been utilized to optimize the pharmacokinetics of insulin. Insulin was coupled to myristate which associates with albumin and thus gained extended half-life.[84–88] Slow dissociation from albumin increased the duration of the therapeutic effect. The half-life of an anticoagulant peptide has been dramatically increased in rabbits by addition of phosphate ester tags to the amino terminus that induces binding to albumin.[89,90]

GENETIC FUSION OF THERAPEUTIC PROTEINS TO ALBUMIN

A number of reports exist that describe genetic fusion between albumin and a therapeutic protein. Examples are hirudin,[91] CD4,[92] insulin (Albulin),[93] growth hormone (Albutropin),[94] granulocyte colony-stimulating factor (Albugranin),[95] and interferon α and β (Albuferon).[96–99] All have shown improved pharmacokinetics compared to nonfused counterparts. Recombinant interferon α2a has a short half-life of 4 hours in humans. In initial studies, interferon α2a was conjugated to PEG, and the increase in MW significantly improved their half-life 10-fold (40 hours).[100] It was also fused to albumin, which further improved the half-life to 141 hours.[96,98] Albumin-fused interferon α2b is now undergoing Phase III trials,[98] and the example pinpoints albumin fusion as a successful platform to generate improved *in vivo* efficiency of small therapeutic proteins currently in the clinic. In addition, a favorable feature of genetic fusion is that it allows a simple one-step synthesis process with no need for *in vitro* chemical cross-linking steps.

FUSION OF Ab FRAGMENTS TO ALBUMIN

Ab fragments can be expressed at high levels in microbial systems, but such fragments have limited therapeutic value due to rapid elimination from the circulation as the molecular weight is below 60 kDa, which leads to renal filtration and accumulation. Several strategies using *in vitro* PEGylation to extend half-life have been described,[9,101–104] as well as chemical cross linking of Fab to rat albumin, which has been demonstrated to extend serum persistence in rats comparable to that observed for nonfused rat albumin.[105] Furthermore, genetic fusion of antitumor necrosis factor (TNF) α scFv to human albumin generated a molecule that had the same half-life as nonfused human albumin in rats,[105] although the half-life of both was only about half of that seen for rat albumin.

The first albumin fusion in antibody-based imaging involved genetic fusion of anti-carcinoembryonic antigen (CEA) scFv to human albumin ("immunobumin"). Increased half-life and specific tumor uptake comparable with "naked" svFc was demonstrated in mice bearing human colorectal carcinoma xenografts.[106]

Bispecific IgGs have been described that direct T lymphocytes to tumor cells and thus induce tumor cell destruction.[107] Recently, a novel approach was explored using bispecific single-chain diabodies (scDb), scFv and tandem svFv (taFv) that were directed against CEA, and the T cell receptor complex molecule CD3. Each was genetically fused to human albumin (Figure 20.1D-F).[108] All variants retained binding to both CEA and CD3, and all showed extended serum half-life in mice compared with parental fragments that were not fused to albumin. Importantly, effector T cell activation was influenced by the format. The albumin-scDb fusion was the most effective in terms of cytotoxicity.[108] Further studies are needed to evaluate whether they may be translated into improved anticancer therapy.

Taken together, a spectrum of Ab fragments may be genetically fused to albumin and produced in high quantities as single polypeptide products without the need for *in vitro* chemical modifications before *in vivo* administration. Importantly, albumin fusion may be an attractive alternative if Fc-mediated side effects are undesirable. The recent generation of recombinant albumin mutants with altered stability, half-life, and organ deposition is interesting.[109–111] In the future, the pharmacokinetics of albumin may be tailored by attenuating or enhancing the albumin-FcRn interaction to fit clinical goals, in a manner similar to that already described for the IgG-FcRn interaction.[41–46] Furthermore, whether FcRn binding, and thereby the pharmacokinetics, is affected by how Ab fragments are fused to albumin (carboxyl or amino terminal) is unknown. In this regard, it is interesting that the half-life of interferon α2b is extended from only 2–3 hours to 6 days after albumin fusion.[97,98] This is still far from the regular half-life of albumin in humans of 19 days.[48]

TARGETING ALBUMIN AS AN ALTERNATIVE ROUTE

An alternative to genetic fusion to albumin is to target endogenous albumin by non-covalent association. One example is bispecific F(ab')$_2$ against rat albumin and TNF. The construct had improved half-life in rats compared with a monospecific anti-TNF F(ab')$_2$.[105] Once injected, the anti-albumin arm may bind strongly to circulating albumin. The complex will then persist in the bloodstream, to allow the anti-TNF arm to encounter and bind TNF. If the anti-albumin Fab is not interfering with albumin-FcRn binding, the complex may be recycled.

Furthermore, peptide phage display technology has been utilized to isolate a variety of peptides that bind serum albumin from multiple species.[112] Affinity maturation gave rise to peptides with a core sequence (DICLPRWGCLW) that was functionally dependent on a disulfide bridge between the two cysteine residues. One of the selected peptides (SA21) had a half-life of 2.3 hours in rabbits that was significantly longer than the 7.3 minutes for an unrelated peptide with similar size.[112]

An anti-tissue factor-specific Fab (D3H44)[113] genetically fused through the carboxy terminal end of the light chain to a sequence related to SA21 (SA08; Figure 20.1G) bound both albumin and antigen simultaneously and had a 26- or 37-fold increased half-life compared to nonfused D3H44 in mice and rabbits, respectively.[112] Using albumin binding peptides with a wide range of affinities[112] fused to a Fab, with specificity for the tumor marker human epidermal growth factor receptor 2 (HER2) (AB.Fab4D5) derived from the clinically approved trastuzumab (Herceptin), a correlation between albumin affinity and serum half-life was clearly demonstrated, as fusions with peptides of low affinity were eliminated more rapidly than fusions with strong binders.[114] Thus, the pharmacokinetics of albumin-binding Fab (AB.Fab) with any antigenic specificity may be tailored as a function of albumin affinity. Furthermore, the peptides may be genetically added to other Ab fragment formats or any recombinant therapeutic protein of interest to increase their *in vivo* efficacy.

To increase half-life without a dramatic increase in total size is a great advantage in tumor imaging and therapy. While radiolabeled intact mAbs diffuse slowly into tumor tissues and accumulate in normal tissue, Ab-derived fragments show enhanced tumor penetration and rapid clearance from the circulation. However, less reach the tumor sites and the fragments accumulate in the kidneys.[115–118] To investigate the properties of AB.Fab in this regard, AB.Fab4D5[119] was tested for and its ability to target tumors overexpressing HER2 in mouse/HER2 allograft models evaluated.[120] AB.Fab4D5 rapidly targeted tumors and was eliminated from the circulation faster than trastuzumab. This led to significantly improved tumor to normal tissue ratios and effective localization to tumor sites within 2 hours post administration, while 24 hours passed before the same levels were reached for trastuzumab. Interestingly, whereas Fab4D5 accumulates in the kidneys, AB.Fab4D5 did not, showing that the fused albumin-targeting peptide had a great impact on the biodistribution and organ deposition. The extended half-life of AB.Fab4D5 and other anti-albumin Ab constructs may be explained by the increase in size above the threshold for renal clearance; in addition, FcRn may indeed be able to recycle the complexes in a manner similar to that described for albumin.[16,18]

TARGETING USING BACTERIAL ALBUMIN BINDING DOMAINS

Several bacterial strains have evolved to express surface proteins with high specificity for IgG and albumin.[121] For instance, Streptococcus strain G148 expresses protein G that contains sites for albumin and IgG binding on two separate domains, which permits binding of both ligands simultaneously. Furthermore, protein G binds albumin and IgG from a broad range of species.[122,123] Thus, truncated recombinant variants of protein G have been extensively used as laboratory tools for affinity purification of IgG and albumin from serum or growth medium.

Two proteins, soluble complement receptor 1 (sCR1) and soluble CD4, have been genetically fused to the albumin-binding domain of protein G (ABD). The half-lives of both increased and were found to be 2.9–5 hours in mice for sCR1-ABD and 15–24 hours in rats for CD4-ABD.[124,125] Recently, the approach was translated into an Ab format, and anti- HER2 Fab4D5 genetically fused via its light chain carboxy terminal end to ABD (Figure 20.1H). In this case, the half-life increased to 21 hours compared to 2 hours for the nonfused Fab4D5 in mice,[126] comparable to that obtained with Fab4D5 fused to albumin-targeting peptides.[114] ABD-fused Fab4D5 accumulated in the kidneys to a lesser extent than "naked" Fab4D5.[126]

Tolmachev et al.[127] studied a divalent anti-HER2 Affibody ($Z_{HER2:342}$) genetically fused to ABD (ABD-$(Z_{HER2:342})_2$; Figure 20.1I) in preclinical tumor imaging experiments. An affibody is a small domain (~7 kDa) from the IgG binding domain of staphylococcal protein A that is used as a scaffold for construction of combinatorial libraries and target selections.[128] The anti-HER2 $Z_{HER2:342}$ was extensively evaluated using several labeling technologies and was found to give high tumor to normal tissue ratios.[129–132] Interestingly, high and specific tumor uptake of radiolabeled ABD-$(Z_{HER2:342})_2$ was demonstrated in HER2 positive microxenograft mice as well as a 25-fold reduction in kidney accumulation. Thus, non-covalent association with albumin may be used to redistribute $Z_{HER2:342}$ to avoid high kidney accumulation, an observation similar to that obtained with AB.Fab4D5.[120]

ABD has also been added to a bispecific scDb (scDbCEACD3-ABD; Figure 20.1J) developed for retargeting of cytotoxic T cells via CD3 to CEA-expressing tumors.[133] The scDbCEACD3-ABD bound all three antigens simultaneously, but the activity measured by interleukin 2 secretion from retargeted T cells showed retained but reduced bioactivity compared to "naked" scDb, although scDbCEACD4-ABD showed 5–6-fold increased half-life in mice.[133]

Whether FcRn binds albumin associated with ABD has not yet been investigated. However, peptide mapping has indicated that ABD binds mainly to a segment located to DII and DIII (amino acids 330–446) of human albumin.[123] Crystallographic data from the co-crystal of human albumin in complex with an ABD homologue from *Finegoldia magna*, albumin-binding protein (PAB), revealed that the binding site is located to domain II.[134] The binding site for FcRn on albumin is localized to DIII,[17] but so far, no site-directed interaction mapping has been done. Thus, FcRn and ABD fused proteins may well bind albumin on separate sites that allow recycling of the complex. A fundamental prerequisite for optimal FcRn recycling of IgG and albumin is the pH dependency described above. Importantly, if anti-albumin peptide or ABD-fused Ab fragments should be properly recycled by FcRn, they must retain albumin-binding ability at acidic pH. This important issue was addressed for both scDbCEACD4-ABD and selected albumin-binding peptides and the albumin-binding capacities were unaffected at pH 6.0 in both cases.[112,133]

Furthermore, several ABD variants with a spectrum of different affinities for albumin have been engineered,[135] and these variants may be used to fine-tune the biodistribution of radiotherapy agents or to tailor the half-life of potentially important protein pharmaceuticals.

CONCLUDING REMARKS

The remarkably long half-life of recombinant IgG mAbs (21 days) has greatly contributed to their usefulness as therapeutics.[2,3] However, a main obstacle in the manufacturing of such mAbs as drugs is costly mammalian production.[7] On the other hand, high levels of Ab fragments can easily be produced in microbial expression systems and genetic fusion directly to albumin or by targeting circulating endogenous albumin can significantly increase their half-life. This may be explained by the extraordinary capacity of FcRn to rescue albumin from degradation. However, no studies have so far directly addressed the role of FcRn in extending the half-life of albumin fused or targeted proteins.

The strategies described may be translated into reengineering of existing recombinant protein therapeutics that are currently used in the clinic or are undergoing preclinical trials. For instance, different classes of novel engineered ligand-binding proteins such as domain antibodies (dAbs),[136] anticalins,[137,138] affibodies,[139,140] designed ankyrin repeat proteins (DARPins),[141] nanobodies,[142] and other scaffolds[143] may be directly genetically fused to albumin, albumin-binding Ab fragments, peptides, or ABD variants as an approach to modulate *in vivo* pharmacokinetics. Eventually, the scaffolds may themselves be promising candidates for selection of new binders that target albumin or FcRn.

Preclinical pharmacokinetic evaluation of albumin mutants, albumin fused, or targeting molecules is often performed in rodents. Since FcRn has been shown to be the major regulator of serum level and half-life of both IgG and albumin,[14,16,25,50,144] cross-species experiments may not directly be used to extrapolate half-life and organ-specific deposition. The affinity of the ligand-FcRn interaction of the species used must be taken into consideration. This is exemplified by the fact that mouse IgGs do not interact with human FcRn[145] and the short half-life of 15 hours of human albumin measured in rats compared to 49 hours of rat albumin in rats.[105] In line with this is the observation that recombinant soluble rat FcRn was not able to interact with human albumin coupled to sepharose.[18] Thus, cross-species interaction with FcRn may have great impact on preclinical evaluations. Furthermore, the half-life of endogenous albumin in mice and rats is only about 1.5 and 2.5 days, respectively, compared to 19 days in humans.[18,48,146,147] Such issues should be addressed in future evaluations of albumin-based therapeutics.

Jan Terje Andersen was supported by grants from the Steering Board for Research in Molecular Biology, Biotechnology and Bioinformatics (EMBIO) at the University of Oslo.

REFERENCES

[1] Spiegelberg, H.L. and B.G. Fishkin, The catabolism of human G immunoglobulins of different heavy chain subclasses. 3. The catabolism of heavy chain disease proteins and of Fc fragments of myeloma proteins. *Clin Exp Immunol*, 1972. **10**(4): pp. 599–607.

[2] Waldmann, T.A. and W. Strober, Metabolism of immunoglobulins. *Prog Allergy*, 1969. **13**: pp. 1–110.

[3] Adams, G.P. and L.M. Weiner, Monoclonal antibody therapy of cancer. *Nat Biotechnol*, 2005. **23**(9): pp. 1147–57.

[4] Carter, P.J., Potent antibody therapeutics by design. *Nat Rev Immunol*, 2006. **6**(5): pp. 343–57.

[5] Reichert, J.M., Monoclonal antibodies in the clinic. *Nat Biotechnol*, 2001. **19**(9): pp. 819–22.

[6] Schrama, D., R.A. Reisfeld, and J.C. Becker, Antibody targeted drugs as cancer therapeutics. *Nat Rev Drug Discov*, 2006. **5**(2): pp. 147–59.

[7] Scott, C.T., The problem with potency. *Nat Biotechnol*, 2005. **23**(9): pp. 1037–9.

[8] Roopenian, D.C. and S. Akilesh, FcRn: the neonatal Fc receptor comes of age. *Nat Rev Immunol*, 2007. **7**(9): pp. 715–25.

[9] Chapman, A.P., et al., Therapeutic antibody fragments with prolonged in vivo half-lives. *Nat Biotechnol*, 1999. **17**(8): pp. 780–3.

[10] Burmeister, W.P., et al., Crystal structure at 2.2 A resolution of the MHC-related neonatal Fc receptor. *Nature*, 1994. **372**(6504): pp. 336–43.

[11] Burmeister, W.P., A.H. Huber, and P.J. Bjorkman, Crystal structure of the complex of rat neonatal Fc receptor with Fc. *Nature*, 1994. **372**(6504): pp. 379–83.

[12] West, A.P., Jr. and P.J. Bjorkman, Crystal structure and immunoglobulin G binding properties of the human major histocompatibility complex-related Fc receptor. *Biochemistry*, 2000. **39**(32): pp. 9698–708.

[13] Hammer, G.E., T. Kanaseki, and N. Shastri, The final touches make perfect the peptide-MHC class I repertoire. *Immunity*, 2007. **26**(4): pp. 397–406.

[14] Akilesh, S., et al., Neonatal FcR expression in bone marrow-derived cells functions to protect serum IgG from catabolism. *J Immunol*, 2007. **179**(7): pp. 4580–8.

[15] Andersen, J.T., J. Dee Qian, and I. Sandlie, The conserved histidine 166 residue of the human neonatal Fc receptor heavy chain is critical for the pH-dependent binding to albumin. *Eur J Immunol*, 2006. **36**(11): pp. 3044–51.

[16] Anderson, C.L., et al., Perspective – FcRn transports albumin: relevance to immunology and medicine. *Trends Immunol*, 2006. **27**(7): pp. 343–8.

[17] Chaudhury, C., et al., Albumin binding to FcRn: distinct from the FcRn-IgG interaction. *Biochemistry*, 2006. **45**(15): pp. 4983–90.

[18] Chaudhury, C., et al., The major histocompatibility complex-related Fc receptor for IgG (FcRn) binds albumin and prolongs its lifespan. *J Exp Med*, 2003. **197**(3): pp. 315–22.

[19] Vaughn, D.E. and P.J. Bjorkman, Structural basis of pH-dependent antibody binding by the neonatal Fc receptor. *Structure*, 1998. **6**(1): pp. 63–73.

[20] Vaughn, D.E., et al., Identification of critical IgG binding epitopes on the neonatal Fc receptor. *J Mol Biol*, 1997. **274**(4): pp. 597–607.

[21] Brambell, F.W., The transmission of immunity from mother to young and the catabolism of immunoglobulins. *Lancet*, 1966. **2**(7473): pp. 1087–93.

[22] Brambell, F.W., W.A. Hemmings, and I.G. Morris, A theoretical model of gamma-globulin catabolism. *Nature*, 1964. **203**: pp. 1352–4.

[23] Fahey, J.L. and A.G. Robinson, Factors controlling serum gamma-globulin concentration. *J Exp Med*, 1963. **118**: pp. 845–68.

[24] Halliday, R., The production of antibodies by young rats. *Proc R Soc Lond B Biol Sci*, 1957. **147**(926): pp. 140–4.

[25] Ghetie, V. and E.S. Ward, Multiple roles for the major histocompatibility complex class I-related receptor FcRn. *Annu Rev Immunol*, 2000. **18**: pp. 739–66.

[26] Simister, N.E. and K.E. Mostov, An Fc receptor structurally related to MHC class I antigens. *Nature*, 1989. **337**(6203): pp. 184–7.

[27] Story, C.M., J.E. Mikulska, and N.E. Simister, A major histocompatibility complex class I-like Fc receptor cloned from human placenta: possible role in transfer of immunoglobulin G from mother to fetus. *J Exp Med*, 1994. **180**(6): pp. 2377–81.

[28] Medesan, C., et al., Delineation of the amino acid residues involved in transcytosis and catabolism of mouse IgG1. *J Immunol*, 1997. **158**(5): pp. 2211–7.

[29] Christianson, G.J., et al., Beta 2-microglobulin-deficient mice are protected from hypergammaglobulinemia and have defective antibody responses because of increased IgG catabolism. *J Immunol*, 1997. **159**(10): pp. 4781–92.

[30] Ghetie, V., et al., Abnormally short serum half-lives of IgG in beta 2-microglobulin-deficient mice. *Eur J Immunol*, 1996. **26**(3): pp. 690–6.

[31] Israel, E.J., et al., Requirement for a beta 2-microglobulin-associated Fc receptor for acquisition of maternal IgG by fetal and neonatal mice. *J Immunol*, 1995. **154**(12): pp. 6246–51.

[32] Israel, E.J., et al., Increased clearance of IgG in mice that lack beta 2-microglobulin: possible protective role of FcRn. *Immunology*, 1996. **89**(4): pp. 573–8.

[33] Junghans, R.P. and C.L. Anderson, The protection receptor for IgG catabolism is the beta2-microglobulin-containing neonatal intestinal transport receptor. *Proc Natl Acad Sci USA*, 1996. **93**(11): pp. 5512–6.

[34] Roopenian, D.C., et al., The MHC class I-like IgG receptor controls perinatal IgG transport, IgG homeostasis, and fate of IgG-Fc-coupled drugs. *J Immunol*, 2003. **170**(7): pp. 3528–33.

[35] Bitonti, A.J., et al., Pulmonary delivery of an erythropoietin Fc fusion protein in non-human primates through an immunoglobulin transport pathway. *Proc Natl Acad Sci USA*, 2004. **101**(26): pp. 9763–8.

[36] Dumont, J.A., et al., Delivery of an erythropoietin-Fc fusion protein by inhalation in humans through an immunoglobulin transport pathway. *J Aerosol Med*, 2005. **18**(3): pp. 294–303.

[37] Kanaya, K., et al., Combined gene therapy with adenovirus vectors containing CTLA4Ig and CD40Ig prolongs survival of composite tissue allografts in rat model. *Transplantation*, 2003. **75**(3): pp. 275–81.

[38] Low, S.C., et al., Oral and pulmonary delivery of FSH-Fc fusion proteins via neonatal Fc receptor-mediated transcytosis. *Hum Reprod*, 2005. **20**(7): pp. 1805–13.

[39] Shen, Y., B. Young, and M.L. Lipman, Suppression of the cell-mediated immune response by a Fas-immunoglobulin fusion protein. *Transplantation*, 2006. **81**(7): pp. 1041–8.

[40] Ghetie, V., et al., Increasing the serum persistence of an IgG fragment by random mutagenesis. *Nat Biotechnol*, 1997. **15**(7): pp. 637–40.

[41] Hinton, P.R., et al., Engineered human IgG antibodies with longer serum half-lives in primates. *J Biol Chem*, 2004. **279**(8): pp. 6213–6.

[42] Hinton, P.R., et al., An engineered human IgG1 antibody with longer serum half-life. *J Immunol*, 2006. **176**(1): pp. 346–56.

[43] Dall'Acqua, W.F., P.A. Kiener, and H. Wu, Properties of human IgG1s engineered for enhanced binding to the neonatal Fc receptor (FcRn). *J Biol Chem*, 2006. **281**(33): pp. 23514–24.

[44] Medesan, C., et al., Localization of the site of the IgG molecule that regulates maternofetal transmission in mice. *Eur J Immunol*, 1996. **26**(10): pp. 2533–6.

[45] Kenanova, V., et al., Tailoring the pharmacokinetics and positron emission tomography imaging properties of anti-carcinoembryonic antigen single-chain Fv-Fc antibody fragments. *Cancer Res*, 2005. **65**(2): pp. 622–31.

[46] Hornick, J.L., et al., Single amino acid substitution in the Fc region of chimeric TNT-3 antibody accelerates clearance and improves immunoscintigraphy of solid tumors. *J Nucl Med*, 2000. **41**(2): pp. 355–62.

[47] Schultze, H.E. and Heremans, J.F., *Molecular Biology of Human Proteins: With Special Reference to Plasma Proteins. Vol. 1: Nature and Metabolism of Extracellular Proteins*. Elsevier, 1966.

[48] Peters, T.J., *All about Albumin: Biochemistry, Genetics, and Medical Applications*. Academic Press, 1996.

[49] Waldmann, T.A. and W.D. Terry, Familial hypercatabolic hypoproteinemia. A disorder of endogenous catabolism of albumin and immunoglobulin. *J Clin Invest*, 1990. **86**(6): pp. 2093–8.

[50] Wani, M.A., et al., Familial hypercatabolic hypoproteinemia caused by deficiency of the neonatal Fc receptor, FcRn, due to a mutant beta2-microglobulin gene. *Proc Natl Acad Sci USA*, 2006. **103**(13): pp. 5084–9.

[51] Borvak, J., et al., Functional expression of the MHC class I-related receptor, FcRn, in endothelial cells of mice. *Int Immunol*, 1998. **10**(9): pp. 1289–98.

[52] Ward, E.S., et al., Evidence to support the cellular mechanism involved in serum IgG homeostasis in humans. *Int Immunol*, 2003. **15**(2): pp. 187–95.

[53] Blumberg, R.S., et al., A major histocompatibility complex class I-related Fc receptor for IgG on rat hepatocytes. *J Clin Invest*, 1995. **95**(5): pp. 2397–402.

[54] Telleman, P. and R.P. Junghans, The role of the Brambell receptor (FcRB) in liver: protection of endocytosed immunoglobulin G (IgG) from catabolism in hepatocytes rather than transport of IgG to bile. *Immunology*, 2000. **100**(2): pp. 245–51.

[55] Haymann, J.P., et al., Characterization and localization of the neonatal Fc receptor in adult human kidney. *J Am Soc Nephrol*, 2000. **11**(4): pp. 632–9.

[56] McCarthy, K.M., Y. Yoong, and N.E. Simister, Bidirectional transcytosis of IgG by the rat neonatal Fc receptor expressed in a rat kidney cell line: a system to study protein transport across epithelia. *J Cell Sci*, 2000. **113**(Pt 7): pp. 1277–85.

[57] Antohe, F., et al., Expression of functionally active FcRn and the differentiated bidirectional transport of IgG in human placental endothelial cells. *Hum Immunol*, 2001. **62**(2): pp. 93–105.

[58] Ellinger, I., et al., IgG transport across trophoblast-derived BeWo cells: a model system to study IgG transport in the placenta. *Eur J Immunol*, 1999. **29**(3): pp. 733–44.

[59] Firan, M., et al., The MHC class I-related receptor, FcRn, plays an essential role in the maternofetal transfer of gamma-globulin in humans. *Int Immunol*, 2001. **13**(8): pp. 993–1002.

[60] Kristoffersen, E.K., Human placental Fc gamma-binding proteins in the maternofetal transfer of IgG. *APMIS* Suppl, 1996. 64: pp. 5–36.

[61] Leach, J.L., et al., Isolation from human placenta of the IgG transporter, FcRn, and localization to the syncytiotrophoblast: implications for maternal-fetal antibody transport. *J Immunol*, 1996. **157**(8): pp. 3317–22.

[62] Radulescu, L., et al., Neonatal Fc receptors discriminates and monitors the pathway of native and modified immunoglobulin G in placental endothelial cells. *Hum Immunol*, 2004. **65**(6): pp. 578–85.

[63] Simister, N.E., et al., An IgG-transporting Fc receptor expressed in the syncytiotrophoblast of human placenta. *Eur J Immunol*, 1996. **26**(7): pp. 1527–31.

[64] Sachs, U.J., et al., A variable number of tandem repeats polymorphism influences the transcriptional activity of the neonatal Fc receptor alpha-chain promoter. *Immunology*, 2006. **119**(1): pp. 83–9.

[65] Vidarsson, G., et al., FcRn: an IgG receptor on phagocytes with a novel role in phagocytosis. *Blood*, 2006. **108**(10): pp. 3573–9.

[66] Zhu, X., et al., MHC class I-related neonatal Fc receptor for IgG is functionally expressed in monocytes, intestinal macrophages, and dendritic cells. *J Immunol*, 2001. **166**(5): pp. 3266–76.

[67] Ober, R.J., et al., Exocytosis of IgG as mediated by the receptor, FcRn: an analysis at the single-molecule level. *Proc Natl Acad Sci USA*, 2004. **101**(30): pp. 11076–81.

[68] Ober, R.J., et al., Visualizing the site and dynamics of IgG salvage by the MHC class I-related receptor, FcRn. *J Immunol*, 2004. **172**(4): pp. 2021–9.

[69] Ward, E.S., et al., From sorting endosomes to exocytosis: association of Rab4 and Rab11 GTPases with the Fc receptor, FcRn, during recycling. *Mol Biol Cell*, 2005. **16**(4): pp. 2028–38.

[70] Prabhat, P., et al., Elucidation of intracellular recycling pathways leading to exocytosis of the Fc receptor, FcRn, by using multifocal plane microscopy. *Proc Natl Acad Sci USA*, 2007. **104**(14): pp. 5889–94.

[71] Sugio, S., et al., Crystal structure of human serum albumin at 2.5 A resolution. *Protein Eng*, 1999. **12**(6): pp. 439–46.

[72] Website: http://www.albumin.org.

[73] Andersen, J.T. and I. Sandlie, A Receptor-Mediated Mechanism to Support Clinical Observation of Altered Albumin Variants. *Clin Chem*, 2007. **53**(12): pp. 2216.

[74] Chuang, V.T., U. Kragh-Hansen, and M. Otagiri, Pharmaceutical strategies utilizing recombinant human serum albumin. *Pharm Res*, 2002. **19**(5): pp. 569–77.

[75] Chuang, V.T. and M. Otagiri, Recombinant human serum albumin. *Drugs Today (Barc)*, 2007. **43**(8): pp. 547–61.

[76] Kobayashi, K., Summary of recombinant human serum albumin development. *Biologicals*, 2006. **34**(1): pp. 55–9.

[77] Stehle, G., et al., Plasma protein (albumin) catabolism by the tumor itself – implications for tumor metabolism and the genesis of cachexia. *Crit Rev Oncol Hematol*, 1997. **26**(2): pp. 77–100.

[78] Bolling, C., et al., Phase II study of MTX-HSA in combination with cisplatin as first line treatment in patients with advanced or metastatic transitional cell carcinoma. *Invest New Drugs*, 2006. **24**(6): pp. 521–7.

[79] Herman, R.A., et al., Pharmacokinetics of low-dose methotrexate in rheumatoid arthritis patients. *J Pharm Sci*, 1989. **78**(2): pp. 165–71.

[80] Kratz, F., K. Abu Ajaj, and A. Warnecke, Anticancer carrier-linked prodrugs in clinical trials. *Expert Opin Investig Drugs*, 2007. **16**(7): pp. 1037–58.

[81] Vis, A.N., et al., A phase II trial of methotrexate-human serum albumin (MTX-HSA) in patients with metastatic renal cell carcinoma who progressed under immunotherapy. *Cancer Chemother Pharmacol*, 2002. **49**(4): pp. 342–5.

[82] Wunder, A., et al., Albumin-based drug delivery as novel therapeutic approach for rheumatoid arthritis. *J Immunol*, 2003. **170**(9): pp. 4793–801.

[83] Curry, S., P. Brick, and N.P. Franks, Fatty acid binding to human serum albumin: new insights from crystallographic studies. *Biochim Biophys Acta*, 1999. **1441**(2–3): pp. 131–40.

[84] Brunner, G.A., et al., Pharmacokinetic and pharmacodynamic properties of long-acting insulin analogue NN304 in comparison to NPH insulin in humans. *Exp Clin Endocrinol Diabetes*, 2000. **108**(2): pp. 100–5.

[85] Klein, O., et al., Albumin-bound basal insulin analogues (insulin detemir and NN344): comparable time-action profiles but less variability than insulin glargine in type 2 diabetes. *Diabetes Obes Metab*, 2007. **9**(3): pp. 290–9.

[86] Kurtzhals, P., et al., Albumin binding and time action of acylated insulins in various species. *J Pharm Sci*, 1996. **85**(3): pp. 304–8.

[87] Markussen, J., et al., Soluble, fatty acid acylated insulins bind to albumin and show protracted action in pigs. *Diabetologia*, 1996. **39**(3): pp. 281–8.

[88] Soran, H. and N. Younis, Insulin detemir: a new basal insulin analogue. *Diabetes Obes Metab*, 2006. **8**(1): pp. 26–30.

[89] Koehler, M.F., et al., Albumin affinity tags increase peptide half-life in vivo. *Bioorg Med Chem Lett*, 2002. **12**(20): pp. 2883–6.

[90] Zobel, K., et al., Phosphate ester serum albumin affinity tags greatly improve peptide half-life in vivo. *Bioorg Med Chem Lett*, 2003. **13**(9): pp. 1513–5.

[91] Syed, S., et al., Potent antithrombin activity and delayed clearance from the circulation characterize recombinant hirudin genetically fused to albumin. *Blood*, 1997. **89**(9): pp. 3243–52.

[92] Yeh, P., et al., Design of yeast-secreted albumin derivatives for human therapy: biological and antiviral properties of a serum albumin-CD4 genetic conjugate. *Proc Natl Acad Sci USA*, 1992. **89**(5): pp. 1904–8.

[93] Duttaroy, A., et al., Development of a long-acting insulin analog using albumin fusion technology. *Diabetes*, 2005. **54**(1): pp. 251–8.

[94] Osborn, B.L., et al., Albutropin: a growth hormone-albumin fusion with improved pharmacokinetics and pharmacodynamics in rats and monkeys. *Eur J Pharmacol*, 2002. **456**(1–3): pp. 149–58.

[95] Halpern, W., et al., Albugranin, a recombinant human granulocyte colony stimulating factor (G-CSF) genetically fused to recombinant human albumin induces prolonged myelopoietic effects in mice and monkeys. *Pharm Res*, 2002. **19**(11): pp. 1720–9.

[96] Bain, V.G., et al., A phase 2 study to evaluate the antiviral activity, safety, and pharmacokinetics of recombinant human albumin-interferon alfa fusion protein in genotype 1 chronic hepatitis C patients. *J Hepatol*, 2006. **44**(4): pp. 671–8.

[97] Balan, V., et al., Modulation of interferon-specific gene expression by albumin-interferon-alpha in interferon-alpha-experienced patients with chronic hepatitis C. *Antivir Ther*, 2006. **11**(7): pp. 901–8.

[98] Subramanian, G.M., et al., Albinterferon alpha-2b: a genetic fusion protein for the treatment of chronic hepatitis C. *Nat Biotechnol*, 2007. **25**(12): pp. 1411–9.

[99] Sung, C., et al., An IFN-beta-albumin fusion protein that displays improved pharmacokinetic and pharmacodynamic properties in nonhuman primates. *J Interferon Cytokine Res*, 2003. **23**(1): pp. 25–36.

[100] Glue, P., et al., Pegylated interferon-alpha2b: pharmacokinetics, pharmacodynamics, safety, and preliminary efficacy data. Hepatitis C Intervention Therapy Group. *Clin Pharmacol Ther*, 2000. **68**(5): pp. 556–67.

[101] Kubetzko, S., et al., PEGylation and multimerization of the anti-p185HER-2 single chain Fv fragment 4D5: effects on tumor targeting. *J Biol Chem*, 2006. **281**(46): pp. 35186–201.

[102] Lee, L.S., et al., Prolonged circulating lives of single-chain Fv proteins conjugated with polyethylene glycol: a comparison of conjugation chemistries and compounds. *Bioconjug Chem*, 1999. **10**(6): pp. 973–81.

[103] Kitamura, K., et al., Chemical engineering of the monoclonal antibody A7 by polyethylene glycol for targeting cancer chemotherapy. *Cancer Res*, 1991. **51**(16): pp. 4310–5.

[104] Chapman, A.P., PEGylated antibodies and antibody fragments for improved therapy: a review. *Adv Drug Deliv Rev*, 2002. **54**(4): pp. 531–45.

[105] Smith, B.J., et al., Prolonged in vivo residence times of antibody fragments associated with albumin. *Bioconjug Chem*, 2001. **12**(5): pp. 750–6.

[106] Yazaki, P.J., et al., Biodistribution and tumor imaging of an anti-CEA single-chain antibody-albumin fusion protein. *Nucl Med Biol*, 2008. **35**(2): pp. 151–8.

[107] Muller, D. and R.E. Kontermann, Recombinant bispecific antibodies for cellular cancer immunotherapy. *Curr Opin Mol Ther*, 2007. **9**(4): pp. 319–26.

[108] Muller, D., et al., Improved pharmacokinetics of recombinant bispecific antibody molecules by fusion to human serum albumin. *J Biol Chem*, 2007. **282**(17): pp. 12650–60.

[109] Iwao, Y., et al., Oxidation of Arg-410 promotes the elimination of human serum albumin. *Biochim Biophys Acta*, 2006. **1764**(4): pp. 743–9.

[110] Iwao, Y., et al., Changes of net charge and alpha-helical content affect the pharmacokinetic properties of human serum albumin. *Biochim Biophys Acta*, 2007. **1774**(12): pp. 1582–90.

[111] Kragh-Hansen, U., et al., Effect of genetic variation on the thermal stability of human serum albumin. *Biochim Biophys Acta*, 2005. **1747**(1): pp. 81–8.

[112] Dennis, M.S., et al., Albumin binding as a general strategy for improving the pharmacokinetics of proteins. *J Biol Chem*, 2002. **277**(38): pp. 35035–43.

[113] Presta, L., et al., Generation of a humanized, high affinity anti-tissue factor antibody for use as a novel antithrombotic therapeutic. *Thromb Haemost*, 2001. **85**(3): pp. 379–89.

[114] Nguyen, A., et al., The pharmacokinetics of an albumin-binding Fab (AB.Fab) can be modulated as a function of affinity for albumin. *Protein Eng Des Sel*, 2006. **19**(7): pp. 291–7.

[115] Wu, A.M. and P.J. Yazaki, Designer genes: recombinant antibody fragments for biological imaging. *Q J Nucl Med*, 2000. **44**(3): pp. 268–83.

[116] Wu, A.M. and P.D. Senter, Arming antibodies: prospects and challenges for immunoconjugates. *Nat Biotechnol*, 2005. **23**(9): pp. 1137–46.

[117] Kashmiri, S.V., Multivalent single-chain antibodies for radioimaging of tumors. *J Nucl Med*, 2001. **42**(10): pp. 1528–9.

[118] Borsi, L., et al., Selective targeting of tumoral vasculature: comparison of different formats of an antibody (L19) to the ED-B domain of fibronectin. *Int J Cancer*, 2002. **102**(1): pp. 75–85.

[119] Perry, C.M. and L.R. Wiseman, Trastuzumab. *BioDrugs*, 1999. **12**(2): pp. 129–35.

[120] Dennis, M.S., et al., Imaging tumors with an albumin-binding Fab, a novel tumor-targeting agent. *Cancer Res*, 2007. **67**(1): pp. 254–61.

[121] Navarre, W.W. and O. Schneewind, Surface proteins of gram-positive bacteria and mechanisms of their targeting to the cell wall envelope. *Microbiol Mol Biol Rev*, 1999. **63**(1): pp. 174–229.

[122] Nygren, P.A., et al., Species-dependent binding of serum albumins to the streptococcal receptor protein G. *Eur J Biochem*, 1990. **193**(1): pp. 143–8.

[123] Falkenberg, C., L. Bjorck, and B. Akerstrom, Localization of the binding site for streptococcal protein G on human serum albumin. Identification of a 5.5-kilodalton protein G binding albumin fragment. *Biochemistry*, 1992. **31**(5): pp. 1451–7.

[124] Makrides, S.C., et al., Extended in vivo half-life of human soluble complement receptor type 1 fused to a serum albumin-binding receptor. *J Pharmacol Exp Ther*, 1996. **277**(1): pp. 534–42.

[125] Nygren, P.A., Flodby P., Andersson R., Wigzell H., and Uhlen M., In vivo stabilization of a human recombinant CD4 derivative by fusion to a serum albumin-binding receptor. Cold Spring Harbor Laboratory Press, New York, 1991. *Vaccines 91, Modern Approaches to Vaccine Development:* pp. 363–368.

[126] Schlapschy, M., et al., Fusion of a recombinant antibody fragment with a homo-amino-acid polymer: effects on biophysical properties and prolonged plasma half-life. *Protein Eng Des Sel*, 2007. **20**(6): pp. 273–84.

[127] Tolmachev, V., et al., Radionuclide therapy of HER2-positive microxenografts using a 177Lu-labeled HER2-specific Affibody molecule. *Cancer Res*, 2007. **67**(6): pp. 2773–82.

[128] Nord, K.,et al., Binding proteins selected from combinatorial libraries of an alpha-helical bacterial receptor domain. *Nat Biotechnol*, 1997. **15**(8): pp. 772–7.

[129] Orlova, A., et al., Tumor imaging using a picomolar affinity HER2 binding affibody molecule. *Cancer Res*, 2006. **66**(8): pp. 4339–48.

[130] Mume, E., et al., Evaluation of ((4-hydroxyphenyl)ethyl)maleimide for site-specific radiobromination of anti-HER2 affibody. *Bioconjug Chem*, 2005. **16**(6): pp. 1547–55.

[131] Orlova, A., et al., Comparative in vivo evaluation of technetium and iodine labels on an anti-HER2 affibody for single-photon imaging of HER2 expression in tumors. *J Nucl Med*, 2006. **47**(3): pp. 512–9.

[132] Tolmachev, V., et al., 111In-benzyl-DTPA-ZHER2:342, an affibody-based conjugate for in vivo imaging of HER2 expression in malignant tumors. *J Nucl Med*, 2006. **47**(5): pp. 846–53.

[133] Stork, R., D. Muller, and R.E. Kontermann, A novel tri-functional antibody fusion protein with improved pharmacokinetic properties generated by fusing a bispecific single-chain diabody with an albumin-binding domain from streptococcal protein G. *Protein Eng Des Sel*, 2007. **20**(11): pp. 569–76.

[134] Lejon, S., et al., Crystal structure and biological implications of a bacterial albumin binding module in complex with human serum albumin. *J Biol Chem*, 2004. **279**(41): pp. 42924–8.

[135] Linhult, M., et al., Mutational analysis of the interaction between albumin-binding domain from streptococcal protein G and human serum albumin. *Protein Sci*, 2002. **11**(2): pp. 206–13.

[136] Holt, L.J., et al., Domain antibodies: proteins for therapy. *Trends Biotechnol*, 2003. **21**(11): pp. 484–90.

[137] Schlehuber, S. and A. Skerra, Anticalins as an alternative to antibody technology. *Expert Opin Biol Ther*, 2005. **5**(11): pp. 1453–62.

[138] Schlehuber, S. and A. Skerra, Anticalins in drug development. *BioDrugs*, 2005. **19**(5): pp. 279–88.

[139] Nilsson, F.Y. and V. Tolmachev, Affibody molecules: new protein domains for molecular imaging and targeted tumor therapy. *Curr Opin Drug Discov Devel*, 2007. **10**(2): pp. 167–75.

[140] Tolmachev, V., et al., Affibody molecules: potential for in vivo imaging of molecular targets for cancer therapy. *Expert Opin Biol Ther*, 2007. **7**(4): pp. 555–68.

[141] Stumpp, M.T. and P. Amstutz, DARPins: a true alternative to antibodies. *Curr Opin Drug Discov Devel*, 2007. **10**(2): pp. 153–9.

[142] Revets, H., P. De Baetselier, and S. Muyldermans, Nanobodies as novel agents for cancer therapy. *Expert Opin Biol Ther*, 2005. **5**(1): pp. 111–24.

[143] Binz, H.K., P. Amstutz, and A. Plückthun, Engineering novel binding proteins from nonimmunoglobulin domains. *Nat Biotechnol*, 2005. **23**(10): pp. 1257–68.

[144] Kim, J., et al., Kinetics of FcRn-mediated recycling of IgG and albumin in human: pathophysiology and therapeutic implications using a simplified mechanism-based model. *Clin Immunol*, 2007. **122**(2): pp. 146–55.

[145] Ober, R.J., et al., Differences in promiscuity for antibody-FcRn interactions across species: implications for therapeutic antibodies. *Int Immunol*, 2001. **13**(12): pp. 1551–9.

[146] Peters, T., Jr., Serum albumin. *Adv Protein Chem*, 1985. **37**: pp. 161–245.

[147] Stevens, D.K., R.J. Eyre, and R.J. Bull, Adduction of hemoglobin and albumin in vivo by metabolites of trichloroethylene, trichloroacetate, and dichloroacetate in rats and mice. *Fundam Appl Toxicol*, 1992. **19**(3): pp. 336–42.

PART IX

INNOVATIVE IMMUNOTHERAPEUTIC APPROACHES

A Stem Cell–Based Platform for the Discovery and Development of Antitumor Therapeutic Antibodies to Novel Targets

Jennie P. Mather, Claudia Fieger, Tony W. Liang, Kathleen L. King, Jonathan Li, Peter Young, Claude Beltejar, Beverly Potts, Monica Licea, and Deryk Loo

The majority of therapeutic monoclonal antibodies (mAbs) on the market and in development focus primarily on a limited set of targets selected on the basis of a few well-studied pathways. Truly novel targets (and their corresponding therapeutic mAbs) are rare and carry increased risk and challenges to develop because they, or the pathways they are involved in, are often neither well characterized nor extensively validated. The Raven therapeutic mAb discovery platform is especially efficient in discovering novel targets. Because the platform utilizes intact, living cells as the immunogen – and thus targets antigens present on the membrane of living cells – it is not biased upfront toward a particular protein, protein family, or signaling pathway. In addition, the presentation of these membrane targets in their fully processed and modified configuration and orientation in the living cell enables the discovery of mAbs to conformational epitopes as well as post-translationally modified epitopes. These epitopes may have greater tumor specificity and antitumor activity than those raised from less biologically relevant input such as purified or recombinant proteins and peptides. These epitopes can include binding sites on carbohydrates or lipids as well as conformational epitopes. In fact, the ability to discover these specific and active epitopes, not obvious when looking at mRNA or protein sequences, may open an entirely new class of antibody targets for cancer and other diseases. RAV12 is one example of a mAb that targets a carbohydrate epitope. The preclinical development of RAV12 has been completed and the mAb is currently in clinical development. We will outline the discovery and development program at Raven and highlight many of the challenges of mAb therapeutics to novel targets primarily using the RAV12 mAb and target as an example.

THE mAb/TARGET DISCOVERY PLATFORM

The general outline of the Raven antibody/target discovery platform is shown in Figure 21.1. One of the critical components of the Raven mAb discovery platform is the source of the immunizing cells. Over the past several years we have developed

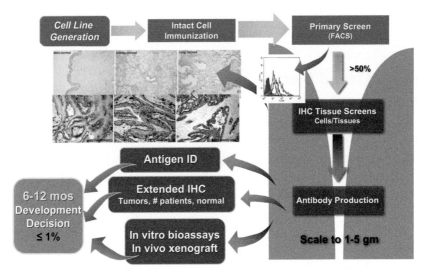

Figure 21.1. Raven antibody discovery platform. Raven-derived human tissue progenitor cell lines and cancer stem cell lines are used as input into the platform. Following immunization and hybridoma generation, the hybridoma supernatants are screened by flow cytometry – greater than 50% of hybridomas typically bind to the cell surface of the immunizing cell line and pass to the immunohistochemical tissue screens on a subset of human normal and tumor tissue samples. Hybridomas that pass this screen for differential expression on tumor tissues are scaled up to generate purified antibody for retesting and expanded immunohistochemistry, as well as antigen identification and bioactivity assays. This process filters out greater than 99% of the antibodies and yields a data package within 6 to 12 months to guide developmental decisions. [See color plate.]

a series of defined serum-free culture media that select for, and support the growth of, tissue-specific progenitor cells from multiple different tissues. To date we have generated more than 15 independent tissue-specific fetal progenitor cell lines from multiple organs including, kidney, colon, pancreas, ovary, lung, liver, stomach, testis, bladder, salivary gland, and skin. Importantly, having laid the foundation by developing tissue-specific serum-free defined culture media, we have extended our cell line development efforts and adapted these culture media to isolate and establish cell lines from a diverse set of human primary tumor tissues, including prostate, breast, skin, colorectal, and lung. We have isolated a number of cell lines from a variety of different tumor types that have properties of cancer stem cells, including self-renewal and the ability to form tumors with diverse cell types from a small number of cells. This large panel of diverse cultured human fetal tissue progenitor cell lines and tumor stem cell lines provides a unique set of input immunogens for the drug discovery platform.

A second key component of our discovery platform is the use of non-denaturing adjuvants together with the healthy, intact, input cell lines to elicit antibody responses primarily to exposed epitopes of antigens present on the cell surface. We have determined that the method of immunization and the cells used as immunogens are both critically important in obtaining the yield and types of mAbs described. The use of serum-free media for deriving and carrying our fetal tissue progenitor lines and our cancer stem cell lines eliminates the generation of undesirable antibodies directed toward components present in serum. As part of the development and validation of the platform we have tested American Type Culture Collection (ATCC) cancer cell lines as input into our immunization platform and found that a large number of cell surface-directed mAbs could be generated; however, all of these mAbs failed the initial immunohistochemistry screen due to broad binding to normal tissues. Of note, we have used Raven-derived cell lines as the input immunogen and successfully identified candidate mAbs by performing the primary screen – for cell surface binding on tumor cells – with ATCC cancer cell lines. Therefore, relevant targets are present on ATCC cancer cell lines; however, they appear to be inefficient at eliciting an antibody response or overwhelmed by more immunogenic but broadly expressed antigens, again suggestive of the critical importance of the immunizing cell source.

Our past efforts have focused on identifying and developing mAbs that bind to antigens expressed on the majority of cells within a tumor, reasoning that these mAbs would have the greatest chance of debulking and eliminating the tumor, and allow a clear path to a clinical study. The emerging tumor stem cell hypothesis runs counter to this approach and proposes that solid tumors are comprised mainly of daughter tumor cells with a limited replication span, together with a small subset of parental tumor stem cells that have unlimited proliferation potential – and it is this small population of tumor stem cells that are responsible for disease recurrence and metastasis. Since we have in hand a panel of putative tumor stem cell lines, we are in a unique position to exploit our cell lines and tailor our discovery platform to generate and identify mAbs directed toward tumor stem cell antigens. An initial survey of mAbs generated from tumor stem cell inputs has identified a subset of 23 mAbs that bind to our panel of tumor stem cells.

Hybridomas are produced using standard fusion technologies (Harlow, 1988), and the resultant cell fusion products are plated in soft agar at clonal density. Independent hybridoma clones are picked and expanded to obtain sufficient conditioned medium to initiate preliminary flow cytometry to assess cell surface binding to the input cell line, and immunohistochemical testing on a limited panel of human normal and tumor tissues to assess tumor selectivity. A large percentage of the hybridomas obtained using this approach produce mAbs that bind to the surface of living input cells. The conditioned media from mAb hybridomas that pass the initial flow cytometry binding assay are then tested on a limited panel of frozen human normal and tumor tissues to assess whether the mAbs perform adequately in immunohistochemistry and to get initial guidance on selectivity for binding to tumor tissue.

The hybridomas of mAbs that pass the initial screens are expanded in order to generate purified mAb preparations. The purified mAb candidates are then subjected to an iterative process whereby the mAbs are more thoroughly characterized with respect to tumor tissue binding selectivity, antigen identification, ability to internalize the mAb *in vitro*, and antitumor activity *in vitro* and *in vivo*. We feel it is vital to have an iterative process, rather than a linear process, since any one mAb in a screening panel is unlikely to meet all criteria on a first pass. Through an iterative process we are able to capture initial, promising activities and flag those mAbs for further investigation, rather than discard mAbs based on an initial negative result.

A classic example of the advantage of the screening process is our experience with a mAb directed toward the EphA2 tyrosine kinase receptor. As is the case for the majority of mAbs generated via our platform, testing for bioactivity using our standard monolayer growth assay was initiated prior to knowing the antigen identification. No bioactivity was observed for the mAb in the monolayer growth assay, which, after the antigen was identified as the EphA2 receptor, is consistent with previous reports (Carles-Kinch, 2002). Because the mAb was highly tumor specific it was tested in a subcutaneous xenograft model in spite of the lack of bioactivity in the monolayer growth assay and was found to have potent antitumor activity. After determining the antigen identification, we also tested the mAb in a soft agar-based *in vitro* assay and found the mAb was active against tumor cells in this format, again consistent with previous reports. Had we relied solely on the *in vitro* monolayer growth assay we would have mistakenly discarded a biologically active mAb to an arguably validated cancer target. Thus, at each iteration we can focus on the set of most promising mAbs based on their emerging profiles, and refine and optimize the research program to address the uniqueness of each mAb and corresponding target.

We have raised more than 200,000 hybridomas over a period of 5 years using this platform technology. One of the main advantages of the platform, outlined in Figure 21.1, is the ability to rapidly screen and discard mAbs that do not have the characteristics we are seeking for an antibody therapeutic – for example, that it binds to the exposed portion of a cell surface epitope and is selective for, or more highly expressed on, tumor tissue over normal adult tissues. We routinely discard 50%–90% of all mAbs raised within the first few weeks after fusion because they do not meet our development criteria. This is important because each immunization program typically produces from 100 to 2,000 independent hybridomas that must be quickly culled to a manageable number for subsequent scale-up and analysis. Since at this point in the discovery process we already have a mAb, we can simultaneously use the mAb to (1) purify and identify the target, (2) screen for *in vitro* and *in vivo* bioactivity, (3) assess safety, and (4) begin to develop a preclinical profile to guide clinical development discussions. mAbs with strong preclinical profiles can be quickly cloned and humanized allowing rapid acquisition of safety and efficacy data to support an investigational new drug (IND) filing. Using this approach, the IND for RAV12 was filed 14 months following the decision to move the KID3 murine antibody into preclinical development.

EPITOPE AND mAb PROPERTIES

As mentioned above, the presentation of target antigens in the context of an intact viable cell membrane has distinct advantages as a drug discovery platform. We now have several hundred mAbs that have passed most of the rigorous screening assays. Several generalizations can be drawn when comparing these mAbs to those raised in more traditional fashion (purified protein, recombinant protein, and peptide

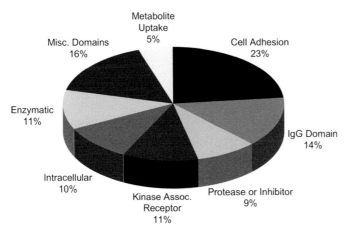

Figure 21.2. Novelty and diversity of targets identified using the Raven discovery platform. The current breakdown of targets recognized by Raven antibodies is illustrated in the pie chart. As shown, Raven antibodies recognize a broad range of protein classes.

immunogens) as assessed from our experience and from the literature. Overall, the mAbs that pass the screens are biased toward binding to nonlinear epitopes, have relatively high affinity binding (nM to pM affinity), work for immunohistochemistry on frozen tissues, and are biologically active by cell internalization and/or other *in vitro* assays. It is interesting to note that a high percentage of mAbs raised using our platform have biological activity compared to other traditional methods of raising mAbs. Overall, approximately 10% of the mAbs that pass the early screens for cell surface binding and differential expression on tumor tissue exhibit some activity *in vitro* or *in vivo*. Approximately 50% of the total are internalized upon binding to tumor cells *in vitro*. The targets recognized cover a broad range of classes of proteins in keeping with not preselecting for any one class or family (Figure 21.2).

Perhaps a more telling statistic is to be gleaned from looking at the Raven mAbs that were generated, via multiple independent immunizations, to a known target for antitumor therapeutics, the epidermal growth factor receptor (EGFR). We chose nine anti-EGFR mAbs based only on passing the first-level flow cytometry and immunohistochemical screens. These mAbs were tested for bioactivity *in vitro* and in binding competition studies. The results are shown in Figure 21.3A. The mAbs fell into three classes based on cross competition. One group cross competes with the commercially approved chimeric anti-EGFR mAb cetuximab for binding to EGFR; two other groups do not cross react with cetuximab or with members of the other group. When these mAbs were tested *in vitro* for activity against EGFR-expressing SW480 tumor cells, eight of the nine mAbs raised had biological activity similar to that of cetuximab. One of the Raven anti-EGFR mAbs was further examined for *in vivo* activity and was also observed to have antitumor activity *in vivo* (Fig. 21.3B). This very high percentage of active mAbs, with varying epitopic specificities, confirms that our immunization process yields panels of mAbs enriched for targeting accessible epitopes on a protein and that our up-front selection process enriches for those that will eventually prove to have biological activity.

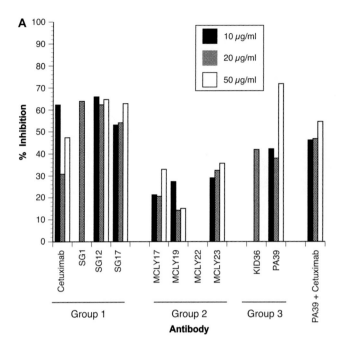

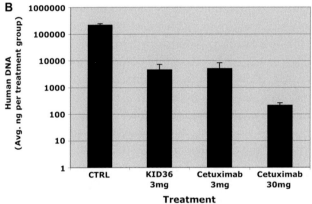

Figure 21.3. Comparison of *in vitro* and *in vivo* growth inhibitory activity of Raven-derived anti-EGFR antibodies with the commercially approved therapeutic antibody cetuximab on SW480 human colon adenocarcinoma cells. (A) Shown are the results from a 4-day monolayer assay measuring cell viability and plotted as percent inhibition relative to control, untreated cells. The anti-EGFR mAbs are divided into three epitope classes: SG1, SG12, and SG17 recognize an epitope that overlaps with cetuximab; MCLY17, MCLY19, MCLY22, and MCLY23 recognize an overlapping epitope that is distinct from cetuximab; KID36 and PA39 also recognize an overlapping epitope that is distinct from cetuximab and also distinct from the epitope recognized by the MCLY set of mAbs. Eight of the nine Raven-derived anti-EGFR mAbs exhibited activity similar to that of cetuximab. (B) Comparison of *in vivo* antitumor activity of the Raven-derived anti-EGFR antibody KID36 with the commercially approved therapeutic antibody cetuximab on SW40 human colon adenocarcinoma cells. 5×10^5 SW480 tumor cells cultured overnight in a collagen button were placed under the mouse kidney capsule and allowed to establish for two days as previously described (Loo, Pryer et al. 2007; Parmar, Young et al. 2002). The mice were then treated twice-weekly over the course of 3 weeks, and tumors were removed for analysis 2 days following the final treatment. Tumors were analyzed by quantitative PCR to quantitate the amount of human DNA, as a surrogate for tumor burden, as described (Loo, Pryer et al. 2007). As shown in the figure, KID36 exhibited potent antitumor activity in the model at a level equivalent to cetuximab.

To date there do not appear to be immuno-dominant proteins or epitopes arising from any single cell line. Typically 10–100 independent mAbs to different protein targets pass the initial screen from each immunization. We have generated multiple mAbs to some targets (e.g., transferrin receptor, carcinoembryonic antigen, and EGFR); however, the mAbs tend to recognize different epitopes within a target and have arisen from immunizations with different cell lines, including normal fetal tissue progenitor cell lines and tumor stem cell lines. As an example, we have immunized with one cell line, the fetal kidney progenitor cell line, 11 times and have obtained 152 mAbs that passed the early screens. We continue to generate mAbs to new targets with each immunization, and thus have yet to exhaust the potential of even this single cell line for obtaining new targets. Two mAbs generated from the kidney progenitor cell line immunizations – KID3 (anti-RAAG12 mAb; parent to RAV12) and KID24 (an anti-ADAM9 mAb) – are in clinical and preclinical development, respectively. Since we have developed a large panel of normal fetal tissue progenitor and cancer stem cell lines at Raven, and some of these have been used for immunization only once, we are confident that there is great potential for the discovery of additional novel therapeutic targets using this platform. Additionally, alternate screening strategies to target specific cancer types and/or biological activities may also be integrated into the platform to bias the system toward specific desirable properties.

As previously mentioned, RAV12 is the chimeric form of the murine antibody KID3. KID3 was generated from an immunization with the fetal kidney tissue progenitor cell line and was chosen as a development candidate based on the novelty and expression profile of the antigen, its potent antitumor activity *in vitro* and *in vivo*, its multiple mechanisms of action, and its preclinical safety profile. The epitope recognized by RAV12 is a novel N-linked carbohydrate epitope, or glycotope, that we have designated RAAG12. The minimal structure required for mAb binding is shown in Figure 21.4 and consists of Galβ1 – 3GlcNAcβ1 – 3Gal. Although this sugar structure bears some homology to Lewis-a, a member of the Lewis family of antigens, as shown in the figure, it is distinct. RAAG12 is found associated with a broad range of proteins in cancer cells but does not require the presence of protein for binding. It is thought to be difficult to obtain high affinity, IgG isotype mAbs to carbohydrate antigens. However, both the original murine mAb (KID3) and the chimerized RAV12 are high-affinity, IgG1 isotype mAbs. The extreme high affinity of RAV12, as measured by biacore analysis, is primarily due to the inability to measure a K_{off}, which may be related to the fact that there are multiple binding sites per antigen molecule.

RAV12 is primate restricted and does not bind to most normal tissues, including cardiovascular, endocrine, neuromuscular, hematopoietic, and nervous system tissue. RAAG12 is found on the surface of some proportion of most adenocarcinomas and on virtually all colorectal, gastric, esophageal, and pancreatic cancers. In the case of gastrointestinal cancers, expression is strong and uniform and encompasses the whole cell membrane. In other adenocarcinomas there was a continuum of expression from weak to very strong. Many normal exocrine epithelial cells express RAAG12, but the distribution of antigen in these cells is distinct from cancer tissue,

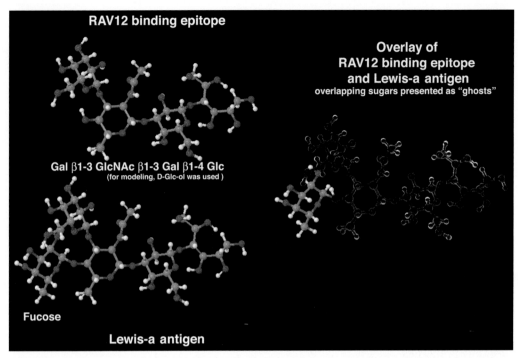

Figure 21.4. The RAAG12 glycotope, the target for the RAV12 antibody, is an N-linked carbohydrate distinct from known cancer glycotopes. The minimal RAV12 binding region encompasses Galβ1 – 3GlcNAcβ1 – 3Gal as determined using synthetic carbohydrate analogs. This epitope is similar to Lewis-a antigen, a member of the Lewis blood group antigens. As can be seen, the two structures are very similar (modeled Galβ1 – 3GlcNAcβ1 – 3Gal on top, as labeled, and modeled Lewis-a antigen on bottom, as labeled). The difference resides in the terminal α1–4 linked fucose found on the Lewis-a antigen. This is accentuated in the overlaid model shown on the right. The overlapping carbohydrate structures are "ghosted" out, highlighting the fucose, the difference between the two structures, and the structure that determines RAV12 specificity. [See color plate.]

with expression localized largely in the cytoplasm and on the luminal surface of polarized epithelial cells. For a complete discussion of the pathophysiology of RAAG12 refer to Loo et al. (Loo, 2008).

SAFETY AND CHOOSING *IN VIVO* TOXICOLOGY MODEL

When using intact stem cells and our immunization technique, a very high percentage of the resultant mAbs work as reagents for immunohistochemistry (IHC). Since these are murine mAbs they can be used directly for staining human tissues, and their binding can be visualized using a labeled anti-murine mAb second reagent. We can thus, very early in the discovery process, determine the extent of expression and tissue and subcellular localization of the target. This screening is done in an iterative fashion. The initial screen is performed on three to six normal tissues and the mAbs ranked as tier 1 (no strong staining on any normal tissue); tier 2 (some staining of normal tissue – further broken down into 2a, b, or c depending on extent and tissue type); or tier 3 (extensive staining on normal tissues). Raven mAbs to EGFR and HER2 are ranked as 2c and 2b, respectively. Tier 3 mAbs are not tested further, while tier 1 and 2 mAbs advance to further screens, including more extensive IHC screening on normal tissues and screening for binding to a range of cancer cell lines, including the NCI 60 collection of tumor lines and the Raven cancer stem cell lines. When a mAb is selected for preclinical development, a series of tissues from rats, mice, cats, dogs, guinea pigs, pigs, and several primate species are screened for cross-reactivity of the mAb. We then select the species where the tissue distribution of the target most closely resembles that in the human for preclinical pharmacology and safety studies. Interestingly, we have not yet seen any mAb generated using this platform that cross-reacts with any species but primate – this includes RAV12 whose target is a glycotope. We have had two mAb candidates that were held from development because we could not find a suitable model for safety testing. One had no cross-reactivity with any species other than human, and the other had more extensive expression of the target in primate tissues than human, making toxicology testing in these species not possible. Having the mAb in hand early allows this go–no go decision to be made early in the discovery/development process before there has been a great investment of resources in the program.

We have found that it is very informative to be able to use the therapeutic mAb itself for screening for tissue binding. We have observed quite distinct tissue binding patterns and bioactivity profiles from families of mAbs to a given single protein target due to differences in their epitopic specificity. By selecting the mAb to the most tumor-specific epitope, we can maximize the relative difference in binding between normal and cancer tissue and thus provide the greatest possible margin of safety. For example, two anti-transferrin receptor (TfR) mAbs raised by our platform have nonoverlapping epitope specificities and exhibit different binding to normal tissues. The LUCA31 mAb exhibits significantly less binding than the OVCA26 mAb to liver, pancreas, and colon, three critical tissues, while both mAbs bind equally strongly to tumors. Additionally, LUCA31 is very active as a naked antibody *in vitro* and *in vivo* in a leukemia xenograft model (Figure 21.5), whereas we have not observed potent bioactivity with OVCA26. Thus, the epitope specificity, not just target specificity, can have a profound influence on the therapeutic attractiveness of a mAb.

In the case of RAV12, immunohistochemical analysis provided additional information relevant to target specificity and safety considerations. As previously noted, RAV12 binds to some cells in the normal exocrine epithelium, especially polarized epithelium in the gut; however, the cellular localization of this binding is distinct from that seen in tumor cells derived from these tissues. In the normal gut, RAAG12 is primarily localized within the cytoplasm and on the luminal surface of the polarized epithelial cells, while in the tumors RAAG12 is predominantly membrane-associated and distributed more evenly around the whole cell membrane (Loo, 2007; Loo, 2008). Beyond differential expression, the number and types of proteins decorated with the RAAG12 glycotope may vary between normal tissue and tumor tissue, and also across individual tumors or tumor types. Thus, the subcellular location of RAAG12, as well as the composition of RAAG12-associated proteins or lipids, may influence the bioactivity and safety profile of RAV12.

Although immunohistochemical analysis of antigen expression on normal human tissues gives important guidance with respect to possible tissue sensitivities, tissue

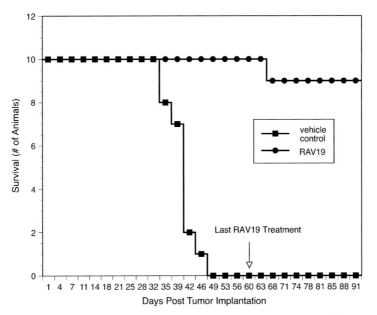

Figure 21.5. *In vivo* antitumor activity of RAV19 antibody, the chimeric form of LUCA31, in a CCRF-CEM human acute T lymphoblastic leukemia model. 10^7 CCRF-CEM tumor cells were inoculated into the tail veins of athymic mice, and then animals were treated twice weekly (intraperitoneal route) for 9 weeks with RAV19 at 50 mg/kg/dose. Animals were assessed for predesignated survival end points. Shown in the graph is a plot of animal survival over time. RAV19 significantly prolonged the survival of mice bearing CCRF-CEM tumors compared to vehicle control.

cross-reactivity has not been consistently correlated with toxicity. As outlined in the previous paragraph, the predictive value of the immunohistochemistry data may be limited since one can not accurately predict the influence of such factors as subcellular localization of antigen, epitope specificity, the composition of the target(s), and the cellular context of the target (e.g., do normal and tumor cells have the same antigen-associated functional pathways?). Thus, in order to best evaluate the safety profile of a mAb, studies must be carried out in experimental animals. Since the mAbs generated by our platform are generally primate restricted, we rely on primate toxicology models for evaluating preclinical safety and pharmacology. Primate models might also be expected to more closely reflect human physiology than rodent models.

In the case of RAV12, three independent studies were performed with cynomologous monkeys: (1) a single dose acute toxicity and pharmacokinetic study examining RAV12 at three doses (10, 30, and 100 mg/kg), (2) a repeat dose study examining RAV12 at doses of 10, 30, and 100 mg/kg, administered once weekly for 5 weeks, with a 4-week recovery period, and (3) a long-term study examining RAV12 at doses of 3, 20, and 60 mg/kg, administered once weekly for 26 weeks, with a 6-week recovery period. The initial single-dose study was performed in order to obtain an early read on possible acute toxicities and to generate preliminary pharmacokinetic data to guide dosage selection for subsequent repeat dose studies. No RAV12-related adverse events were reported in this study and animals appeared healthy throughout the duration of the study. The 5-week study was undertaken to support the initial

IND filing and support our proposed 4 once-weekly treatment regimen for the Phase I study in patients with relapsed adenocarcinoma. RAV12 was well tolerated, and the no adverse event level (NOAEL) was established at 30 mg/kg for 5 weekly doses in primates based on limited microscopic pathologic findings at the 100 mg/kg level. No corresponding changes in serum chemistries were noted. The 26-week study was subsequently conducted to allow extended treatment in the Phase I study for patients who exhibit signs of stable disease in response to RAV12 treatment. RAV12 was well tolerated in the 26-week study. Dose-dependent vomiting was seen in all RAV12 dose groups early in the study, which did not persist, and transient and sporadic increases in serum liver chemistries were observed. As expected, since the human/mouse chimeric protein is foreign to cynomologous monkeys, hypersensitivity occurred in approximately half of the RAV12-treated animals, which developed clinical signs or pathological evidence of anaphylaxis, often in the context of monkey antichimeric antibody formation. Of note, no RAV12-associated pathological findings were observed.

IN VITRO AND *IN VIVO* ANTITUMOR mAb EFFICACY: THE CHALLENGE OF SELECTING THE APPROPRIATE, PREDICTIVE MODELS

One challenge in screening for activity of potential cancer therapeutics is the historical poor correlation between the antitumor activity demonstrated in these models and clinical activity. Analysis of the results from extensive small molecule screening on the NCI 60 cells at the National Cancer Institute (Johnson, 2001) showed that activity against a specific tumor cell type did not predict activity against that same cancer type in the clinic. However, compounds that were active against multiple cell lines *in vitro* did tend to be active in the clinic in some setting. Antibody therapeutics present both advantages and different challenges when compared to small molecule development. One can assume that the lack of target would predict inactivity, but not the converse. To complicate matters, target expression in tumor tissues and in cell lines derived from these tumors frequently is not identical. Given that many of the established tumor lines have undergone alterations during extensive passage in serum (which provides a selective influence and promotes genetic instability [Loo, 1987]) and/or in animals, or by deliberate mutagenesis, it is not surprising that these lines differ significantly from the *in vivo* tumor type from which it was derived. In addition, different *in vivo* xenograft models can give differing, often contradictory, results for any one test agent. There are, however, some advantages with the existing models for testing mAbs for antitumor agents. The availability of immune deficient rodents has enabled the implantation of human tumor xenografts in order to examine the effect of test agents directly on relevant human tumor cell masses *in vivo*. This is especially critical for mAb therapeutics when there is often limited or no cross-reactivity between rodent and human targets. However, this very lack of cross-reactivity precludes obtaining efficacy and safety data concurrently in the same animal model.

We have developed a strategy to address these limitations in three different ways: (1) by incorporating multiple *in vitro* and *in vivo* tumor models of efficacy, with the requirement that candidate development mAbs be active in more than one model; (2) by developing new tumor-derived cell lines using specifically tailored defined culture media, which allows the isolation of cells with the characteristics of cancer stem cells, and using these cell lines for *in vitro* and *in vivo* efficacy screens; and (3) by developing an *in vivo* rodent tissue toxicology model with matured normal human tissues that allows an initial toxicology read on relevant human tissues in a mouse model. Each of these will be discussed.

The process of selecting and screening antibodies/targets should ideally yield a bioactive mAb. Our strategy is to assess mAbs for three *in vitro* bioactivities – antitumor activity as a naked mAb, the ability to be internalized by tumor cells expressing the target antigen, and the ability to recruit host cell effector functions. The first property, antitumor activity as a naked mAb, can be achieved via a cytostatic mechanism (e.g., cell cycle control) or a cytotoxic mechanism (apoptosis, oncosis, mitotic catastrophe, etc.). Our initial *in vitro* bioactivity screen is a 4-day monolayer growth assay, using the indicator dye Alamar Blue as a measure of cell number. This assay is run in a nonoptimized moderately high-throughput format, with the goal of rapidly identifying bioactive mAbs within a set of mAbs from an immunization that have passed the initial screens for cell surface binding and cancer specificity. mAbs are typically tested on multiple tumor cell lines that express the target antigen, and under varying culture conditions, to confirm or rule out bioactivity. When bioactive mAbs are identified, the generic monolayer assay can be optimized to capture the bioactivity of specific mAbs.

In the case of RAV12, we observed only a 15% reduction in cell number in the initial monolayer growth assay screen; however, after optimizing the assay we were able to observe much greater bioactivity, up to 90% inhibition, with an ED_{50} of 7 ug/ml (Loo, 2007). As mentioned earlier, our screening process is iterative, and new information learned about a mAb or its target often helps to guide additional efforts. In addition to the monolayer assay we have incorporated a soft agar-based growth assay, a cellular ATP content assay, apoptosis assays, cell adhesion/migration assays, and cytokine release assays in order to maximize our ability to capture bioactivity. The second property we examine is the ability of mAbs to be internalized by target cells, which is important for assessing the value of a toxin- or radiolabeled mAb approach. The third property we examine, which is a unique feature of antibody therapeutics, is the ability of mAbs to recruit aspects of the host immune system to attack tumor cells expressing the target (i.e., effector function). Two of the effector function activities – antibody-dependent cellular cytotoxicity (ADCC) and complement-dependent cytotoxicity (CDC) – have been implicated as mechanisms of action for several mAb therapeutics, including trastuzumab and rituximab (Adams, 2005; Johnson, 2003; Smith, 2003). The ability of a mAb to elicit host effector functions will be influenced by the isotype of the mAb, the mAb production system, and whether the mAb has been engineered to modulate effector functions, as well as the nature of the target.

Results from *in vitro* bioactivity assays, together with antigen profiling data, help to guide our *in vivo* efficacy studies. We have used the industry standard subcutaneous (SC) implantation of human tumor cells as one model with intravenous (i.v.) or intraperitoneal (i.p.) injection of mAb. Tumor xenografts are typically implanted in the hind flank of mice, and growth can be assessed using calipers to measure tumor size in living animals. This has the advantage that multiple time points can be obtained from the same animal over the course of the study, which allows for visualization of the rate of tumor growth or inhibition. Tumor growth tends to be quite variable from animal to animal in SC studies; therefore large sample groups are needed (N greater than or equal to 10) to generate statistically meaningful results. In addition to utilizing large sample groups, preselecting for cells that grow more rapidly *in vivo* and develop more uniform sized can greatly reduce the variability in these models. One potential drawback of preselecting for tumor cells with these *in vivo* characteristics is that these selected cells are, by definition, different from the original tumor cells and should be carefully checked to see that the target expression and other relevant phenotypic characteristics are not dramatically altered by the selection method. Selecting for rapidly growing tumors also may further remove the phenotype of these models from that of the original human tumor. An additional constraint can be added to reduce variability by allowing the tumors to grow and become established in all animals for a preset time or to a predetermined average tumor size, eliminating the animals with the largest and smallest tumors, then randomly sorting the animals into designated control and treatment groups. The results obtained from SC models can also be influenced by the site of tumor implantation (e.g., behind the neck or on the flank), the time of initiation of treatment (and, of course the dose and schedule), and the input cells, which may differ significantly from laboratory to laboratory even though they originally came from the same source (typically, American Type Cell Culture, ATCC). In addition, some models initiate the xenografts from cells or tumor tissue fragments that have been carried and passaged through animals rather than initiated from *in vitro* cell cultures. The results obtained from these animal passage models can vary significantly from those obtained using cultured cells to inoculate tumors.

Not all tumor cell lines grow, or can be adapted to grow, in an SC setting. An alternate xenograft model, the subrenal capsule model (SRC) was developed in order to efficiently establish and propagate human tumor tissues in immune deficient mice (Parmar, 2002). The SRC model has been adapted at Raven to enable the growth of tumor cell lines, some of which do not grow in the SC setting *in vivo*, and provide a rapid model to assess the antitumor activity of our mAbs. The SRC model is a much more laborious model since it requires delicate surgery to inoculate the tumor cells under the renal capsule membrane, and subsequently requires the removal of the tumor mass for measurement by either volume or weight at the end of the study. An obvious advantage of the SRC model is that no preselection is required for establishment and growth of most tumor cells in the SRC setting and suggests that the SRC setting might better reflect the in situ tumor environment, a suggestion that is supported by the ability of small pieces of primary tumor to more readily establish and grow when implanted directly into the SRC.

One of the limitations of the SRC model is that the end point readout of tumor volume or weight is prone to artifact because the measurement does not take into

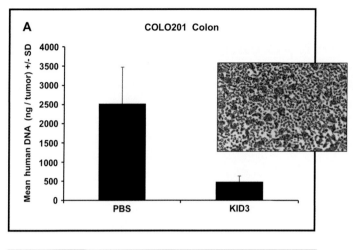

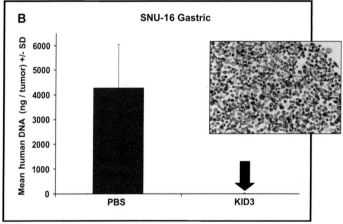

Figure 21.6. *In vivo* antitumor activity of KID3 antibody, and the chimeric form RAV12, in a series of subrenal capsule human tumor xenograft studies. In all four studies, 5 x 10^5 tumor cells were suspended in collagen and surgically implanted beneath the renal capsule of athymic mice and allowed to establish for 2 days. Animals were then treated i.p. twice weekly for 2 weeks and animals were sacrificed on day 16 and tumors were analyzed by quantitative PCR for human DNA to quantify tumor mass. (A) COLO 201 colon tumor cells treated with 50 mg/kg/dose KID3 antibody. (B) SNU-16 gastric tumor cells treated with 50 mg/kg/dose KID3 antibody. (C) A549 lung tumor cells treated with 50 mg/kg/dose KID3 antibody. (D) COLO 201 colon tumor cells treated with KID3 or RAV12 antibody at the indicated doses. RAAG12 expression of the tumor cell lines shown in the inset was performed on frozen cell pellets.

account necrotic cores within tumors or build-up of fluid within tumors, and also because it is technically difficult to separate the tumor from the murine kidney tissue since the tumors are relatively small and tumor cells may invade the host kidney. In order to circumvent this limitation, we have developed a quantitative PCR (QPCR) assay in which human DNA can be specifically quantitated in the presence of excess mouse DNA. This method is very sensitive so small tumors can be accurately measured and thus one can obtain quantitative results after only a short growth period (2–3 weeks) without the need to select for tumor cells with rapid tumor growth characteristics. We have found that using QPCR to quantify human DNA in the tumors (as a surrogate for number of living tumor cells) can decrease animal-to-animal

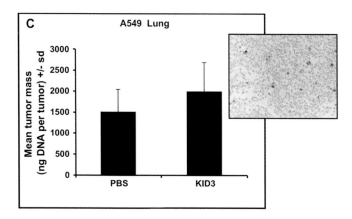

C   A549 Lung

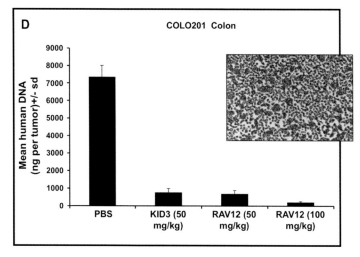

D   COLO201 Colon

variability and provide a more accurate assessment of human tumor burden. This measurement, however, requires termination of the animals and thus is currently an end point analysis only. Importantly, the SRC model also may be utilized to test for bioactivity in a setting of spontaneous metastasis. A number of our cancer stem cell lines spontaneously metastasize from the SRC to a number of organs, including the mesentary, liver, lung, and pancreas over the course of several weeks. Interestingly, we have not seen metastases with the same cancer stem cell lines when grown SC (in those cancer stem cell lines that can be grown SC). This difference in metastatic potential between the two models is likely influenced by environmental factors (e.g., vascularization potential of the implantation site, contribution of local stroma via cell-cell interactions, and production of paracrine factors). We are currently investigating the feasibility of incorporating imaging techniques in order to better characterize the growth of the implanted tumor throughout the study, and also to visualize small, spontaneously arising metastatic lesions in living animals.

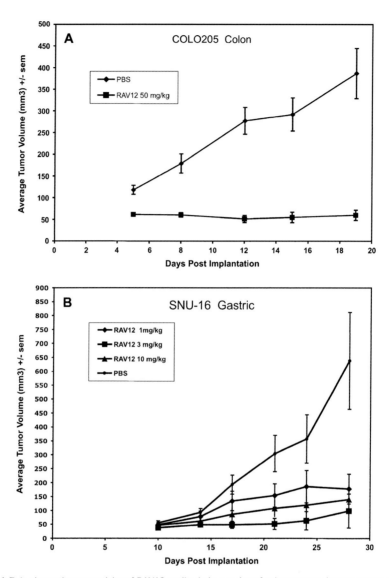

Figure 21.7 *In vivo* antitumor activity of RAV12 antibody in a series of subcutaneous human tumor xenograft studies. (A–C) Athymic mice were implanted subcutaneously with 5×10^6 of the indicated tumor cells in Matrigel and treated with RAV12 twice weekly at the indicated doses, beginning on the day of tumor implantation. (D) Experiment performed as above on COLO 205 tumor xenografts, except treatment with RAV12 began after the tumors reached an average of 250 mm^3. (E) 35 to 40 mg fragments of COLO 205 tumor cells, propagated in an *in vivo* passage, were implanted subcutaneously and allowed to grow to ~100 mg in weight (~100 mm^3 in size). Animals were then treated (beginning on day 9) i.p. with RAV12 twice weekly for 4 weeks at the indicated dose.

Comparisons of data obtained from SC and SRC models with high RAAG12-expressing human tumor cell lines treated with KID3 or RAV12 are shown in Figures 21.6 and 21.7. Initial studies using KID3 showed that it was highly efficacious in the SRC model, exhibiting a statistically significant reduction, and in many animals the elimination of COLO201 cells by the end of the study (Figure 21.6A). KID3 also

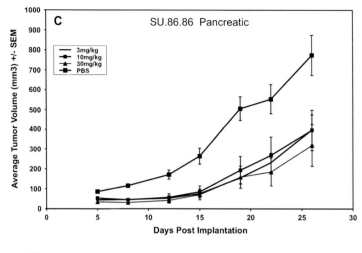

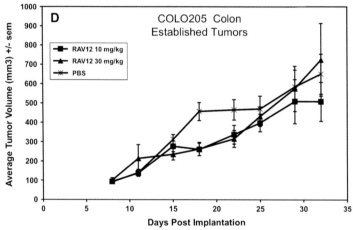

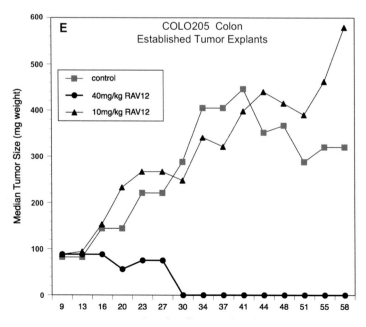

exhibited potent antitumor activity toward SNU-16 gastric tumor cells in this model
(Figure 21.6B), but did not show activity toward A549 lung tumor cells which express
little RAAG12 (Figure 21.6C). Upon generation of the chimeric antibody RAV12, a
side-by-side comparison was done in the SRC model using COLO201 tumor cells to
confirm that the chimeric antibody retained the antitumor activity observed with
KID3 (Figure 21.6D). RAV12 was also efficacious toward RAAG12-positive tumor cell
lines in the SC model. RAV12 exhibited potent antitumor activity toward COLO205
(colon), SNU-16 (gastric), and SU.86.86 (pancreatic) tumor cell xenografts when
administered beginning on the day of tumor cell implantation (preventive model;
Figure 21.7A, B, and C); conversely, RAV12 was not efficacious toward COLO205
tumor cells in the SC model when administration began after the tumors were
established and had reached a mean volume of 250 mm^3 (established model; Figure
21.7D). It is of interest that in a second established tumor model using COLO205
tumor cells carried as *in vivo* transplantable tumors (rather than in culture) there
was a marked effect of RAV12 even when treatment was initiated in animals with
large tumors (Figure 21.7E). Additionally, in another SC model using SNU-16 gastric
tumor cells, RAV12 exhibited potent antitumor activity toward 150–200 mm^3 established tumors (Loo, 2007) – highlighting the importance of surveying multiple *in vivo*
models and modes of mAb administration.

As noted previously, while IHC with candidate mAbs on normal human tissues is
both informative, and required to register a mAb for entry into clinical trials, the
presence of the target on normal tissue is inadequate to predict toxicity. For example, HER2, the target of the commercially approved mAb trastuzumab, is strongly
expressed in the normal human kidney, but no renal toxicity has been reported in
the clinic (Ewer, 2007). We have extended the SRC model for tumor growth to
provide a murine xenograft model, which may help predict toxicity of mAbs in
normal human tissues. Since many mAbs are primate restricted, this model is useful
for getting an early readout on possible toxicities in normal human tissues that
express the target. In this model, normal human fetal tissue fragments are implanted
under the kidney capsule (or other site) of severe combined immunodeficient mice
(Mather, 2004). These animals are then maintained and the tissues allowed to grow
and mature for 2 to 10 months, until the tissue of interest has matured to resemble
that of the adult tissue histologically, biochemically, and with respect to expression of
the target of interest. Following maturation of the fetal tissue, tumor cells can be
implanted under the contralateral kidney capsule and allowed to establish for a few
days. The animal may then be treated systemically with mAb via i.p. or i.v. administration. Difference in the effect of the mAb on the tumor tissue relative to normal
tissue is hypothesized to reflect the therapeutic window for that mAb candidate. An
experiment of this type using a toxin-conjugated mAb is shown in Figure 21.8. We
chose a mAb that had slight *in vivo* activity as a naked mAb and whose target was
expressed on several normal tissues, including pancreatic acinar cells. After toxin
conjugation, potent antitumor activity of the toxin-conjugated mAb was seen toward the DU-145 prostate tumor xenograft, with activity observed at the lowest dose
of 3 mg/kg. Conversely, while no effect on normal tissues was seen with unconjugated
mAb, the toxin conjugated mAb was toxic toward the matured fetal pancreatic

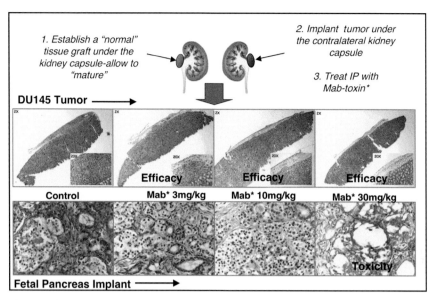

Figure 21.8. *In vivo* human tissue toxicology model. Human fetal pancreatic tissue was implanted under the renal capsule of athymic mice and allowed to mature for 5.5 months until it resembled that of the adult pancreas. 5×10^5 DU145 prostate tumor cells, which express the antigen of interest, were subsequently implanted under the contralateral renal capsule and allowed to establish for 2 days. The animals were then treated with a toxin-conjugated antibody twice weekly for 2 weeks, and the xenografts were analyzed histologically on day 16. Toxicity of the matured pancreatic tissue implant was observed at 30 mg/kg/dose, whereas antitumor efficacy was observed with doses as low as 3 mg/kg. [See color plate.]

implant, which also expresses the target. This toxicity was only observed at the highest dose of 30 mg/kg, suggesting a 10-fold or greater therapeutic window for the toxin-conjugated mAb. While this is clearly a first approximation of the efficacy/ toxicity profile of a candidate mAb, it does provide an early look at possible toxicities toward human tissue in the context of an antitumor efficacy readout, and enables one to make go–no go development decisions, or to better direct animal safety studies should toxicity be observed. However, this type of model might be considered a more relevant readout for mAbs than for small molecules where the differences in metabolism of the drug by mice and man might affect both activity and toxicity.

MECHANISMS OF ACTION

We focus on antitumor activity to validate a mAb and its target, which may involve a cytostatic mechanism (e.g., cell cycle control) or a cytostatic mechanism (apoptosis, oncosis, mitotic catastrophe, etc.). The monolayer assay is able to capture both of these activities; however, it cannot distinguish between them. In the case of RAV12, the initial observation of bioactivity came from an *in vitro* monolayer assay measuring COLO205 tumor cell number following treatment with RAV12 for 4 days. Subsequent studies showed that RAV12 is directly cytotoxic to COLO205 cells

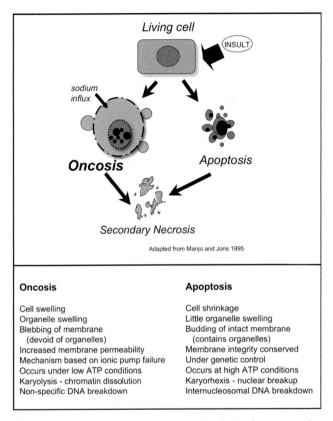

Figure 21.9. Oncosis is a cell death mechanism distinct from apoptosis.

in vitro via an oncotic mechanism. Oncosis has been observed in numerous human diseases, including myocardial infarction, stroke, and acute renal and liver failure (Liu, 2004). This mechanism is distinct from the more familiar apoptotic mechanism of cell death, and the key differences of the two cell death mechanisms reported to date are outlined in Figure 21.9. Oncosis is energy independent and so does not require synthesis of new mRNA or protein. In some cases, oncosis has been shown to result from decreased levels of ATP and dysregulated membrane ion channels, which leads to sodium influx, cell swelling, and lysis (Barros, 2001). In the case of RAV12, oncosis begins within a few hours of adding RAV12, which makes this mechanism more challenging to study than apoptosis. However, this is a physiologically relevant mechanism (Barros, 2001; Liu, 2004; Majno, 1995), and at least two other mAbs (Ma, 2001; Matsuoka, 1995) and a small molecule (Suarez, 2003) have been shown to act via this pathway. It is also possible that some of the agents said to have "caspase-independent" cytotoxicity, or necrotic cytotoxicity, may also act via oncosis (Barros, 2001; Trump, 1997).

RAV12 is also interesting in that the cancer cells that have high levels of RAAG12 on their surface seem to accomplish this by putting this glycotope on a large number of different proteins, including growth factor receptors (Li, 2007), as shown in Figure 21.10. The decoration of cell surface growth factor receptors with

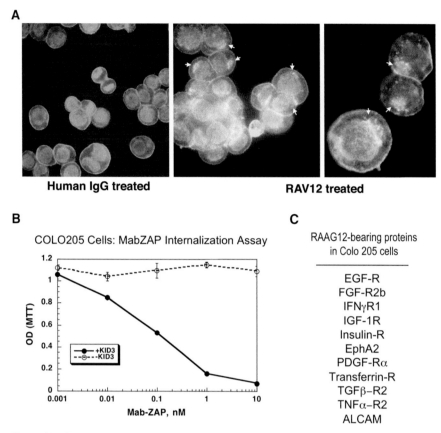

Figure 21.10. KID3 binds to RAAG12-bearing cell surface proteins and is rapidly internalized. (A) COLO 205 tumor cells were treated with RAV12 antibody or human IgG for 48 hours (see figure label) then applied human IgG Fc was visualized by fluorescent microscopy. The treatment with RAV12, which binds strongly to the cell surface, results in capping and internalization of the RAV12 antibody (red, Cy3-conjugated antihuman IgG Fc – see arrows). Capping and internalization of RAV12 could be observed within 1 hour of antibody treatment. Capping and internalization was not observed in conditions where cells were treated with control human IgG. Unbound RAAG12 was stained using fresh KID3 antibody (green, FITC-conjugated anti-mouse IgG Fc) and is membrane specific on both RAV12 treated and untreated cells. (B) *In vitro* internalization of KID3 antibody by COLO 205 tumor cells measured by internalization of a toxin-conjugated anti-mouse secondary antibody (mAb-ZAP). A differential decrease in cell viability in the KID3 condition relative to the control condition (no KID3 present), as measured by MTT, indicates antibody internalization. (C) A partial list of cell surface proteins that are decorated with RAAG12 in COLO 205 cells. [See color plate.]

carbohydrate structures has been shown to play a role in the function and regulation of these receptors. As an example, the cell surface growth factor receptors ErbB1 and ErbB2 have been reported to be decorated with the Lewis Y carbohydrate on human breast and epidermoid tumor cells, and anti-Lewis Y mAbs can block EGF- and heregulin-mediated signaling events in these cells (Klinger, 2004). As the antigen-mAb complex is internalized, these receptors would be depleted on the cell surface and the effects of their respective growth factors, including survival signals, would be diminished. Thus a secondary direct effect of mAb binding might be to decrease the accessibility of necessary growth factors for tumor cells. Finally RAV12 has also been shown to recruit host immune effector function, leading to tumor cell cytotoxicity via both ADCC and CDC *in vitro*.

RAV12 also has additive or synergistic effects with a number of chemotherapeutic agents *in vitro* and *in vivo*. Additivity or synergy of mAbs with chemotherapeutic agents seems to be a common property of most therapeutic antibodies, including toxin-conjugated mAbs, which one would expect should kill virtually every cell that internalizes them. While arguments have been made for mechanism-based synergies with some mAb/chemotherapy combinations, an intriguing suggestion is that the benefit of adding two such therapies together lies partially, or completely, in the chemotherapeutic agent causing sufficient damage to the tumor that the vasculature becomes compromised and enables macromolecules to leak into and out of the vasculature. This may benefit a mAb therapeutic by allowing trapped shed antigen, which could bind and inactivate the mAb, to leak out, thus decreasing mAb binding by soluble antigen in the tumor (Zhang, 2007).

To date there is still a great deal to be learned about the biological activity of even well-studied and marketed mAbs to very well-studied targets such as EGFR and HER2. Our experience has been that, even looking only at the external part of a target molecule, the epitope recognized by the mAb on a given target may play a role in the biological function of the mAb including modulation of biological activity *in vitro* and *in vivo*, internalization, phosphorylation of the target molecule, and pattern of IHC binding to tumor and normal tissue. In many cases these activities are independent so that, for instance, *in vivo* activity cannot always be predicted by *in vitro* activity even when the mAbs bind to the same protein. Until more is understood of this biological complexity we are left with the necessity of using a fairly large number of assays and looking at the entire set of data to select the "best" mAb for a specific application. Undoubtedly this situation will improve as more clinical experience is accumulated with mAbs.

CONCLUSION

The use of mAbs for the treatment of cancer and other diseases is still in its infancy, with just a little over a decade of experience with approved antibodies. The field of antibody engineering has provided a host of new antibody formats and conjugates. The experience at Raven suggests that there are a large number of novel mAb targets and novel epitopes on known proteins yet to be discovered. Experience with many mAbs in the clinical setting has led to the adoption of combination therapies, combining small molecule and mAb therapeutics to increase the efficacy of these therapeutics without increasing toxicity. Additionally, treatment with mAbs at earlier stages of disease progression has proven advantageous in some cancers (Dinh, 2007). It seems likely that this field will continue to grow as we identify new targets and develop better ways of using these mAbs clinically. The Raven platform can contribute to this progress by discovering important new targets and therapeutic antibodies for the treatment of cancer which have new mechanisms of action and improved safety profiles. The first mAb from the Raven platform, RAV12, is currently in Phase II clinical trials. The combination of engineered antibodies, novel targets, and improved clinical administration should significantly improve patient outcome in cancer and a number of other diseases in the decades to come.

REFERENCES

Adams, G.P. and L.M. Weiner (2005). "Monoclonal antibody therapy of cancer." *Nat Biotechnol* **23**(9): 1147–57.

Barros, L.F., T. Hermosilla, et al. (2001). "Necrotic volume increase and the early physiology of necrosis." *Comp Biochem Physiol A Mol Integr Physiol* **130**(3): 401–9.

Carles-Kinch, K., K.E. Kilpatrick, et al. (2002). "Antibody targeting of the EphA2 tyrosine kinase inhibits malignant cell behavior." *Cancer Res* **62**(10): 2840–7.

Dinh, P., E. de Azambuja, et al. (2007). "Trastuzumab for early breast cancer: current status and future directions." *Clin Adv Hematol Oncol* **5**(9): 707–17.

Ewer, M.S. and J.A. O'Shaughnessy (2007). "Cardiac toxicity of trastuzumab-related regimens in HER2-overexpressing breast cancer." *Clin Breast Cancer* **7**(8): 600–7.

Harlow, E. and D. Lane (1988). *Antibodies: a laboratory manual*, Cold Spring Harbor Laboratory Press.

Johnson, J.I., S. Decker, et al. (2001). "Relationships between drug activity in NCI preclinical in vitro and in vivo models and early clinical trials." *Br J Cancer* **84**(10): 1424–31.

Johnson, P. and M. Glennie (2003). "The mechanisms of action of rituximab in the elimination of tumor cells." *Semin Oncol* **30**(1 Suppl. 2): 3–8.

Klinger, M., H. Farhan, et al. (2004). "Antibodies directed against Lewis-Y antigen inhibit signaling of Lewis-Y modified ErbB receptors." *Cancer Res* **64**(3): 1087–93.

Li, J.C. and R. Li (2007). "RAV12 accelerates the desensitization of Akt/PKB pathway of insulin-like growth factor I receptor signaling in COLO205." *Cancer Res* **67**(18): 8856–64.

Liu, X., T. Van Vleet, et al. (2004). "The role of calpain in oncotic cell death." *Annu Rev Pharmacol Toxicol* **44**: 349–70.

Loo, D., M. Armanini, et al. (2008). "The RAV12 monoclonal antibody recognizes the N-linked glycotope RAAG12; expression in human normal and tumor tissue." *Arch Pathol and Lab Medicine*. In press.

Loo, D., N. Pryer, et al. (2007). "The glycotope-specific RAV12 monoclonal antibody induces oncosis in vitro and has antitumor activity against gastrointestinal adenocarcinoma tumor xenografts in vivo." *Mol Cancer Ther* **6**(3): 856–65.

Loo, D.T., J.I. Fuquay, et al. (1987). "Extended culture of mouse embryo cells without senescence: inhibition by serum." *Science* **236**(4798): 200–2.

Ma, F., C. Zhang, et al. (2001). "Molecular cloning of Porimin, a novel cell surface receptor mediating oncotic cell death." *Proc Natl Acad Sci USA* **98**(17): 9778–83.

Majno, G. and I. Joris (1995). "Apoptosis, oncosis, and necrosis. An overview of cell death." *Am J Pathol* **146**(1): 3–15.

Mather, J.P. and P.F. Young, inventors; Raven Biotechnologies, Inc., assignee. Animal model for toxicology and dose prediction. *United States patent US* **20**,040,045,045. 2004 March 4.

Matsuoka, S., Y. Asano, et al. (1995). "A novel type of cell death of lymphocytes induced by a monoclonal antibody without participation of complement." *J Exp Med* **181**(6): 2007–15.

Parmar, H., P. Young, et al. (2002). "A novel method for growing human breast epithelium in vivo using mouse and human mammary fibroblasts." *Endocrinology* **143**(12): 4886–96.

Smith, M.R. (2003). "Rituximab (monoclonal anti-CD20 antibody): mechanisms of action and resistance." *Oncogene* **22**(47): 7359–68.

Suarez, Y., L. Gonzalez, et al. (2003). "Kahalalide F, a new marine-derived compound, induces oncosis in human prostate and breast cancer cells." *Mol Cancer Ther* **2**(9): 863–72.

Trump, B.F., I.K. Berezesky, et al. (1997). "The pathways of cell death: oncosis, apoptosis, and necrosis." *Toxicol Pathol* **25**(1): 82–8.

Zhang, Y., L. Xiang, et al. (2007). "Immunotoxin and Taxol synergy results from a decrease in shed mesothelin levels in the extracellular space of tumors." *Proc Natl Acad Sci USA* **104**(43): 17099–104.

Antibody Directed Enzyme Prodrug Therapy (ADEPT)

Helen L. Lowe, Surinder K. Sharma, Kenneth D. Bagshawe, and Kerry A. Chester

In antibody-directed enzyme prodrug therapy (ADEPT), an antibody is used to target an enzyme to tumor. After tumor localization and deactivation or clearance of enzyme from blood and other normal tissue, a prodrug is given. The prodrug is converted into a toxic chemotherapeutic by the pretargeted enzyme at the tumor site (Figure 22.1). The ADEPT system, originally conceived in 1987,[1] has a number of potential advantages over standard chemotherapy or the use of antibody-toxin conjugates. If a relatively nontoxic prodrug is used and there is no significant conversion of prodrug in nontarget organs, toxicity is restricted to the tumor site, allowing highly potent and specific treatments. Moreover, since one enzyme is able to turn over many prodrug molecules, the tumor essentially becomes a factory for generating its own means of destruction. Importantly, active drug can also diffuse to nearby cells, creating a local bystander effect where antigen negative cells and tumor-supportive stromal elements are destroyed.

ADEPT is a complex system that can be influenced by many components. These components, outlined in Figure 22.2, have been investigated by various workers over the last 2 decades and the results provide a platform of understanding for future applications of the treatment. Here we describe the progress of ADEPT since the first proofs-of-principle[1-3] to recent advances in the clinic.

ADEPT SYSTEMS

Prodrugs

Most of the prodrugs used in ADEPT have been designed for conversion into cytotoxic drugs that are already licensed for clinical use. The difference in toxicity between prodrug and drug determines how much prodrug can be given. For instance, if the toxicity differential is 100-fold, then up to a 100-fold times more prodrug can be given than the corresponding toxic drug. Half-life of active drug is also important. Optimal $t_{1/2}$ is yet to be established; however, it has been shown that a drug with $t_{1/2}$ of only 30 minutes could leak back into the blood from tumor sites and cause myelosuppression.[4] Most licensed cytotoxic agents have half-lives that are several hours in duration and it is possible that only drugs with a very short half-life would restrict cytotoxic action to tumor sites.

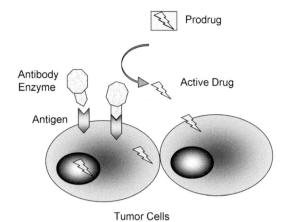

Figure 22.1. Schematic diagram of ADEPT. An antibody-enzyme localizes to the tumor site. Once the protein is cleared from normal tissue a prodrug is administered. The prodrug is converted to toxic drug at the site of the tumor and a bystander effect can be seen on tumor cells that do not express the targeting antigen.

Many of the prodrugs that have been applied in ADEPT systems are represented in Table 22.1. However, although the design and production of prodrugs for conversion to active drug by specific enzymes is an important component of ADEPT, the development of prodrugs in its wider context is largely beyond the scope of this review; the reader is referred to several excellent publications covering this field.[5–7]

ADEPT ENZYME OVERVIEW

Antibodies have been used to target a number of enzymes for utility in ADEPT systems and a wide variety of these enzymes have shown promising results. These

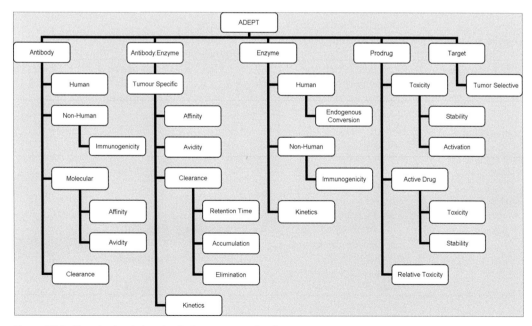

Figure 22.2. Organizational chart for the key concepts of antibody directed enzyme prodrug therapy (ADEPT).

TABLE 22.1. Summary of ADEPT systems

Enzyme	Antibody	Format	Active drug	References
Alkaline phosphatase	IgG2a antibody to carbohydrate antigen on carcinomas	Chemical conjugate	Etoposide, mitomycin C, doxorubicin, phenol mustard,	[3,8,9] [10,11]
Carboxypeptidase A	Monoclonal antibody to human lung adenocarcinoma		Methotrexate	[12,13]
	Monoclonal antibody to glycosylated surface protein on human ovarian teratocarcinoma			[14]
	Monoclonal antibody to Ep-CAM			[15]
Carboxypeptidase A1 mutant (human)	Monoclonal antibody to EpCAM			[16]
	scFv to seminoprotein	Fusion protein		[17]
Carboxypeptidase G2	hCG antibody	Chemical conjugate	Nitrogen mustard	[2,18,19]
	CEA F(Ab′)2			[20,21] [22,23] [24,25]
	CEA scFv	Fusion protein		[26,27] [28,29] [30]
Cytosine deaminase	IgG2a to carcinoma	Chemical conjugate	5-Fluorouracil	[31,32] [33,34]
	scFv to gpA33 antigen in colon cancers	Fusion protein		[35,36]
B-Galactosidase	Monoclonal antibody	Chemical conjugate		[37]
B-Glucuronidase	Monoclonal antibody to carcinomas		Daunorubicin and doxorubicin	[38–40]
	IgG2a antibody expressed on AS-30D cell line		Phenol mustard	[41]
	CEA	Fusion protein	Doxorubicin	[42,43]
B-Glucuronidase (human)	scFv to EpCAM			[44]
	F(Ab′)2 to a tumor necrosis antigen			[45]
B-Lactamase	IgG2a F(Ab′)2 to carbohydrate antigen on carcinomas	Chemical conjugate	Nitrogen mustard	[46,47]
	dsFv to p185^{HER2}	Fusion	Doxorubicin	[48]
	scFv to melanotransferrin p97	Protein	Nitrogen mustard	[49,50]

Enzyme	Antibody	Format	Active drug	References
	scFv to melanoma		Paclitaxel	[51]
	scFv to TAG72 carbohydrate epitope		Melphalan	[52]
	Nanobody to CEA		Nitrogen mustard	[53]
Penicillin-G-amidase	IgG2a Monoclonal antibody to carcinoma cells	Chemical conjugate	N-(4-hydroxyphenyl-acetyl) palytoxin, doxorubicin, melphalan	[54,55]
Penicillin V amidase	IgG2a antibody to carbohydrate antigen on carcinomas		Doxorubicin and melphalan	[56]
Prolyl endopeptidase (human)	Monoclonal antibody to EDB domain of fibronectin		Methotrexate, cephalosporin analogs and melphalan	[57]

include alkaline phosphatase,[3,8–11] carboxypeptidase A,[12–17] carboxypeptidase G2,[2,18–30] cytosine deaminase,[31–36] β-galactosidase,[37] β-glucuronidase,[38–45] β-lacta-mase,[46–53] penicillin amidase,[54–56] and prolyl endopeptidase.[57] The first enzymes investigated were alkaline phosphatase and carboxypeptidase G2 (CPG2). CPG2 is the only ADEPT enzyme to be tested in clinical trials and is discussed separately later in the chapter. Alkaline phosphatase hydrolyzes esters of phosphoric acid and therefore dephosphorylates prodrugs for conversion into active drug. The enzyme has been used successfully in preclinical ADEPT systems using prodrugs such as etoposide phosphate,[3] mitomycin phosphate,[9] and doxorubicin phosphate.[9] For example, an etoposide phosphate prodrug was successfully converted by alkaline phosphatase into an etoposide drug that was 100-fold more toxic than its prodrug counterpart.[58] The antibody-alkaline phosphatase conjugates used in these studies were also shown to be stable and free from aggregates. Furthermore, *in vivo* experiments demonstrated better responses with conjugate and prodrug than with either drug or prodrug alone.[58] Similarly, when a monoclonal antibody-alkaline phosphatase conjugate was used with a phenol mustard prodrug, the targeted therapy showed a much greater response than with prodrug alone or with the use of a nonspecific antibody.[11]

Essentially, the use of alkaline phosphatase in ADEPT enables a large number of prodrug systems to be explored because the enzyme lacks substrate specificity and the addition of a phosphate group dramatically reduces the toxicity of many drugs. This is thought to be due to the reduced cellular uptake of phosphorylated drugs.[7] The downside to use of alkaline phosphatase is that its human counterpart is found in many tissues and this could cause unwanted toxicity by off-target conversion of prodrug by endogenous enzyme in blood and other tissues.

The enzymes and ADEPT systems employed with these enzymes are shown in Table 22.1. The majority of these enzymes are of bacterial origin as this reduces or eliminates the possibility of endogenous conversion of prodrug, although human enzymes have also been employed (see the section of this chapter entitled Modifying T Cell Epitopes). The most developed bacterial enzymes are β-lactamase and CPG2.

β-Lactamase

β-Lactamase enzyme hydrolyses the β-lactam (C-N) bond in β-lactam antibiotics and has been used successfully to convert many prodrugs into nitrogen mustards, doxorubicin, mitomycin, paclitaxel, and platinum reagents. These prodrugs all contain β-lactam rings which are cleaved to form the active drugs (as reviewed by Senter and Springer[6]).

β-Lactamase ADEPT systems have shown preclinical success with a variety of antibody formats. For instance, with a F(ab′)2 antibody fragment chemically conjugated to β-lactamase and used in combination with a cephalosporin mustard prodrug.[46] In this case, the prodrug showed a 50-fold increase in toxicity when converted to active drug by the conjugated β-lactamase and only when the specific antigen was present on cells.[46] In vivo the prodrug was less toxic than the active drug and an antitumor ADEPT effect was observed with the F(ab′)2–β-Lactamase conjugate but not with conjugate or prodrug alone.[47]

A humanized disulphide linked Fv antibody fragment, whose parent antibody has been used in clinical trials for targeting p185[HER2] in breast cancer, has also been used for ADEPT as a genetic fusion with β-lactamase.[48] The fusion protein was used with a doxorubicin prodrug and it retained antigen-binding and kinetic activity, and cleared rapidly from circulation in nude mice.[48] This fusion protein was an important step forward in ADEPT as genetic fusions are more readily reproduced than chemical conjugations and are more appropriate for use in a regulatory environment.

A β-lactamase fusion protein has also been shown to be superior to a chemical conjugate in a side-by-side comparison of ADEPT using Fab fragments or single chain Fv antibody fragments (scFvs) of a monoclonal antibody that binds to the p97 antigen on melanomas and carcinomas.[49] The Fab-enzyme conjugate and scFv-enzyme fusion were both able to elicit cures in two in vivo models. However, the fusion protein localized to the tumor much faster and cleared more rapidly from the circulation than the Fab conjugate, enabling a more favorable therapeutic window for prodrug administration.[49]

β-Lactamase has also been used for ADEPT as a fusion protein with a "nanobody" reactive with carcinoembryonic antigen (CEA). Nanobodies are naturally occurring single VHH domain antibody fragments found in the camel immune system. The nanobody-β-lactamase protein was expressed in bacteria and was highly promising in preclinical in vivo biodistribution and therapy studies, where tumor remissions and some complete cures were reported in xenograft models.[53]

Excellent results have also been reported using β-lactamase as a fusion protein with an scFv to TAG-72, a carbohydrate epitope exposed and overexpressed in many solid malignancies. The fusion protein showed a tumor retention time of 36.9 hours in vivo with tumor:blood ratios of 1000:1. When combined with a melphalan prodrug that was designed to enhance the solubility of the prodrug there was significant efficacy in a xenograft tumor model.[52]

Clearly, β-lactamase ADEPT systems show great potential. The main drawback with this enzyme, and indeed the downside to using foreign enzymes, is that it is most likely to be immunogenic in humans. However, for β-lactamase this has been addressed to some extent (see Modifying T Cell Epitopes).

Carboxypeptidase G2 (CPG2)

Carboxypeptidase G2 (CPG2) is a bacterial, dimeric zinc-dependent exopeptidase enzyme that acts by cleaving the glutamic acid moiety from folic acid and folate analogs such as the chemotherapeutic agent methotrexate. As with β-lactamase, CPG2 does not have a human equivalent in terms of substrate specificity, allowing use of prodrugs that will not be subjected to unwanted conversion to potent active drug by endogenous enzymes. All published clinical ADEPT trials to date have utilized the CPG2 enzyme, although there have been variations in format developed through close feedback with preclinical research as described later in the chapter.

The first reported *in vivo* studies using CPG2-based ADEPT used a xenograft model for choriocarcinoma with an antibody directed toward human chorionic gonadotrophin (hCG).[2] Since there is a large pool of hCG in the blood, the mice showed accelerated clearance of the conjugate from the blood and the benzoic acid prodrug could be administered between 56 and 72 hours after the conjugate. This resulted in the eradication of 9 out of 12 tumors that were resistant to conventional chemotherapy[19] and demonstrated the exciting potential of this enzyme for ADEPT.

In later studies, a CEA-binding F(ab′)2 fragment of the A5B7 murine monoclonal antibody was chemically conjugated to CPG2 and tested for efficacy in mice bearing LS174T human colon adenocarcinoma xenografts. However, in this case, clearance of conjugate from plasma was slow, possibly due to low circulating levels of CEA. As a result, it was necessary to delay prodrug injection for up to 6–7 days to avoid toxicity, with the consequence that no therapeutic benefit occurred.[59] To increase the speed with which the conjugate cleared, an antibody (SB43) directed to the active site of CPG2 was used to inactivate the circulating enzyme.[60] This enzyme inactivating antibody was also galactosylated to accelerate clearance of conjugate from blood via receptors in the liver[61] without affecting enzyme levels in the tumor. It was found that the prodrug, 4-[2-chloroethyl-(2 mesyloxyethyl)amino]benzoyl-L-glutamic acid (CMDA)[18] could be given within 24 hours after the conjugate without toxicity and resulted in significant growth delay of the human colon and ovarian tumor xenografts.[62,63] Following this success with this three-phase ADEPT system, a pilot clinical trial of ADEPT was initiated.[20]

F(ab′)2-CPG2 Clinical Trial

The first clinical trial of ADEPT used the three-phase system described earlier, that is, an anti-CEA F(ab′)2-CPG2 conjugate followed by an inactivating galactosylated antibody to CPG2 and subsequently by the CMDA prodrug. The trial demonstrated that this ADEPT system could achieve high tumor levels of enzyme and low amounts in normal tissues in humans. The 17 patients treated had advanced stage metastatic colorectal cancer and the study was also set up to investigate the prodrug escalation. Remarkable results were obtained from the eight patients who received the highest doses of prodrug; four had partial responses and one a mixed response.[20–22] Most patients suffered myelosuppression and it was suspected that the drug had leaked back from tumor sites into the blood.

The same system was subsequently used by Napier et al. to investigate a lower dose of antibody enzyme conjugate. One patient achieved a partial response and most of the other patients had stable disease for several months.[24] This study included the use of liver biopsies from metastatic sites taken once the enzyme inactivating antibody had been administered. The tumor:blood ratios were in excess of 10,000:1 and it is therefore thought that the myelosuppressive effects seen in patients did not result from the conversion of prodrug to active drug in the blood but was probably due to the leak back of the drug from tumors. The drug derived from CMDA had a half-life of approximately 30 minutes.[27] It was concluded from these studies that ideally, the generated drug should have a very short half-life to avoid toxicity due to the leak back effect.

A new bis-iodo-phenol mustard prodrug with a short half-life active drug was synthesized to address potential toxicity.[64] Together with the F(ab′)2 fragment chemically conjugated to CPG2, the new prodrug system gave impressive cell kill data *in vivo*.[23] However, in a later trial designed to simplify the system, the use of the clearing antibody step was omitted and there was no evidence of efficacy.[25] Without using a clearing antibody the conjugate took too long to be eliminated from the blood and at the point of prodrug administration there was not sufficient enzyme present in the tumor.[25]

ScFv-CPG2 Recombinant Fusion Protein

A scFv-CPG2 fusion protein was designed to combine the advantage of recombinant technology with those of CPG2 ADEPT using the bis-iodo-phenol mustard prodrug MFE-23; a clinically validated phage-derived anti-CEA scFv was used and the resultant fusion protein, MFE23::CPG2, produced in *E. coli*.[65] The fusion protein was dimeric due to the natural homodimeric structure of CPG2 and was shown to localize effectively in CEA-positive LS174T human colon adenocarcinoma tumor xenografts after intravenous injection into nude mice.[26] Enzyme activity, demonstrated by excision of tissues and measurement of ability to catalyze methotrexate, was found to be substantially higher in tumor than normal tissues – for example, 371:1 (tumor to liver), 450:1 (tumor to lung), 562:1 (tumor to kidney), 1,477:1 (tumor to colon). However, tumor to plasma ratios did not exceed 19:1 (48 hr).[26] These data were promising but plasma clearance was considered to be too slow for safe clinical use.

To improve clearance, the MFE23::CPG2 fusion protein was produced in the yeast *Pichia pastoris* where it was shown to be glycosylated with branched mannose at two of three potential glycosylation sites.[27] This led to clearance via human and mouse mannose receptors, predominantly in the liver.[28] The enhanced clearance from

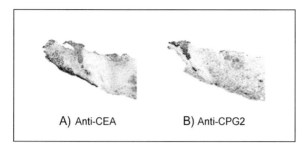

A) Anti-CEA   B) Anti-CPG2

Figure 22.3. Biopsy of liver metastasis from a patient on the MFECP1 ADEPT clinical trial. The biopsy was taken 4.5 hours after the end of infusion of MFECP1. (A) Immunostaining with anti-CEA antibody confirms the presence of CEA within the tumor. (B) Immunohistochemistry with an anti-CPG2 antibody shows the presence of fusion protein within the tumor (Image adapted with kind permission from *Clinical Cancer Research Journal*).

blood resulted in high tumor:normal tissue ratios without using a clearing antibody. *In vivo* testing of the fusion protein was carried out using xenografts of two human colonic adenocarcinoma cell lines LS174T and SW1222 in nude mice. Functional enzyme was found localized in tumors and rapid clearance from plasma was observed within 6 hours, resulting in tumor:plasma ratios of 1400:1 in the LS174T xenograft model and 339:1 in the SW1222 xenograft model.[29] A single ADEPT cycle gave reproducible tumor growth delay in both models, and multiple ADEPT cycles significantly enhanced the therapeutic effect of a single cycle in the xenografts with minimal toxicity. These studies gave the background research for the next stage in clinical development of ADEPT[29] and formed the basis of a Phase I/II clinical trial of ADEPT using the mannosylated fusion protein and the bis-iodo-phenol mustard prodrug.

ScFv-CPG2 Fusion Protein Clinical Trial

The recombinant fusion protein was produced according to good manufacturing practice (GMP).[66,67] Clinical-grade fusion protein was named MFECP1. This trial successfully established the optimal conditions for single administration of MFECP1, the timing for safe clearance of fusion protein from normal tissues, and the dose escalation of prodrug. Of the 28 patients evaluable for response, 11 had stable disease and one patient had a 10% reduction in tumor diameter. Enzyme was confirmed to be in the tumor (Figure 22.3) and DNA interstrand cross links were present in the tumor, indicating that the prodrug had in fact been converted to active drug at the tumor site.[30] A study testing repeat treatment is under way.

IMMUNOGENICITY

Immune Responses in the Clinic

One of the main challenges for ADEPT is the immune response to the antibody-enzyme moiety. For example, a single dose of the anti-CEA F(ab′)2 -CPG2 conjugate in patients receiving ADEPT elicited an immune response to both the murine antibody (100%) and the bacterial CPG2 enzyme (96%).[68] The MFECP1 fusion protein was less immunogenic, although 36% (11 of 30) of patients still developed antibodies to CPG2 after a single administration.[30]

Many established and novel methods are available for addressing the immunogenicity of recombinant antibodies as described in earlier chapters of this book. However, reducing the immunogenicity of enzymes is more troublesome, and reliable methods to achieve this are much required.

Modifying B Cell Epitopes

One approach is to mutate or modify B cell epitopes, and there is some evidence of success of this approach in the clinic, where a reduced immune response to CPG2 was thought to be partly due to the addition of a hexa-His-tag at the C-terminus.[69] It was proposed that the tag masked a conformational B cell epitope[69] that had been previously identified by a novel method of epitope mapping.[70] It is possible that this mutation of immunodominant B cell epitopes would render foreign enzymes less immunogenic. However, an argument often used against this strategy is that repeated administration with the modified protein may elicit an antibody response to a different set of epitopes on the same molecule. Thus, removing antigenic B cell epitopes may not necessarily reduce overall immunogenicity.

Modifying T Cell Epitopes

Another approach to reduce immunogenicity of ADEPT is to focus on modification of T cell epitopes. This is based on the rationale that T cell help is required to mount a long-lived, isotype switched and high-affinity antibody response. The concept of preventing the interaction between APC and T cells by identifying and modifying T cell epitopes has been extensively reviewed in other chapters (see also references 71 and 72).

The T cell epitope modification approach is attractive as it could provide a fundamental solution to the problem of immunogenicity and it has already been successful with β-lactamase isolated from *Enterobacter cloacae*. Here, mapping indicated the presence of four T cell epitopes, two of which were successfully changed with a single point mutation at each site. The new variant significantly reduced T cell proliferative responses and retained stability and activity of the enzyme.[73]

Using Human Enzymes

Immunogenicity can also be reduced by using human enzymes for ADEPT, although if native human enzymes are used, the danger of endogenous inactivation or unwanted prodrug conversion must be considered. Early preclinical successes have been reported with this approach – for example, the first fully human ADEPT system described[44] that utilized a fusion protein of human β-glucuronidase and an anti-EpCAM scFv. β-glucuronidase is found intracellularly in microsomes and lysosomes and there is no detected activity in blood. This enzyme is able to convert a hydrophilic doxorubicin prodrug, which is unable to cross cell membranes, to doxorubicin. It was established that the prodrug was completely converted to active drug *in vitro* using tissue culture techniques, and a bystander effect was demonstrated by seeding 10% antigen-positive cells and 90% antigen-negative cells.[40,74] *In vivo* data for this ADEPT system fusion protein are awaited.

Another potentially interesting enzyme is human prolyl endopeptidase (PEP), a highly active serine endopeptidase that cleaves peptide bonds on the carboxyl side of proline in peptides. PEP is a cytosolic enzyme with low activity in human blood and it is proposed that this should prevent nonspecific conversion of prodrug.[57] When PEP was expressed in *E. coli* it was found to be unstable at 37°C; however, a single point mutation improved protein stability giving a half-life of 16 hr at 37°C in phosphate buffer. PEP also has the advantage that it is possible to make prodrugs with any cytotoxic that contains a primary amine moiety – for example, methotrexate, cephalosporin analogs, and melphalan. When the stable PEP mutant was conjugated to the human antibody L19, which is specific to the EDB domain of fibronectin, the resulting immunoconjugate retained both enzyme activity and antigen-binding capacity. As with the β-glucuronidase ADEPT system, *in vivo* studies with PEP ADEPT are yet to be reported.

One way of preventing unwanted activation of prodrug by human enzymes is mutating them to activate prodrugs that will not be recognized by their wild-type human equivalent. A prodrug is then designed to make use of the "new" enzyme. This is an extremely attractive approach and has been shown in principle to be possible with the T268G mutant of human carboxypeptidase A1 (hCPA1), which has been modified to activate prodrugs of methotrexate *in vitro*.[16] The mutated enzyme remained more than 99% human and therefore it is predicted that it would not be immunogenic. The hCPA1 mutant was attached to an anti-EpCAM antibody and *in vivo* data showed that the conjugate targeted tumor, and the enzyme was active. Unfortunately, in this instance there was no tumor reduction in the mouse model.[16]

Another way of adapting human enzymes is to mutate the enzyme in such a way as to reduce the affinity for the natural substrate and at the same time retain the enzyme's natural active site. This has been achieved with human pancreatic ribonuclease by converting the positively charged lysine 66 residue in the substrate binding pocket to a negatively charged glutamic acid. This single mutation reduced the affinity for its natural substrate, RNA, and enabled design of a prodrug with relative specificity for this "reverse polarity" mutant.[75] Fusion proteins of the mutant enzyme with sm3E, a high-affinity humanized anti-CEA scFv,[76] are currently being evaluated for potential with this ADEPT system.

Abzymes

A less exploited way to achieve foreign enzyme specificity with human proteins is to use human catalytic antibodies (also known as abzymes), which as their name suggests are antibodies that act like enzymes. The first abzymes were polyclonal or monoclonal antibodies created by immunizing them with analogs of transition states of the substrate.[77,78] Abzymes created in this way are thought to function by interacting to stabilize the transition state, in a similar manner to enzymes. The efficacy of abzymes has been shown with a number of substrates.[77,78]

Abzymes have potential for use in ADEPT as they have already shown promise in enzyme-prodrug therapy of cancer. For example, Kakinuma et al.[79] used a vitamin B6 phosphonate transition state analog and the antibodies obtained were able to convert several prodrugs that had been derived from esterification with vitamin B6. These prodrugs were resistant to degradation by natural endogenous enzymes in serum due to steric hindrance.[79]

Another successful abzyme system reported is the aldolase antibody 38C2, which converts prodrugs of etoposide.[80] *In vitro* this prodrug was 100-fold less toxic than the active drug and drug activity was restored with addition of the abzyme.[80] Mice with neuroblastoma xenografts received one intratumoral injection of 38C2 and then intra-peritoneal (systemic) injections of prodrug illustrated a 75% reduction in tumor growth with no effect shown with either prodrug or antibody alone. Importantly, when mice were treated with a 30-fold higher dose of prodrug than the maximum tolerated dose of etoposide they showed no signs of prodrug toxicity; therefore, it can be deduced that the prodrug is not activated by endogenous enzymes. Given the potential of current antibody technology to create recombinant human abzymes,[81] it is entirely possible that bispecific antitumor/abzyme molecules could eventually provide an entirely nonimmunogenic approach for ADEPT.

Future Perspectives

In vitro experiments, preclinical testing and Phase I/II clinical trials have now identified the key elements for successful ADEPT as the following:

- Appropriate tumor-selective antibody-enzyme moiety, produced stably in reproducible form using a process feasible for bulk manufacture.
- Effective prodrug conversion, low toxicity for prodrug, and high toxicity for active drug with optimal half-life and diffusion properties.
- Tumor localization and retention to give high tumor enzyme level *in vivo*.
- Little or no enzyme in normal tissue at the time of prodrug administration.
- Nonimmunogenic system for repeated therapy.

If these are successfully implemented, it is most likely that ADEPT will become a potent and nontoxic therapy for cancer treatment, with specifically designed antibodies and prodrugs available for treatment of many solid tumors.

REFERENCES

[1] Bagshawe, K.D. (1987) *Br. J. Cancer* **56**, 531–532.
[2] Bagshawe, K.D., Springer, C.J., Searle, F., Antoniw, P., Sharma, S.K., Melton, R.G., and Sherwood, R.F. (1988) *Br. J. Cancer* **58**, 700–703.

[3]   Senter, P.D., Saulnier, M.G., Schreiber, G.J., Hirschberg, D.L., Brown, J.P., Hellstrom, I., and Hellstrom, K.E. (1988) *Proc. Natl. Acad. Sci. U.S.A* **85**, 4842–4846.

[4]   Martin, J., Stribbling, S.M., Poon, G.K., Begent, R.H., Napier, M., Sharma, S.K., and Springer, C.J. (1997) *Cancer Chemother. Pharmacol.* **40**, 189–201.

[5]   Niculescu-Duvaz, D., Niculescu-Duvaz, I., and Springer, C.J. (2004) *Methods Mol. Med.* **90**, 161–202.

[6]   Senter, P.D. and Springer, C.J. (2001) *Adv. Drug Deliv. Rev.* **53**, 247–264.

[7]   Burke, P.J. (1996) *Adv. Drug Deliv. Rev.* **22**, 331–340.

[8]   Haisma, H.J., Boven, E., Van, M.M., De, V.R., and Pinedo, H.M. (1992) *Cancer Immunol. Immunother.* **34**, 343–348.

[9]   Senter, P.D., Schreiber, G.J., Hirschberg, D.L., Ashe, S.A., Hellstrom, K.E., and Hellstrom, I. (1989) *Cancer Res.* **49**, 5789–5792.

[10]   Senter, P.D. (1990) *FASEB J.* **4**, 188–193.

[11]   Wallace, P.M. and Senter, P.D. (1991) *Bioconjug. Chem.* **2**, 349–352.

[12]   Haenseler, E., Esswein, A., Vitols, K.S., Montejano, Y., Mueller, B.M., Reisfeld, R.A., and Huennekens, F.M. (1992) *Biochemistry* **31**, 891–897.

[13]   Vitols, K.S., Haag-Zeino, B., Baer, T., Montejano, Y.D., and Huennekens, F.M. (1995) *Cancer Res.* **55**, 478–481.

[14]   Perron, M.J. and Page, M. (1996) *Br. J. Cancer* **73**, 281–287.

[15]   Smith, G.K., Banks, S., Blumenkopf, T.A., Cory, M., Humphreys, J., Laethem, R.M., Miller, J., Moxham, C.P., Mullin, R., Ray, P.H., Walton, L.M., and Wolfe, L.A., III (1997) *J. Biol. Chem.* **272**, 15804–15816.

[16]   Wolfe, L.A., Mullin, R.J., Laethem, R., Blumenkopf, T.A., Cory, M., Miller, J.F., Keith, B.R., Humphreys, J., and Smith, G.K. (1999) *Bioconjug. Chem.* **10**, 38–48.

[17]   Hao, X.K., Liu, J.Y., Yue, Q.H., Wu, G.J., Bai, Y.J., and Yin, Y. (2006) *Prostate* **66**, 858–866.

[18]   Springer, C.J., Antoniw, P., Bagshawe, K.D., Searle, F., Bisset, G.M., and Jarman, M. (1990) *J. Med. Chem.* **33**, 677–681.

[19]   Springer, C.J., Bagshawe, K.D., Sharma, S.K., Searle, F., Boden, J.A., Antoniw, P., Burke, P.J., Rogers, G.T., Sherwood, R.F., and Melton, R.G. (1991) *Eur. J. Cancer* **27**, 1361–1366.

[20]   Bagshawe, K.D., Sharma, S.K., Springer, C.J., Antoniw, P., Boden, J.A., Rogers, G.T., Burke, P.J., Melton, R.G., and Sherwood, R.F. (1991) *Dis. Markers* **9**, 233–238.

[21]   Bagshawe, K.D., Sharma, S.K., Springer, C.J., and Antoniw, P. (1995) *Tumour Targeting* **1**, 17–30.

[22]   Bagshawe, K.D. and Begent, R.H. (1996) *Adv. Drug Deliv. Rev.* **22**, 365–367.

[23]   Blakey, D.C., Burke, P.J., Davies, D.H., Dowell, R.I., East, S.J., Eckersley, K.P., Fitton, J.E., McDaid, J., Melton, R.G., Niculescu-Duvaz, I.A., Pinder, P.E., Sharma, S.K., Wright, A.F., and Springer, C.J. (1996) *Cancer Res.* **56**, 3287–3292.

[24]   Napier, M.P., Sharma, S.K., Springer, C.J., Bagshawe, K.D., Green, A.J., Martin, J., Stribbling, S.M., Cushen, N., O'Malley, D., and Begent, R.H. (2000) *Clin. Cancer Res.* **6**, 765–772.

[25]   Francis, R.J., Sharma, S.K., Springer, C., Green, A.J., Hope-Stone, L.D., Sena, L., Martin, J., Adamson, K.L., Robbins, A., Gumbrell, L., O'Malley, D., Tsiompanou, E., Shahbakhti, H., Webley, S., Hochhauser, D., Hilson, A.J., Blakey, D., and Begent, R.H. (2002) *Br. J. Cancer* **87**, 600–607.

[26]   Bhatia, J., Sharma, S.K., Chester, K.A., Pedley, R.B., Boden, R.W., Read, D.A., Boxer, G.M., Michael, N.P., and Begent, R.H. (2000) *Int. J. Cancer* **85**, 571–577.

[27]   Medzihradszky, K.F., Spencer, D.I., Sharma, S.K., Bhatia, J., Pedley, R.B., Read, D.A., Begent, R.H., and Chester, K.A. (2004) *Glycobiology* **14**, 27–37.

[28]   Kogelberg, H., Tolner, B., Sharma, S.K., Lowdell, M.W., Qureshi, U., Robson, M., Hillyer, T., Pedley, R.B., Vervecken, W., Contreras, R., Begent, R.H., and Chester, K.A. (2007) *Glycobiology* **17**, 36–45.

[29]   Sharma, S.K., Pedley, R.B., Bhatia, J., Boxer, G.M., El-Emir, E., Qureshi, U., Tolner, B., Lowe, H., Michael, N.P., Minton, N., Begent, R.H., and Chester, K.A. (2005) *Clin. Cancer Res.* **11**, 814–825.

[30]   Mayer, A., Francis, R.J., Sharma, S.K., Tolner, B., Springer, C.J., Martin, J., Boxer, G.M., Bell, J., Green, A.J., Hartley, J.A., Cruickshank, C., Wren, J., Chester, K.A., and Begent, R.H. (2006) *Clin. Cancer Res.* **12**, 6509–6516.

[31]   Senter, P.D., Su, P.C., Katsuragi, T., Sakai, T., Cosand, W.L., Hellstrom, I., and Hellstrom, K.E. (1991) *Bioconjug. Chem.* **2**, 447–451.

[32]   Kerr, D.E., Garrigues, U.S., Wallace, P.M., Hellstrom, K.E., Hellstrom, I., and Senter, P.D. (1993) *Bioconjug. Chem.* **4**, 353–357

[33]   Wallace, P.M., MacMaster, J.F., Smith, V.F., Kerr, D.E., Senter, P.D., and Cosand, W.L. (1994) *Cancer Res.* **54**, 2719–2723.

[34]   Aboagye, E.O., Artemov, D., Senter, P.D., and Bhujwalla, Z.M. (1998) *Cancer Res.* **58**, 4075–4078.

[35]   Deckert, P.M., Renner, C., Cohen, L.S., Jungbluth, A., Ritter, G., Bertino, J.R., Old, L.J., and Welt, S. (2003) *Br. J. Cancer* **88**, 937–939.

[36]   Coelho, V., Dernedde, J., Petrausch, U., Panjideh, H., Fuchs, H., Menzel, C., Dubel, S., Keilholz, U., Thiel, E., and Deckert, P.M. (2007) *Int. J. Oncol.* **31**, 951–957.

[37]   Abraham, R., Aman, N., von, B.R., Darsley, M., Kamireddy, B., Kenten, J., Morris, G., and Titmas, R. (1994) *Cell Biophys.* **24–25**, 127–133.

[38]   Haisma, H.J., Boven, E., van Muijen, M., de Jong, J., van der Vijgh, W.J., and Pinedo, H.M. (1992) *Br. J. Cancer* **66**, 474–478.

[39]   Houba, P.H., Boven, E., and Haisma, H.J. (1996) *Bioconjug. Chem.* **7**, 606–611.

[40]   Houba, P.H., Boven, E., van der Meulen-Muileman, I.H., Leenders, R.G., Scheeren, J.W., Pinedo, H.M., and Haisma, H.J. (2001) *Int. J. Cancer* **91**, 550–554.

[41]   Wang, S.M., Chern, J.W., Yeh, M.Y., Ng, J.C., Tung, E., and Roffler, S.R. (1992) *Cancer Res.* **52**, 4484–4491.

[42]   Bosslet, K., Czech, J., Seemann, G., Monneret, C., and Hoffmann, D. (1994) *Cell Biophys.* **24–25**, 51–63.

[43]   Florent, J.C., Dong, X., Gaudel, G., Mitaku, S., Monneret, C., Gesson, J.P., Jacquesy, J.C., Mondon, M., Renoux, B., Andrianomenjanahary, S., Michel, S., Koch, M., Tillequin, F., Gerken, M., Czech, J., Straub, R., and Bosslet, K. (1998) *J. Med. Chem.* **41**, 3572–3581.

[44]   de Graaf, G.M., Boven, E., Oosterhoff, D., van der Meulen-Muileman, I.H., Huls, G.A., Gerritsen, W.R., Haisma, H.J., and Pinedo, H.M. (2002) *Br. J. Cancer* **86**, 811–818.

[45]   Biela, B.H., Khawli, L.A., Hu, P., and Epstein, A.L. (2003) *Cancer Biother. Radiopharm.* **18**, 339–353.

[46]   Svensson, H.P., Kadow, J.F., Vrudhula, V.M., Wallace, P.M., and Senter, P.D. (1992) *Bioconjug. Chem.* **3**, 176–181.

[47]   Vrudhula, V.M., Svensson, H.P., Kennedy, K.A., Senter, P.D., and Wallace, P.M. (1993) *Bioconjug. Chem.* **4**, 334–340.

[48]   Rodrigues, M.L., Presta, L.G., Kotts, C.E., Wirth, C., Mordenti, J., Osaka, G., Wong, W.L., Nuijens, A., Blackburn, B., and Carter, P. (1995) *Cancer Res.* **55**, 63–70.

[49]   Kerr, D.E., Vrudhula, V.M., Svensson, H.P., Siemers, N.O., and Senter, P.D. (1999) *Bioconjug. Chem.* **10**, 1084–1089.

[50]   Siemers, N.O., Kerr, D.E., Yarnold, S., Stebbins, M.R., Vrudhula, V.M., Hellstrom, I., Hellstrom, K.E., and Senter, P.D. (1997) *Bioconjug. Chem.* **8**, 510–519.

[51]   Vrudhula, V.M., Kerr, D.E., Siemers, N.O., Dubowchik, G.M., and Senter, P.D. (2003) *Bioorg. Med. Chem. Lett.* **13**, 539–542.

[52]   Alderson, R.F., Toki, B.E., Roberge, M., Geng, W., Basler, J., Chin, R., Liu, A., Ueda, R., Hodges, D., Escandon, E., Chen, T., Kanavarioti, T., Babe, L., Senter, P.D., Fox, J.A., and Schellenberger, V. (2006) *Bioconjug. Chem.* **17**, 410–418.

[53]   Cortez-Retamozo, V., Backmann, N., Senter, P.D., Wernery, U., De, B.P., Muyldermans, S., and Revets, H. (2004) *Cancer Res.* **64**, 2853–2857.

[54]   Bignami, G.S., Senter, P.D., Grothaus, P.G., Fischer, K.J., Humphreys, T., and Wallace, P.M. (1992) *Cancer Res.* **52**, 5759–5764.

[55]   Vrudhula, V.M., Senter, P.D., Fischer, K.J., and Wallace, P.M. (1993) *J. Med. Chem.* **36**, 919–923.

[56] Kerr, D.E., Senter, P.D., Burnett, W.V., Hirschberg, D.L., Hellstrom, I., and Hellstrom, K.E. (1990) *Cancer Immunol. Immunother.* **31**, 202–206.

[57] Heinis, C., Alessi, P., and Neri, D. (2004) *Biochemistry* **43**, 6293–6303.

[58] Senter, P.D. (1990) *Front Radiat. Ther. Oncol.* **24**, 132–141.

[59] Bagshawe, K.D. (1989) *Br. J. Cancer* **60**, 275–281.

[60] Sharma, S.K., Bagshawe, K.D., Burke, P.J., Boden, R.W., and Rogers, G.T. (1990) *Br. J. Cancer* **61**, 659–662.

[61] Sharma, S.K., Bagshawe, K.D., Burke, P.J., Boden, J.A., Rogers, G.T., Springer, C.J., Melton, R.G., and Sherwood, R.F. (1994) *Cancer* **73**, 1114–1120.

[62] Sharma, S.K., Bagshawe, K.D., Springer, C.J., Burke, P.J., Rogers, G.T., Boden, J.A., Antoniw, P., Melton, R.G., and Sherwood, R.F. (1991) *Dis. Markers* **9**, 225–231.

[63] Sharma, S.K., Boden, J.A., Springer, C.J., Burke, P.J., and Bagshawe, K.D. (1994) *Cell Biophys.* **24–25**, 219–228.

[64] Springer, C.J., Dowell, R., Burke, P.J., Hadley, E., Davis, D.H., Blakey, D.C., Melton, R.G., and Niculescu-Duvaz, I. (1995) *J. Med. Chem.* **38**, 5051–5065.

[65] Michael, N.P., Chester, K.A., Melton, R.G., Robson, L., Nicholas, W., Boden, J.A., Pedley, R.B., Begent, R.H., Sherwood, R.F., and Minton, N.P. (1996) *Immunotechnology.* **2**, 47–57.

[66] Tolner, B., Smith, L., Begent, R.H., and Chester, K.A. (2006) *Nat. Protoc.* **1**, 1213–1222.

[67] Tolner, B., Smith, L., Begent, R.H., and Chester, K.A. (2006) *Nat. Protoc.* **1**, 1006–1021.

[68] Sharma, S.K., Bagshawe, K.D., Melton, R.G., and Sherwood, R.F. (1992) *Cell Biophys.* **21**, 109–120.

[69] Mayer, A., Sharma, S.K., Tolner, B., Minton, N.P., Purdy, D., Amlot, P., Tharakan, G., Begent, R.H., and Chester, K.A. (2004) *Br. J. Cancer* **90**, 2402–2410.

[70] Spencer, D.I., Robson, L., Purdy, D., Whitelegg, N.R., Michael, N.P., Bhatia, J., Sharma, S.K., Rees, A.R., Minton, N.P., Begent, R.H., and Chester, K.A. (2002) *Proteomics.* **2**, 271–279.

[71] Chirino, A.J., Ary, M.L., and Marshall, S.A. (2004) *Drug Discov. Today* **9**, 82–90.

[72] De Groot, A.S., Rayner, J., and Martin, W. (2003) *Dev. Biol. (Basel)* **112**, 71–80.

[73] Harding, F.A., Liu, A.D., Stickler, M., Razo, O.J., Chin, R., Faravashi, N., Viola, W., Graycar, T., Yeung, V.P., Aehle, W., Meijer, D., Wong, S., Rashid, M.H., Valdes, A.M., and Schellenberger, V. (2005) *Mol. Cancer Ther.* **4**, 1791–1800.

[74] Bosslet, K., Czech, J., and Hoffmann, D. (1995) *Tumour Target* **1**, 45–50.

[75] Taylorson, C.J. (1999) Taylorson et al. (UCL) 1999 US Patent #5: 985,281.

[76] Graff, C.P., Chester, K., Begent, R., and Wittrup, K.D. (2004) *Protein Eng. Des. Sel.* **17**, 293–304.

[77] Nevinsky, G.A. and Buneva, V.N. (2003) *J. Cell Mol. Med.* **7**, 265–276.

[78] Xu, Y., Yamamoto, N., and Janda, K.D. (2004) *Bioorg. Med. Chem.* **12**, 5247–5268.

[79] Kakinuma, H., Fujii, I., and Nishi, Y. (2002) *J. Immunol. Methods* **269**, 269–281.

[80] Shabat, D., Lode, H.N., Pertl, U., Reisfeld, R.A., Rader, C., Lerner, R.A., and Barbas, C.F., III (2001) *Proc. Natl. Acad. Sci. U.S.A* **98**, 7528–7533.

[81] Cesaro-Tadic, S., Lagos, D., Honegger, A., Rickard, J.H., Partridge, L.J., Blackburn, G.M., and Pluckthun, A. (2003) *Nat. Biotechnol.* **21**, 679–685.

CHAPTER TWENTY-THREE

Immune Privilege and Tolerance – Therapeutic Antibody Approaches

Daron Forman, Paul Ponath, Devangi Mehta, Joe Ponte,
Jessica Snyder, Patricia Rao, Herman Waldmann, and
Michael Rosenzweig

The discovery of monoclonal antibodies by Kohler and Milstein in 1975 sparked the generation of novel drugs that could be used to antagonize functional receptors of the immune system. The anti-CD3 antibody, OKT3, was the first of these drugs to be exploited clinically in the treatment of acute allograft rejection.[1,2] Although the antibody was efficacious, neutralizing immunogenicity[3,4] and, in particular, the often severe "flu-like" cytokine-release syndrome[5,6] associated with initial doses of the antibody limited its application to other indications. As a consequence, the emergence of other immune-modulating CD3 or T cell-directed antibodies as therapeutics took a surprisingly long time. Three scientific developments rekindled interest in immune-modulating therapeutic antibodies resulting in many more antibody candidates entering clinical trials. The first development was the discovery that co-receptor CD4 antibodies could be used to tolerize to other proteins,[7,8] thus establishing tolerance as a therapeutic paradigm. The second development was the discovery that rodent antibodies could be reengineered or reshaped to minimize their immunogenicity.[9] Finally, the third development was the discovery that transplantation tolerance induced by co-receptor blockade was "dominant" and dependent on the induction of CD4$^+$ regulatory T cells through so-called infectious tolerance.[10] These findings together suggested that antibodies might be used sparingly to recruit the host's own tolerance mechanisms without evoking neutralizing responses.

Further studies in transplant models indicated that anti-CD4 therapeutic antibodies alone were insufficient when CD8$^+$ T cells were also involved. In those circumstances, antagonism of CD8 function was also required. Targeting of both co-receptors was shown to restore transplantation tolerance not only in primed mice but also in mice well into the rejection process.[11] Many subsequent studies in mice have demonstrated that a wide variety of blocking antibodies can induce such dominant tolerance, not only in transplantation but also in autoimmune disease. The possible mechanisms underlying induction of regulation and infectious tolerance have been discussed fully elsewhere.[12]

Co-receptor blockade with anti-CD4 antibodies proved very effective in preventing diabetes in the nonobese diabetic (NOD) mouse;[13] however, it was less effective in reversing established disease. This was most likely due to residual activity of CD8$^+$ T cells.[14] Currently, the clinical application of a combination of anti-CD4 and anti-CD8 antibodies to autoimmune disease is simply impracticable, until a representative of each is licensed and available for therapy. In contrast, short-term therapy with an anti-CD3 antibody targeting the T cell receptor complex of all T cells did reverse auto-immune diabetes in the NOD mouse.[15] Just as for anti-CD4 antibodies, a functional Fc region was not essential for the therapeutic effect as F(ab')$_2$ fragments could mediate remission.[15]

In order to render anti-CD3 antibodies more useful for immunomodulatory therapy, we generated the first humanized anti-CD3 antibody with substantially reduced ability to induce cytokine release. Initially, we attempted to reduce or eliminate cytokine-related side effects by engineering a monovalent form of the rodent antibody.[16] As this antibody appeared both efficacious and safe, we subsequently generated a novel, monovalent, humanized form of the antibody,[17] but clinical-scale manufacturing and development of this molecule appeared impractical. As an alternative, we created an Fc-disabled antibody by amino acid substitution so as to eliminate the N-linked glycosylation site.[18] By a variety of *in vitro* assays, this antibody was shown to be nonmitogenic and far less capable of eliciting cytokine release, and was consequently selected for clinical development. In a small Phase I study in patients undergoing renal allograft rejection episodes, the side effect profile of this humanized antibody appeared much superior to that reported for OKT3, while therapeutic efficacy remained comparable.[19] Based on these studies, the Belgian Diabetes Registry (BDR) assessed the effects of short-term therapy with the Fc-disabled CD3 antibody in a randomized, placebo-controlled study in subjects with type 1 diabetes. The 18-month efficacy data were reported and clear benefit of therapy established.[20] However, immunogenicity and cytokine release (albeit less than OKT3) were still observed, as was a transient loss of EBV control. This necessitated a more detailed analysis of how benefit could be maintained while the undesirable effects were eliminated. In short, how could the antibody be used to maintain efficacy, while minimizing cytokine release and immunogenicity?

GENERATION AND HUMANIZATION OF OTELIXIZUMAB

The rat hybridoma, YTH12.5, was produced by immunization of Dark Agouti (DA) rats with normal human T cells and was characterized as secreting an IgG2b, λ mAb specific for human CD3 epsilon antigen.[17,21–25] The YTH12.5 variable heavy (VH) and variable light (VL) chain genes were cloned as described.[26,27] A database search was performed to identify human variable region genes with the highest degree of sequence similarity to YTH12.5. In selecting the human variable region sequences upon which to base the humanization, we gave preferences to sequences with framework and CDR lengths (as defined by Kabat et al.[28]) closest to those of the parental rat gene. The frameworks from human VH type III gene, VH26-D-J (Genebank Accession No. M17746), were chosen for humanization of the VH.[29] Humanization of the YTH12.5 VH gene was performed by the method of framework grafting based on the procedure of Orlandi et al.[26] PCR-mediated oligonucleotide site-directed mutagenesis was performed with mutagenic oligonucleotides complementary to the sequence of the cloned rat VH gene. The resulting humanized VH region gene was subcloned together with the human γ-1 constant region derived from the wild-type G1m (1,17) gene.[30] To disrupt antibody binding to Fc receptors as well as complement fixation, a single amino acid substitution (N297A) was introduced in the Fc region of the heavy chain, eliminating the site of N-linked glycosylation.

Sequencing of the YTH12.5 VL gene confirmed serological analysis indicating that the YTH12.5 light chain was of the λ subclass. However, the amino acid sequence was markedly different from published rat and mouse sequences, having only about 49% and 52% sequence identity at the nucleic acid and amino acid levels, respectively.[17] The light chain of YTH12.5 was thus chimerized by attaching the rat YTH12.5 light chain variable region to the human Kern⁻Oz⁻ lambda light chain constant region.[31] The antibody, otelixizumab, is thus comprised of an Fc-disabled, humanized heavy chain and a chimeric light chain.

The heavy chain and light chain genes encoding the otelixizumab antibody were cloned into an expression vector under the control of EF1α promoters. Stable transfectants were generated in Chinese hamster ovary (CHO) cells, and the antibody produced by hollow fiber fermentation. The antibody was purified from culture supernatants by protein A affinity chromatography, followed by ion exchange chromatography, nanofiltration, and size exclusion chromatography.

PHARMACODYNAMIC EFFECTS OF OTELIXIZUMAB *IN VITRO*

Otelixizumab is being developed for the treatment of auto-immune disorders in which activated T cells play a dominant role, including type 1 diabetes, psoriasis, and rheumatoid arthritis. To date, several *in vitro* experiments have been performed examining the response of human CD3⁺ T cells to otelixizumab with regard to TCR saturation and modulation, T cell proliferation, cytokine release, and inhibition of mixed lymphocyte cultures. These studies have provided insights into the possible mechanisms of action of otelixizumab and are discussed below.

CD3/TCR Saturation and Modulation

Anti-CD3 antibodies bind to the CD3/TCR complex with variable effects on T cell activation and function.[32] For example, anti-CD3 antibodies that bind with high avidity and dissociate slowly result in phosphorylation and internalization of CD3/TCR from the cell surface that is both dose and time dependent.[33] Although the mechanism of action of anti-CD3 antibodies is complex, it has been shown to depend at least partly on CD3/TCR down-modulation.[5–7]

Saturation and modulation of CD3/TCR by otelixizumab was examined by monitoring the CD3/TCR complex by 3 methods: (1) cell surface bound otelixizumab was monitored with antihuman IgG-FITC; (2) free CD3/TCR sites were monitored with

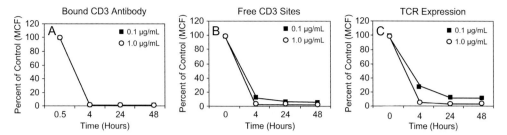

Figure 23.1. Otelixizumab modulation and saturation of the CD3/TCR complex. Peripheral blood mononuclear cells (PBMC) were incubated at 37°C with 0, 0.1 μg/mL, or 1 μg/mL of otelixizumab in RPMI media with 10% human serum. (A) At the indicated times, samples were stained with antihuman IgG-FITC to detect cell-bound otelixizumab. Control cells were first stained with a saturating amount of each antibody to determine the maximum mean channel fluorescence (MCF) of bound antibody. (B) Free, unbound CD3 sites were detected with FITC-conjugated otelixizumab. For each staining condition, the MCF of the antibody-treated cells was compared with the MCF of the control cells to determine the percentage of the control level of expression for each reagent. (C) Additional samples were also stained with BMA031, an anti-TCRαβ antibody that does not compete with otelixizumab for binding to CD3 at serum levels below 1 μg/mL. Modulation can be detected as a decrease in the MCF of bound antibody with a decrease in TCR expression and a lack of free CD3 sites on cells. Data shown are the cumulative mean values with SD obtained from three separate individuals.

otelixizumab-FITC; and (3) cell surface CD3/TCR complex was monitored with the noncompeting anti-TCRαβ mAb, BMA031. Both a subsaturating concentration of 100 ng/mL and a saturating concentration of 1 μg/mL of otelixizumab resulted in modulation of the CD3/TCR complex by 4 hours and lasted for at least 48 hours (Figure 23.1).

Mitogenicity

Most anti-CD3 antibodies are mitogenic for human T cells *in vitro*.[34,35] Anti-CD3 antibody-mediated activation of T cells requires binding of the anti-CD3 antibody to the CD3/TCR complex as well as Fc receptor-mediated cross linking of the antibody. The aglycosyl Fc modification of otelixizumab greatly reduces its binding affinity for human Fc receptors rendering it nonmitogenic (Figure 23.2).

Cytokine Release

Activation of T cells by anti-CD3 antibodies results in the release of a variety of cytokines.[5,6] To examine the effects of the aglycosyl Fc modification on otelixizumab-induced cytokine release, cell culture supernatants were collected 48 hours after exposure of PBMC to either the parental rat anti-CD3 antibody, YTH12.5, or otelixizumab and cytokines quantitated. YTH12.5 induced the release of all cytokines examined with the exception of TGF-β1. In contrast, otelixizumab induced no significant release of these cytokines but did induce low levels of TGF-β1 (Table 23.1).

Dose-Dependent CD3/TCR Modulation and Inhibition of Mixed Lymphocyte Cultures by Otelixizumab

Anti-CD3 antibodies are reported to inhibit proliferation of mixed lymphocyte cultures.[22,36] To examine in detail the effect of otelixizumab on T cell proliferation

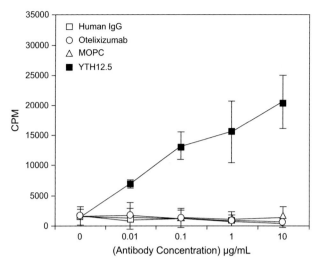

Figure 23.2. Otelixizumab is nonmitogenic. PBMC were cultured in RPMI media with 10% human serum in the presence of the indicated concentrations of antibody in triplicate. Cultures were fed on day 4 with media containing ^{3}H-thymidine to label proliferating cells. Eighteen hours later, cultures were harvested, and ^{3}H-thymidine incorporation was measured by scintillation counting. YTH12.5, the parental rat monoclonal antihuman CD3 antibody, was used as a positive control. MOPC (mouse IgG1) and human IgG were used as the isotype controls for YTH12.5 and otelixizumab, respectively. Data shown are the mean CPM values with SD obtained from three separate individuals.

in mixed lymphocyte cultures and to determine a dose-response correlation with CD3/TCR modulation, otelixizumab (0.001–1.0 µg/mL) was added at the initiation of mixed lymphocyte cultures. After incubation for 4–120 hours, cultures were washed thoroughly and re-cultured in media without antibody. At the end of 5 days, cultures were harvested and CD3/TCR expression assessed. Otelixizumab significantly decreased the number of free CD3 sites when T cells were exposed to at least 0.1 µg/mL of antibody for greater than 48 hours (Figure 23.3A). Whereas exposure with 0.1 µg/mL antibody for 24 hours or less decreased free CD3 sites by 30%–38%, exposure for greater than 48 hours decreased free CD3 sites by 56%–94%. Maximum saturation of CD3 sites was observed with exposure of at least 0.5 µg/mL of otelixizumab for 120 hours. Expression of TCR followed essentially identical kinetics when cells were exposed to the same level of antibody (Figure 23.3B).

Similar cultures were harvested at the end of 5 days and proliferation assessed by ^{3}H-thymidine incorporation. Proliferation was inhibited by approximately 90% in mixed lymphocyte cultures exposed to at least 0.1 µg/mL of otelixizumab for at least 48 hours, whereas exposure for less than 48 hours in 0.1 µg/mL of antibody inhibited proliferation by 36%–44% (Figure 23.4). These data indicate that exposure of human PBMC for 48 hours or more to at least 0.1 µg/mL of otelixizumab markedly reduces TCR expression and free CD3 sites with a corresponding increase in the inhibition of primary mixed lymphocyte cultures. 0.1µg/mL of otelixizumab for 48 hours induced approximately a 50% reduction in CD3 and TCR expression and a 90% inhibition of

TABLE 23.1. Otelixizumab induced cytokine release

Cytokine	Otelixizumab	YTH12.5
IL-1α	0	583
IL-1β	0	426
IL-2	1	12
IL-4	0	7
IL-5	0	13
IL-6	6	1200
IL-8	−4151	230159
IL-10	−1	162
IL-12p40	3	24
IL-12p70	0	3
IL-13	0	340
GM-CSF	1	799
IFNγ	0	556
TGFβ1	3061	−2309
TNFα	7	895

Note: PBMC were cultured in RPMI media with 10% human serum in the presence of 10 μg/mL otelixizumab. YTH12.5, the parental rat monoclonal antihuman CD3 antibody, was used as a positive control. Supernatants were removed from the cultures after 48 hours and tested for cytokines using SearchLight Multiplexed assay technology (Endogen). Unstimulated cells in the same media and media alone were also tested for cytokine content. Cytokine release was calculated from the mean of the levels produced by each individual after subtraction of cytokine present in the absence of antibody. Data shown are the cumulative mean values in pg/mL obtained from six separate individuals.

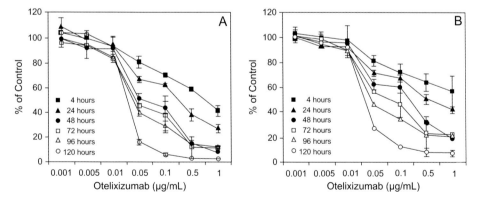

Figure 23.3. Effect of otelixizumab incubation time on free CD3 sites (A) and TCR expression (B). PBMC were incubated with 0.001–1.0 μg/mL of otelixizumab for 4–120 hours in RPMI media with 10% human serum. (A) After 5 days, free, unbound CD3 sites present on cells were detected with FITC-conjugated otelixizumab. (B) In addition, samples were stained with BMA031, an anti-TCRαβ antibody demonstrated not to compete with otelixizumab for binding to CD3. For each staining condition, the mean channel fluorescence (MCF) of antibody treated cells was compared with the MCF of control cells to determine the percentage of control level of expression for each reagent. Modulation was detected as a decrease in TCR expression and a reduction in free CD3 sites. Data shown are the mean with SD from 4 individuals.

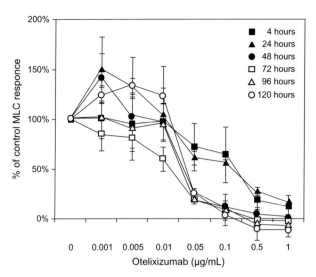

Figure 23.4. Otelixizumab inhibits proliferation of mixed lymphocyte cultures. PBMC were isolated by Ficoll density gradient centrifugation, and nonresponding stimulator cells were prepared by treatment with mitomycin C. Primary mixed lymphocyte cultures were established by combining equal numbers of responder and stimulator cells in RPMI media with 10% human serum and otelixizumab at the specified concentrations (0.001–1.0 μg/mL). Cultures were incubated in the presence of otelixizumab for the length of time indicated in the legend (4–120 hours). On day 5, cultures were fed with media containing ^{3}H-thymidine. Proliferation was assessed by ^{3}H-thymidine incorporation after 18 hours. Results are expressed as the percentage of ^{3}H-thymidine incorporation in antibody treated wells relative to untreated control wells. Data shown are the mean values with SD from 6 individuals.

proliferation suggesting that complete CD3/TCR modulation is not necessary to inhibit a mixed lymphocyte culture.

Effect of Otelixizumab on the Generation of Memory Responses

To examine the effect of otelixizumab on memory T cell responses, the recall response of cells previously sensitized to alloantigen in a primary response was assessed. Addition of otelixizumab to these secondary mixed lymphocyte cultures blocked the recall response by approximately 80%, whereas addition of YTH12.5 resulted in only an insignificant reduction in proliferation compared to control (Figure 23.5A).

Although otelixizumab blocked alloantigen-stimulated proliferation of lymphocytes when added to primary mixed lymphocyte cultures, such inhibition does not necessarily preclude sensitization or differentiation of some lymphocyte subsets. To assess the effect of antibody treatment on these processes, secondary mixed lymphocyte cultures were established by restimulating cells from otelixizumab- or YTH12.5-treated primary cultures with original stimulator cells in the absence of antibody (Figure 23.5B). The proliferative response of cells previously treated with YTH12.5 was variably diminished in the secondary cultures, but the reduction was not statistically significant. However, the secondary proliferative response of cells previously treated with otelixizumab was consistently reduced by greater than 90%. To determine whether the lack of secondary proliferative response was the

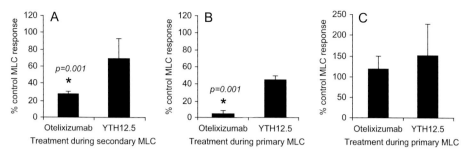

Figure 23.5. Otelixizumab blocks the generation of memory responses. Otelixizumab inhibits proliferation of secondary mixed lymphocyte cultures (MLC) more effectively than YTH12.5. (A) PBMC were sensitized to an unrelated donor in a primary MLC. After sensitization, rested cells were re-stimulated with donor cells from the original stimulator source in the presence of no antibody or 1 µg/ml of otelixizumab or YTH12.5. Otelixizumab significantly inhibited proliferation of the secondary response (p = 0.001, paired t-test, n = 3). (B, C) Primary MLC were established in the presence of no antibody or 1 µg/mL of otelixizumab or YTH12.5. After sensitization, rested cells were washed to remove any remaining antibody and re-stimulated with donor cells from the original stimulator source (B) or cells from a new, third party donor (C). No antibody was added to the re-stimulated cultures. Proliferation was measured by uptake of ^{3}H-thymidine added to cultures 3 days after re-stimulation. Data shown are the mean of three independent experiments.

result of a dysfunction in all T cells following otelixizumab treatment, cultures were restimulated with cells from a new, unrelated donor. Despite a poor proliferative response to original stimulator cells, cells treated previously with otelixizumab responded as well as untreated, control cells to third party stimulation (Figure 23.5C).

Effect on CD4⁺FoxP3⁺ and CD8⁺FoxP3⁺ Cells

The ability of otelixizumab to bind to the CD3/TCR complex and block T cell activation, proliferation, and cytokine release suggests that the antibody may beneficially modulate detrimental autoimmune responses by preventing the activation and function of autoreactive T cells. Indeed, clinical studies have confirmed that aglycosyl anti-CD3 antibodies exhibit potent immunomodulatory activity in both transplant[19] and autoimmune disease[20] settings without inducing significant cytokine release syndrome.

In vivo models have demonstrated a role for regulatory T cells in the long-term maintenance of anti-CD3 antibody-mediated remission of autoimmune disease (reviewed in[37]). One intriguing possibility is that otelixizumab treatment results in the induction or expansion of regulatory T cells. Several types of regulatory T cells have been characterized. Naturally occurring, thymic-derived regulatory T cells (nTregs) are characterized phenotypically by expression of CD25 and FoxP3 (forkhead box P3) and functionally by suppression of T cell activation in a contact-dependent manner.[38,39] Adaptive regulatory T cells are similarly CD25⁺FoxP3⁺ and functionally suppressive but are generated in the periphery from CD25⁻ lymphocytes stimulated in the presence of TGF-β.[40,41] The importance of Tregs in controlling autoimmunity has been shown in both mice and humans, where mutations in FoxP3 promote autoimmunity (reviewed in[37]). Defective regulatory T cell function has been reported in humans with autoimmune disease, including diabetes.[42] Interestingly, anti-CD3 antibodies have been shown to induce adaptive Tregs in mouse models in which nTregs are absent.[43]

To examine the effects of otelixizumab on Treg cells, human PBMC were incubated with otelixizumab and FoxP3 expression was assessed in CD4$^+$ and CD8$^+$ T cells by flow cytometry. No change in CD4$^+$FoxP3$^+$ cells was detected on day 1 and day 3. Interestingly, CD4$^+$FoxP3$^+$ cells were increased approximately threefold on day 7 in otelixizumab-treated cultures when compared to untreated control cultures (Figure 23.6A). Preliminary studies with these CD4$^+$FoxP3$^+$ cells from day 7 cultures demonstrated that these cells possess suppressive function (unpublished observations, D. Forman). Interestingly, an increase in CD4$^+$FoxP3$^+$ cells was also detected in the peripheral blood of subjects with type 1 diabetes treated with otelixizumab (unpublished observation). The increase in CD4$^+$FoxP3$^+$ cells detected *in vivo* occurred two weeks after dosing, once otelixizumab had cleared from the circulation (data not shown), suggesting that other mechanisms may also be responsible for the increase of CD4$^+$FoxP3$^+$ cells *in vivo* as compared to what was observed *in vitro*.

An examination of CD8$^+$ T cells showed no changes in FoxP3$^+$ cells in either untreated or otelixizumab-treated cultures, with the exception of a slight increase on day 1 (Figure 23.6B). Moreover, an increase in CD8$^+$FoxP3$^+$ cells was not detected in the peripheral blood of type 1 diabetic subjects treated with otelixizumab (unpublished observations).

The increase in CD4$^+$FoxP3$^+$ cells observed in PBMC cultures after exposure to otelixizumab could be due to the conversion of CD4$^+$FoxP3$^-$ cells into CD4$^+$FoxP3$^+$ cells, or, alternatively, to the expansion of CD4$^+$FoxP3$^+$ cells. In order to distinguish between these two possibilities, human PBMC were depleted of CD25$^+$ cells by magnetic bead depletion to eliminate FoxP3$^+$ cells prior to culture with otelixizumab. Whereas untreated PBMC once again showed an increase in CD4$^+$FoxP3$^+$ cells,

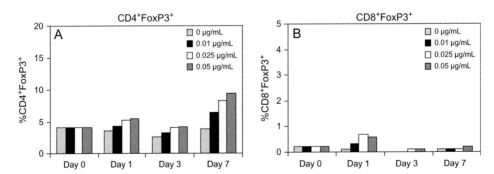

Figure 23.6. Effect of otelixizumab on CD4$^+$FoxP3$^+$ and CD8$^+$FoxP3$^+$ cells. PBMC were incubated with 0–0.05 µg/mL of otelixizumab for up to 7 days in RPMI media with 0.5% human serum. At the specified time points, cultures were harvested and surface stained with fluorescently conjugated CD4 and CD8 antibodies. After two washes, cells were fixed and permeabilized overnight followed by staining with anti-FoxP3 mAb (Clone PCH101, Ebiosciences) according to the manufacturer's suggestions. Dead cells were eliminated from analysis based on forward and side scatter. Effect of otelixizumab on (A) CD4$^+$FoxP3$^+$ cells and (B) CD8$^+$FoxP3$^+$ cells are representative of experiments from three separate individuals.

no increase in CD4$^+$FoxP3$^+$ cells was observed in cultures depleted of CD25$^+$ (FoxP3$^+$) cells prior to culture, suggesting that otelixizumab itself does not directly convert CD4$^+$CD25$^-$FoxP3$^-$ cells into CD4$^+$FoxP3$^+$ cells (data not shown).

OTELIXIZUMAB AND ANTIGEN-SPECIFIC MEMORY RESPONSES

Effect on EBV-Specific Memory T Cell Responses

A recent clinical study with ChAglyCD3 (otelixizumab) in new onset type 1 diabetes resulted in a transient loss of EBV control in the majority of patients treated.[20] To examine the effects of otelixizumab on EBV-specific memory cells, PBMC were cultured with various concentrations of otelixizumab for 24 or 48 hours. Following treatment with otelixizumab, PBMC were washed to remove residual antibody and stimulated with EBV-specific peptide pools from either the lytic or latent phase of the viral replication cycle.[44] Both peptide pools stimulated IFNγ expression as measured by ELISPOT. The number of IFNγ-producing cells was decreased in otelixizumab-treated cultures in a dose-dependent manner beginning at 0.1 µg/mL of antibody (Figure 23.7A and B), indicating that otelixizumab has an inhibitory effect on the CD8$^+$ memory T cell population. As CD8$^+$ T cells are the major IFNγ-producing effector cell population generated in response to EBV infection, otelixizumab inhibition of CD8$^+$ T cells may contribute to the transient loss of EBV control. It is important to note, however, that inhibition of EBV-specific memory responses in otelixizumab-treated cultures is not completely ablated even at the highest concentrations tested. These data are consistent with the findings from otelixizumab-treated patients, where those subjects developing a transient loss of EBV control were able to subsequently generate an effective EBV-specific cellular immune response and control the virus.[20] Thus, while otelixizumab partially

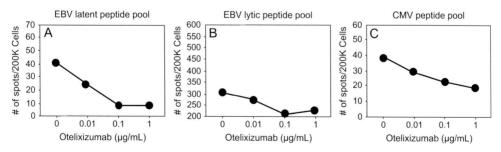

Figure 23.7. Otelixizumab inhibits EBV- and CMV-specific memory T cell responses in a dose dependent manner. PBMC were isolated and cultured with varying concentrations of otelixizumab (0–1 µg/mL) in RPMI media with 10% human serum for 24 hours. PBMC were then washed and stimulated with 20 µg/mL EBV-specific peptides (latent or lytic peptide pool) or 10 µg/mL CMV-specific peptides for 24 hours. IFN-γ production was measured by ELISPOT with 200,000 cells per well. A representative of three experiments is shown.

inhibits EBV specific memory responses, this inhibition is transient as appropriate cellular responses to an active infection are rapidly generated when otelixizumab is cleared.

When otelixizumab was tested for its ability to inhibit CMV memory responses *in vitro* using the ELISPOT methods described earlier, it inhibited CMV-specific memory responses in a dose-dependent manner (Figure 23.7C) similar to its effects on the EBV response. However, while *in vivo* a transient loss of EBV control was seen in otelixizumab-treated patients, there was no similar loss of CMV control. This suggests that factors other than, or in addition to, the direct suppressive effects of otelixizumab on T cells plays a role in the transient loss of EBV control.

Role of Cytokines on EBV Viral Responses

We investigated the possibility that cytokines could exacerbate the transient loss of EBV control seen in otelixizumab-treated patients by culturing PBMC with the antibody in the presence of TNFα, IL-6, IFNγ, and IL-10 in various combinations. A dose-dependent induction of these cytokines is associated with administration of anti-CD3 antibodies in both rodent models[45–47] and clinical studies.[5,6] In summary, the addition of cytokines to otelixizumab-treated PBMC had no measurable effect on CD8$^+$ T cell memory responses as measured by IFNγ production (data not shown) and suggests that otelixizumab-mediated cytokine release is unlikely to be a contributing factor to the transient loss of EBV control by direct impairment of T cell responses. These assays, however, only assess the direct effect of cytokine induction on T cell anti-viral responses, and the role of cytokine-mediated effects such as the effect on the cellular host of EBV, the B cell, remains to be determined.

Otelixizumab Directly Inhibits EBV-Specific CD8 T Cell Responses

Thus far, all experiments measuring CD8$^+$ memory response have utilized PBMC, a mixture of lymphocytes and accessory cells. In order to determine whether the otelixizumab-mediated inhibition of CD8$^+$ memory responses was a direct effect on the CD8$^+$ T cell or instead an indirect effect through another immune cell type, CD8$^+$ T cells were purified and cultured in the presence or absence of otelixizumab and then stimulated with EBV peptides to measure IFNγ production. As expected, cultures lacking CD8$^+$ T cells showed no significant production of IFNγ (data not shown). In purified CD8$^+$ T cell cultures, otelixizumab treatment resulted in an inhibition of IFNγ production in response to EBV peptides. These data demonstrate that otelixizumab-mediated inhibition of EBV-specific CD8$^+$ T cell responses is a direct effect and not one mediated through accessory cells.

Otelixizumab-Mediated Inhibition of EBV-Specific Memory CD8 T Cell Responses Is Reversible

We have shown that $CD8^+$ T cell memory responses are partially inhibited when stimulated with viral antigen peptides in the presence of otelixizumab. We next wanted to determine whether this inhibition is a permanent effect or a transient and reversible response. In addition, we wanted to correlate the amount of CD3/TCR modulation with the effect of otelixizumab on $CD8^+$ T cell function, that is, IFNγ production. As shown previously, treatment of PBMC with otelixizumab for 24 hours results in inhibition of IFNγ production by memory $CD8^+$ T cells in response to EBV-specific viral peptides (Figure 23.8A and B) and in parallel, a complete down-regulation of CD3/TCR expression (data not shown).

When these otelixizumab-treated PBMC were further cultured in the absence of otelixizumab for 1 week, the percentage of CD3/TCR-expressing cells returned to pretreatment levels, while the intensity of staining (mean channel fluorescence, MCF) remained diminished by 20% (data not shown). When memory $CD8^+$ T cell function was measured in response to EBV-specific viral peptides, like the 24-hour post-treatment time-point, IFNγ production was still impaired (Figure 23.8A and B). However, if otelixizumab-treated PBMC are cultured in the absence of

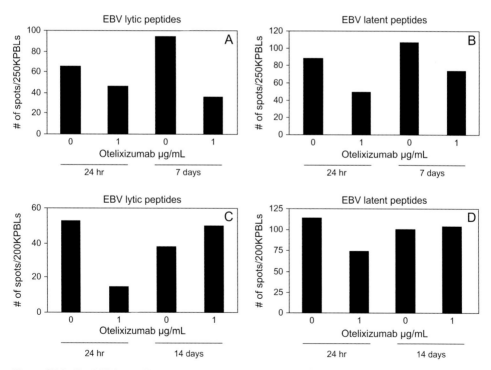

Figure 23.8. The inhibitory effect of otelixizumab on memory $CD8^+$ T cell responses to EBV-specific viral peptides is reversible. PBMC were isolated and cultured in the presence or absence of otelixizumab (1 μg/mL) in RPMI media with 10% human serum for 24 hours. Cultures were then washed and either stimulated or further cultured for up to 2 weeks and then stimulated with 20 μg/mL EBV-specific peptides (lytic (A and C) or latent (B and D) peptide pools) for 24 hours. IFN-γ production was measured by ELISPOT with 200,000–250,000 cells per well.

otelixizumab for 2 weeks after treatment, the percentage of CD3/TCR-expressing cells as well as the intensity of staining returns to pretreatment levels (data not shown). When tested for their ability to respond to EBV viral peptides, the CD8$^+$ T cell memory response had recovered and levels of IFNγ as high as those produced by untreated memory cells were produced (Figure 23.8C and D). The percentage of CD8$^+$ T cells in the 2-week cultures was also measured and shown to be equivalent to untreated cultures (data not shown) indicating that normalization of CD8$^+$ T cell responses was not due to an increased percentage of CD8$^+$ T cells but rather a recovery of function by the otelixizumab-treated CD8$^+$ T cells. Again, these data are consistent with findings from otelixizumab-treated patients who were able to mount a cellular immune response against EBV within a short time after their last treatment.[20] Overall, the data demonstrate that otelixizumab-mediated inhibition of the EBV-specific memory CD8$^+$ T cell response is the consequence of transient CD3/TCR modulation.

IMMUNOGENICITY OF OTELIXIZUMAB

Immunogenicity of therapeutic proteins remains an issue for this class of drugs.[48] Immune responses to therapeutic proteins are common, and this has resulted in a number of strategies directed at mitigating such responses.[49] Many of these efforts have focused on engineering these proteins in such a way as to make them less foreign. Such strategies have resulted in the engineering of antibodies to derive chimeric, humanized, or fully-human constructs. It was hypothesized that this approach would reduce the potential immunogenicity of these proteins; however, review of the literature reveals that reduced immunogenicity is not necessarily the outcome when proteins are engineered to be more humanlike.[48,49] This observation has resulted in an understanding that the immune response to therapeutic proteins may be influenced by a number of additional factors including formulation, route of administration, dose, and dosing regimen. Furthermore, the function of the protein itself may induce changes such as pro-inflammatory cytokine release or cell activation that may increase the immunogenicity of these proteins.

Initial studies conducted by the BDR in subjects with type 1 diabetes administered 48 mgs of otelixizumab over a 6-day course of treatment. The observed immunogenicity rate in this study was approximately 75%.[20] Single-dose studies with between 1 and 4 mgs of otelixizumab in subjects with psoriasis showed similar rates of immunogenicity (unpublished observation). Increases in circulating cytokines, particularly IL-6 and TNFα, were observed shortly after dosing in both studies (data not shown). In subsequent studies we have modified the dosing regimen in an effort to reduce cytokine release and interestingly, this has also resulted in greatly reduced immunogenicity of otelixizumab. In these studies, doses lower than those in the BDR study were administered, and this decrease in dose could certainly have contributed to a mitigation of immunogenicity. Using this dosing regimen, we have observed a significant decrease in immunogenicity at cumulative doses similar to those administered to subjects in the psoriasis study. We have thus concluded that dose, dosing regimen, and cytokine release all contribute to the potential for immunogenicity of otelixizumab. Thus, as a fortunate consequence of developing a dosing regimen designed to reduce cytokine release, a decrease in immunogenicity has also been observed. This decrease in immunogenicity may open up the possibility of re-treatment of subjects if necessary with subsequent doses of otelixizumab.

DISCUSSION

To alleviate the cytokine-related adverse side effects associated with anti-CD3 antibody therapy, a number of anti-CD3 monoclonal antibodies, including otelixizumab, have been modified to disrupt Fc receptor binding and significantly reduce T cell activation and its ensuing cytokine release.[22,50–53] *In vitro* studies have demonstrated that Fc receptor binding by the aglycosyl human $\gamma1$ heavy chain used in the construction of otelixizumab is sufficiently diminished to render the antibody nonmitogenic and substantially reduce the induction of cytokine release.[22] Studies in mice with a number of Fc-modified anti-CD3 antibodies have demonstrated that Fc receptor binding and severe cytokine release syndrome are separable from therapeutic efficacy.[15,54–59] Indeed, disruption of Fc receptor binding did not affect the ability of otelixizumab to inhibit proliferation of mixed lymphocyte cultures, suggesting that the antibody would still function *in vivo* to disrupt T cell-mediated immune responses. Furthermore, clinical studies have confirmed that aglycosyl anti-CD3 antibodies retain potent immunomodulatory activity in both transplant[19] and autoimmune disease[20] settings without inducing significant cytokine release syndrome.

Other studies have demonstrated that FcR-binding and FcR-nonbinding anti-CD3 antibodies differentially affect specific T cell subsets.[32,55,60–63] For example, FcR-nonbinding anti-CD3 F(ab')$_2$ fragments have been shown to preferentially deplete CD4$^+$ T cells by inducing susceptibility to Fas-mediated apoptosis of cycling T cells.[64,65] This effect appears to target polarized Th1 cells, and not Th2 cells, thus skewing the repertoire of antigen-activated T cells toward the Th2 phenotype.[55,61,65] Consistent with these findings, mice treated with anti-CD3 F(ab')$_2$ also show a marked reduction in the ability of T helper cells to secrete IL-2 and IFNγ, but not IL-4, when challenged *in vitro* with mitogen or alloantigen.[55,61,65]

Although both otelixizumab and the parental rat antibody, YTH12.5, block proliferation of primary mixed lymphocyte cultures, our data show that these antibodies differ in their immunomodulatory effects *in vitro*. Addition of YTH12.5 to primary mixed lymphocyte cultures resulted in a small reduction in secondary proliferation in the absence of any anti-CD3 antibody. The reduction was not, however, statistically significant, when compared to the proliferation of control cultures, indicating that memory cells capable of proliferation to recall antigen were generated even though proliferation was blocked during the period of original antigen presentation. Further studies have shown that addition of IL-2 to the secondary mixed lymphocyte cultures completely rescues this otherwise diminished proliferative response of cells primed in the presence of YTH12.5 (data not shown), indicating that clonal anergy was induced in at least a portion of the alloantigen-specific cells during the primary culture. In contrast to YTH12.5, the secondary proliferative response of cells primed in the presence of otelixizumab remained almost completely abolished (>90%) and provision of exogenous IL-2 was unable to restore proliferation of these cells (data not shown). Third party stimulation of cells primed in the presence of either YTH12.5 or otelixizumab resulted in proliferative responses identical to that of untreated, control cell cultures demonstrating that the attenuated secondary responses were antigen-specific. Induction of alloantigen-specific nonresponsiveness of human T cells has been reported with other Fc receptor-nonbinding or nonmitogenic anti-CD3 antibodies.[36,66] The results presented here with otelixizumab are most similar to those reported by Anasetti et al.[36] In that report, antigen-specific non-responsiveness was induced in naïve, unprimed T cells, but not memory T cells, by the addition of nonmitogenic murine anti-CD3 mAbs to mixed lymphocyte cultures.

One possible explanation for the loss of alloantigen-specific responsiveness induced by otelixizumab is the selective depletion of activated cells, as reported with some other Fc receptor-nonbinding anti-CD3 antibodies.[60,64,67] The almost complete loss of recall antigen responses together with the absence of effect on responses to new, third party antigens would be consistent with the elimination of alloantigen responsive cells. However, we have been unable to detect any significant increase in the number of dead cells or in the number of cells undergoing apoptosis in otelixizumab-treated mixed lymphocyte cultures over that observed in control cultures or YTH12.5-treated cultures (unpublished observation). Nevertheless, this mechanism remains a possibility, as the previous studies reporting FcR-nonbinding anti-CD3 induced apoptosis of activated T cells utilized nonspecific pre-activation of T cells with plate bound CD3 antibody[60] or immunized TCR transgenic mice with TCR-specific antigen,[64,67] thereby greatly increasing the number of activated T cells in the experimental models. In our studies, by contrast, the absolute number of alloantigen-specific T cells present in primary cultures is likely to be extremely small and, therefore, any increase in the number of dead or apoptotic cells resulting from specific effects of antibody treatment on these cells may be difficult to detect against the background level in control cultures.

A second possible mechanism that could explain the alloantigen-specific non-responsiveness of otelixizumab-treated mixed lymphocyte cultures is the induction or expansion of a highly effective, antigen-specific regulatory T cell population. However, additional work is needed to evaluate this possibility. Nevertheless, we have investigated the direct effect of otelixizumab on Treg cells as defined by FoxP3 expression. Although an increase in CD8$^+$FoxP3$^+$ cells was not observed, a threefold increase in CD4$^+$FoxP3$^+$ cells was observed in PBMC cultures after 7 days. This increase in CD4$^+$FoxP3$^+$ cells after a short delay is consistent with the reports of other investigators.[68] Preliminary functional studies with these CD4$^+$FoxP3$^+$ cells from day 7 cultures demonstrate that these cells also possess suppressive capabilities (unpublished observations, D. Forman).

Our studies on the effects of otelixizumab on CD8$^+$ antigen-specific memory cells indicates that antibody treatment may result in a slight reduction in the number of CD8$^+$ antigen-specific memory cells probably as a result of apoptosis. However, the most significant suppressive effects of otelixizumab on CD8$^+$ cells appear to result from the modulation of CD3/TCR. Our *in vitro* studies demonstrate, however, that this effect is both transient and reversible as CD8$^+$ cell effector functions as measured by IFNγ production return to pretreatment levels with the return of cell surface CD3/TCR expression. These data suggest, as has been demonstrated in clinical studies, that preservation of the memory responses to previously encountered pathogens should protect patients receiving otelixizumab from opportunistic infection and reactivation of chronic viral infections.

Although a number of issues remain to be resolved regarding the otelixizumab mechanism of action, our results and those from studies utilizing other Fc-modified anti-CD3 antibodies allow proposal of a model that involves two phases: induction and maintenance.[69] During the induction or treatment phase with otelixizumab, autoimmune inflammation is rapidly restrained. This is accomplished by (1) CD3/TCR blockade and modulation from the cell surface; (2) induction of anergic T cells either directly by otelixizumab or indirectly through modulation of sufficient numbers of CD3/TCR molecules from the cell surface; and (3) induction of apoptosis of activated, effector T cells. The induction phase is followed by maintenance of autoimmune quiescence by regulatory T cells. Our *in vitro* results suggest that otelixizumab treatment may result in the expansion of preexisting regulatory T cells, and this is consistent with observations in rodent models.[70] In addition, otelixizumab treatment may also result in *de novo* generation of regulatory T cells from FoxP3$^-$ cells as has been reported in some models with other Fc-modified anti-CD3 antibodies.[43] Although we have not observed otelixizumab-induced conversion of FoxP3$^-$ to FoxP3$^+$, this may reflect the *in vitro* nature of our studies. *De novo* induction of FoxP3$^+$ cells may be an indirect consequence of otelixizumab treatment and result from down-modulation of CD3/TCR below the threshold required for activation. Alternatively, anergic T cells, which we have observed to be induced by exposure to otelixizumab *in vitro*, could compete with naïve T cells for both antigen and cytokine at the antigen-presenting cell interface in the lymph node and prevent activation of T cells.

REFERENCES

[1] Cosimi, A.B., et al., Treatment of acute renal allograft rejection with OKT3 monoclonal antibody. *Transplantation*, 1981. **32**(6): pp. 535–9.

[2] Cosimi, A.B., et al., Use of monoclonal antibodies to T-cell subsets for immunologic monitoring and treatment in recipients of renal allografts. *N Engl J Med*, 1981. **305**(6): pp. 308–14.

[3] Chatenoud, L., et al., Restriction of the human in vivo immune response against the mouse monoclonal antibody OKT3. *J Immunol*, 1986. **137**(3): pp. 830–8.

[4]   Jaffers, G.J., et al., Monoclonal antibody therapy. Anti-idiotypic and non-anti-idiotypic antibodies to OKT3 arising despite intense immunosuppression. *Transplantation*, 1986. **41**(5): pp. 572–8.

[5]   Abramowicz, D., et al., Release of tumor necrosis factor, interleukin-2, and gamma-interferon in serum after injection of OKT3 monoclonal antibody in kidney transplant recipients. *Transplantation*, 1989. **47**(4): pp. 606–8.

[6]   Chatenoud, L., et al., Systemic reaction to the anti-T-cell monoclonal antibody OKT3 in relation to serum levels of tumor necrosis factor and interferon-gamma [corrected]. *N Engl J Med*, 1989. **320**(21): pp. 1420–1.

[7]   Wofsy, D., et al., Inhibition of humoral immunity in vivo by monoclonal antibody to L3T4: studies with soluble antigens in intact mice. *J Immunol*, 1985. **135**(3): pp. 1698–701.

[8]   Benjamin, R.J., et al., Tolerance to rat monoclonal antibodies. Implications for serotherapy. *J Exp Med*, 1986. **163**(6): pp. 1539–52.

[9]   Riechmann, L., et al., Reshaping human antibodies for therapy. *Nature*, 1988. **332**(6162): pp. 323–7.

[10] Qin, S., et al., "Infectious" transplantation tolerance. *Science*, 1993. **259**(5097): pp. 974–7.

[11] Cobbold, S.P., et al., Reprogramming the immune system for peripheral tolerance with CD4 and CD8 monoclonal antibodies. *Immunol Rev*, 1992. **129**: pp. 165–201.

[12] Waldmann, H., et al., Infectious tolerance and the long-term acceptance of transplanted tissue. *Immunol Rev*, 2006. **212**: pp. 301–13.

[13] Hutchings, P., et al., The use of a non-depleting anti-CD4 monoclonal antibody to re-establish tolerance to beta cells in NOD mice. *Eur J Immunol*, 1992. **22**(7): pp. 1913–8.

[14] Cooke, A., J.M. Phillips, and N.M. Parish, Tolerogenic strategies to halt or prevent type 1 diabetes. *Nat Immunol*, 2001. **2**(9): pp. 810–5.

[15] Chatenoud, L., et al., Anti-CD3 antibody induces long-term remission of overt autoimmunity in nonobese diabetic mice. *Proc Natl Acad Sci USA*, 1994. **91**(1): pp. 123–7.

[16] Abbs, I.C., et al., Sparing of first dose effect of monovalent anti-CD3 antibody used in allograft rejection is associated with diminished release of pro-inflammatory cytokines. *Ther Immunol*, 1994. **1**(6): pp. 325–31.

[17] Routledge, E.G., et al., A humanized monovalent CD3 antibody which can activate homologous complement. *Eur J Immunol*, 1991. **21**(11): pp. 2717–25.

[18] Routledge, E.G., et al., The effect of aglycosylation on the immunogenicity of a humanized therapeutic CD3 monoclonal antibody. *Transplantation*, 1995. **60**(8): pp. 847–53.

[19] Friend, P.J., et al., Phase I study of an engineered aglycosylated humanized CD3 antibody in renal transplant rejection. *Transplantation*, 1999. **68**(11): pp. 1632–7.

[20] Keymeulen, B., et al., Insulin needs after CD3-antibody therapy in new-onset type 1 diabetes. *N Engl J Med*, 2005. **352**(25): pp. 2598–608.

[21] Clark, M., et al., The improved lytic function and in vivo efficacy of monovalent monoclonal CD3 antibodies. *Eur J Immunol*, 1989. **19**(2): pp. 381–8.

[22] Bolt, S., et al., The generation of a humanized, non-mitogenic CD3 monoclonal antibody which retains in vitro immunosuppressive properties. *Eur J Immunol*, 1993. **23**(2): pp. 403–11.

[23] McMichael A.J., Beverly, P.C.L., Cobbold, S., Crumpton, M.J., Gilks,, W., Gotch, F.M., Hogg, N., Horton, M., Ling, N., MacLennan, I.C.M., Mason, D.Y., Milstein, C., Spiegelhalter, D., Waldmann, H., eds., *Leukocyte Typing III: White Cell Differentiation Antigens*, 1987, Oxford, UK: Oxford University Press.

[24] Knapp, W., Dorken, B., Gilks, W.R., Rieber, E.P., Schmidt, R.E., Stein, H., von dem Borne, A.E.G. Kr., eds., *Leucocyte Typing IV: White Cell Differentiation Antigens*, 1989, Oxford, UK: Oxford University Press.

[25] Cobbold, S.P. and H. Waldmann, Therapeutic potential of monovalent monoclonal antibodies. *Nature*, 1984. **308**(5958): pp. 460–2.

[26] Orlandi, R., et al., Cloning immunoglobulin variable domains for expression by the polymerase chain reaction. *Proc Natl Acad Sci USA*, 1989. **86**(10): pp. 3833–7.

[27] Steen, M.L., L. Hellman, and U. Pettersson, The immunoglobulin lambda locus in rat consists of two C lambda genes and a single V lambda gene. *Gene*, 1987. **55**(1): pp. 75–84.

[28] Kabat, E., *Sequences of proteins of immunological interest.* 4th ed, ed. N.I.o.H.U.D.o.R. Resources. 1987, Bethesda, MD: US Department of Health and Human Services, Public Health Service, National Institutes of Health.

[29] Dersimonian, H., et al., Relationship of human variable region heavy chain germ-line genes to genes encoding anti-DNA autoantibodies. *J Immunol*, 1987. **139**(7): pp. 2496–501.

[30] Takahashi, N., et al., Structure of human immunoglobulin gamma genes: implications for evolution of a gene family. *Cell*, 1982. **29**(2): pp. 671–9.

[31] Rabbitts, T.H., A. Forster, and J.G. Matthews, The breakpoint of the Philadelphia chromosome 22 in chronic myeloid leukaemia is distal to the immunoglobulin lambda light chain constant region genes. *Mol Biol Med*, 1983. **1**(1): pp. 11–9.

[32] Smith, J.A., et al., Nonmitogenic anti-CD3 monoclonal antibodies deliver a partial T cell receptor signal and induce clonal anergy. *J Exp Med*, 1997. **185**(8): pp. 1413–22.

[33] Yu, X.Z., et al., Lck is required for activation-induced T cell death after TCR ligation with partial agonists. *J Immunol*, 2004. **172**(3): pp. 1437–43.

[34] Tax, W.J., et al., Fc receptors for mouse IgG1 on human monocytes: polymorphism and role in antibody-induced T cell proliferation. *J Immunol*, 1984. **133**(3): pp. 1185–9.

[35] Clement, L.T., A.B. Tilden, and N.E. Dunlap, Analysis of the monocyte Fc receptors and antibody-mediated cellular interactions required for the induction of T cell proliferation by anti-T3 antibodies. *J Immunol*, 1985. **135**(1): pp. 165–71.

[36] Anasetti, C., et al., Induction of specific nonresponsiveness in unprimed human T cells by anti-CD3 antibody and alloantigen. *J Exp Med*, 1990. **172**(6): pp. 1691–700.

[37] Baecher-Allan, C. and D.A. Hafler, Human regulatory T cells and their role in autoimmune disease. *Immunol Rev*, 2006. **212**: pp. 203–16.

[38] Takahashi, T., et al., Immunologic self-tolerance maintained by CD25+CD4+ naturally anergic and suppressive T cells: induction of autoimmune disease by breaking their anergic/suppressive state. *Int Immunol*, 1998. **10**(12): pp. 1969–80.

[39] Thornton, A.M. and E.M. Shevach, CD4+CD25+ immunoregulatory T cells suppress polyclonal T cell activation in vitro by inhibiting interleukin 2 production. *J Exp Med*, 1998. **188**(2): pp. 287–96.

[40] Chen, W., et al., Conversion of peripheral CD4+CD25-naive T cells to CD4+CD25+ regulatory T cells by TGF-beta induction of transcription factor Foxp3. *J Exp Med*, 2003. **198**(12): pp. 1875–86.

[41] Cobbold, S.P., et al., Induction of foxP3+ regulatory T cells in the periphery of T cell receptor transgenic mice tolerized to transplants. *J Immunol*, 2004. **172**(10): pp. 6003–10.

[42] Lindley, S., et al., Defective suppressor function in CD4(+)CD25(+) T-cells from patients with type 1 diabetes. *Diabetes*, 2005. **54**(1): pp. 92–9.

[43] Belghith, M., et al., TGF-beta-dependent mechanisms mediate restoration of self-tolerance induced by antibodies to CD3 in overt autoimmune diabetes. *Nat Med*, 2003. **9**(9): pp. 1202–8.

[44] Woodberry, T., et al., Differential targeting and shifts in the immunodominance of Epstein-Barr virus–specific CD8 and CD4 T cell responses during acute and persistent infection. *J Infect Dis*, 2005. **192**(9): pp. 1513–24.

[45] Ferran, C., et al., Cytokine-related syndrome following injection of anti-CD3 monoclonal antibody: further evidence for transient in vivo T cell activation. *Eur J Immunol*, 1990. **20**(3): pp. 509–15.

[46] Alegre, M., et al., Hypothermia and hypoglycemia induced by anti-CD3 monoclonal antibody in mice: role of tumor necrosis factor. *Eur J Immunol*, 1990. **20**(3): pp. 707–10.

[47] Ferran, C., et al., Cascade modulation by anti-tumor necrosis factor monoclonal antibody of interferon-gamma, interleukin 3 and interleukin 6 release after triggering of the CD3/T cell receptor activation pathway. *Eur J Immunol*, 1991. **21**(10): pp. 2349–53.

[48] Chamberlain, P., Immunogenicity of therapeutic proteins. *Regulatory Review*, 2002. **5**(5): pp. 4–9.

[49]   Amin, T.C., G., Immunogenicity issues with therapeutic proteins. *Current Drug Discovery*, 2004: pp. 20–24.

[50]   Alegre, M.L., et al., A non-activating "humanized" anti-CD3 monoclonal antibody retains immunosuppressive properties in vivo. *Transplantation*, 1994. **57**(11): pp. 1537–43.

[51]   Alegre, M.L., et al., Effect of a single amino acid mutation on the activating and immunosuppressive properties of a "humanized" OKT3 monoclonal antibody. *J Immunol*, 1992. **148**(11): pp. 3461–8.

[52]   Cole, M.S., C. Anasetti, and J.Y. Tso, Human IgG2 variants of chimeric anti-CD3 are non-mitogenic to T cells. *J Immunol*, 1997. **159**(7): pp. 3613–21.

[53]   Cole, M.S., et al., HuM291, a humanized anti-CD3 antibody, is immunosuppressive to T cells while exhibiting reduced mitogenicity in vitro. *Transplantation*, 1999. **68**(4): pp. 563–71.

[54]   Alegre, M.L., et al., An anti-murine CD3 monoclonal antibody with a low affinity for Fc gamma receptors suppresses transplantation responses while minimizing acute toxicity and immunogenicity. *J Immunol*, 1995. **155**(3): pp. 1544–55.

[55]   Hughes, C., et al., Induction of T helper cell hyporesponsiveness in an experimental model of autoimmunity by using nonmitogenic anti-CD3 monoclonal antibody. *J Immunol*, 1994. **153**(7): pp. 3319–25.

[56]   Herold, K.C., et al., Prevention of autoimmune diabetes with nonactivating anti-CD3 monoclonal antibody. *Diabetes*, 1992. **41**(3): pp. 385–91.

[57]   Parlevliet, K.J., et al., In vivo effects of IgA and IgG2a anti-CD3 isotype switch variants. *J Clin Invest*, 1994. **93**(6): pp. 2519–25.

[58]   Hirsch, R., et al., Anti-CD3 F(ab′)2 fragments are immunosuppressive in vivo without evoking either the strong humoral response or morbidity associated with whole mAb. *Transplantation*, 1990. **49**(6): pp. 1117–23.

[59]   Vossen, A.C., et al., Fc receptor binding of anti-CD3 monoclonal antibodies is not essential for immunosuppression, but triggers cytokine-related side effects. *Eur J Immunol*, 1995. **25**(6): pp. 1492–6.

[60]   Carpenter, P.A., et al., Non-Fc receptor-binding humanized anti-CD3 antibodies induce apoptosis of activated human T cells. *J Immunol*, 2000. **165**(11): pp. 6205–13.

[61]   Smith, J.A., Q. Tang, and J.A. Bluestone, Partial TCR signals delivered by FcR-nonbinding anti-CD3 monoclonal antibodies differentially regulate individual Th subsets. *J Immunol*, 1998. **160**(10): pp. 4841–9.

[62]   Woodle, E.S., S. Hussein, and J.A. Bluestone, In vivo administration of anti-murine CD3 monoclonal antibody induces selective, long-term anergy in CD8+ T cells. *Transplantation*, 1996. **61**(5): pp. 798–803.

[63]   Hirsch, R., J. Archibald, and R.E. Gress, Differential T cell hyporesponsiveness induced by in vivo administration of intact or F(ab′)2 fragments of anti-CD3 monoclonal antibody. F(ab′)2 fragments induce a selective T helper dysfunction. *J Immunol*, 1991. **147**(7): pp. 2088–93.

[64]   Yu, X.Z., et al., Induction of apoptosis by anti-CD3 epsilon F(ab′)2 in antigen receptor transgenic murine T cells activated by specific peptide. *J Immunol*, 1996. **157**(8): pp. 3420–9.

[65]   Yu, X.Z. and C. Anasetti, Enhancement of susceptibility to Fas-mediated apoptosis of TH1 cells by nonmitogenic anti-CD3epsilon F(ab′)2. *Transplantation*, 2000. **69**(1): pp. 104–12.

[66]   Popma, S.H., D.E. Griswold, and L. Li, Anti-CD3 antibodies OKT3 and hOKT3gamma1(Ala-Ala) induce proliferation of T cells but impair expansion of alloreactive T cells; aspecifc T cell proliferation induced by anti-CD3 antibodies correlates with impaired expansion of alloreactive T cells. *Int Immunopharmacol*, 2005. **5**(1): pp. 155–62.

[67]   Yu, X.Z., et al., Anti-CD3 epsilon F(ab′)2 prevents graft-versus-host disease by selectively depleting donor T cells activated by recipient alloantigens. *J Immunol*, 2001. **166**(9): pp. 5835–9.

[68]   Cao, O., et al., Induction and role of regulatory CD4+CD25+ T cells in tolerance to the transgene product following hepatic in vivo gene transfer. *Blood*, 2007. **110**(4): pp. 1132–40.

[69] Chatenoud, L., CD3-specific antibody-induced active tolerance: from bench to bedside. *Nat Rev Immunol*, 2003. **3**(2): pp. 123–32.

[70] Peng, Y., et al., TGF-beta regulates in vivo expansion of Foxp3-expressing CD4+CD25+ regulatory T cells responsible for protection against diabetes. *Proc Natl Acad Sci USA*, 2004. **101**(13): pp. 4572–7.

PART X

MARKET OVERVIEW AND OUTLOOK

CHAPTER TWENTY-FOUR

Antibody Therapeutics: Business Achievements and Business Outlook

Christophe Bourrilly

It has become a business truism to highlight the contribution of monoclonal antibodies (mAbs) to the drug arsenal of physicians and to the revenues of the pharmaceutical industry. They have become mainstays of therapies for major inflammatory disorders and for a range of hematological and solid tumors. In 2007, mAbs had revenues of $24.8 billion, as estimated by ABN AMRO.

MAbs have outperformed as drug development candidates by showing attractive therapeutic indices in diseases with complex underlying molecular etiologies. They were also a compelling value proposition to the medical affairs departments of large pharmaceutical companies ("Big Pharma"), which first saw their potential for multiple indications and for pricing leverage, later for immunity to patent expiry. Time will tell to what extent mAbs can be protected by manufacturing patents or trade secrets and can thwart generic competition sustainably. It takes many levels of "robustness" for new technology to translate into billion-dollar products. These multiple dynamics have here been taken into account in attempting to describe the growth of the market for mAbs.

The success of the first generation of mAbs offers an interesting road map to the current wave of antibody and antibody fragment companies. I have therefore included a snapshot of these technology markets where so many entrepreneurial initiatives are already undergoing "robustness tests," and give a perspective on the new research and development frontiers that the private sector is tackling.

MONOCLONAL ANTIBODIES: 10 YEARS OF BLOCKBUSTER DRUG CLASS

Currently Marketed Monoclonal Antibodies

The current market for mAbs has grown from $6.9 billion in 2003 to an estimated $24.8 billion in 2007 according to ABN AMRO. This represents an average annual growth rate of 38% over the 2004–2007 period. In 2007 alone, growth was impacted by the launch of only one mAb (eculizumab, branded Soliris® by Alexion Pharmaceuticals), yet amounted to 27%. MAbs have become a well-validated new drug development approach and are an icon of the success of biotechnologies, in the footsteps of major

I thank Melvyn Little at Affimed Therapeutics AG (Affimed) for giving me the opportunity to write on this subject and participate in this book. I also thank my senior and junior colleagues at ABN AMRO for freeing-up time or resources to facilitate this contribution.

protein drugs such as recombinant insulin or Amgen's Epogen®/ Neupogen®. The first mAb, muromonab (OrthoClone OKT3; Johnson & Johnson), was approved by the Federal Food and Drug Administration (FDA) in 1986 and sales of early murine or chimeric antibodies remained low for a long period of time. In reality, success comes from a handful of key products in auto-immune disease and cancer, as shown in Table 24.1.

The physician target population for mAbs is comparatively small and, as a result, physician penetration in developed economies, whether these are oncologists, rheumatologists, or gastroenterology specialists, is already significant. Growth and magnitude of sales of certain mAb categories, such as anti-CD20 or anti-TNF-α mAbs, are likely to be comparable to the performance achieved by several major drug classes, such as proton pump inhibitors, statins, biphosphonates, or anthracyclines. However, adjusted for the annual price of a treatment or protocol, patient population penetration remains comparatively modest and potential for growth still exists.

According to ABN AMRO, currently approved mAbs, to which we added motavizumab (Numax®, Medimmune, now part of AstraZeneca) to offset Synagis® cannibalization, are expected to grow to $38.8 billion in sales by 2010. Physician adoption in the United States and spreading from the United States to other developed countries is one growth factor. Beyond geographic expansion, the growth of currently approved mAbs is expected to continue as the pharmaceutical industry expands the scope of their applications. All major mAbs are currently the subjects of large Phase IV studies, aimed at demonstrating their benefits in more "senior" positions in treatment protocols and guidelines – for instance, as second-line therapies instead of third- or even first-line combination therapies – or leading to approval in larger population pools of patients or in other disease areas. For instance, based on data showing that the vascular endothelial growth factor (VEGF) may play a broad role in a range of cancers, a global development program for Avastin® currently includes more than 300 clinical trials in 20 different tumor types, according to Genentech. Avastin® is being evaluated in Phase III clinical trials for its potential use in adjuvant and metastatic colorectal, renal cell, breast, pancreatic, non-small-cell lung, prostate, and ovarian cancers. Avastin® is also being evaluated in Phase I/II trials as a potential therapy in a variety of other solid tumors and hematological malignancies, and is being studied in combination with other targeted therapy agents in the absence of chemotherapy.

Growth has indeed resulted, not only from organic adoption by physicians but also from approvals in multiple indications. The case of anti-TNF-α mAbs is exemplified in Table 24.2.

Growth has also resulted from off-label use by opinion-leading physicians. In oncology in particular, where regulatory authorities may tolerate it more than in other therapeutic areas, off-label use or compassionate use programs are systematic. While the reimbursement prices of mAbs may limit such uses, clinical practices frequently provide insights to medical affairs teams as to future clinical development and study designs. Our discussions with prominent oncologists in the United States have revealed that cetuximab (Erbitux®, Bristol-Myers Squibb/ImClone Systems), for instance, was experimented with in head and neck cancer patients as early as 2001, although it was approved by the FDA for colorectal cancer in February 2004 and head and neck cancer in May 2006.

TABLE 24.1. Key FDA-approved monoclonal antibodies

Brand	Generic	Target	Marketer(s)/ originator	Indications	Launch year	Sales (in $millions) 2006	2007	2010e
Orthoclone OKT3®	muromonab-CD3	CD3	Johnson & Johnson	Transplant	1986	10	10	10
ReoPro®	Abciximab	Glycoprotein IIb/IIIa platelet r.	Lilly/Centocor (J&J)	Hemostasis	1995	260	260	250
Rituxan®/ MabThera®	rituximab	CD20	Genentech/ Biogen Idec/Chugai/ Roche	NHL/RA	1997	3,810	4,300	6,300
Zenapax®	daclizumab	IL-2	Roche	Transplant	1997	10	10	10
Herceptin®	trastuzumab	HER-2	Roche (ROW)/ Genentech (US)	Breast cancer	1998	3,092	3,800	4,700
Remicade®	infliximab	TNF-α	Centocor (US)/ Tanabe Seiyaku/ Schering-Plough (ROW)	RA, PA, Crohn's, AS, UC	1998	4,440	5,050	5,550
Simulect®	basiliximab	IL-2	Novartis	Transplant	1998	20	20	20
Synagis®	palivizumab	Human RSV Fusion glycoprotein	MedImmune (AZ)	RSV disease	1998	1,091	1,100	70
MyloTarg®	gemtuzumab	CD33	UCB/Wyeth	AML	2000	35	40	60
Campath®	alemtuzumab	CD52	Genzyme (ROW)/ Schering (Asia & Japan)	CLL	2001	59	90	150

(continued)

TABLE 24.1 *(continued)*

Brand	Generic	Target	Marketer(s)/ originator	Indications	Launch year	Sales (in $millions)		
						2006	2007	2010e
Zevalin®	ibritumomab tiuxetan	CD20	Cell Th./Bayer Schering (ROW)	NHL	2002	16	20	20
Bexxar®	tositumomab-1131	CD20	GSK	NHL	2003	20	20	20
Erbitux®	cetuximab	EGF	ImClone Systems/BMS (US, Canada, Japan)/Merck KGaA (ROW)	Colon, head, & neck cancers	2003	1,080	1,350	2,600
Humira®	adalimumab	TNF-α	Abbott	RA, PA, Crohn's, AS	2003	2,044	2,900	5,500
Raptiva®	efalizumab	CD11a	Xoma/ Genentech (US)/Serono (ROW)	Psoriasis	2003	146	200	250
Xolair®	Omalizumab	IgE	Genentech (US)/Novartis (US+ROW)	Asthma	2003	526	650	950
Avastin®	bevacizumab	VEG	Genentech (US)/Roche (ROW)	Solid tumors	2004	2,332	3,200	7,300
Lucentis®	ranibizumab	VEG	Genentec (US)/ Novartis (ROW)	Acute macular degeneration	2006	380	1,150	2,100

Brand	Generic	Target	Marketer(s)/ originator	Indications	Launch year	Sales (in $millions)			
						2006	**2007**	**2010e**	
Tysabri®	natalizumab	CD49	Elan (50% of US) /Biogen Idec (50% US +ROW)	Multiple sclerosis	2004	51	330	1,200	
Soliris™	eculizimab	C5	Alexion	PNH	2007	0	50	450	
Vectibix®	panitumumab	EGF	Amgen	Colorectal cancer	2006	39	180	150	
Actemra®	Tocilizumab	IL-6	Roche/Chugai	Castleman's disease	2005 (Jap)	3	25	450	
Numax®	Motevizumab	Human RSV Fusion glycoprotein	MedImmune (AZ)	RSV disease	2009	0	0	1,300	
					Total:	**19,484**	**24,755**	**39,410**	

Source: Company data. ABN AMRO estimates.

TABLE 24.2. Indications of infliximab, adalimumab, and tocilizumab

First FDA Approval	24 August 1998	31 December 2002	See below
U.S. indications	■ Rheumatoid arthritis ■ Psoriatic arthritis ■ Ankylosing spondylitis ■ Crohn's disease (adult and pediatric); ■ Fistulizing Crohn's disease ■ Ulcerative colitis ■ Psoriasis	■ Rheumatoid arthritis ■ Psoriatic arthritis ■ Ankylosing spondylitis ■ Crohn's disease	■ See below
EU indications	■ Rheumatoid arthritis ■ Crohn's disease ■ Ankylosing spondylitis ■ Psoriatic arthritis ■ Ulcerative colitis ■ Psoriasis	■ Rheumatoid arthritis ■ Psoriatic arthritis ■ Ankylosing spondylitis	■ See below
Japan indications	■ Rheumatoid arthritis ■ Crohn's disease	■ See below	■ Castleman's disease
Indications in development	■ Juvenile rheumatoid arthritis (Phase III) ■ COPD (Phase II) ■ Cancer related cachexia (Phase II)	■ Rheumatoid arthritis (December 2005 filing in Japan) ■ Crohn's disease (September 2006 filing in the EU) ■ Psoriasis (April 2007 filing) ■ Juvenile rheumatoid arthritis (May 2007 filing) ■ Ulcerative colitis	■ Crohn's disease (May 2006 filing) ■ Rheumatoid arthritis (Phase III completed) ■ Psoriasis (phase II)

Source: Company data; FDA; EMEA.

Pipeline of Monoclonal Antibodies

More impressive than the currently available mAbs perhaps is the pipeline of mAbs in clinical or preclinical developments. Few targets have been addressed through mAbs at present and over 80% of sales are coming from a few solid and hematological tumors and a few inflammatory diseases (see Figure 24.1).

ABN AMRO estimates that there are currently more than 350 mAb preclinical or clinical development projects ongoing. Table 24.3 includes the later stage projects. Interestingly, 50% of the projects in Phase III target antigens where the clinical utility has already been validated, such as CD20 or TNF-α, as market practice has underscored areas of product improvement. New diseases expected to be addressed by mAbs primarily include certain poorly addressed cancers that offer attractive regulatory routes. Examples include melanoma or renal cell carcinoma. New targets are also being explored through mAbs for several inflammatory diseases, including

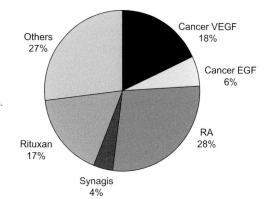

Figure 24.1. 2007 sales breakdown of monoclonal antibodies.
Source: Company data. ABN AMRO estimates.

TABLE 24.3. Monoclonal antibodies in late-stage clinical development

Brand	Target	Marketer/originator(s)	Type	Stage	Estimated peak sales (in $ millions)
Inflammation					
Cimzia™ (certolizumab pegol)	TNF-α	Nektar/UCB	Humanized	Filed	820
Ticilimumab	CTLA-4	Pfizer	Human	Ph III	Na
Denosumab (AMG 162)	RANKL	Amgen	Human	Ph III	3,000
CNTO 1275 (Ustekinumab)	IL12 / IL23	Medarex/ Centocor	Human	Ph III	680
CNTO 148 (Golimumab)	TNF-α	Centocor (US) /Janssen Pharma/ Schering-Plough	Human	Ph III	2,300
Infectious diseases					
Numax® (Motavizumab)	RSV	MedImmune/ Abbott	Humanized	Ph III	1,700
TNX-355	CD4	Biogen Idec/ Tanox	Humanized	Ph III	Na
Aurograb	Staphylococcus aureus	Novartis/ NeuTec	Human	Ph III	Na
Oncology					
Ipilimumab (+MDX-1379)	CTLA-4	Medarex/ BMS	Human	Ph III	185
Humax CD4 (Zanolimumab)	CD4 / EGFr	Genmab/ Medarex	Human	Ph III	250
Humax CD20 (ofatumumab)	CD20	Genmab/ GSK	Human	Ph III	2,040
Rencarex (WX-G250)	MN / CAIX	Esteve/Wilex	Chimeric	Ph III	400
LymphoCide (epratuzumab)	CD22	Immunomedics/ Amgen	Humanized	Ph III	Na

Note: Na: not available.

Source: Company data. ABN AMRO estimate.

asthma; for non-Hodgkin's lymphomas, where the patient population refractory to Rituxan® is an attractive target; for other forms of hematological tumors; and to fight bacterial infections.

Market Valuation of Monoclonal Antibody Companies

Figure 24.2 provides the stock price performance of leading antibody players and a translation of mAbs' commercial success into market values on international stock exchanges.

The success of "mAb stocks" on Nasdaq or European stock exchanges mirrors the general interest of investors in new technology penetration and their logical focus on companies with outstanding sales and earnings momentum.

Stock price performance and high equity market valuations (see Figure 24.3) have, however, also reflected the powerful value propositions offered by mAb companies in the universe of pharmaceutical or life sciences companies.

- The high price of mAbs, negotiated with reimbursement authorities out of their breakthrough clinical data and their high cost of goods, has guaranteed a quick path to profitability to mAb companies even at low penetration rates.
- The substantial backing by Big Pharma through discovery, development, and commercialization collaboration of multiple sizes and formats (see also Table 24.10 later in the chapter) has provided validation for public investors in quest of value signals, and has provided mAb companies with the financial support necessary to cope with costly clinical developments, manufacturing, and commercialization.
- The historical ability of mAb companies to retain commercialization rights on their mAbs has allowed them to transform into full commercial organizations. The history of Genentech is interesting from that viewpoint. Genentech was founded in 1976 and completed its initial public offering in 1980, raising $35 million to bridge the launch of its recombinant insulin, together with Lilly, in 1982. Roche Holding acquired a 60% stake in Genentech in 1990, at an unfavorable time. However, that dilution may have been more than offset by Roche's backing and may have provided Genentech with the stability required to develop its current capabilities.
- MAbs offer a greater degree of intellectual property protection than small molecules. Patent expiry of several blockbuster small molecule drugs of the late 1990s has had a considerable impact on the stock prices and valuation of Big Pharma stocks. The absence of regulatory guidelines for the approval of generic, bioequivalent mAbs, combined with the complexity of manufacturing and the potential presence of manufacturing trade secrets, makes the emergence of generic mAbs remote at present. As a result, exposure to mAbs has translated into premium public valuations. Possibly, the outperformance of Roche Holding within the Big Pharma universe is the most representative of that particular long-term value contribution of mAb companies (Figure 24.4).

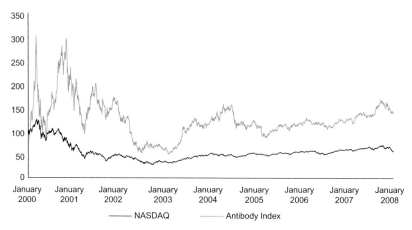

Figure 24.2. Stock price performances of leading antibody companies versus Nasdaq Index – 2000 to present. *Source:* Datastream (Note: Antibody Index composed of ImClone Systems, Alexion Pharmaceuticals, Genentech, Xoma, Dyax, Biogen Idec, and Medarex).

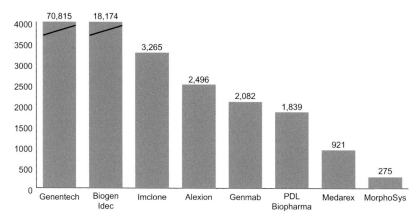

Figure 24.3. Technology values of leading mAb companies (in $ millions). *Source:* Company data. Share prices as of January 28, 2007.

Beyond technology excellence and innovation, capital markets have rewarded concrete business achievements. Technology values, as of December 31, 2007, of mAb companies that have remained technology providers or pursue yet to be validated targets reached an average of $217 million, as shown in Figure 24.5.

MONOCLONAL ANTIBODIES: FACTORS DRIVING MARKET ADOPTION

Fundamental Impact on Treatment Paradigms: MAbs Address Large Unmet Medical Needs

MAbs' target specificity and predictable pharmacokinetics have translated into attractive therapeutic indices, allowing either greater efficacy with the same toxicity or comparable efficacy with lower toxicity depending on the disease. MAbs, particularly those available through subcutaneous injection, have also proven to have

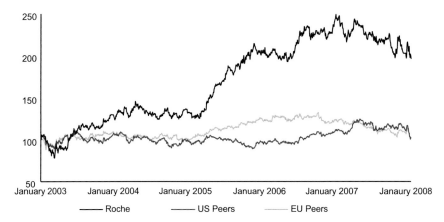

Figure 24.4. Roche Holding stock price performance versus peers – 2003 to present. *Source:* Datastream (Note: U.S. peers composed of Abbott Laboratories, Bristol-Myers Squibb, Eli Lilly & Co., Merck & Co., Pfizer, Schering-Plough, and Wyeth; EU peers composed of AstraZeneca, GlaxoSmithKline, Novartis, Roche Holding, and Sanofi-Aventis).

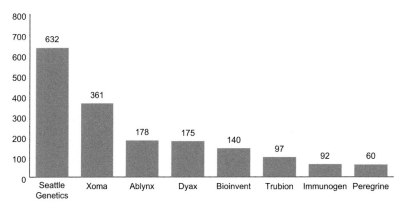

Figure 24.5. Technology value of selected antibody companies (in $ millions). *Source:* Company data. Share prices as of January 28, 2007.

potential for greater patient compliance. The representation of mAbs' contribution is distorted by their success in several highly prevalent and lethal cancers where they have slowed down disease progression and/or increased survival times. The timeline in Table 24.5 (later in the chapter) reminds us of the landmark clinical studies when Avastin® demonstrated survival advantages over standard chemotherapeutic cocktails of 30% to 33% in metastatic colorectal cancer, and of 19% in metastatic non-small-cell lung cancer.

MAbs have become cornerstones of treatment protocols in complex, nonlethal diseases where clinical outcome was capped by older drugs with relatively low target specificities and less attractive therapeutic indices. In rheumatoid arthritis, for instance, the immediate, direct contribution of biologics has been a breakthrough improvement, measured by ACR50 scores in studies, that has translated into greater quality of life and slower disease progression for many. The indirect contribution of mAbs, however, goes far beyond the benefits to rheumatoid arthritis patients. Their introduction has opened new avenues for better treatment combinations and

TABLE 24.4. Main phage display selection technology platforms

	Cambridge Antibody Technology	Morphosys	Dyax	Affitech
Date created	1990	1992	1995*a*	1997
Key patents	■ McCafferty patents	■ HuCal (combinatorial libraries)	■ Ladner patents	■ Breitling patents
	■ Griffiths patents	■ Cysdisplay (display of proteins on phages using disulfide bonds)		
	■ Winter II and Winter/House/ Lerner patents			
Equity market value (in millions)	£702*b*	€289	$211	Private
Key collaborations	■ AstraZeneca	■ Novartis		■ Roche Holding
	■ Abbott Laboratories	■ Roche		■ Peregrine
	■ Human Genome Sciences			

a Formed through merger of Biotage and Protein Engineering.

b Represents purchase price for 100% of the equity at AstraZeneca's offer price.

Source: Company data.

algorithms, has led to more relevant patient stratification and orphan markets, elicited the use of complementary clinical trial end points and shorter regulatory routes, and created insights into new biological targets that provided the scientific rationales for new drug developments. Moreover, their high reimbursement levels have "re-priced" entire segments of the drug industry, thereby providing the economic rationale to large and start-up companies to invest in research and development in a range of inflammatory, gastrointestinal and autoimmune disorders.

Advances toward Antibody Humanization

It was rapidly found that the application of the original murine antibodies was limited because it caused immunogenicity reactions, known as human anti-mouse antibodies (HAMA) response, as the murine antibody is recognized as foreign by the human immune system. In 1984, the first chimeric antibody, in which 30%–35% of the molecule is derived from mouse antibody sequences and 65%–70% from human antibody sequences, was reported (see Chapter 1, Humanization of Recombinant Antibodies, by José Saldanha). Chimeric antibodies represent the main achievement in antibody engineering, as measured by historical sales. Rituximab (Rituxan®/Mab-Thera®, Genentech/Roche Holding/Biogen Idec) and infliximab (Remicade®, Johnson & Johnson/Schering-Plough) have proven extraordinarily successful antibody therapeutics.

TABLE 24.5. Avastin® landmark dates

1989	Napoleone Ferrara, M.D., and his team at Genentech clone VEGF and publish in *Science* some of the first evidence that a specific angiogenic growth factor exists.
1993	Ferrara and his team publish a study in *Nature* demonstrating that an anti-VEGF antibody can suppress angiogenesis and tumor growth in preclinical models.
1997	Genentech submits an investigational new drug (IND) application to the FDA and begins a Phase I trial of Avastin®.
1998	Phase II trials of Avastin® begin.
2000	A Phase III trial of Avastin® in first-line metastatic colorectal cancer (in combination with the IFL [5-FU/leucovorin/CPT-11] regimen) begins.
May 2003	A Phase III trial of Avastin® and the IFL chemotherapy regimen in first-line metastatic colorectal cancer exceeds its primary end point of improving overall survival and meets its secondary end points of progression-free survival, response rate, and duration of response.
September 2003	Genentech submits a Biologics License Application (BLA) to the FDA for Avastin® in metastatic colorectal cancer under the FDA's Fast Track program. The FDA grants Priority Review (a 6-month review of the application).
February 2004	FDA approves Avastin® in combination with intravenous 5FU-based chemotherapy for the first-line treatment of patients with metastatic carcinoma of the colon or rectum, making Avastin the first approved anti-angiogenesis treatment for cancer
April 2004	The NCCN, an alliance of 19 of the world's leading cancer centers, updates their Colorectal Clinical Practice Guidelines and adds Avastin® in combination with intravenous 5FU-based regimens – including those using oxaliplatin or irinotecan – to its list of first-line treatment options for advanced colon or rectal cancer.
May 2005	A Phase III trial of Avastin® plus paclitaxel and carboplatin chemotherapies in first-line non-squamous, NSCLC meets its primary efficacy end point of improving overall survival. A Phase III trial of Avastin® plus paclitaxel chemotherapy in first-line metastatic breast cancer exceeds its primary efficacy end point of improving progression-free survival, compared to chemotherapy alone.
October 2005	The NCCN updates its Clinical Practice Guidelines in Oncology and adds Avastin® in combination with chemotherapy to its list of first-line therapy for advanced NSCLC.
June 2006	FDA approves Avastin® in combination with intravenous 5-FU-based chemotherapy for patients with second-line metastatic colorectal cancer.
October 2006	FDA approves Avastin® in combination with carboplatin and paclitaxel for the first-line treatment of patients with unresectable, locally advanced, recurrent or metastatic non-squamous, NSCLC.
December 2007	Genentech receives negative FDA ruling to expand Avastin® label to breast cancer because of its lack of impact on overall survival.

Source: Genentech.

The next technological development was humanization technology. In a humanized antibody, 90%–95% of the sequences are of human origin and the complement determining region (CDR), typically determining binding specificity and strength, remain of murine origin. PDL Biopharma, through its SMART® humanization patents, has become the main provider of humanization technology and claims today royalty on several leading humanized antibodies. According to PDL Biopharma, there are nine humanized antibodies currently on the market, including bevacizumab (Avastin®, Genentech/Roche Holding), trastuzumab (Herceptin®, Genentech/Roche Holding), and omalizumab (Xolair®, Genentech/Novartis), and more than 40 in clinical development.

Fully human antibodies – for instance, those engineered by Medarex or Abgenix through their UltiMab® and XenoMouse®/XenoMax® respective transgenic mice technology platforms (see Chapter 7 by Aya Jakobovits on the XenoMouse technology) – can be derived from mice whose immune system genes were replaced with human antibody encoding genes. When immunized, these mice react by producing human antibodies. The incidence of immunogenicity is believed to correlate only loosely with the rate of humanization (see chapters on immunogenicity by Philippe Stas and Frank Carr). However, at present, we estimate that over the 2009–2011 period, between 70% and 80% of all mAbs potentially approved will be fully human mAbs. The shift toward fully human antibodies reflects the pharmaceutical industry's natural bias for products with a lower clinical development risk.

High Diversity and High Affinity

Two main methods have been historically used for the generation of diversity in mAb drug discovery:

- The generation of "native" antibody libraries from the insertion and ultimate expression in an organism, such as transgenic mice or bacteria, of a human antibody gene repertoire. Diversity in the binding domains is achieved through the random combination of variable heavy chain domains and variable light chain domains.
- The generation of "synthetic" antibody libraries from the insertion of randomized amino-acid sequences into a backbone scFv or Fab segment, and ultimate expression in a bacterial cell.

Using these technologies and their variants, mAb companies have been able to offer libraries counting billions of mAbs, a number that is incomparably higher than any of the small molecule libraries of Big Pharma. As the best approximation for natural antibodies, these mAbs are characterized by a very high level of target affinity and resulting binding strength.

In parallel with manufacturing and humanization technology, further advances have enabled the selection *in vitro* of antibodies with high affinity. Phage display technologies (Table 24.4) are the best known of the high throughput methods to generate assays to screen for target affinity and to isolate the mAb with highest binding strength. Phage display involves the engineering and further expression of bacteriophages (viruses that infect bacteria) that lead to the display on the phage surfaces of mAbs. Libraries of phages are then screened against immobilized target antigens and later washed away to select the most strongly binding antibody structures. Further experiments lead to selection and isolation of a subset of potential lead candidates with optimal binding strength.

ANTIBODY MANUFACTURING

Therapeutic antibodies are required in much larger volumes than proteins and demand can exceed one ton per year. Remicade®, for instance, is typically administered in 5 mg/kg every 8 weeks, giving an average annual requirement of 2g per patient. Assuming 500,000 patients per year receive Remicade®, Centocor needs to manufacture at least 1 ton of infliximab per year. The importance of manufacturing capabilities to ensure market penetration was illustrated by Immunex's issues in launching Enbrel® over 2000–2002. Inadequate planning of capacity led to sales shortage of $700 million and created an opportunity for Amgen to take over Immunex.

The mastering of mammalian cell culture for production of mAbs, together with a ramp-up in capacity, both from biotechnology companies and contract manufacturers like Lonza Biologics, have removed the manufacturing bottlenecks from the mAb sector. The yield and cost of manufacturing, on the other hand, have superseded the initial under-capacity issue in manufacturing.

Mammalian cell cultures remain the most widely used means of manufacturing mAbs. Although they are difficult and expensive to grow, they are more suitable than cheaper bacterial systems that cannot reproduce the glycosylation, folding, and other structural features of human proteins. The most commonly used cells are recombinant Chinese hamster ovary (CHO) cells, recombinant myelomas, or hybridomas. Indeed, the hybridoma discovery was very much an advance that allowed for mAbs' manufacturability. Batch manufacturing is the most common practice in commercial scale manufacturing. Under batch manufacturing protocols, a master cell line is cultured in a nutrient-rich medium in 10,000-liter to 15,000-liter bioreactors. After 2 weeks, the medium is removed and the antibodies undergo a purification process, the most costly step in the process, averaging 1.5 times to 2.3 times the initial cost of batch production. After purification, the bioreactor can be recycled for another production batch. Under continuous perfusion protocols, different kinds of bioreactors are designed so as to feed cell lines continuously with fresh media. Reportedly, continuous perfusion generates yields of up to 600 mg/liter/day, which is several times the yield of larger batch manufacturing reactors. These basic manufacturing techniques are under continuous improvements as cost of goods is a major preoccupation. Time will tell whether a new generation of production vehicles, such as transgenic animal systems or plant systems, can reduce the manufacturing cost of mAbs with the same level of reliability and safety.

CONCLUSIONS

The most remarkable aspect of mAbs' emergence has perhaps been the speed of their clinical development. We believe that mAb technologies have empowered drug discovery departments with a unique tool capable of generating sufficient diversity and specificity to address the targets from the genomic discoveries. While medicinal chemistry campaigns require 2 to 4 years of iterations in which drug discovery must monitor all pharmacological parameters in parallel, constantly arbitraging between selectivity or potency and other properties, the mAb engine allows for the generation in 6 months to 1 year of leads with unprecedented target specificity and sub-nanomolar potencies and straightforward mechanism of action. MAbs also come from known scaffolds, primarily human or humanized IgG, which adds to the predictability of their pharmacokinetics. Adding 1 year to profile a mAb's antigenicity and similar times for preclinical profiling and toxicology, preclinical development times of mAbs can be at least 33% shorter than those traditionally observed in drug development.

Few statistics exist on the comparative risk of mAb clinical development versus small molecules. The time lag that has separated the approval of tyrosine kinase inhibitors from mAbs is possibly the best metric that may explain mAbs' past and ongoing success. The case of Avastin®, whose development is well known for its short approval time, is quite revealing. It highlights how quickly regulatory authorities can endorse a new data package under Fast Track status and through priority review (see Table 24.5). There are counter-examples just as notorious of delayed regulatory reviews (e.g., Xolair®, Eribitux®), however, and late-stage clinical development is not a ground for correlating media or drug classes and clinical development risks. Even so, the Avastin® discovery time line shown earlier in the chapter is evidence of the potential speed of antibody design and path to an investigational new drug (IND).

Adoption by Big Pharma

Big Pharma's endorsement is a guarantee of continuity in the emergence of mAbs. Big Pharma's investment in mAb projects or capabilities has, however, taken time as their large organizations have not seen the benefit of biotechnology in their traditional markets. One could argue also that organizational focus on established research protocols, revolving around the small molecule discovery approach to new targets, manufacturing expertise as well as the existence of successful small molecule series and well validated mechanisms of action not amenable to mAbs, have initially distracted Big Pharma's senior management from investing massively in mAbs capabilities. The earliest bets on owning mAb engines have been Roche Holding, and Johnson & Johnson, through its 1998 acquisition of Centocor for $5.3 billion.

However, a high number of target-based collaborations and single-project licensing ventures were entered into over the last 20 years. Table 24.6 shows only a subset of major capabilities-driven or project-driven collaborations.

More recently, Big Pharma has accelerated its investment in mAb engines through an unprecedented wave of acquisitions. We believe the catalysts have included strategic and operational considerations. Acquisitions, at valuations far in excess of those paid by historical investors, have been first motivated by the long-term lower patent exposure of mAbs relative to small molecules. The same motivation has been observed in certain M&A transactions in the vaccine industry.

TABLE 24.6. Partnerships and M&A in monoclonal antibodies

Collaboration	Year	Deal size (Mio)	Equity (Mio)	Description
OncoMed/ GlaxoSmithKline (GSK)	2007	$1,400	–	OncoMed will use its xenograft cancer models to identify mAbs against cancer stem cells and develop them through Phase II proof of concept studies in multiple indications. The deal includes OncoMed's lead candidate, OMP-21M18, which is expected to start Phase I in solid tumor patients in 2008. OncoMed will receive an undisclosed upfront payment and equity investment and is eligible for up to $1.4 billion in milestones, plus double-digit royalties. In addition, GSK has an option to invest in OncoMed in a future initial public offering.
Regeneron/ Sanofi-Aventis	2007	$1,122	$312	Partnership to discover, develop and commecialize human therapeutic antibodies using Regeneron's VelociSuite® technologies, including its VelocImmune® mAb technology. Sanofi-Aventis will pay $312 million to increase its stake in Regeneron to 19.5% (from its current holding of 4.0%), $85 million in upfront payment and up to $475 million in research funding over the five-year deal. Regeneron is also eligible for $250 million in sales milestones.
MorphoSys/ Novartis	2007	$1,000	–	Extension of a 2004 agreement to use MorphoSys' HuCAL GOLD® library to jointly discover and optimize an increased number of antibodies against a number of targets provided by Novartis. MorphoSys to receive more than $600 million in research and development funding and up to $400 million in milestones and technology access fees over 10 years and is eligible for royalties.
BioInvent/Genentech	2007	$190	–	Partnership to co-develop and commercialize BI-204, in North America, for the treatment of multiple cardiovascular conditions. BioInvent receives $15 million in upfront payment and is eligible for up to $175 million in milestones and royalties on North American sales.

Collaboration	Year	Deal size (Mio)	Equity (Mio)	Description
Seattle Genetics/ Genentech	2007	$860	–	Genentech receives exclusive worldwide license to develop and commercialize Seattle Genetics' SGN-40, a humanized ADC mAb targeting CD40. Seattle Genetics is eligible for $60 million upfront and more than up to $800 million in milestones, plus double-digit royalties.
Genmab/ GlaxoSmithKline (GSK)	2006	$2,059	$357	Licensing deal in which GSK receives exclusive global rights to co-develop and commercialize Genmab's ofatumumab for cancer and auto-immune diseases. Genmab receives a DKK582 million upfront licensing fee, a DKK2 billion equity investment, and is eligible for up to DKK9 billion in milestones and double-digit royalties
Trubion/Wyeth	2006	$800	–	Trubion grants Wyeth worldwide rights to TRU-015 and other Small Modular Immunopharmaceuticals (SMIPs™) targeting CD20 to treat inflammatory diseases and cancer. Trubion receives $40 million in upfront payment and is eligible for up to $760 million in milestones, plus royalties and co-promotion fees.
AstraZeneca/CAT[a]	2006	£574	£702	AstraZeneca's acquisition of CAT follows from the two companies' existing partnership to develop antibody therapies using CAT's leading fully human antibody engineering platforms. Acquisition values CAT at £702 million (excluding net cash of £128 million). AstraZeneca already owned c. 20% of CAT from previous partnerships.
Amgen/Abgenix[a]	2005	$2,367	$2,200	Amgen acquired Abgenix to gain full ownership of one of its most important advanced pipeline products, panitumumab (Vectibix®). The acquisition also created additional value to Amgen by eliminating a tiered royalty that Amgen might have paid to Abgenix on future sales of denosumab (formerly AMG162), which was created using Abgenix's XenoMouse® antibody technology.

(continued)

TABLE 24.6 *(continued)*

Collaboration	Year	Deal size (Mio)	Equity (Mio)	Description
PDL BioPharma/ Biogen Idec	2005	$800	$100	Partnership to develop and commercialize three of PDL BioPharma's antibodies: daclizumab, a humanized anti-CD25 antibody; volociximab (M200), an antibody against integrin α5β1; and HuZAF fontolizumab, a humanized antibody against IFN-γ. PDL BioPharma receives $40 million in upfront payment, a $100 million equity investment, is eligible for up to $660 million in milestones, plus royalties.
Medarex/Bristol-Myers Squibb	2004	$530	$25	Partnership to develop Medarex's MDX-010 anti-CTLA-4 antibody and MDX-1379 gp100 peptide vaccine to treat melanoma. Medarex receives $25 million in upfront payment, a $25 million equity investment, and is eligible for up to $480 million in regulatory and sales milestones plus royalties.
Medarex/Pfizer	2004	$510	$30	10-year deal covering the discovery and development of up to 50 antibodies using MEDX's UltiMAb® human antibody technology. Medarex receives $80 million in upfront payment, a $30 million in equity investment and is eligible for more than $400 million in milestones.
ImClone Systems/ Bristol-Myers Squibb	2001	$2,007	$1,007	Major partnership to co-develop and co-promote IMC-C225 (Erbitux®) in the United States, Canada, and Japan. Under the agreement ImClone is eligible to receive upfront and milestone payments of up to $1,000 million in addition to an equity investment of $1,007 million. Delay in Erbitux® approval led to renegotiations of certain terms of the deal in favor of Bristol-Myers Squibb.

[a] Indicates M&A transactions.
Source: ABN AMRO.

They come actually at a time when a number of key umbrella patents from mAb pioneers are running out of protection themselves, providing immediate intellectual property leverage to Big Pharma owners. Presumably also, the management of complex collaboration agreements between organizations with different agendas and locations has also been a motivation in seeking full control over assets.

The two most recent antibody collaborations shown in Table 24.6 may be, if not early signs of a new trend, a late return toward transactions that are closer in nature to Roche Holding or American Home Products taking stakes in Genentech and drug development and commercialization from Immunex, respectively. Acquisition is in several instances more advantageous than a collaboration as it provides a more straightforward control over project developments and a faster path to generation of INDs. Nevertheless, several Big Pharma companies have also expressed concerns about losing the most creative minds in the biotechnology organizations they would acquire. From that perspective, the Sanofi-Aventis/Regeneron and Novartis/MorphoSys transactions may be optimal solutions for Big Pharma and biotechnology shareholders in the long term.

Big Pharma have also been aggressive at buying out from venture capitalists several early stage next generation antibody, antibody fragment, or antibody-analog protein (NGA) companies. From that standpoint, the history of the NGA companies differs materially from the first generation. In the third part of this chapter, we look at the NGA companies, attempting to explain the burgeoning of these companies on the private and public capital markets and the application, or not, of the lessons from the mAb wave to their growth pathways and commercial successes.

NEXT-GENERATION ANTIBODY, ANTIBODY FRAGMENT, OR ANTIBODY-ANALOG (NGA) THERAPEUTICS

Despite their well-known virtues, mAbs have nevertheless shown limits, largely owing to the inherent biophysical properties and complex molecular composition of immunoglobulins. These limits have created rationales for the development of several small molecule drugs acting on the same target family or pathway. In particular,

- MAbs' size and format do not make them amenable to a large number of targets. Furthermore, they cannot penetrate cells or bind to targets in the cytoplasm or in the nucleus.
- MAbs' pharmacokinetics can also be a limiting factor in certain instances. IgG molecules have a long half-life. Nonetheless, their half-lives may be too short to exert a prolonged therapeutic effect on certain targets or in certain tissues and address certain chronic disorders optimally. Or alternatively, it may be too long to treat flares or acute disorders. In addition, the tissue penetration of mAbs is an important limiting factor, both in absolute terms and when compared to small molecules. MAbs do not cross the blood-brain barrier, or only in minute quantities, which makes them irrelevant for central nervous system applications. They also have a limited ability to penetrate tumoral tissues in depth.
- MAbs' invasive modes of administration, through intravenous or subcutaneous injections, are also a competitive disadvantage over certain small molecules and a limit in many diseases.
- MAbs are difficult to produce and their cost of goods remains one of the highest in the pharmaceutical industry.

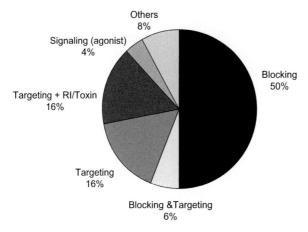

Figure 24.6. Antibody therapeutics (Phase I to launched) per mechanism of action. *Source:* Chugai Pharmaceuticals.

The possible mechanisms of action of antibody as therapeutics are diverse, yet designing "neutralizing" or "blocking" antibodies has been the main objective at hand of the research and development efforts (Figure 24.6). Several constraints have hindered the design of antibodies with alternative modes of action – for example, signaling, opsonizing, and targeting, with potential direct or indirect therapeutic effects.

These shortcomings have legitimately stimulated public and private creativity. For a long time already, in parallel with first-generation mAbs, a number of platforms have evolved to enhance mAb efficacy, such as radiolabeled Zevalin® or payload-antibody Mylotarg®. Exploiting mAbs' superior target specificity, payload antibody companies have brought several drug candidates into clinical studies, as illustrated in Table 24.7. Payload antibodies, however, have remained unproven so far and the number of such mAb candidates in development is small.

In the case of treatment of rheumatoid arthritis, patients have benefited first from intravenously administered Remicade® and subsequently from subcutaneously administered Humira®. In 2006, UCB Celltech filed certolizumab pegol, brand-named Cimzia™, as the first pegylated antibody fragment. Following a first setback with regulatory authorities in March 2007, Cimzia's approval is now expected for 2009. The potential expected benefits of Cimzia include prolonged maintenance of remission (up to 18 months) in patients with Crohn's disease and rheumatoid arthritis as well as its subcutaneous injection administration. Cimzia is the first success of a new format in the trade-off between pharmacokinetics, potency, and antibody-like specificity. However, only recently have a new wave of antibody and antibody fragment companies emerged that try to address the main mAb limits while preserving, or even trying to increase, their affinity.

The Intellectual Property Challenges

Antibody therapeutics has historically been a field for deleterious patent disputes and famous settlements. Several are well known:

TABLE 24.7. Payload antibody leaders – Seattle Genetics and Immunogen

	Seattle Genetics	Immunogen
Equity market value	$724 millions	$146 millions
Platform/Key technologies	Antibody-drug conjugates (ADC)	Tumor-activated prodrug (TAP)
		IMGN242 (gastric cancer) Phase II
		Trastuzumab DM1 (breast cancer) Phase I/II
	SGN-40 (BCL/multiple myeloma) Phase II/Phase I	IMGN901 (SCL cancer/multiple mycloma) Phase II
	SGN-33 (AML/MDS) Phase II/Phase I	IMGN242 (solid tumors) Phase I
	SGN-35 (HL) Phase I	AVE9633 (AML) Phase I
	SGN-30 (HL/ALCL) Phase II	AVE1642 (solid tumors) Phase I
		SAR3419 (NHL) Phase I
Key collaborations	Genentech	Sanofi-Aventis, Genentech
Established	1997	1981
Number of employees	180	213

Source: Company data. Share prices as of January 28, 2007. Number of employees as of last 10-K.

- Genentech and Celltech on the "New Cabilly" patents, which covers the co-expression of heavy and light chains using recombinant DNA technology.
- Cambridge Antibody Technology and MorphoSys on Cambridge Antibody Technology's McCafferty and Griffiths patents, covering, respectively, the process by which antibodies are displayed on phage surfaces and methods of selecting antibodies targeting a certain antigen from libraries, and the use of phage display technology to isolate human "anti-self" antibodies that bind to molecules found in the human body.
- Cambridge Antibody Technology and Dyax on a conflict over Dyax's Ladner patents covering the practice of display technologies, including display of antibodies, peptides, and proteins on any cell, spore, or virus, including bacteriophages.
- Dyax and Affitech on Affitech's Breitling patents, covering key elements of phage display technology.

A number of these patents will fall in the public domain in the foreseeable future. However, other patent derivatives or improvements continue to represent barriers to entry for users. Significant intellectual property positions also exist in antibody expression in yeast or mammalian cells and in manufacturing processes. The development of new antibody formats, generation platforms, and engineering techniques as well as the generation of entire classes of antibody-analog proteins is in part solely motivated by a search for freedom to operate or by attempts to create new, independent patent positions. The future will tell how much intellectual property conflict exists between these various new technologies and between these new and the old ones. A number of the NGA companies have actually preempted potential future issues by entering into licensing or cross-licensing agreements with the incumbent companies. While developing its proprietary NGA formats and building its semi-synthetic libraries, Affimed, for instance, has already avoided future potential issues and spent the early years of its existence nurturing its proprietary mAb library and antibody format technology base while entering into the necessary licensing agreements with several incumbent companies.

The Availability of Capital

The first generation of mAb companies has offered a clear road map to business success in biotechnology, and NGAs can be seen, in comparison with other ventures, as attractive prospects for shareholder value creation. Venture capital investments in mAbs have also to be observed against the backdrop of relative biopharmaceutical successes, on U.S. stock exchanges primarily, and of a recent surge in acquisitions by Big Pharma companies (see Table 24.8). Table 24.10 (shown later in the chapter) shows the bets placed by leading venture capital firms in the United States.

European venture capitalists have been even more prolific in supporting NGAs. Table 24.9 shows a number of national champions and their financial sponsors.

The Next-Generation Value Propositions

The experience gained in operating with synthetic libraries has generated multiple novel approaches to the design of high-specificity antibody-like molecules harnessing scaffolds that are smaller than IgG and have certain pharmacological and manufacturing advantages. In parallel, significant progress has been made in the understanding of antibody-dependent cell cytotoxicity and on the molecular structure that enhances it on the Fc region of antibodies. The value propositions of the NGA companies mirror the main limits of mAbs. Each NGA company has been articulating its contribution through one or several of the following key axes.

Enhanced Pharmacodynamic Properties

Antibody format engineering has focused on the size, as measured by their molecular weight, of antibody fragments as well as their valence, in order to improve their ability to bind to more relevant epitopes or bind with greater avidity to the target antigen. NGA companies also aim at increasing certain tissue penetration, such as solid tumor tissues. Antibody fragments, single-chain antibodies or Nanobodies™, to name a few of the new formats, are tools to reach less accessible targets or target epitopes, such as certain receptor cavities or enzyme-binding pockets. Multivalent antibody formats or antibody analogs seek to enhance binding avidity and mimic the strength of native polyclonal antibodies. Table 24.10 shows benchmarks for sizes of NGA compared to the IgG molecule backbone used in mAbs.

The majority of NGA companies make claims on the benefits of their formats, as a better tool to design a trade-off between affinity and other variables.

TABLE 24.8. Venture capital investment in selected U.S. next-generation antibody companies

	Alta P.	Atlas V.	Flagship V.	Frazier H.	HealthCare V.	InterWest P.	MPM Cap.	Orbimed Ad.	Oxford Bio	Polaris V.	Sofinnova V.	Venrock	Others
Adnexus		★											★
Agensys	★		★					★		★			★
Biorexis													★
GlycoFi										★			★
Kalobios							★				★		★
Macrogenics	★					★	★	★					★
Rinat Neur.							★						★
Trubion				★					★			★	★
Xencor					★				★				★

Note: Shading indicates M&A exit.
Source: Company data.

TABLE 24.9. Venture capital investment in selected European next-generation antibody companies

	3i	Abingworth	Alta P.	Atlas V.	Biomedinvest	Clarus V.	Forbion Cap.	Glide H.	GIMV	GLSV	HBM	Healthcap	LSP	Orbimed Ad.	MVM	Sofinnova P.	TVM Cap.	Others[a]
4-Antibody			*										*					*
Ablynx		*							*							*		*
Affibody								*				*						*
Affimed					*								*	*				*
Affitech	*																	*
Domantis															*			*
Esbatech					*	*					*							*
F-star				*														*
GlycArt							*	*		*								*
Glycotope							*											*
Micromet[b]							*	*									*	*
Pangenetics							*											*
Pieris							*	*	*									*

Note: Shading indicates M&A exit.

[a] Includes other major European venture capital funds such as Aescap, Credit Agricole Private Equity, Index Ventures, or Novo.

[b] Micromet was acquired by CancerVax in exchange for shares representing a majority interest in CancerVax's capital.

Source: Company data.

TABLE 24.10. Antibody therapeutic formats – Valence and molecular weight

	IgG	Fab	scFv	(scFV)2	Diabody	SMIP™	TandAb®	Nanobody®
Valence	Bi	Mono	Mono	Bi	Bi	Mono	Tetra	Mono
Molecular weight	159kD	60kD	29kD	58kD	50kD	40–50kD	105kD	15kD

Source: Affimed, Ablynx, Trubion.

Ability to Trigger an Antibody-Dependent Cell Cytoxic (ADCC) Response

We find these approaches particularly interesting as mAbs have primarily been "neutralizing" antibodies to date and have not played the natural role to recruit effector cells of the immune system to eliminate their targets. They are particularly relevant in this book entitled *Recombinant Antibodies for Immunotherapy*. The few platforms in development in this field, at the border between antibody therapeutics and immunotherapy, can be divided into two sets of approaches. Bispecific antibodies are a first approach whereby the NGA targets its antigen while also binding to a receptor on cytotoxic T cells or natural killer cells. Such recruitment of the effector cells then facilitates a subsequent immune response. Heidelberg-based Affimed is possibly the most advanced company in this field.

The other approaches have revolved around the engineering of sugar motives present on the Fc region of antibodies. Sugar motives, including the ones obtained through glycosylation or sialylation, catalyze ADCC mechanisms; they also influence other pharmacodynamic and pharmacokinetic properties. The control of their design is seen as an exciting area in NGA development. Several companies, including Biowa, a subsidiary of Kyowa Hakko Kogyo; GlycoFi, now part of Merck & Co.; GlycArt, now part of Roche Holding; and Glycotope, are leaders in this field.

Improved Pharmacokinetics

NGA companies claim to be able to modulate the half-lives of mAbs both in relation to their sizes and in line with their therapeutic objectives. Small antibody-like molecules have a greater tissue penetration but lose in serum half-life compared to IgG scaffolds. NGA companies are working on increasing the half-life of the smaller NGA formats and are exploiting a few of the main technologies, such as PEGylation® or albumin-binding linkers, in order to increase the half-life of their drug candidates. The majority of antibody fragment companies, such as Ablynx, Domantis (a subsidiary of Glaxo-SmithKline), Esbatech, or recently founded F-Star, make claims of improving tissue penetration or offering platforms where serum half-life can be modulated.

Improved Manufacturing Processes and Lower Cost of Goods

Unlike mAbs, several antibody fragments or antibody-analogs can be manufactured in *E. coli* or other organisms at a fraction of the cost of goods from current mammalian cell cultures. Allegedly, immunogenicity may be a bottleneck compared to today's fully human antibodies, as the final molecule will be of nonhuman nature or will have been altered by engineering. Furthermore, production capacity is today concentrated in a few companies, with Roche Holding, Genentech, and Chugai Pharmaceuticals together accounting for more than 25% of the world capacities, according to Chugai Pharmaceuticals. New manufacturing processes are therefore also a path to freedom to operate.

Diagnostic Applications

The high specificity and affinity of monoclonal antibodies have led to applications in many diagnostic platforms. The performance of NGA applications in diagnostics will be measured against the sensitivity and specificity achieved with current reagents, consisting primarily of monoclonal antibodies made out of mouse hybridomas. For diagnostics, long shelf-life and high level of bacterial expression, all translating into low production costs, will be of critical importance. Certain NGAs, particularly antibody-like proteins, are believed to have potential in diagnostic imaging applications.

Affibody and Pieris have major programs applying their Affibody® and Anticalin® platforms for diagnostic imaging applications, underpinned by collaborations with industry leader GE Healthcare. While all teams currently have significant know-how in antibody design and development, Table 24.11. summarizes the value propositions put forward by selected NGA companies at the time this chapter was written and based on public information available.

OUTLOOK

Few data points on serum half-life, tissue penetration, tissue-to-blood ratios, or immunogenicity of NGAs are available. A few NGAs, such as Ablynx's ALX-0081 or Adnexus' Angiocept, have now reached proof of concept through to Phase I studies and are progressing in efficacy studies. These early data are critical validation points given the claims that are made and were key catalysts of M&A transactions in the sector.

There are various views on the actual benefits and levels of differentiation between the platforms developed by NGA companies. One view in particular is to focus on the novelty and utility of the targets pursued rather than on the features of the toolbox. The extent to which an NGA addresses that target better than a mAb or a small molecule is likely to be the determinant of success. The claims that are made, the biological targets that are actually pursued, and the resulting pipelines are first arguments to source financing from the venture capital and pharmaceutical community prior to being promises of medical breakthroughs. Several NGA companies have been validating their approaches by developing NGAs to known targets, such as receptors in the VEGF-receptor family or TNF-α. Pursuing these targets with alternative scaffolds has allowed them to reach Phase I studies in an expedited manner and provided immunogenicity, pharmacokinetic, and sometimes early efficacy data that could be benchmarked against mAbs. Even though the level of disclosure on

TABLE 24.11. Technology focus of selected antibody therapeutics companies

| | Main platform toolbox | | | | | Key platform claims | | | | | |
	New Ab format	New protein scaffold	Fc region engineering	Affinity engineering	Target focus/tech agnostic	Affinity/Target amenability	PK	ADCC enhancement	Manufacturing	Diagnostic	Development data
4-Antibody					**	**					Preclinical
Ablynx	**			*		*	*		*		Phase I
Adnexus		**				*	*		*		Phase I/II
Affibody		**							*	**	Preclinical
Affimed	**			*		*		**			Preclinical
Affitech				**	*	**		*			Preclinical
Agensys					**						Na
Avidia	**					*	*		*		Na
Bioinvent					**	*					Phase I/II
Biowa			**			*	*	**	*		Na
Biorexis		**				*	*		*		Na
Domantis	**		*	*		*	**		*		Phase I/II
F-Star			**	**		*	*	*	*		Preclinical
Glycotope			**	*		*		**			Preclinical
Kalobios			**	**		**			*		Phase I
Macrogenics	*		**			**		**			Phase II
Micromet	**		**			**		**			Phase I/II
Oncomed					**	*					Preclinical
Pangenetics					**						Preclinical
Pieris	**					*	*		*	**	Preclinical
Raven					**	*	**				Phase I
Rinat Neuro.	**				**		*				Na
Trubion	**					*	*				Phase II
Wilex					**					*	Phase III
Xencor	*	**				**	**				Preclinical

Note: Na: Not available. Single asterisk indicates the platform toolbox and claims for the company; double asterisks indicate a major feature of the firm.
Source: Company data; ABN AMRO.

targets is limited, Table 24.12 shows that NGA companies have a primary focus on novel targets, especially in the cancer space.

Beyond the need for early technology validation, NGA companies pursue largely unvalidated targets, several of which are pursued by mAbs as well. Certain companies, like Raven Biotechnologies or Oncomed, have even put the discovery of novel cancer antigens and the generation, through an immunization stress, of antibodies to new cell surface-receptor antigens on proprietary cell lines from tumor tissues, the core of their research strategy. For these reasons, the time to market for NGAs may actually be significantly longer than expected. We believe their success, both as new media and as media that compete with mAbs, will depend on their ability to translate into drugs on these novel targets. In fact, certain companies have followed a technology-agnostic approach, basing their value only on target novelty and level of validation, and on their management's team experience in developing commercially relevant antibody therapeutics. Agensys, for instance, has actually focused on discovery and validation of targets in cancer, based on their biology engine, and obtained XenoMouse®/XenoMax® licenses to generate a pipeline (see Table 24.13). Pangenetics, run by former senior members of Cambridge Antibody Technology's management, has in-licensed mAbs to partially validated targets such as CD40 or new targets such as Nerve Growth Factor. It is also our view that the critical success factor, as demonstrated by the history of mAb companies, may reside in the clinical content and medical capabilities of the antibody companies rather than on technology fine-tuning.

Interestingly, the number of technology licenses or discovery collaborations entered into by NGA companies is limited when compared to the number of such agreements entered into by mAb companies. The history of mAb companies has shown the low economic value of monetization of technology through royalty-bearing agreements and target-based discovery and development collaborations. Using the lessons of the past, NGA companies have been focusing their financial and human resources on advancing their technologies to proof of concept.

This strategy so far has been lucrative for NGA companies' shareholders and stock option holders. The few arguments developed earlier are key to rationalizing the number of acquisitions of NGA companies completed by Big Pharma over the last 3 years. These acquisitions are motivated by Big Pharma's experience in mAb development and their corporate purpose of staying at the edge of biomedical research. They also come at a time when Big Pharma pipelines are massively exposed to patent expiries of blockbuster small molecule drugs of the 1980s and 1990s. Financing through development and commercialization partnerships have not been ruled out, as exemplified by Ablynx's 1.3 billion collaboration with Boehringer Ingelheim entered into in September 2007. However, M&A has been so far a more natural evolution for NGA companies that have largely kept development and commercialization rights to their pipelines. M&A is also a logical aspiration of their shareholders that arbitrage between immediate exit and exiting at far higher valuations by shouldering the risk and financing requirements of deploying clinical expertise and manufacturing and commercial capabilities.

TABLE 24.12. Target focus of NGA companies

	Oncology		Inflammation			Anti-infectives	Others	Target focus		Development data
Oncology	Solid tumors	Hematology	Rheumatoid arthritis	Asthma	Others			Validated targets	New targets	
4-Antibody										
Ablynx	✓		✓		✓		✓	*	**	Phase I
Adnexus	✓	✓			✓		✓	**	**	Phase I/II
Affibody							**		*	Preclinical
Affimed	✓	✓		✓	✓		✓	**	*	Preclinical
Affitech	✓	✓							**	Preclinical
Agensys	✓	✓							**	Preclinical
Avidia	✓	✓								
Bioinvent	✓	✓					✓	*	**	Phase I/II
Biowa	✓	✓	✓	✓			✓	**	**	Phase I
Biorexis							✓	**		Phase I/II
Domantis	✓				✓					Preclinical
F-Star										
Glycotope	✓	✓	✓		✓			*	**	Preclinical
Kalobios			✓	✓	✓	✓		*	*	
Macrogenics	✓		✓		✓			*	**	Phase II
Micromet	✓	✓			✓			*	*	Phase II
Oncomed	✓	✓								Preclinical
Pangenetics	✓		✓		✓		✓		**	Preclinical
Pieris	✓	✓		✓			✓	**		Preclinical
Raven	✓									Phase I
Rinat Neuro.							✓		**	
Trubion	✓	✓	✓		✓			**	*	Phase II
Wilex	✓	✓						**	**	Phase III
Xencor	✓	✓	✓	✓	✓			**	*	Preclinical

Note: Single asterisk denotes whether a firm is working with validated or new targets (or both); double asterisks indicate a major focus.

Source: Company data; ABN AMRO.

TABLE 24.13. Partnerships and M&A in next-generation antibodies

Announcement date	Target	Acquirer	Transaction value (in millions)	Key assets
November 07	Agensys	Astellas	$537[a]	Antibody programs based on proprietary targets and on a XenoMouse®/XenoMax® license from Abgenix
October 07	Haptogen	Wyeth	Na	Protein therapeutics
March 07	Morphotek	Eisai	$325	Morphodoma™ and Libridoma™ platform for high-affinity mAbs
February 07	Biorexis	Pfizer	Na	Transferrin-based protein therapeutics and Trans-bodies™
December 06	Domantis	GlaxoSmithKline	£230	Domain antibody (dAbs®) platform
September 06	Avidia	Amgen	$450	Avimer™ platform and programs
May 06	GlycoFi	Merck & Co.	$400	Glycosylation platform
May 06	Abmaxis	Merck & Co.	$80	In-silico mAb engineering platform
April 06	Rinat Neurosciences	Pfizer	Na	BBB – Crossing mAb therapeutics
July 05	GlycArt	Roche Holding	Sfr. 235	Glycosylation platform

Note: Na: not available.

[a] Includes a $150 million earn-out payment.

Source: Company data.

Index

Printed in the United States
by Baker & Taylor Publisher Services